SOMATIC DYSFUNCTION IN OSTEOPATHIC FAMILY MEDICINE

WRITTEN UNDER THE AUSPICES
OF THE AMERICAN COLLEGE
OF OSTEOPATHIC FAMILY PHYSICIANS

Editor
Kenneth E. Nelson, DO, FAAO, FACOFP
Professor, Departments of Osteopathic
Manipulative Medicine, Family
Medicine, and Biochemistry
Chicago College of Osteopathic Medicine
Midwestern University, Downers Grove, Illinois

Associate Editor
Thomas Glonek, PhD
Professor, Department of Osteopathic Manipulative Medicine
Chicago College of Osteopathic Medicine
Midwestern University, Downers Grove, Illinois
Chicago Osteopathic Family Practice
Michael Reese Hospital, Chicago, Illinois

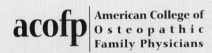

acofp American College of Osteopathic Family Physicians

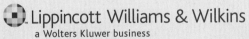

Lippincott Williams & Wilkins
a Wolters Kluwer business
Philadelphia · Baltimore · New York · London
Buenos Aires · Hong Kong · Sydney · Tokyo

Acquisitions Editor: Nancy Anastasi Duffy
Managing Editor: Kelly Horvath
Marketing Manager: Emilie Linkins
Production Editor: Julie Montalbano
Designer: Terry Mallon
Compositor: International Typesetting and Composition
Printer: R.R. Donnelley & Sons—Crawfordsville

351 West Camden Street
Baltimore, MD 21201

530 Walnut Street
Philadelphia, PA 19106

Printed in the United States of America

Library of Congress Cataloging-in-Publication Data

Somatic dysfunction in osteopathic family medicine / sponsored by the American College of Osteopathic Family Medicine; editor, Kenneth E. Nelson; associate editor, Thomas Glonek.
    p. ; cm.
  Includes bibliographical references.
  ISBN-13: 978-1-4051-0475-3
  ISBN 1-4051-0475-9
 1. Osteopathic medicine.   2. Manipulation (Therapeutics)   I. Nelson, Kenneth E., DO.
II. Glonek, Thomas.   III. American College of Osteopathic Family Medicine.
  [DNLM: 1. Manipulation, Osteopathic.   2. Family Practice.   3. Patient-Centered Care.   4. Physician-Patient Relations.   WB 940 S693 2007]
RZ342.S66 2007
615.5'33—dc22

2006019403

The publishers have made every effort to trace the copyright holders for borrowed material. If they have inadvertently overlooked any, they will be pleased to make the necessary arrangements at the first opportunity.

To purchase additional copies of this book, call our customer service department at **(800) 638-3030** or fax orders to **(301) 223-2320**. International customers should call **(301) 223-2300.**

Visit Lippincott Williams & Wilkins on the Internet: http://www.LWW.com. Lippincott Williams & Wilkins customer service representatives are available from 8:30 am to 6:00 pm, EST.

07 08 09 10
2 3 4 5 6 7 8 9 10

Dedicated to Andre V. Gibaldi, DO, FACOFP, family physician, educator, colleague, mentor, and friend.

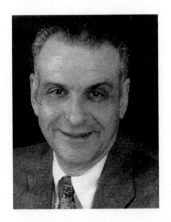

Preface

As osteopathic medicine has grown and taken its rightful place in the mainstream of medical practice, the isolated environment in which we once taught our students and residents has given way to open-staffed hospitals. Consequently, our clinical educators are now as apt to be allopathic as they are to be osteopathic physicians. At this same time, and in part because of this progress, there has developed a need to demonstrate what we have that is distinctly osteopathic. The American Osteopathic Association has mandated that our residents demonstrate seven core competencies; the first of those competencies is osteopathic philosophy and osteopathic manipulative medicine.

Thus, there has arisen a need for a clinically oriented text that addresses the distinctive aspects of osteopathic medicine. In an attempt to fill that need, this text presents a contemporary understanding of the fundamentals of osteopathic philosophy and the applied diagnosis and treatment of somatic dysfunction throughout the practice of family medicine. It is not intended to be a review of general medical practice. There are many such texts. Nor is it intended to be a manual of osteopathic manipulative treatment (OMT) procedures, although many examples of applicable procedures are provided throughout the book. Again, many excellent and more complete procedure manuals are available. Rather, this text provides medical students, residents, and physicians in practice with a description of how their patients may be empowered to take an active part in the establishment and maintenance of health; how the diagnosis and treatment of somatic dysfunction fosters a holistic, patient-oriented approach to health care; how somatic dysfunction affects the patient's health status; and the clinical logic for the use of OMT in the care of those patients with examples of possible procedural choices.

All too often individuals consider OMT as an appropriate treatment only for musculoskeletal pain. Although this is one area in which the modality is effective, it is but a single application. Early osteopaths employed OMT to treat patients with all manner of medical conditions. These pioneers were frequently criticized for their practices, for inappropriately treating cholecystitis or a myocardial infarction with OMT. This, of course, was not the case. Rather, these clinicians were treating the patient, attempting to alleviate the effects of somatic dysfunction upon the individual's overall ability to respond to the illness. They were addressing the effects of somatic dysfunction upon their patients mechanically as well as the effect it exerted upon circulation and neurophysiology.

Following in that original tradition, this text is focused upon the advantages of the diagnosis and treatment of somatic dysfunction in all types of patients, of all ages, with all manner of clinical conditions. The specific conditions discussed are used as examples of the clinical approach to broad categories of illness, and the reader is encouraged to generalize. After all, there is consistency in the ways somatic dysfunction affects an individual mechanically and physiologically, whether the infirmity is gastrointestinal or upper respiratory. The answer to how I would "osteopathically" treat a patient with hypertension is . . . the same way I would treat a patient with diabetes. The focus is upon the patient, in the context of his or her given illness, but still (pun intended) *upon* the patient. Recognition of the inherent reliability of human anatomy and the universality of the presence and effects of somatic dysfunction fosters this approach.

This approach is possibly one of the most difficult concepts for clinicians who practice disease-focused medicine. Certainly, the specific disease process affecting the patient must be diagnosed and treated appropriately, but always in the context of the total function of the individual. Such a patient-focused approach paradigm, once mastered, proves to be significantly less frustrating to the clinician than is a disease-focused approach, especially when the problem being addressed falls into the broad and often ambiguous category of functional illnesses. This is why osteopathic medicine is applied so naturally to the practice of family medicine.

This text is divided into four areas: philosophy and principles of patient care, categories of patients encountered, categories of clinical conditions encountered, and practice issues. Within these categories, the chapters that deal with the middle two begin with a discussion of the patient or clinical condition and are followed, in each case, with examples of the OMT procedures that could be applicable. We have attempted to provide examples from all categories of OMT. The procedures selected are for the most part representative of what the author of a given chapter has found to be effective in his or her experience. Consequently, we have most assuredly failed to include procedures that other clinicians prefer. This text—it must again be stressed—is not intended as an OMT procedures manual. Further, the reader must realize that the examples of OMT provided are just that: examples. They do not represent the exact procedure to be employed at all times for a given condition. OMT must be individually applied. After all, we are treating the patient, and every patient is a unique individual, as is every physician. Although the dysfunctional areas manipulated can be expected to demonstrate some consistency for a given condition, the procedures that prove most effective for a given condition will differ from patient to patient as well as from clinician to clinician.

For further inquiry into osteopathic medicine, we have included chapter references, which, though often old, should not be considered dated. This literature continues to be pertinent—not to mention important—because if we do not yet have "scientific" studies supporting our position, at least we can demonstrate that it is a longstanding one.

This text would not have come to light if it were not for the inspiration and tireless effort of many individuals. It began as a request from Andre V. Gibaldi, DO, FACOFP, then Chair of the Department of Family Medicine at the Chicago College of Osteopathic Medicine, for a series of lectures for postdoctoral education. Then a student and now a contributor to this project, Anette Mnabhi observed that the materials would lend themselves well to a textbook of clinical practice. This end product is the result of the clinical experience and much didactic research on the part of the contributing authors, overseen by the members of the American College of Osteopathic Family Practice (ACOFP), Committee for Osteopathic Principles and Practice, and a number of other conscriptees, who acted as peer reviewers.

Gratitude must be expressed to the leadership of the ACOFP and Mr. Peter Schmelzer, executive director of the ACOFP, for their support in this project. Gratitude must also be expressed to Patricia Nuccio, RN, who as educational manager for the ACOFP coordinated resources and materials and maintained communications (took the heat) throughout this effort.

Finally, thanks beyond measure must be extended to Tom Glonek, PhD, the associate editor for this text, without whose broad-based knowledge and experience and long hours of dedicated effort, this book would have never been completed.

Respectfully submitted,
K. E. Nelson
June 7, 2005

Contributors

Zachary J. Comeaux, DO, FAAO
Associate Professor
Division of Osteopathic Philosophy and Practice
West Virginia School of Osteopathic Medicine
Lewisburg, West Virginia

David M. Driscoll, DO
Assistant Clinical Professor of Medicine
Tufts University School of Medicine
Boston, Massachusetts
Director of Inpatient Services, Department of Internal Medicine
Lahey Clinic
Peabody, Massachusetts

David B. Fuller, DO
Assistant Professor, Department of Family Medicine
Chicago College of Osteopathic Medicine
Midwestern University
Downers Grove, Illinois
Attending Family Physician
North Baldwin Infirmary
Bay Minette, Alabama

Thomas Glonek, PhD
Professor, Department of Osteopathic Manipulative Medicine
Chicago College of Osteopathic Medicine
Midwestern University
Downers Grove, Illinois
Chicago Osteopathic Family Practice
Michael Reese Hospital
Chicago, Illinois

Ann L. Habenicht, DO, FAAO, FACOFP
Professor, Department of Osteopathic Manipulative Medicine
Chicago College of Osteopathic Medicine
Midwestern University
Downers Grove, Illinois
Senior Staff, Department of Family Medicine
Palos Community Hospital
Palos Heights, Illinois

Kurt Heinking, DO
Associate Professor and Chairman
Department of Osteopathic Manipulative Medicine
Chicago College of Osteopathic Medicine
Midwestern University
Downers Grove, Illinois

Jan Lei Iwata, MS, PharmD, DO
Adjunct Clinical Instructor
Department of Osteopathic Manipulative Medicine
Midwestern University
Chicago College of Osteopathic Medicine
Midwestern University
Downers Grove, Illinois

Douglas J. Jorgensen, DO, CPC
Adjunct Assistant Professor of Community and Family Medicine
Dartmouth Medical School
Hanover, New Hampshire
Osteopathic Manipulation and Pain Management
Manchester Osteopathic Healthcare
Jorgensen Consulting, LLC
Manchester, Maine

Raymond T. Jorgensen, MS, CPC
President and Co-Founding Partner
Priority Management Group, Inc.
Pawtucket, Rhode Island

Janet M. Krettek, DO, FACOS, NMM/OMM
Clinical Assistant Professor, Department of Surgery
Kansas City University of Medicine and Biosciences
Kansas City, Missouri
General Surgeon, North Baldwin Infirmary
Bay Minette, Alabama

James Laub, MS, DO, MPH, FACPM
Attending Physician
Family Practice and Osteopathic Manipulative Medicine
Grandview Medical Center
Dayton, Ohio

Andrew Lovy, DO, FACN
Past Chairman, Department of Psychiatry
Chicago College of Osteopathic Medicine
Midwestern University
Downers Grove, Illinois
Psychiatric Consultant
Northeast Missouri Health Council
Kirksville, Missouri

John McPartland, DO, MS
Associate Professor
Unitec School of Health
Auckland, New Zealand

Anette Karin Schilling Mnabhi, RN, MSN, DO
Adjunct Clinical Faculty
Department of Osteopathic Manipulative Medicine
Midwestern University
Downers Grove, Illinois
Staff, Department of Family Medicine
Rush Copley Medical Center
Aurora, Illinois

Kenneth E. Nelson, DO, FAAO, FACOFP
Professor, Departments of Osteopathic Manipulative Medicine,
    Family Medicine, and Biochemistry
Chicago College of Osteopathic Medicine
Midwestern University
Downers Grove, Illinois

Nils Olson, DO, FACOFP
Adjunct Professor of Family Medicine
University of Des Moines College of Osteopathic Medicine
Des Moines, Iowa
Attending Physician, Department of Family Medicine
Marshfield Clinic/Mercer Center
Mercer, Wisconsin
Midwestern University College of Osteopathic Medicine
Chicago, Illinois
Affiliate Staff, Howard Young Medical Center
Woodruff, Wisconsin

Dean Raffaelli, DO
Clinical Assistant Professor
Departments of Family Medicine and Osteopathic Manipulative Medicine
Chicago College of Osteopathic Medicine
Downers Grove, Illinois
Midwestern University
Attending Physician, Chicago Osteopathic Family Practice
Michael Reese Hospital
Chicago, Illinois

Thomas M. Richards, DO, FAAO, CIME
Department of Neuromusculoskeletal Medicine
Marshfield Clinic/Lakeland Center
Minocqua, Wisconsin
Community Preceptor
Kansas City University of Medicine and Biosciences
Kansas City, Missouri
Attending Physician
Primary Care Department
Howard Young Medical Center
Woodruff, Wisconsin

Joey Rottman, DO, FACOOG
Associate Professor and Director of Clinical Clerkship
Department of Obstetrics and Gynecology
University of Medicine and Dentistry of New Jersey
School of Osteopathic Medicine
Stratford, New Jersey
Professor, Department of Obstetrics and Gynecology
Philadelphia College of Osteopathic Medicine
Philadelphia, Pennsylvania
Associate Professor, Department of Obstetrics and Gynecology
Chicago College of Osteopathic Medicine
Midwestern University
Downers Grove, Illinois

Nicette Sergueef, DO (France)
Adjunct Assistant Professor
Department of Osteopathic Manipulative Medicine
Chicago College of Osteopathic Medicine
Midwestern University
Downers Grove, Illinois

Sandra L. Sleszynski, DO, AOBNMM
Adjunct Clinical Assistant Professor
Department of Osteopathic Manipulative Medicine
Chicago College of Osteopathic Medicine
Downers Grove, Illinois

Charles J. Smutny III, DO, FAAO
Assistant Professor, Clinical Osteopathic Medicine
New York College of Osteopathic Medicine
Old Westbury, New York
NMM Residency Director
North Shore LIJ at Plainview
Plainview, New York

Frank C. Walton, Sr., DO, FAAO
Adjunct Associate Professor, Department of Family Medicine
Chicago College of Osteopathic Medicine
Midwestern University
Downers Grove, Illinois
Program Director NMM-OMM Residency
Westview Osteopathic Hospital
Indianapolis, Indiana

Alice J. Zal, DO, FACOFP
Adjunct Faculty, Department of Family Medicine
Philadelphia College of Osteopathic Medicine
Philadelphia, Pennsylvania
Private Practice, Family Medicine Geriatrics
Family Practice Staff
Mercy Suburban Hospital/Montgomery Hospital
Norristown, Pennsylvania

Reviewers

Joseph D. Allgeier, DO
Program Director and Director of Medical Education
Florida Hospital East Orlando
Orlando, Florida

Richard K. Book, DO
Active Medical Staff, Family Medicine
Arkansas Valley Regional Medical Center
La Junta, Colorado

Jeffrey S. Brault, DO
Assistant Professor of Physical Medicine and Rehabilitation
Mayo Clinic
Rochester, Minnesota

Janet M. Burns, DO
Assistant Professor of Osteopathic Manipulative Medicine
Ohio University College of Osteopathic Medicine
Athens, Ohio

Boyd Buser, DO, FACOFP
Professor of OMM
University of New England College of Osteopathic Medicine
Biddeford, Maine

Sarah Cates
Osteopathic Medical Student, 4th year
Virginia College of Osteopathic Medicine
Virginia Polytechnic Institute and State University
Blacksburg, Virginia

Robert S. Dolansky, Jr., DO
Director of Medical Education
St. Luke's Hospital, Allentown Campus
Allentown, Pennsylvania

Mary E. Franz, DO, FACOFP
Private Practice, Family Medicine
Topeka, Kansas

Dan C. Galloway, DO, FACOFP
Private Practice, Family Medicine
Seasons Health Center
Crown Point, Indiana

Ann L. Habenicht, DO, FAAO, FACOFP
Professor, Department of Osteopathic Manipulative Medicine
Chicago College of Osteopathic Medicine
Midwestern University
Downers Grove, Illinois
Senior Staff, Department of Family Medicine
Palos Community Hospital
Palos Heights, Illinois

Patrick J. Hanford, DO, FACOFP
Private Practice, Kings Park Urgent Care Center
Lubbock, Texas

Wilbur T. Hill, DO, FACOFP
Private Practice, Family Medicine (Retired)
Liberty, Missouri

Howard H. Hunt, DO, FACOFP
Professor of Family Medicine (Retired)
West Virginia School of Osteopathic Medicine
Lewisburg, West Virginia

Douglas J. Jorgensen, DO, MS, CPC
Adjunct Assistant Professor of Community and Family Medicine
Dartmouth Medical School
Hanover, New Hampshire
Osteopathic Manipulation and Pain Management
Jorgensen Consulting, LLC
Manchester, Maine

John N. Kasimos, DO, FCAP, FASCP, FAOCP
Chair and Professor of Pathology
Chicago College of Osteopathic Medicine
Midwestern University
Downers Grove, Illinois

Brian Loveless, DO
Private Practice, Family Medicine
Chino Valley Medical Center
Chino, California

Barbara Peterson, DLitt
Adjunct Associate Professor, Department of Internal Medicine
Chicago College of Osteopathic Medicine
Midwestern University
Downers Grove, Illinois

Thomas M. Richards, DO, FAAO, CIME
Department of Neuromusculoskeletal Medicine
Marshfield Clinic/Lakeland Center
Minocqua, Wisconsin
Community Preceptor
Kansas City University of Medicine and Biosciences

Kansas City, Missouri
Attending Physician
Primary Care Department
Howard Young Medical Center
Woodruff, Wisconsin

J. Jerry Rodos, DO, DSc, FAANP
Clinical Professor, Department of Behavioral Medicine
Chicago College of Osteopathic Medicine
Midwestern University
Downers Grove, Illinois

Steven F. Rubin, DO, FACOFP dist
Adjunct Clinical Professor, Departments of Osteopathic
    Manipulative Medicine and Family Medicine
University of Medicine and Dentistry of New Jersey,
    School of Osteopathic Medicine
Stratford, New Jersey
Private Practice, Family Medicine
Fair Lawn, New Jersey

George T. Sawabini, DO, FACOFP
Private Practice, Family Medicine
Farmington Village, Michigan

Frank R. Serrecchia, DO, RDH
Adjunct Assistant Professor, Department of Osteopathic
    Manipulative Medicine
Chicago College of Osteopathic Medicine
Midwestern University
Downers Grove, Illinois

William H. Stager, DO, FACOFP
Clinical Assistant Professor of Family Medicine and
    Osteopathic Manipulative Medicine
NOVA Southeastern University College of Osteopathic Medicine
Fort Lauderdale, Florida

Marline A. Wager, DO
Professor of Family Medicine
West Virginia School of Osteopathic Medicine
Lewisburg, West Virginia

Earle Noble Wagner, DO, FACOFP
Private Practice, Family Medicine
Cheltenham, Pennsylvania

Elaine M. Wallace, DO, MSc
Chair and Professor of Osteopathic Principles and Practice
NOVA Southeastern University College of Osteopathic Medicine
Fort Lauderdale, Florida

Anthony M. Will, DO
Assistant Clinical Professor, Pre-clinical Division
Arizona College of Osteopathic Medicine
Midwestern University
Glendale, Arizona

Alice J. Zal, DO, FACOFP
Adjunct Faculty, Department of Family Medicine
Philadelphia College of Osteopathic Medicine
Philadelphia, Pennsylvania
Private Practice, Family Medicine Geriatrics
Family Practice Staff
Mercy Suburban Hospital/Montgomery Hospital
Norristown, Pennsylvania

Contents

List of Abbreviations

A-A, atlantoaxial (joint)

AACOM, American Association of Colleges of Osteopathic Medicine

AAFP, American Academy of Family Physicians

AAO, American Academy of Osteopathy

ABG, arterial blood gas

ACL, anterior cruciate ligament

ACOFP, American College of Osteopathic Family Physicians

ACTH, adrenocorticotropic hormone, corticotropin

ADLs, activities of daily living

AEA, anandamide, arachidonylethanolamine

2-AG, 2-arachidonylglycerol

AIDS, acquired immune deficiency syndrome

ALT, alanine amino transferase

AMA, American Medical Association

ANA, antinuclear antibody (panel)

ANS, autonomic nervous system

AOA, American Osteopathic Association

AP curve, anteroposterior curve

ART, articulatory treatment

ASIS, anterior superior iliac spine

AST, aspartate transaminase

AVM, arteriovenous malformation

BA, body areas

BLT, balanced ligamentous tension/ligamentous articular strain

BMI, body mass index

BMT, balanced membranous tension

BPH, benign prosthetic hypertrophy

BTS, British Thoracic Society

C2, 3, etc., cervical vertebral segments

CAE, certified association executive

CAM, complementary and alternative medicines

CAP, Clinical Assessment Program

CAP, community acquired pneumonia

CBC, complete blood count

CC, chief complaint

CCK, cholecystokinin

CCR5, chemokine chemotaxis receptor

CDC, Centers for Disease Control and Prevention

CDROM, compact disk read-only memory

CFIDS, chronic fatigue and immune dysfunction syndrome

CFS, chronic fatigue syndrome

CHF, congestive heart failure

CME, continuing medical education

CMS, Center for Medicare Standards

cNOS, constitutive NO-synthase

CNS, central nervous system

CN X, cranial nerve X

COMT, catechol O-methyl transferase

COPD, chronic obstructive pulmonary disease

CPC, Certified Professional Coder

CPM, continuous passive motion

CPT, current procedural terminology

CR, cranial, cranial osteopathy (see also OCF)

CRH, corticotrophin-releasing hormone

CRI, cranial rhythmic impulse

CS, counterstrain

CSF, cerebrospinal fluid

CT, cervical-thoracic (junction)

CT, computed tomography

CV-4, compression of the fourth ventricle

DAs, dopamine agonists

DASH, dietary approaches to stop hypertension

DBP, diastolic blood pressure

DBS, deep brain stimulation

DECIDA (also DISIDA), technetium-99m diisopropyl iminodiacetic
   acid hepatobiliary scintigraphy

DIR, direct (treatment)

DIT, diiodotyrosine

DJD, degenerative joint disease

DNR, do not resuscitate

DO, Doctor of Osteopathy, Doctor of Osteopathic Medicine

DSM-IV-TR, Diagnostic and Statistical Manual of Mental Disorders:
   4th Text Revision

DVD, digital video disk

E&M, evaluation and management

EEG, electroencephalogram

EENT, eyes, ears, nose, throat

EKG, electrocardiogram

EMG, electromyogram

EMR, electronic medical record

EMS, electrical muscle stimulation

ENT, ears, nose, throat

EPF, expanded-problem-focused

eSOAP, electronic SOAP Note Form

ESR, erythrocyte sedimentation rate

EV-4, expansion of the fourth ventricle

FACOFP, Fellow of the American College of Osteopathic Family
   Physicians

FAAO, Fellow of the American Academy of Osteopathy

FM, fibromyalgia

FPR, facilitated positional release

GAS, general adaptive syndrome

GERD, gastroesophageal reflux disease

GH, growth hormone

GHAA, Group Health Association of America

GI, gastrointestinal

GMS, general multi-system (examination)

GVA, general visceral afferent neuron

H&P, history and physical

HCFA, Health Care Financing Administration

HCPCS, HCFA's Common Procedural Coding System (pronounced
   "hickpicks")

HDL, high density lipoprotein

HEENT, head, eyes, ears, nose, throat

HIDA, hepato nuclear medicine biliary tract scans

HIPAA, Health Insurance Portability and Accountability Act

HIV, human immunodeficiency virus

HLA, human leukocyte antigen

HPA, hypothalamic-pituitary adrenal (axis)

HPI, history of present illness

HS CRP, high sensitivity C-reactive protein

HVLA, high-velocity, low-amplitude

ICD-9CM, International Classification of Disease, Ninth Clinical Modification

ICHD-2, International Classification of Headache Disorders, 2nd ed.

ID, internal derangement

IDET, intradiscal electrothermal therapy

IGE, immunoglobulin-E

IL-1, -6, and so on, interleukin

ILA, inferior lateral angle (sacrum)

IND, indirect (treatment)

INR, integrated neuromuscular release

IT, Information Technologies (Department)

JNC 7, Seventh Report of the Joint National Committee on High Blood Pressure

KOH, potassium (kalium) hydroxide

L1, 2, etc., lumbar vertebral segments

LAS, ligamentous articular strain/balanced ligamentous tension

LBORC, Louisa Burns Osteopathic Research Committee

LC-NE, locus ceruleus-norepinephrine axis

LHRH, leuteinizing hormone releasing hormone

MA, Medical Assistant

MAO-B, monoamine oxidase B

MD, doctor of medicine

MDM, medical decision-making

ME, myalgic encephalopathy

ME, muscle energy

MFR, myofascial release

MIT, monoiodotyrosine

MODEMS, Musculoskeletal Outcomes Data Evaluation and Management System

MPD, myofascial pain dysfunction

MRI, magnetic resonance imaging

MSA, multiple system atrophy

NADH, nicotinamide adenine dinucleotide (reduced form)

NC, noncontributory

NK, natural killer (cells)
NO, nitric oxide
NOS, NO synthase
NSAID, non-steroidal anti-inflammatory drugs
OA, occipitoatlantal (joint)
OCF, osteopathy in the cranial field
OMM, osteopathic manipulative medicine
OMT, osteopathic manipulative treatment
OPTI, osteopathic post-graduate training institutions
OS, organ systems
OTH, other treatments used
PAG, periaquaductal gray (region)
PAH, pulmonary artery hypertension
PAN, peripheral afferent nociceptors
PC, personal computer
PCP, phencyclidine
PD, Parkinson's disease
PET, positron emission tomography
PFSH, past family, medical, and social history
PhD, doctor of philosophy
PI, pelvic index
PIPIDA, para-isopropyl acetanilido-iminodiacetic acid
PMH, past medical history
PNI, psychoneuroimmunology
PTSD, post-traumatic stress disorder
PPD, (tuberculin) purified protein derivative
PSIS, posterior superior iliac spines
PSP, progressive supranuclear palsy
PSS, pelvic side shift
PT, physical therapy
PTU, propylthiouracil
RA, rheumatoid arthritis
RAIU, radioactive iodine uptake
ROM, range of motion
REM, rapid eye movement
RF, rheumatoid factor
RICEM (principle), rest, ice, compress, elevate, medicate

RN, registered nurse

ROS, review of systems

RPR, rapid plasma reagin

SARS, severe acute respiratory syndrome

SBP, systolic blood pressure

SBS, sphenobasilar synchondrosis

SF36, Rand 36-Item Health Survey

SI, sacroiliac (joint)

SNS, sympathetic nervous system

SOAP, subjective, objective, assessment, plan

SOQ, Specialized Osteopathic Questionnaire

SOS, Single Organ System (SOAP note form)

SPECT, single photon emission computed tomography

SS, sphenosquamous

SSRI, selective serotonin reuptake inhibitor

ST, soft tissue (treatment)

STDA, soft-tissue, deep articulation

SP, substance P

T1, 2, etc., thoracic vertebral segments

T_3, triiodothyronine

T_4, thyroxine

TART, tissue texture change, asymmetry, range of motion, tenderness

TENS, transcutaneous electrical nerve stimulation (unit)

TRH, thyrotropin releasing hormone

TIA, transient ischemic attack

TMJ, temporomandibular joint

TNF, tumor necrosis factor

TRH, thyrotropin-releasing hormone

TSH, thyroid-stimulating hormone

UPDRS, Unified Parkinson's Disease Rating Scale

VIP, vasoactive intestinal polypeptide

WHO, World Health Organization

Philosophy and Principles of Patient Care

CHAPTER 1

Patient Empowerment

James L. Laub

INTRODUCTION

After years working in a variety of hospitals and clinics in the military, facilities where medical doctors and doctors of osteopathic medicine worked side by side, occasionally a patient newly assigned to the installation would ask when first checking in to the medical facility, "Do you have any DOs on the staff?" I thought I knew why, so I never—nor did any of the other staff members—ask why the patient requested an osteopathic physician. One day in my clinic, I had an allopathic medical student shadowing me for the afternoon. The patient, who had more than 20 years of military service and whom I had seen on several previous visits, struck up a short conversation with the student while I was finishing the note in the chart. In the conversation, he mentioned that he always preferred osteopathic physicians and sought them out at every opportunity. When the student asked why, his answer surprised me a bit: "Because they listen better." Mine was a neuromusculoskeletal medicine clinic. More than 90% of the treatment I gave was OMT (osteopathic manipulative treatment). My patients were all referred from their primary care physician. This patient was assigned at a nearby military installation and drove 50 miles to see me for his chronic myofascial pain, which was showing marked improvement. But his number one reason for seeking my counsel as a physician apparently was that my osteopathic colleagues and I were known to him to be good listeners. Moreover, I believe he was saying that his osteopathic physician was listening at the level needed to understand him and thereby showed respect for his perspectives concerning his health care.

Respecting patients' perspectives makes them part of the treatment team and establishes the basis for empowering them actively to seek solutions to their own medical issues. The empowered patient is not just the sufferer; the empowered patient is a collegial member of the team seeking the most effective therapeutic plan. As with any form of participative management, the patient is a stakeholder in the success of the therapeutic plan, not the subject of it. This starts with good listening, but it is necessary to do more than just good listening to make patient empowerment work. Healing occurs from within; the first step to assisting patients to get past the barriers to their own healing power is for them to develop a personal commitment to the therapeutic plan for their own recovery. The most effective way to secure that commitment is to ensure that patients are partners in the plan's development. Their partnership in the process is most easily done through a patient-centered medical practice. The next few paragraphs explore and contrast the patient-centered medical practice model with what is perhaps the more familiar physician-centered model. Later on the chapter addresses how the patient-centered model is the cornerstone of effective patient empowerment.

The physician-centered model is a parent-child transaction[1] in which the patient is expected to be passive and dependent on the doctor's advice in an unequal relationship. Teaching is designed to keep information simple to facilitate retention. The health professional holds valued medical information and conveys it to the patient, who is expected to absorb it uncritically. The chief issue in the physician-centered model is the patient who is unable to understand or to retain the information or who lacks the motivation to comply. The model assumes that a rational argument is sufficient to persuade patients they need to change their behavior to accommodate the health message. In this relationship, the primary reason for failure is the bad, noncompliant patient who just wouldn't do what the doctor said. Also, in this relationship, a patient who gathers outside information challenges the veracity of the health professional and is often admonished or criticized for doing so. Therefore, the energy to improve this system is expended in getting patients to comply. Metrics (e.g., weight, laboratory values, blood pressure) are used for judgment.

The patient-centered model is an adult-adult transaction[1] in which the patient participates as an equal partner with the professional to make informed judgments and develop a personal therapeutic plan. This model seeks to elicit and satisfy patients' expressed needs as a first step toward taking greater control over their own health. Patients' involvement in decision making is the key part of the educational process itself. Use of the patient-centered model develops our patients' understanding and encourages self-reliance, with access to information necessary to exercise control over their own body. The energy to improve this system is spent encouraging patients to share and reflect upon their existing understanding as a basis for future learning. Metrics are used for self-evaluation.

Patients have the capability to monitor the performance of their body continuously. When they assess something and find it awry, they attempt to make a determination as to what may be the problem from their knowledge, ability, and experience (diagnosis). They go on to decide what to do about it, again from their knowledge, ability, and experience (treatment). And finally, they watch for their expected outcome (follow-up). Patients seek counsel when the problem is outside of their knowledge, ability, or experience to diagnose or treat or when there is no improvement at follow-up. I submit that doctors of osteopathic medicine go through the same process with patients. And if treatment fails, clinicians do the same thing: seek the counsel of a specialist and call it a referral. True primary care medicine occurs before the patients even are present. Osteopathic physicians show patients a desire to understand by consulting patients as they would a referring physician. It is necessary to respect the fact that patients have exceeded their level of expertise and exchange information collegially, discuss courses of action, what outcomes to expect, and when they should occur. In addition, when patients gather information on their condition from outside sources, they are providing more data to draw upon. No one's knowledge is infinite, and when a colleague shares knowledge, it has the potential to contribute to better decision making. An inquiring patient is not challenging the physician's veracity but participating in an effort to achieve a successful therapeutic decision from the team. And that participation also enfranchises the patient as a stakeholder in the success of the therapeutic plan.

Not long after osteopathic physicians attained full practice rights, the search was on to find out what makes them distinct. Apparently with full practice rights comes the loss of the osteopathic equivalent of the Holy Grail. In an excellent 1993 article, J. F. Peppin lists six potential activities for osteopathic distinction.[2] After discrediting each, he suggests that touch is a better candidate. Peppin includes a statement from an osteopathic physician who claims "true" osteopathic medicine no longer exists in the United States and a statement from another who suggests it is not any one of his six factors but the collection together that makes osteopathic medicine distinct, an osteopathic collage.[2] While pursuing this search is beyond the scope of this chapter, one irrefutable item does bind all osteopathic physicians the letters "DO" after one's name. Fewer than 5% of physicians in the United States have an osteopathic professional degree. As with any minority, the actions of one frequently speak for many. The action of a medical physician usually only speaks to how the patient population regards that one individual. But the action of an osteopathic physician frequently speaks to how the patient population regards osteopathic physicians collectively. Thus, doctors of osteopathic medicine entrust part of their reputation to each other and should do their best for one another.

Patient empowerment is not anything that's uniquely osteopathic. Patients will hold the empowering allopathic physician in high regard, also. But the empowering osteopathic physician may well engender a positive reflection on our entire profession. I always felt a sense of pride when a family transferred into our military installation and requested to see a DO. It told me one or more of my osteopathic colleagues had left them with an identifiably positive experience. The pride continued along with a profound sense of responsibility when the staff chose to send that family to me to continue their care in that same identifiably positive way. Regardless of the chosen specialty, it is necessary to continue the legacy, listen well, practice patient-centered medicine, and empower patients.

The material in this chapter comes from a collection of concepts that I have taken and tested in the laboratory of life. Certainly, the concept of empowerment is not new and is easily traceable in both the clinical and management literature over 50 years.[3,4] I received my original exposure to participative management concepts in the mid-1970s as a graduate student at the University of Utah. Especially significant to me were the writings of Douglas McGregor[5] and Abraham Maslow,[6] along with the lectures and writings of Frederick Hertzberg.[7,8] There I also had the good fortune to take a course in social psychology from Martin Chemers. Since at the time I was a military officer, I could easily take a collage of academic concepts and test them from my positions as a manager and leader. From this empirical immersion, my use of and confidence in empowerment evolved. Later, when I embarked on my quest to study osteopathic medicine, I discovered

I had learned some tools to describe what some of my clinician mentors had discovered apparently by trial and error. Empowerment, whether in a clinic or at a worksite, has a demonstrated history of success. Thomas Gordon[4] has an excellent description of his experiences in the preface of *Making the Patient Your Partner*, including his exposure to the clinical work of Carl Rogers in clinical psychology in the 1950s. I recommend the book by Gordon and Edwards[4] to any clinician who wants to learn more in this area.

Later, after my osteopathic internship, I reentered the military and was exposed to the work of W. Edwards Deming[9] in quality management. I now was reenergized to expand the empowerment concepts from my management background into my clinic. I learned from both coworkers and patients; my appreciation for the value of empowerment continued to evolve. In preparing for this chapter, I came across the work of Carl E. Schneider,[10] *The Practice of Autonomy*, in which he discusses the development of autonomy as a sociological movement in our society. Thus, the use of empowerment concepts in a population whose desire for autonomy is on the rise is a terrific combination for success. Additionally, I recently came upon the work of Daniel Fisher[11] and his use of empowerment as the basis for success with schizophrenic patients. At least on the surface, empowerment appears to be just a portion of a larger sociological movement. And I, as a subject in this movement, have merely read, listened, tried, and learned. If anyone feels I've encroached upon his or her intellectual property, I humbly beg forgiveness.

Where I believe this treatise fits in osteopathic literature is perhaps in the revered stature the osteopathic profession gives to physicians who have engendered empowerment in the practice of osteopathic medicine. Despite the profession's inability heretofore to codify what those revered osteopathic physicians do, the profession subjectively embraces them. Reverence begets emulation, and emulation begets a culture (treat the person, not the disease).

HOW TO BE ON A TEAM WITH AN EMPOWERED PATIENT

Teams can take one of three basic forms. The first is the synergistic team. The synergistic team exploits the ideas and participation from each of its members and seeks to reach a set of conclusions that is superior to what any individual on the team could do alone. The second is the leader–follower team. The leader–follower team designates one member as the expert who autonomously selects the set of conclusions for the team. The third is the antagonistic team. The antagonistic team is one in which internal conflict, personal interest, and politicking usually attempt a compromise set of conclusions that often are inferior to what many of the members could have accomplished individually.

If we wish to be part of a synergistic team as we empower our patients, here are two basic rules:

There is no room for ego in clinical encounters. This is easier to understand in concept than to accomplish in fact. Ego challenges cause a visceral reaction. That reaction has to be recognized for what it is and discarded at the same emotional level it enters, before the physician can continue with the patient interaction.

Empowering the patient does not abrogate the responsibility of the clinician. No two combinations of patient and illness are the same. Each will require a unique interplay among the decision team members. Each will demand a contribution from the clinician at some level given the situation.

References

1. Berne E. What Do You Say After You Say Hello? New York: Grove, 1972.
2. Peppin JF. The osteopathic distinction: fact or fancy? J Med Humanit 1993;14(4):203–222.
3. Siegal B, August Y. Help Me to Heal. Carlsbad, CA: Hay House, 2003.
4. Gordon T, Edwards WS. Making the Patient Your Partner. Westport, CT: Auburn House, 1995.
5. McGregor D. The Human Side of Enterprise. 25th Anniversary Printing. New York: McGraw Hill, 1985.
6. Maslow A. Motivation and Personality. 2nd ed. New York: Harper & Row, 1970.
7. Hertzberg F. Work and the Nature of Man. London: Harper Collins, 1966.
8. Hertzberg F. Motivation to Work. Somerset, NJ: Transaction, 1993.
9. Deming WE. The New Economics for Industry, Government, Education. 2nd ed. Cambridge, MA: MIT, 2000.
10. Schneider CE. The Practice of Autonomy. New York: Oxford University Press, 1998.
11. Fisher D. National Empowerment Center. Available at *http://www.power2u.org*. Accessed February 20, 2005.

CHAPTER 2

Osteopathic Distinctiveness

Kenneth E. Nelson

INTRODUCTION

Osteopathic medicine is a success. With the new millennium, this nineteenth century medical reactionary movement is well established within the mainstream of contemporary medicine. Success, however, has come with a price. Mainstream acceptance has resulted in the assimilation of the allopathic model of practice by osteopathic physicians to the detriment of their reactionary heritage.

The osteopathic profession is being challenged to demonstrate its unique qualities and thereby justify its existence as an independent institution within American health care. To do so, osteopathic distinctiveness must be identified, measured, and validated. The responsibility to prove osteopathic distinctiveness ultimately belongs to the osteopathic academic community, basic scientists and clinicians alike.

Since contemporary osteopathic medicine has become mainstream, it is logical to look to its origin to identify its distinctiveness. The philosophy of osteopathic medicine is based on four key principles:[1]

1. The body is a unit; the person is a unit of body, mind, and spirit.
2. The body is capable of self-regulation, self-healing, and health maintenance.
3. Structure and function are reciprocally interrelated.
4. Rational treatment is based upon an understanding of the principles of body unity, self-regulation, and the interrelationship of structure and function.

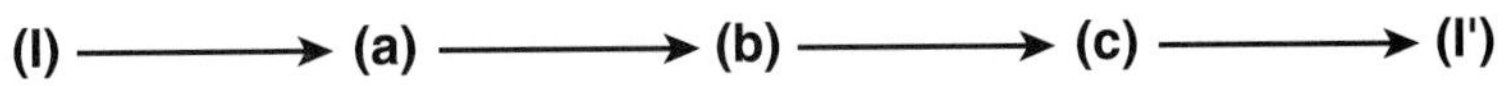

(I) ⟶ (a) ⟶ (b) ⟶ (c) ⟶ (I')

FIGURE 2.1   A schematic representing cause-and-effect logic.

These individual principles, however, are not necessarily unique to osteopathic medicine, and they are extremely difficult to quantify.

Consistent with principle 1, contemporary osteopathic physicians claim to be holistic. This is an admirable trait, but it is not distinctly osteopathic. Holism has been all but usurped by contemporary alternative medicine, and increasing numbers of practitioners are approaching their patients in this manner.

Consistent with principle 2, contemporary osteopathic physicians claim to be patient oriented (as opposed to disease oriented). Although allopathic medicine focuses upon the diagnosis and treatment of disease, the practice of medicine is acknowledged to be highly personal.[2] With the progressive understanding of the role of the immune system, much of the contemporary treatment of disease is focused on assisting the patient's ability to respond to the illness.

An apparent difference (consistent with principle 3) is the diagnosis and treatment of dysfunction in the musculoskeletal system. Yet many doctors of osteopathic medicine do not use osteopathic manipulation, and a number of medical doctors, most notably in physical medicine and rehabilitation, employ manual therapy.

Principle 4 appears to identify the distinction by combining the first three principles to form a system for clinical practice. If osteopathic medicine is distinctive and the understanding of somatic dysfunction in the context of the patient's level of wellbeing occupies a pivotal position in that distinctiveness, then it is the appreciation of the significance of dysfunction of the neuromusculoskeletal system that offers osteopathic physicians a uniquely holistic system of clinical logic.

HOLISTIC LOGIC

The logic of Western science, and consequently Western medicine, is Aristotelian (Fig. 2.1). It seeks to understand systems by reducing them to the sequential relationship of their smallest parts *(atomos)*. Therefore, in Figure 2.1, the sequence could represent an individual (I) who gets caught in the rain (a), which lowers his resistance (b). He is exposed to a virus (c), which causes him to catch a cold (I').

Comparatively, holistic logic may at first appear to be an oxymoron. Holism is an acceptance of the totality and indivisibility of a system. It is nonlinear. It is exemplified by the Taoist philosophy of ancient China. Such a nonlinear system might be illustrated (Fig. 2.2) as the determination of a resultant vector. As multiple forces act upon the individual (I), the resultant vector or outcome (I') is the development of disease or the maintenance of health.

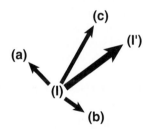

FIGURE 2.2   A schematic representing holistic logic.

STRUCTURE, FUNCTION, AND DYSFUNCTION

The third principle, describing the relationship between structure and function, gives rise to the recognition of somatic dysfunction. The diagnosis and treatment of somatic dysfunction differentiate osteopathic medicine from allopathic medicine. Somatic dysfunction is impaired function of fundamentally normal anatomy. It is not pathology. Rather, it is thought to predispose to and, once established, maintain pathology.

The mechanics of somatic dysfunction have been described.[1,3–5] Somatic dysfunction may occur as functional impediment due to altered soft tissue (muscular, ligamentous, fascial) tensions, articular motion restriction, or any combination of these components. Articular dysfunction of typical spinal segments (adjacent vertebrae possessing zygapophyseal joints and intervertebral discs) may occur as group dysfunctions composed of three or more consecutive segments, or as segmental dysfunctions composed of two adjacent segments. Articular dysfunction of atypical spinal segments and appendicular joints is determined by their unique anatomy.

The response of the axial musculoskeletal system to the force of gravity is nearly always asymmetric. Most individuals have unequal leg length, with resultant pelvic unleveling.[3] Therefore, everyone is predisposed to compensatory group and segmental spinal dysfunction.[5] Add to this the asymmetry imposed by dominance (left- and right-handedness), stresses from activities of daily living, and trauma (micro and macro), and it is understandable that musculoskeletal problems are so widespread. Somatic dysfunction, both group and segmental dysfunctions, occur in response to side-bending forces.[4]

The physiology of somatic dysfunction has been extensively studied.[6–9] The greater body of scientific literature has been reviewed and compared to the proposed mechanisms of somatic dysfunction.[10,11]

Van Buskirk[12] offers a nociceptively rooted model for spinal somatic dysfunction as follows:

1. A peripheral focus of irritation results in activation of nociceptive neurons. These may be somatosensory or general visceral afferent neurons.
2. These primary afferent neurons synapse in the dorsal horn of the spinal cord with internuncial neurons.
3. Ongoing afferent stimulation of insufficient intensity to reach firing potential results in the establishment of a state of irritability (facilitation) of the internuncial neurons.
4. Additional afferent activity from any source results in a segmental response to significantly less stimulus than would normally be required.
5. Such activity from internuncial neurons, which synapse with ventral horn motor neurons, results in segmentally related myospasticity. Stimulation of internuncial neurons, which synapse in the intermediolateral cell column of the thoracic and upper lumbar cord, will produce a segmentally related sympathetic response (somatic and/or visceral). The same response to stimulation applies to the parasympathetic efferent system. Moreover, internuncial neurons travel up and down the spinal cord for several segments and further synapse with the spinothalamic tract. These neurons are, thus, capable of initiating a broad response.

SPINAL SOMATIC DYSFUNCTION AS A FOCAL POINT FOR HOLISM

A focus of irritation producing spinal facilitation can affect structures in segmentally related dermatomes, myotomes, sclerotomes, and viscerotomes. If the peripheral focus of irritation is the result of vertebral articular dysfunction, the paravertebral myospasticity and sensitivity found with spinal dysfunction result. If a peripheral somatic focus of irritation (dysfunction or pathology) produces a ventral horn motor response, the result is a somatosomatic reflex. If the somatic focus of irritation produces a response in the intermediolateral cell column or a parasympathetic nucleus, the result may be a somatovisceral or a (sympathetic) somatosomatic reflex. In a similar fashion, general visceral afferent activity is capable of producing viscerosomatic and viscerovisceral reflexes. As such, the spinal cord links seemingly unrelated systems and structures in a manner that fosters a clinical system of logic, rendering it more inclusive or holistic.

Clinical Example

A patient presents with dysesthesia of the palmar surface of the right hand consistent with a diagnosis of carpal tunnel syndrome of uncertain etiology.

Upper extremity complaints have been specifically linked to upper thoracic somatic dysfunction.[13] Although the involved somatosensory innervation, the median nerve, should result in somatosomatic reflex findings paravertebrally from C6 to T1, such findings are more typically encountered in the upper thoracic region. The sympathetic innervation of the upper extremity arises from T1 to T4. Autonomic nerves contain afferent as well as efferent neurons. Therefore, "sympathetic afferent" neurons from the right upper extremity are capable of producing facilitation in the upper thoracic region lateralizing to the right.

Facilitation, lateralizing to the right in the upper thoracic region, may be the result of primary spinal dysfunction. Spinal segmental dysfunction with facilitation also can result from postural accommodation to pelvic unleveling or from environmental stresses with resultant symptoms referable to the right hand.

Viscerosomatic and/or somatovisceral mechanisms may also be present. The high thoracic region receives general visceral afferent input from myocardium, lungs, and esophagus.[14] Pathology in any of these organs is capable of producing high thoracic facilitation. Facilitation of upper thoracic spinal segments can result in a reflex visceral response. Tachycardia through the sympathetic innervation of the sinoatrial node of the heart is an example.

Further, somatic dysfunction of minor intensity may be amplified through central facilitation by emotional stress.

Spinal segmental facilitation has been shown to result in segmentally related soft tissue edema.[15] Edema of the contents of the carpal tunnel can compress the median nerve. Thus, the upper thoracic spinal segmental facilitation, of whatever etiology, can produce or maintain carpal tunnel syndrome.

As such, the symptoms of carpal tunnel syndrome may be the result of organic pathology of the wrist. They may be a manifestation of a somatosomatic reflex from upper thoracic somatic dysfunction, either primary or as postural accommodation, or they may be a reflex from visceral pathology. Finally, the entire situation may be increased by the patient's mental status.

Conversely, carpal tunnel syndrome may result in spinal facilitation with secondary (reflex mediated) spinal somatic dysfunction and untold effect upon segmentally related viscera.

DISCUSSION

From this description of the mechanics and physiology of spinal somatic dysfunction, it can be seen how seemingly unrelated structures are linked through the axial central nervous system. A logical argument can be made as to how one might alleviate a tachyarrhythmia by treating carpal tunnel syndrome or how a proton pump inhibitor might be employed to decrease the inflammation of reflux esophagitis (viscerosomatic reflex T3, right), thereby reducing the median nerve compression of a right-sided carpal tunnel syndrome.

These are, of course, hypothetical proposals, presented merely to illustrate how the appreciation of somatic dysfunction leads to the development of a distinctive form of clinical logic that is unique to osteopathic medicine. The basic science is sound, but much more should be done in the areas of functional anatomy, biochemistry, and physiology. The preceding discussion deals superficially with only the mechanics and neurophysiology of somatic dysfunction. No mention is made of the effect of somatic dysfunction upon circulation, the immune system, and homeostasis.

From the perspective of clinical research, such complex problems are best pursued as outcome studies, for which massive amounts of data are necessary. The development of such a database is predicated upon effective data gathering. The American Osteopathic Association (AOA) requires that a musculoskeletal examination be incorporated into the medical record. In the hospital, this is typically recorded in the admitting history and physical examination. It is, therefore, imperative that this portion of the medical record be completed with particular diligence. The American Academy of Osteopathy (AAO) has developed and validated a series of outpatient osteopathic SOAP (subjective, objective, assessment, plan) note forms for outpatient use (see Chapter 31).[16–18] The Des Moines College of Osteopathic Medicine and Surgery is developing an Internet-mediated central database for purposes of electronically gathering information pertaining to the practice of osteopathic medicine. The validity of the degree of osteopathic physicians rests to a significant extent upon the results of this future research and consequently upon the efficacy with which they participate in these projects.

References

1. Ward RC, ed. Foundations for Osteopathic Medicine. 2nd ed. Philadelphia: Lippincott Williams & Wilkins, 2002.
2. Fauci AS, ed. Harrison's Principles of Internal Medicine. 14th ed. New York: McGraw Hill, 1998;1.
3. Schwab WA. Principles of Manipulative Treatment: The Low Back Problem. 1965 Yearbook. Vol 2. Indianapolis: American Academy of Osteopathy, 1965;95.
4. Fryette HH. Principles of Osteopathic Technique. Indianapolis: American Academy of Osteopathy, 1954, 1980.
5. Nelson KE. The management of low back pain: Short leg syndrome/postural balance. AAO J 1999;9(1):33–39.
6. Beal MC, ed. Louisa Burns, DO, Memorial. 1994 Yearbook. Indianapolis: American Academy of Osteopathy, 1994.
7. Beal MC, ed. Selected papers of John Stedman Denslow, DO. 1994 Yearbook. Indianapolis: American Academy of Osteopathy, 1994.
8. Peterson B, ed. The Collected Papers of Irvin M. Korr. Indianapolis: American Academy of Osteopathy, 1979.
9. King HH, ed. The Collected Papers of Irvin M. Korr. Vol 2. Indianapolis: American Academy of Osteopathy, 1997.
10. Patterson MM, Howell JN, eds. The Central Connection: Somatovisceral and Viscerosomatic Interaction. 1989 international symposium. Athens, OH: University Classics, 1992.
11. Willard FH, Patterson MM, eds. Nociception and the Neuroendocrine-Immune Connection. Athens, OH: University Classics, 1994.
12. Van Buskirk RL. Nociceptive reflexes and the somatic dysfunction: a model. J Am Osteopath Assoc 1990;90:792–794, 797–809 [review].

13. Larson NJ. Osteopathic manipulation for syndromes of the brachial plexus. J Am Osteopath Assoc 1972;72:378–384.
14. Van Buskirk RL, Nelson KE. Osteopathic family practice: An application of the primary care model. In: Ward RC, ed. Foundations for Osteopathic Medicine. 2nd ed. Philadelphia: Lippincott Williams & Wilkins, 2002;292.
15. Ramey K et al. MRI assessment of changes in swelling of wrist structures following OMT in patients with carpal tunnel syndrome. AAO J 1999;9:25–31.
16. Nelson KE, Glonek T. Computer/outcomes: Hardcopy SOAP note preliminary report: Family physician. Fam Physician 1999;3:8–10.
17. Sleszynski SL, Glonek T, Kuchera WA. Standardized medical record: A new outpatient osteopathic SOAP note form: Validation of a standardized office form against physician's progress notes. J Am Osteopath Assoc 1999;99:516–529.
18. Sleszynski SL, Glonek T, Kuchera WA. Outpatient osteopathic single organ system musculoskeletal exam form: Training and certification. J Am Osteopath Assoc 2004;104:76–81.

CHAPTER 3

Diagnosing Somatic Dysfunction

Kenneth E. Nelson

INTRODUCTION

Somatic dysfunction is a distinctly osteopathic diagnosis. It is unique in contemporary medicine in that it is considered to be central to the practice of osteopathic medicine, yet it is not organic pathology. It is functional impairment.

Somatic dysfunction is present to a greater or lesser degree in all individuals. It should be part of the approach to the care of any patient to identify the relative importance of somatic dysfunction in the overall clinical presentation and to address it appropriately. Osteopathic manipulative treatment (OMT) is the definitive treatment of somatic dysfunction. The effective use of OMT is predicated upon the effective diagnosis of somatic dysfunction.

"Somatic Dysfunction Defined

A. Somatic dysfunction: Impaired or altered function of related components of the somatic (body framework) system: skeletal, arthrodial, and myofascial structures, and related vascular, lymphatic, and neural elements. Somatic dysfunction is treatable using OMT. The positional and motion aspects of somatic dysfunction are best described using at least one of three parameters: (1) the position of a body part as determined by palpation and referenced to its adjacent defined structure, (2) the directions in which motion between two adjacent structures is freer, and (3) the directions in which motion is restricted. Somatic dysfunction may be primary or secondary.

B. Acute somatic dysfunction: Immediate or short-term impairment or altered function of related components of the somatic (body-framework) system; characterized in early stages by vasodilation, edema, tenderness, pain, and tissue contraction; diagnosed by history and palpatory assessment of tenderness, asymmetry of motion and relative position, restriction of motion, and tissue texture change (TART).

C. Chronic somatic dysfunction: Impairment or altered function of related components of the somatic (body framework) system, characterized by tenderness, itching, fibrosis, paresthesias, tissue contraction; identified by TART.

D. Primary somatic dysfunction: 1. The somatic dysfunction that maintains a total pattern of dysfunction. 2. The initial or first somatic dysfunction to appear temporally.

E. Secondary somatic dysfunction: Somatic dysfunction arising either from mechanical or neurophysiologic response subsequent to or as a consequence of other etiologies."

A. T. Still[1]

Secondary somatic dysfunction may be mechanical, as is seen with sacral dysfunction resulting from unequal leg length, or it may be of neural reflex origin, as a viscerosomatic or somatosomatic reflex.

Because somatic dysfunction is functional impairment and not organic pathology, primary somatic dysfunction is completely reversible when correctly diagnosed and specifically treated with OMT. Secondary somatic dysfunction also responds to OMT, but it will recur unless the primary condition is identified and treated. Somatic dysfunction that is a reflex response to visceral pathology (viscerosomatic reflex) typically does not respond to OMT until the underlying visceral pathology is treated.

Somatic dysfunction independently is responsible for a great deal of discomfort that cannot be attributed to organic cause. Because it manifests through the nervous and vascular systems as well as the musculoskeletal system, it can result in a broad array of symptoms.

Somatic dysfunction also contributes to the effect of organic pathology. Somatic dysfunction of the thoracic spine, ribs, and diaphragm results in decreased thoracic compliance, increasing the severity of existent congestive heart failure. It also exerts deleterious effect upon viscera receiving innervation from the same spinal segment (somatovisceral reflex).

DIAGNOSIS

The physical diagnosis of somatic dysfunction is accomplished by palpation. **TART,** a mnemonic for the four diagnostic criteria of somatic dysfunction, stands for the following:

Tissue texture abnormality
Asymmetry of position
Restriction of motion
Tenderness

The presence of any one of these is justification for the diagnosis of somatic dysfunction.

Palpation for tissue texture abnormality is probably the most efficient screen for somatic dysfunction. The qualitative aspects of tissue texture abnormality, as indicated in the definitions given previously, are used to differentiate acute from chronic somatic dysfunction. The degree of tissue texture abnormality indicates the severity of the somatic dysfunction.

Mechanical somatic dysfunction typically demonstrates asymmetry of position and restriction of motion. Asymmetry of position is stressed in the diagnostic paradigm of muscle energy. Restriction of motion is stressed in the diagnostic paradigm of articular dysfunction.

Tenderness must not be confused with pain. Pain is the subjective awareness of nociceptor activity. Tenderness is pain elicited upon palpation. As such, tenderness is an objective physical finding. Tenderness is often elicited as an involuntary pain response, a muscular twitch or facial wince, to diagnostic palpation, and may be employed to confirm the diagnosis of somatic dysfunction following the observation of tissue texture abnormality.

Like tissue texture abnormality, tenderness is indicative of the severity of somatic dysfunction. Although the site of the patient's pain may demonstrate tenderness, it is fairly common for significant findings of somatic dysfunction to be adjacent to or distant from the site of pain.

Commonly, the motion restriction of somatic dysfunction places compensatory stress upon adjacent structures, with resultant pain in those adjacent structures. The pain, however, may be distant from the etiologic dysfunction, presumably because of shared innervation (often sympathetic). This innervation results in a trigger point at the location of the responsible dysfunction which when palpated reproduces the distant pain.

Tissue texture abnormality and tenderness in the absence of the findings of mechanical somatic dysfunction, particularly restriction of motion, are indicative of somatic dysfunction of reflex origin, that is, viscerosomatic or somatosomatic reflexes.

PROCEDURES

In diagnosis of somatic dysfunction, it is appropriate to begin, when possible, with an overall assessment of the patient's weight-bearing mechanics. A decision can then be made as to what extent postural mechanics contribute to the condition being evaluated.

This is followed by regional assessment of the problem area. It is here that screening for tissue texture abnormality offers an effective method for quickly identifying areas requiring more definitive examination.

Once discrete somatic dysfunction is recognized, it is necessary to precisely identify asymmetry of position and all components of motion restriction (flexion and extension, side bending left and right, rotation left and right, translation anterior and posterior and left and right, with additional motions as appropriate for assessing appendicular dysfunction). To accomplish this, it is useful to be aware of common mechanical patterns of dysfunction.

Spinal somatic dysfunction is defined as type I (neutral, principle 1 of spinal physiologic motion) and type II (nonneutral, principle 2 of spinal physiologic motion).[1,2] These mechanics are found between typical vertebrae, that is, vertebrae possessing zygapophyseal joints and separated by intervertebral discs: the entire spine from C2 upon C3 to L5 upon S1, although the cervical spine demonstrates regionally atypical type I mechanics.

In type I mechanics, a group of three or more vertebrae demonstrate a coupled relationship between side bending and rotation. Under neutral circumstances (absence of spinal flexion or extension engaging the zygapophyseal articulations) when side-bending forces are applied to a group of typical vertebrae, rotation of the entire group will occur toward the side of the produced convexity. Side bending and rotation of the entire group are coupled in opposite directions. In the cervical region, the entire group will demonstrate coupled side bending and rotation in the same direction.

The levels of transitional mechanics within and between group curves are important. The vertebrae of maximum rotation, also where rotational mechanics change direction, is designated the apex of the curve. The conjuncture of two curves, or crossover point, is where side-bending mechanics change direction.

Anterior-posterior (AP) spinal mechanics are affected by type I mechanics. The presence of a group curve increases the existing spinal kyphosis or lordosis. Therefore, a thoracic type I curve will demonstrate increased kyphosis, and a lumbar curve will demonstrate increased lordosis. At a crossover point, the existing AP curve is decreased.

Although type II (nonneutral) somatic dysfunction may affect any two adjacent typical vertebrae, it is often found at the transitional points of group mechanics. Fryette[2] noted that type II dysfunction most commonly occurs when forces decrease the existing AP curve. The preexisting AP flattening at the crossover point therefore makes this area most vulnerable for the development of type 2 mechanics.

Because the AP curve is flattened at the crossover point between two type I curves, the physician would expect to find type II extension dysfunctions in the thoracic region and type II flexion dysfunction in the lumbar region.

The rotational relationship between individual vertebrae changes direction between the apical segment of a group curve and the vertebrae immediately above it. For this reason, the upper half of a group curve behaves as a series of type II dysfunctions. Because a group curve produces an increase in the normal AP curve, type II flexion mechanics might be expected above the apex of a type I thoracic curve and type II extension mechanics above the apex of a type I lumbar curve.

Atypical spinal segments, occiput on C1, C1 on C2, and the sacrum between the ilia, demonstrate dysfunctional mechanics as dictated by their unique anatomy. The occiput on C1 and the sacrum between the ilia become dysfunctional with restriction of side bending and rotation coupled in opposite directions. C1 on C2 becomes dysfunctional with restriction of rotation.

The identification of spinal somatic dysfunction should lead the physician to inquire about segmentally related viscera, thereby identifying the contribution of viscerosomatic and somatovisceral reflexes to the clinical picture. Somatic dysfunction that is the result of a viscerosomatic reflex is primarily of diagnostic value. It is definitively treated by treating the causative visceral pathology. Viscerosomatic reflexes are addressed in Chapter 5.

Somatic dysfunction of areas other than the spine occurs as restricted motion that is dictated by the anatomy of the structures involved. It is common for articular motion restriction to involve the minor motions of the affected area.

Rib dysfunction is often secondary to dysfunction of the respective thoracic spinal segments. Primary rib dysfunction occurs as restriction of inspiratory or expiratory excursion.

When examining for appendicular dysfunction, one should begin by examining the region of complaint, followed by a thorough examination of the areas proximal and distal to the complaint. However, the examination is not complete until related spinal segments have been examined.[3]

Finally, once the mechanical pattern of the somatic dysfunction has been diagnosed, the physician must further decide what is causing it. Is the dysfunction an articular restriction? Is the dysfunction the result of tight muscles or altered fascial tension? It is certain that very few dysfunctions are purely articular, muscular, or fascial in origin. However, more times than not, the physician will feel that one component contributes significantly. Making this decision will help the physician to choose the type of OMT that can best treat the dysfunction.

Examining the Patient

The diagnostic assessment of any patient begins from the focal point of the chief complaint. This allows the physician to prioritize the physical examination. That is not to say that one will necessarily skip parts of the examination, but the physician may emphasize some aspect in one patient and examine the same region less extensively in another. The physician must learn to do this because it is necessary to understand the significance of that component of the physical examination in the context of the patient's condition. It would arguably be logical to perform a more extensive neurological examination upon a patient with a recent onset of seizures than an individual with melena.

The evaluation of the musculoskeletal system for somatic dysfunction as part of the complete physical examination should be performed upon every patient. However, it can be modified to conform to the diagnostic requirements of each patient. To determine how to do this, it is appropriate that the physician answer the following questions:

- Does the somatic dysfunction have a mechanical effect upon the patient? Restriction of the thoracic cage and diaphragm, while detrimental to anyone, will be particularly deleterious to a patient with chronic obstructive pulmonary disease or congestive heart failure. Similarly, does the patient have a pain complaint that is the result of or is compounded by somatic dysfunction? Physicians often become so focused upon the patient's serious illness that they overlook simple problems that contribute greatly to the patient's discomfort.
- Is there facilitation of sympathetic (thoracolumbar) or parasympathetic (high cervical or sacral) components of the spinal cord? (See Chapter 5.) If so, how does it affect the patient? Sympathetic stimulation of the gastrointestinal tract decreases peristalsis, which predisposes the patient to constipation or the development of an ileus. Parasympathetic stimulation increases peristalsis that can produce diarrhea and colic.
- How does venous and/or lymphatic stasis affect the patient? Impaired circulation interferes with the body's natural defenses and with its ability to mount an effective healing process and retards the efficacy of medications.

The diagnosis of somatic dysfunction is best approached in an organized fashion. The examination may have to be modified as dictated by the physical status of the patient. Some patients cannot stand, sit, or even move freely in bed. If physicians keep in mind these questions, they will identify methods of modifying the physical examination to accommodate even the sickest of patients. The only reason not to perform an examination for somatic dysfunction is an emergency that necessitates *immediate* attention.

Begin with an overall screen of the patient's general body pattern. If the patient can stand, assess postural balance. Look for unequal leg length and pelvic and pectoral girdle unleveling. Identify type I spinal mechanics and look at regional mechanics, such as thoracic cage excursion, that will affect the clinical presentation. If the patient cannot stand, ileoileal mechanics and thoracic cage excursion can be assessed while the patient is supine. Examine areas where one would expect to find sympathetic and parasympathetic viscerosomatic reflexes associated with the patient's medical problems. Having identified the overall body pattern, specifically diagnose localized, segmental, dysfunction that is relevant to the presentation of the patient.

The following exercises are intended to demonstrate a systematic approach to diagnosis of the spine. The discussion is limited to the diagnosis of the spine. The appropriate osteopathic texts offer descriptions of appendicular, thoracic cage, and cranial diagnosis.

- Standing structural examination
- Supine structural examination
- Regional and segmental examination
- Palpation for tissue texture abnormality; layer palpation
  - Cervical spine
  - Thoracic spine
  - Lumbar spine
  - Sacrum and pelvis

Standing Structural Examination

The purpose of the examination is to learn as much as possible about the patient's general body mechanics so that findings of local somatic dysfunction can be placed in context. Standing behind the patient, observe for the symmetry of each of these structures (Figure 3.1).

- Mastoid processes
- Shoulder (acromion)
- Inferior angle of scapula
- Iliac crests
- Posterior superior iliac spine (PSIS)
- Greater trochanter of femur

TEST FOR PELVIC SIDE SHIFT (PSS)

From behind, observe the standing patient to see whether the pelvis is deviated toward one side or appears centered. Place one hand on the patient's shoulder. Place your other hand on the patient's opposite hip. Gently push the hip and pelvis medially. Switch your hands to the patient's opposite shoulder and hip and repeat the process. Compare the symmetry of motion between both sides. The pelvic side shift test is positive on the side toward which the pelvis more easily moves.

OBSERVATION FOR LATERAL CURVES

From behind, observe the standing patient as the patient bends forward at the waist. Look for paravertebral prominence resulting from spinal rotation that occurs as one component of the type I mechanics of lateral spinal curves. In the thoracic region, the scapula will appear more posterior on the side toward which the spine is rotated.

OBSERVATION OF THE AP CURVES

From the side, inspect lumbar, thoracic, and cervical AP curves for increased and flattened areas. Determine whether any such areas correspond to the observed lateral curves.

Supine Structural Examination

Although the supine examination does not yield as much information about the postural mechanics of the patient as the standing examination, if this is the only position that the patient can be examined in, it is useful to do so. Assess pelvic, ileoileal, and thoracic cage mechanics by sliding your hands under the patient and palpating for paravertebral tissue texture abnormality. Screen lumbar and thoracic spinal mechanics and look for viscerosomatic reflexes. Examine the cervical region as described later in the chapter.

Spinal Curvature

Anterior/Posterior	I	N	D
Cervical Lordosis:	☐	☐	☐
Thoracic Kyphosis:	☐	☐	☐
Lumbar Lordosis:	☐	☐	☐

I=Increased   N=Normal   D=Decreased

Lateral (Scoliosis)	Exam Position
☐ None	Sitting ☐
☐ Functional	Standing ☐
☐ Mild	Prone/Supine ☐
☐ Moderate	Lat. Recumb ☐
☐ Severe	No Exam ☐

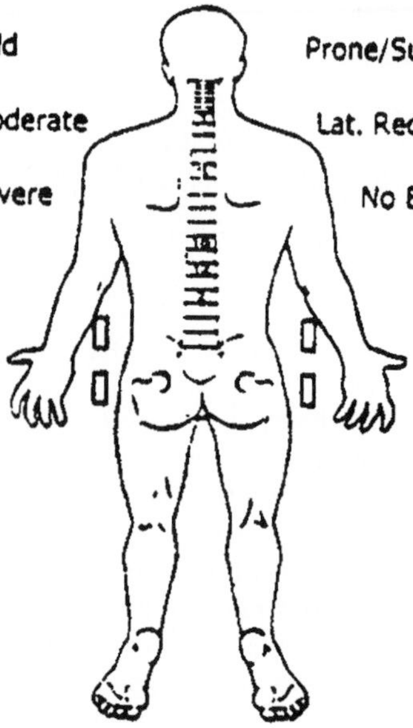

FIGURE 3.1   The recording format for the standing structural examination from the standardized osteopathic SOAP note. (See Chapter 31.)

Palpation for Tissue Texture Abnormality, Layer Palpation

Use layer palpation to gain significant information about tissue texture abnormality in each of the procedure descriptions that follow. Screen each region looking for tissue texture abnormality. When such abnormality is identified, perform a thorough segmental examination.

Place your palpating hand on the skin and make light contact. Palpate for temperature and texture.

Next, evaluate the subcutaneous tissue. Use more palpatory pressure. Sense how thick this area feels. The tissue texture abnormalities found in association with viscerosomatic reflexes cause distinctive changes in subcutaneous tissues that closely mirror the severity of the reflex.

Introduce movement in various directions and notice the directions of loosest and tightest movement. This assesses superficial fascial tension in the region.

To palpate the deep fascial layer, increase palpating pressure until you sense the deeper underlying structures. The deep fascia is generally described as a smooth, firm, and continuous layer. Identify areas of thickening involving the fascia that surrounds the regional musculature.

Palpate through the deep fascia, concentrating on the underlying muscle. Identify individual muscle fibers. Attempt to palpate the direction in which the muscle fibers run. Pay attention to areas of increased musculature tension.

Regional and Segmental Examination of the Cervical Spine (Fig. 3.2)

EXAMINATION OF THE CERVICAL REGION

Patient position: supine. Physician position: seated at the head of the examination table.

This position is not always easily accomplished in the hospital setting. Palpate for tissue texture abnormality and tenderness. After you have appropriately screened the cervical region, with the patient remaining supine, examine the specific segments where you have identified TART findings.

Examination of the Occiput (C0 on C1)

The major motions of this articulation are flexion and extension. The minor motions are rotation and side bending. The most commonly used test for motion is the lateral translation test. Grasp the patient's head, placing your fingertips in contact with the occipitoatlantal (OA) junction. Identify OA side bending by introducing lateral translation to the left and right. Greater ease of lateral translation in one direction is indicative of side bending in the opposite direction.

Once you have identified the side bending, you can extrapolate rotational mechanics because OA rotation and side bending are coupled in opposite directions. That is, side bending to the left of the occiput upon the atlas is associated with rotation to the right, and side bending right is associated with rotation to the left.

Next, introduce OA flexion and extension and observe the symmetry of these motions. This test, along with the location of tissue texture change (and tenderness), is used to identify anterior or posterior occiput dysfunction.

If the occiput translates with greater ease to the right, it indicates that the occiput is sidebent to the left side, and consequently rotated to the right upon the atlas. If the right

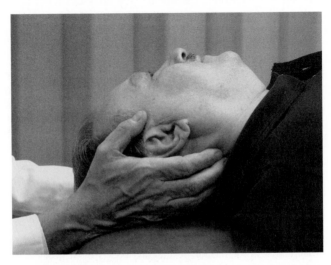

FIGURE 3.2   The supine position may be used for both the regional and segmental examination of the entire cervical spine.

OA joint will not move forward when extension is introduced and the right OA joint has palpable tissue texture change and is tender, the diagnosis is posterior occiput on the right.

If the occiput translates more freely to the right, it indicates that the occiput is sidebent to the left side and rotated to the right on the atlas. If the left OA joint will not move to the posterior when flexion is introduced and the left OA joint has palpable tissue texture change and is tender, the diagnosis is anterior occiput on the left.

Examination of the Atlas (C1 on C2)

The major motion of this articulation is rotation. This articulation is the exception that makes the rule. Atlantoaxial dysfunction involves restriction of the major motion of rotation with little or no minor motion restriction.

With the patient supine, flex the cervical spine. This greatly reduces freedom of rotation from C2 through C7, significantly limiting available rotation to the atlas upon C2. While palpating over the lateral masses of the atlas, rotate the head to the right and then to the left, observing for rotational asymmetry. You may use the nose or chin as a gauge to compare available rotation. Identify the direction of greatest rotation. The dysfunction, posterior on the side toward which rotation occurs most freely or anterior on the side toward which rotation is restricted, is indicated by the side where palpable tissue texture abnormality and tenderness are found.

Segmental Examination of the Cervical Spine (C2 on C3 to C7 on T1)

Palpate the cervical paraspinal tissues from C2 to C7. Look for asymmetric tissue texture abnormality and tenderness and focus motion assessment on these areas. C2 to C7 demonstrates type II (nonneutral) and regionally unique type I (neutral) dysfunctional mechanics.

To test for rotation, hold the head and neck in your hands and place your fingertips posterior to the transverse processes of the cervical segment being examined. Rotate the vertebra to the right and to the left. Observe for restriction of rotation in either direction. Rotation is named for the direction of freer motion. Example: C5 rotates more freely to the right, or left rotation is restricted. C5 is rotated right.

To test for side bending, employ a lateral translation test. Place your fingertips over the lateral edge of the transverse processes of the cervical vertebra being tested. Translate the vertebra to the left and to the right. Translation to the left results in side bending to the right and vice versa. Side bending is also named for the direction of freer motion. Example: C5 translates more freely to the left; it is, therefore, side bent to the right. Using the information gained from the rotational test, C5 is rotated right and side bent right.

To test for forward bending (flexion) and backward bending (extension), introduce flexion and extension between the vertebrae being examined. Decide whether flexion or extension demonstrates the freer motion. To confirm your findings, attempt to rotate the vertebrae being examined after introducing flexion and again after introducing extension. This is application of principle 3 of spinal physiologic motion.[1] In the example, C5 upon C6 is rotated and sidebent to the right (restricted rotation and side bending to the left). If a type II dysfunction is present, rotation will be more restricted in the dysfunctional component of flexion and extension. That is, if C5 is flexed (restricted extension), rotation will be more restricted to the left in extension than in flexion. This dysfunction, named for the unrestricted components of motion, is recorded as C5 sidebent and rotated right flexed.

REGIONAL AND SEGMENTAL EXAMINATION OF THE THORACIC SPINE

Begin by palpating the paravertebral soft tissues. After identifying segmental tissue texture abnormality, assess for motion restriction. This is most easily accomplished from behind the seated patient. Move the patient through a complete range of motion (flexion, extension, side bending, and rotation).

Evaluation of the Upper Thoracic Region (T1–T4) Using the Head and Cervical Region as a Lever

Patient position: seated. Physician position: standing behind patient.

Place your active hand on the patient's head and your monitoring hand on the appropriate thoracic segment.

Flexion and Extension

With your monitoring hand, place the pad of your middle finger in the interspinous space below the segment you wish to evaluate. Allow the index and ring fingers to contact the interspinous spaces above and below. With your active hand, introduce forward bending from above downward until motion is sensed at the spinal level being examined. Note how far and how easily the spinous processes separate. Then introduce backward bending until motion is sensed at this segment. Note how close and how easily the spinous processes approximate.

Side Bending and Rotation

Place your thumb and index finger over the spinous process of the segment you wish to evaluate. Side-bend left and right from above down to the segment being examined. This process may be repeated for rotation. Note asymmetry and quality of motion.

Evaluation of the Upper Thoracic Region (T1–T4) Using the Thumbs to Assess Motion

Patient position: seated. Physician position: standing behind patient. The thumbs of both hands should contact the transverse processes of the thoracic segment being examined.

This procedure is effectively used to assess rotation, flexion, and extension. It is less effective in assessing side bending.

Rotation

Place your thumbs over the transverse processes of the segment to be tested. Allow your fingers to rest over the patient's shoulder area. Motion is introduced by applying pressure anteriorly, alternately through your thumbs. Introduce rotation left and right. Note any restriction of motion. Assess quality and quantity of motion.

Flexion and Extension

Place your thumbs and hands in the same position. Instruct the patient to flex the neck (you should feel flexion localize all the way down to the vertebral segment you are testing). Assess rotation in the manner already described with the patient's neck in flexion. Instruct the patient to extend the neck. Assess rotation in the same manner. Rotation will be more restricted when attempted in the dysfunctional component of flexion and extension.

Example: T2 rotates freely to the right upon T3. Rotation to the left is restricted. When T2 is rotated to the left, the right transverse process appears more prominent underneath your thumb; therefore, T2 is rotated right. With the neck positioned in flexion, T2 has increased rotation to the left (motion still restricted but improved). With the neck extended, T2 has decreased rotation to the left. Flexion results in increased rotation. Extension results in decreased rotation. T2 is therefore rotated right and flexed.

Evaluation of the Lower Thoracic Region (T5–T12): Using the Shoulders as a Lever

Patient position: seated. Physician position: standing behind the patient to the left side.

Drape your left forearm (the active hand) across the patient's posterior cervicothoracic junction, so that your left elbow touches the anterior surface of the patient's left shoulder and your left hand rests comfortably across the right shoulder. Place the thumb and index finger of your right (monitoring) hand on the spinous process of the thoracic segment to be examined.

Side Bending and Rotation

Introduce side bending to the left by using a downward motion through your left arm while monitoring the segment. Move to the patient's right side (switch hand and arm positions) and introduce right side bending. Assess the difference in side bending at that segment.

Return to your original assessment position at the patient's left side. Introduce rotation by applying a posterior motion through your left elbow. Repeat this procedure from the right side and assess the difference in rotation at that segment. Once you become accustomed to this procedure, a combined side bending and rotation movement that is much more efficient can be employed.

Flexion and Extension

Assess flexion and extension by placing the fingers of your monitoring hand over the lower thoracic interspinous spaces. Instruct the patient to cross the arms over the chest. Use your active hand to hold on to the patient's crossed arms. Introduce forward and backward bending from below upward by rocking the patient forward and backward on the ischial tuberosities.

REGIONAL AND SEGMENTAL EXAMINATION OF THE LUMBAR SPINE

Begin by palpating the paravertebral soft tissues. After identifying segmental tissue texture abnormality, assess for motion restriction. This may also be accomplished with the patient seated, using the method described for the low thoracic region already described, or the patient may be examined in the supine position.

Patient position: prone. Physician position: stand at the patient's side.

Place the pads of your thumbs over the transverse processes of a single segment. Wrap the rest of your hands around the lumbar paraspinal area.

Rotation

Use one hand to rotate the vertebra by directing an anterior force through your thumb over one transverse process. This will rotate the vertebra to the opposite side. Repeat the process in the other direction, and compare one side with the opposite side and with the segments above and below.

Side Bending

Assess side bending with your hands in the same position. Use both hands to laterally translate the vertebra to the left and right. Translating the vertebra to the right introduces side bending to the left, and translating the vertebra to the left introduces side bending to the right.

Flexion and Extension

Assess flexion and extension by directing an anterior force over the spinous process with your thumb. Then allow the segment to spring back to its original position. An extended segment will easily move anteriorly and will not spring back properly. The opposite is true for a flexed segment.

Flexion and Extension (Patient on Side)

The patient lies on the side facing you with the knees bent. Place the fingers of your monitoring hand over the interspinous spaces of the vertebrae being tested. Cradle the patient's legs below the knees using your active hand. Assess flexion and extension by introducing these motions through the patient's hips and pelvis up into the lumbar spine.

EXAMINATION OF THE SACRUM AND PELVIS

Sacropelvic articular dysfunction occurs commonly as sacroiliac dysfunction. Ileoileal and global lumbosacropelvic (torsion) mechanics are given significant consideration in the muscle energy approach to pelvic dysfunction. Additionally, pubic symphysis articular dysfunction is occasionally encountered. This discussion focuses upon sacroiliac dysfunction. Diagnosis of sacroiliac dysfunction is a two-step process. First, determine the mechanical pattern of the dysfunction. Second, determine the side of the dysfunctional sacroiliac articulation.

Motion Test for Sacroiliac Articular Dysfunction (Figure 3.3)

Patient position: prone. Physician position: standing at the patient's side near hip level.

Place the pads of the index and middle fingers of your monitoring hand so that one contacts the posterior superior iliac spine and the other rests in the superior portion of the sulcus of the sacroiliac joint. Place the heel of your active hand in contact with the sacral inferior lateral angle (ILA) on the side opposite the monitoring fingers. With your active hand, apply downward (anterior) pressure on the apex and ILA of the sacrum, produce motion, and note freedom or restriction. With your monitoring hand, appreciate posterior motion of the base of the sacrum (reduction in depth of the sulcus) or absence thereof. Assess both quantity and quality of available motion. Repeat this process, examining the opposite sacroiliac joint, and compare the two sides.

Somatic dysfunction can be named in terms of position and in terms of motion restriction. Because anatomic structures vary in their size, shape, and symmetry in the normal population, diagnosis by defining motion restriction is considered to be the superior method.

Pressure over the left ILA of the sacrum with the active hand produces right rotation about the left oblique axis. Conversely, pressure over the right ILA produces left rotation about the right oblique axis. When you palpate these motions, you will commonly note that one rotational pattern occurs with greater ease than the other. It is not readily possible to produce left rotation about the left oblique axis or right rotation about the right oblique axis since this would require directing a posterior force to the anterior surface of the sacrum.

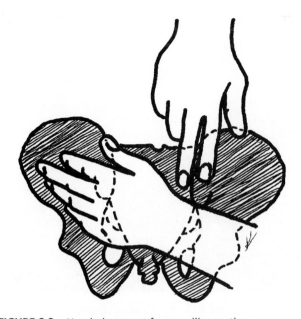

FIGURE 3.3   Hand placement for sacroiliac motion assessment.

Example: Pressure over the left ILA results in unrestricted motion, while pressure over the right ILA is met by significant resistance. Since the unrestricted sacrum can rotate both right and left about either oblique axis and decreased rotation left about the right oblique axis is identified, it is possible to extrapolate that the sacrum is rotated right on the right oblique axis. This motion pattern is consistent with the articular dysfunctions of either an anterior sacrum left or a posterior sacrum right. The mechanical pattern of sacral motion having been identified, the next step is to identify the side of the dysfunctional sacroiliac articulation. The dysfunctional side can be determined by performing the sacral flexion tests (discussed later).

Additional Findings to Assist in Diagnosing an Anterior Sacrum (Upper Pole) Somatic Dysfunction

Look for a deeper sacral sulcus, tissue texture abnormality, tenderness, and decreased posterior motion at the upper pole. Also look for increased gluteal muscle tension on the somatic dysfunction side (the same side as the deep sulcus).

Additional Findings to Assist in Diagnosing a Posterior Sacrum (Lower Pole) Somatic Dysfunction

Look for tenderness of the lower pole and piriformis muscle tension, all on the somatic dysfunction side (side opposite to the deep sulcus, if present). The deep sulcus

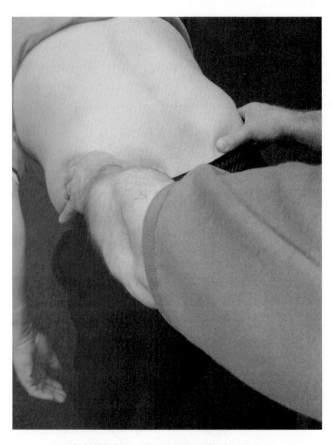

FIGURE 3.4   The standing flexion test.

should become less deep when movement is initiated, that is, not be *stuck* in a deep position.

Standing Flexion Test (Figure 3.4)

Stand behind the standing patient. Place your thumbs over the PSIS. Ask the patient to bend forward. The standing flexion test is positive on the side where the thumb moves further superiorly. This occurs because in the standing position the sacrum rests in a relatively flexed position. With further flexion of the lumbar spine, the sacrum moves without also moving the innominate bones. However, if sacroiliac joint restriction exists, motion of the sacrum will move the innominate bone (hip bone) on the side of the restriction. The innominate will thus move with the sacrum, and the PSIS will shift superiorly on the restricted side. This innominate motion will cause the PSIS monitoring thumb to rise superiorly, indicating a positive standing flexion test on that side. Although usually indicative of sacroiliac joint dysfunction, a positive standing flexion test could also indicate dysfunction anywhere in the ipsilateral pelvis or lower extremity.

Seated Flexion Test (Fig. 3.5)

This test is performed in a manner similar to the standing flexion test. The patient is preferably seated with the feet flat on the floor and asked to bend forward at the waist. The physician monitors for PSIS motion with the thumbs. The seated flexion test is positive on the side where the thumb rises more superiorly. This test is more specific for

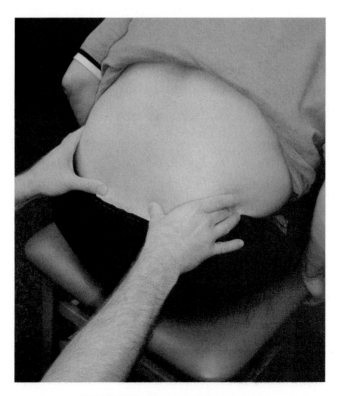

FIGURE 3.5   The seated flexion test.

sacroiliac joint dysfunction than the standing flexion test because the influence of lower extremity dysfunction is effectively removed by sitting down.

References

1. ECOP. Glossary of osteopathic terminology. In: Ward RC, ed. Foundations for Osteopathic Medicine. 2nd ed. Philadelphia: Lippincott Williams & Wilkins, 2002;1229–1253.
2. Fryette HH. Principles of Osteopathic Technique. Indianapolis: American Academy of Osteopathy, 1954, 1980.
3. Strachan WF. Applied anatomy of the pelvis and lower extremities. J Am Osteopath Assoc. 1940;40:59–60.

CHAPTER 4

The Manipulative Prescription

Kenneth E. Nelson

"One must not be a blacksmith only, and only able to hit large bones and muscles with a heavy hammer, but one must be able to use the most delicate instruments of the silversmith in adjusting the deranged, displaced bones, nerves, muscles and remove all obstructions, and thereby set the machinery of life moving. To do this is to be an osteopath."

A. T. Still[1]

As defined by *Stedman's Medical Dictionary*, a prescription is "a written formula for the preparation and administration of any remedy."[2]

When writing a prescription, you must determine which therapy, how much, how often. An example is ampicillin 500 mg every 6 hours.

The same questions must be answered when deciding upon a prescription for osteopathic manipulative treatment (OMT).

OMT is a therapeutic intervention. It is the definitive treatment for somatic dysfunction and is employed to treat primary somatic dysfunction. It is also used to address the effect of somatic dysfunction upon a patient's recuperative abilities from concomitant disease processes. Because it is a therapeutic modality, its dosage must be determined and prescribed. This is defined by the diagnosis of the somatic dysfunction within the context of the individual patient.

DIAGNOSIS

Before one can determine what therapy is to be used, a diagnosis must be made. A diagnosis is a logical conclusion based upon information obtained from the chief complaint, the patient's history, and the physical examination.

The diagnosis of primary somatic dysfunction is often, although not always, associated with musculoskeletal pain. Somatic dysfunction may contribute to the patient's illness, as in the effect of motion restriction of the thoracic cage upon the patient with pneumonia. Consequently, somatic dysfunction should be appropriately treated, even in the absence of musculoskeletal complaint.

The diagnosis of somatic dysfunction is based upon the identification of one or more of the physical findings described as TART: tissue texture abnormality, asymmetry of position, restriction of motion, and tenderness.

Of these, tenderness and tissue texture abnormality may be sought out when screening an area for significant dysfunction. Once a dysfunctional area has been identified, one must specifically define (diagnose) the mechanics of the dysfunction. (See Chapter 3.)

Define the Barrier

The physician examines the patient and precisely identifies asymmetry of position and restriction of motion. Motion restriction is particularly important because the most common goal of OMT is restoration of free movement. The mechanical pattern of the motion restriction determines the mechanics of the therapeutic intervention.

Determine Why the Barrier Is Present

Once the physician has diagnosed the mechanical pattern of the somatic dysfunction, it is necessary to identify what is causing the dysfunction. Is it the result of articular restriction? Is it due to tight muscles or altered fascial tension? Making this decision will help to determine what type of OMT will be selected to treat the dysfunction.

TREATING THE PATIENT

If it is determined that the barrier is the result of articular dysfunction, the procedure should be directed at affecting articular mechanics. Such procedures include high-velocity, low-amplitude (HVLA) thrust and low-velocity, moderate- to high-amplitude articulation procedures.

If the barrier is the result of soft tissue tension, a procedure that is intended to affect soft tissue is chosen (muscle energy, soft tissue stretching, myofascial release).

If the dysfunction is best addressed by attempting to reduce neural reflex activity, counterstrain and facilitated positional release may prove to be the procedures of choice.

Somatic dysfunction that is the result of viscerosomatic reflex activity is specifically treated by treating the underlying visceral pathology. Treatment of the visceral pathology may be facilitated (but not replaced) by manipulating the somatic component (somatovisceral reflex). Procedures chosen under these circumstances should produce somatic relaxation with minimal stimulation. Once the visceral component has been effectively treated, residual somatic dysfunction may be treated using the logic described earlier and that discussed in the following paragraphs.

Patient Tolerance

The physician at this point is almost ready to choose the procedure. There is, however, one more decision-making point to consider: How much can the patient tolerate? Obviously, a healthy 27 year old has greater tolerance than a healthy 90 year old. Also, a healthy 27 year old can tolerate more than the same individual with pneumonia.

Patient tolerance dictates the level of aggressiveness of the procedure chosen. A somewhat artificial continuum of procedures can be created based upon the relative aggressiveness of the procedures.

High-velocity, low-amplitude (HVLA), most aggressive
Articulation (ART)
Soft tissue (ST)
Direct fascial release (DIR)
Muscle energy (ME)
Counterstrain (CS)
Facilitated positional release (FPR)
Indirect fascial release (IND)
Indirect cranial (CR), least aggressive

As stated, this list is quite arbitrary and open to debate, but the idea is valid. The physician should also consider that besides the aggressiveness of a procedure type, the time required for application can affect tolerance. The longer a procedure takes, the more likely the patient cannot tolerate it. As a rule, the more aggressive the procedure, the less time required for its application.

Consideration of the diagnosis of the mechanical pattern of the dysfunction, the anatomic component (articular, muscular, fascial) responsible for the dysfunction, and patient tolerance will identify the most appropriate procedure for the patient.

RESPONSE

How much OMT is enough? Treat the patient until a response occurs.

What kind of response should the physician look for? Relaxation of the soft tissues in the area being treated is a good response, often referred to as a release. Increased muscle spasm during the application of a procedure indicates that the patient's tolerance has been exceeded and that a less aggressive procedure should be selected or that treatment should be stopped and attempted again at a later time. Altered autonomic tone is also an indication of a response. Peripheral vasodilation resulting in increased skin temperature or redness and increased perspiration indicates that it is time to stop. Increased heart or respiratory rate also indicates that one has reached the patient's level of tolerance. If the patient feels that the intervention is too uncomfortable, the physician should stop and choose another approach or wait and try again later.

The overall health status of the patient affects tolerance to whatever procedure is chosen. The sicker the patient, the lower one can expect the tolerance to be. Consequently, a smaller dose of OMT will be necessary to obtain the optimal therapeutic response without exceeding the patient's tolerance.

Individuals at the extremes of age (infants, children, and geriatric patients) generally require lower doses of OMT to obtain a therapeutic response.

How often should the patient be treated? This is not an easy question. It depends upon the patient's response to the initial intervention. It also depends upon whether one is treating primary somatic dysfunction or addressing the contribution of somatic dysfunction to coexistent illness.

Primary Somatic Dysfunction

When treating primary somatic dysfunction that is typically associated with musculoskeletal complaints, such as headache and low back pain, the physician can base a decision upon the following sequence of responses. The dose of the initial treatment is estimated as described earlier, in the discussion of tolerance. After the initial intervention, the patient frequently reports immediate symptom reduction. This relief is occasionally followed by a brief intensification of the original complaint and may be treated with appropriate analgesia. Such a rebound reaction should not last more than 24 hours. If it does, the intensity of the second OMT intervention should be appropriately reduced. As the rebound reaction subsides, a period of resolution typically follows, and the chief complaint is significantly reduced or absent. This period of resolution may last a few hours, or it may be permanent. Ideally the patient should be reevaluated 48 hours after the initial treatment. By this time, the rebound reaction should have subsided, and residual somatic dysfunction can be specifically diagnosed and treated. Symptom resolution should last progressively longer following each application of manipulative treatment, and treatment intervals should be adjusted accordingly.

Failure of this resolution period to increase indicates than an incomplete diagnosis has been made. Contributing causes must be thoroughly explored, identified, and treated.

Contributory Somatic Dysfunction

Somatic dysfunction encountered in patients with established disease processes, whether acute or chronic, contributes to the coexistent illness. The effect upon the patient may be mechanical (i.e., thoracic cage compliance in obstructive pulmonary disease or congestive heart failure), or it may be somatovisceral. The desired response to treatment is related to the status of the respective disease processes. The same principles as described earlier apply; however, the circumstances are more complex. The very sick patient will respond significantly to very little intervention. The duration of the response may be short, however, necessitating repetition of treatment in as little as 4 to 6 hours.

The hospitalized patient is more likely to be aged or very young and will consequently respond differently, as discussed earlier. Geriatric patients respond slowly and may require more time between treatments. (See Chapter 12.) Infants and children respond rapidly and may be treated again after shorter intervals. (See Chapter 8.)

The determination of what kind of OMT, how much, and how often is not as easy as prescribing ampicillin. The physician can base decisions upon the parameters listed earlier, but each consecutive intervention must be individualized to the patient's response to the previous treatment. The dose also must continually be adjusted to the patient's tolerance.

TREATMENT OF TRAUMA PATIENTS

OMT is used specifically to treat somatic dysfunction. In most cases, its use is intended to increase available motion. It is, therefore, inappropriate to manipulate areas of the musculoskeletal system that are structurally unstable. With this caution in mind, the physician should recognize that trauma patients still can benefit greatly from appropriately applied OMT.

Because trauma often results in torn soft tissue and fractures, extreme care must be taken not to apply force through such areas. This said, areas adjacent to traumatic instability frequently demonstrate somatic dysfunction. Appropriate treatment results in less physical stress and increased circulation (tissue perfusion) in the area of instability, decreasing the patient's discomfort.

However, because the condition is the result of exogenous force, it is initially very difficult to estimate the patient's tolerance. A simple approach to this dilemma is to decide how much one believes the patient will tolerate and apply about one-half that dose. Subsequent treatments may then be adjusted as outlined earlier. This is an area where the use of indirect procedures (counterstrain, facilitated positional release, myofascial release, and cranial) can produce impressive results.

Recording in the Progress Note (See Chapter 31)

As noted earlier, in most cases (exceptions to this include lymphatic procedures), OMT is specifically employed to treat somatic dysfunction. As such, the physical findings that justify the diagnosis of somatic dysfunction must be recorded in the *objective* portion of the SOAP note, and the anatomically specific diagnosis of somatic dysfunction must be recorded in the *assessment* portion of the SOAP note.[3–7]

OMT is a procedure. The prescription must be charted in the *plan* portion of the SOAP note.

The OMT prescription consists of the following steps:

1. Select procedure type or types.
2. Indicate the anatomic region to be treated.
3. Indicate frequency of treatment.

Examples of prescriptions follow:

Muscle energy, cervicothoracic, daily
Pedal fascial pump lymphatic mobilization every 8 hours
Rib raising, thoracic cage, every 6 hours

CONCLUSION

A prescription for a therapeutic intervention is determined by the condition to be treated and the requirements and limiting factors of the patient receiving the treatment. A prescription identifies the therapy to be used, and the quantity and frequency of its use. All of these criteria apply whether the therapeutic intervention is ampicillin or OMT.

Use of any therapeutic intervention must be properly recorded in the medical record.

References

1. Still AT. The Autobiography of A. T. Still. Chapter 24. Kirksville, MO: Author, 1908:290.
2. Williams RH, Stedman TL, eds. Stedman's Medical Dictionary. 25th ed. Baltimore: Williams & Wilkins, 1990.
3. Nelson KE, Glonek T. Computer/outcomes: Hardcopy SOAP note preliminary report. Fam Physician 1999;3:8–10.

4. Sleszynski SL, Glonek T, Kuchera WA. Standardized medical record: A new outpatient osteopathic SOAP note form: Validation of a standardized office form against physician's progress notes. J Am Osteopath Assoc 1999;99:516–529.
5. Sleszynski SL, Glonek T, Kuchera WA. Outpatient osteopathic single organ system musculoskeletal exam form: Training and certification. J Am Osteopath Assoc 2004;104:76–81.
6. Sleszynski S, Glonek T, Kuchera WA. Outpatient osteopathic single organ system musculoskeletal exam form series: Validation of the outpatient osteopathic SOS musculoskeletal exam form, a new standardized medical record. J Am Osteopath Assoc 2004;104:423–438.
7. Licciardone JC, Nelson KE, Glonek T, et al. Osteopathic manipulative treatment of somatic dysfunction among patients in the family practice: A retrospective analysis. J Am Osteopath Assoc 2005;105:537–544.

CHAPTER 5

Viscerosomatic and Somatovisceral Reflexes

Kenneth E. Nelson

INTRODUCTION

Osteopathy began in the latter half of the nineteenth century as a holistic approach to medical practice. Fundamental to the earliest osteopathic theory and extending to the present is the concept that dysfunction of the musculoskeletal system affects the health and well being of the remainder of the body. This impact may occur in a directly mechanical fashion. From the earliest years of the profession, however, it was recognized that visceral pathology was reflected along the spine as somatic dysfunction. Additionally, it was recognized that the effect of spinal somatic dysfunction upon the nervous system also applied to segmentally related viscera. This was proposed to occur through what were originally known as spinal centers.[1,2]

These principles, developed through clinical empiricism, were based upon the scientific knowledge of the day. The autonomic nervous system, as described by Claude Bernard,[3] was known to consist of both efferent and afferent neurons. The somatic distribution of sensation and/or referred pain from visceral disease had been thoroughly described.[4–7]

Louisa Burns, possibly the best known of early osteopathic investigators, dedicated much of her career to the study of viscerosomatic and somatovisceral reflexes and of the effect of osteopathic manipulative treatment (OMT) upon these reflexes.[8–10] As early as 1907, her studies on animals and human subjects led her to conclude that (1) "A very important, if not the only, pathway of viscero-sensory impulses enters the

33

spinal cord through its posterior roots." (2) "Somatovisceral reflexes are less circumscribed and less direct than are viscerosomatic reflexes." (3) "Since abnormal conditions of the viscera follow . . . pressure upon somato-sensory nerves as is sufficient to lessen conscious sensation, and since section of the somato-sensory nerve is followed by abnormal conditions of the viscera, it is inferred that normal visceral activity depends in part upon the stimulation derived from the somato-sensory nerves." (4) "The possibility of recognition of abnormal viscerosomatic reflexes as an aid in diagnosis is inferred."[8]

THE PHYSIOLOGY OF VISCEROSOMATIC AND SOMATOVISCERAL REFLEXES

Following upon Burns's pioneering studies, John Stedman Denslow[11] and Irvin M. Korr[12] identified the physiology of spinal segmental facilitation and demonstrated its association with somatic dysfunction. The facilitated spinal segment was shown to occur not just as a result of simple spinal somatic dysfunction but also as the result of segmentally related visceral pathology. Furthermore, it was shown in some instances to be demonstrably present prior to the overt presentation of a clinical complaint.[13] This physiology has been clearly demonstrated to be involved in viscerosomatic and somatovisceral reflex relationships.[14] Van Buskirk[15] proposed a nociceptively initiated model for spinal somatic dysfunction that offers a description of the physiology of viscerosomatic and somatovisceral reflexes. Thus, reflexively mediated spinal somatic dysfunction is thought to occur as follows:

1. A peripheral focus of irritation, in the case of a viscerosomatic reflex from the inflammation associated with visceral pathology, activates general visceral afferent neurons. In the case of a somatovisceral reflex, primary somatic dysfunction results in the activation of somatosensory nociceptive neurons.
2. These primary afferent neurons enter the spinal cord and synapse in the dorsal horn with internuncial neurons.
3. Ongoing afferent stimulation from the focus of irritation, be it visceral or somatic, results in establishment of a state of irritability (facilitation) of the internuncial neurons of that spinal segment.
4. Additional afferent activity from any source results in a spinal segmental response to less stimulus than would be normally required. In the case of a viscerosomatic reflex, this results in tenderness that is proportionate to the degree of visceral pathology, when the area of the associated dermatome or myotome is palpated. If the amount of afferent activity from the offending organ is sufficient to cause spontaneous internuncial firing with the activation of ascending spinal pathways, referred pain results.
5. Such activity from internuncial neurons, which synapse with ventral horn motor neurons, results in segmentally related myospasticity, as seen in primary somatic dysfunction and viscerosomatic reflexes. Activity from internuncial neurons that synapse with neurons in the intermediolateral cell column of the thoracic and upper lumbar cord results in segmentally related somatosomatic, somatovisceral and viscerovisceral reflex sympathicotonia. Similar physiology is thought to occur in the parasympathetically mediated reflexes, although in this instance it is less clearly identified.
6. The degree of segmental irritability that is directly proportionate to the severity of the visceral pathology, and the anatomic relationship between the involved organ and the paravertebral soft tissues that makes the location of the reflex changes consistent from individual to individual, together allow

viscerosomatic reflexes to be of diagnostic value. OMT reduces the facilitated state and thereby provides a therapeutic somatovisceral result.

Viscerosomatic Reflexes

Somatic dysfunction is present, by definition, when any of the criteria (tissue texture change, asymmetry of functional position, restriction of motion, or tenderness) are identified by palpation. Viscerosomatic reflexes are the somatic reflection of visceral pathology. As such, they are somatic dysfunction that is secondary to the segmentally related visceral inflammation and are mediated through the general visceral afferent neurons of the autonomic nervous system. Because they are reflexive in origin and not primary mechanical somatic dysfunction, they may not clearly manifest asymmetry of functional position or restriction of motion. Any motion restriction is commonly generalized and may be without asymmetry. Rather than manifesting a distinctive restrictive barrier, viscerosomatic reflex somatic dysfunction often demonstrates ambiguity of the barrier. However, because tenderness, tissue texture change, and generalized motion restriction are present and can be identified by palpation, viscerosomatic reflexes indicate somatic dysfunction and may be classified according to the appropriate 739 codes listed in the ICD-9CM.[16]

The anatomic reliability of autonomic innervation of the viscera makes the segmental paravertebral location of organ-specific reflexes predictable and consequently of diagnostic value. The intensity of the palpatory findings directly mirrors the severity of the causative visceral pathology, offering additional clinical insight for the clinician with discerning touch. Visceral neoplasia is an exception to this principle. Because neoplasms are typically without innervation, they do not provide general visceral afferent input to the spinal cord. Any afferent neural activity occurs because of the effect of the tumor upon surrounding tissues.

Chapman's reflexes provide another method of recognizing viscerosomatic effects.[17–19] These are small (2–3 mm) nodular masses, palpable in soft tissue, that demonstrate sharp pinpoint nonradiating tenderness. As viscerosomatic reflexes, they are typically found in locations that are segmentally related to visceral innervation. Chapman's reflexes are thought to be the effect of dysfunction of the sympathetic nervous system upon segmentally related lymphatic vasculature.[19] They are commonly located posteriorly in the tissues adjacent to the spine and anteriorly often in segmentally related areas. Traditionally, the anterior points have been employed diagnostically, while the posterior points are treated by applying slow circular pressure.

Diagnosis of Viscerosomatic Reflexes

Viscerosomatic reflexes are identified, as are all other manifestations of somatic dysfunction, by palpation. They are similar in their clinical manifestation to primary somatic dysfunction. They may, as described earlier, present with ambiguity of end feel of the restrictive barrier. Beal[20] recommends that special palpatory attention be directed toward the costotransverse area in the thoracic spine and suggests that viscerosomatic reflexes may be differentiated from primary somatic dysfunction by the involvement of two or more adjacent spinal segments. The initial response may be limited to two adjacent segments, but as the duration or severity of the underlying condition increases, the response will spread to adjacent segments via internuncial connections.[21] Localized skin and subcutaneous tissue texture changes also provide indications as to the severity and acuity or chronicity of the underlying visceral pathology.

Corresponding tissue texture change of muscle is most apparent in the deep paravertebral musculature, multifidi and rotatores, because of their limited segmental innervation as compared to the more superficial paravertebral musculature. The spinal level of the deep muscular involvement consequently most closely corresponds to the spinal level of reflex segmental somatic dysfunction.

Signs of acute viscerosomatic reflex activity similar to those of acute primary somatic dysfunction can be appreciated by palpating sequentially from superficial to deep tissues. The examination should begin with the lightest of touch and progress through increasingly greater palpatory pressure. Increased skin temperature will be present as a result of vasodilation. Red reflex, a visual observation, is a prolonged vasomotor reaction to tactile stimulation that results in dermatomally related cutaneous erythema. The acute sudomotor reaction results in increased sweating. This increases skin drag, the perception of resistance as the examiner slides the hand over the patient's skin. Cutaneous and subcutaneous tissue texture change, a result of increased interstitial fluid, produces skin thickening and subtle subcutaneous edema that once appreciated, may be quantified (mild, moderate, severe) to provide invaluable diagnostic information as to the severity and acuity of the reflex. The segmentally related deep paravertebral musculature will demonstrate active spasm.

The signs of chronic viscerosomatic reflex activity, as might be anticipated, include local vasospasm with resultant decreased skin temperature and reduced sudomotor activity with decreased skin drag because of decreased sweating. Slightly deeper palpation reveals the sensation of subcutaneous fibrosis, while with even deeper pressure the deep paravertebral muscles feel hard and tense and exhibit hypersensitivity to palpation.

Testing for passive motion of the spinal segments involved is performed in a fashion similar to motion testing for primary spinal somatic dysfunction. (See Chapter 3.) Differentiation between primary spinal somatic dysfunction and that of viscerosomatic origin is often difficult. As noted earlier, rather than manifesting a distinctive restrictive barrier, such as that demonstrable with primary spinal somatic dysfunction, viscerosomatic reflex somatic dysfunction often demonstrates ambiguity of the restrictive barrier. Any motion restriction is commonly generalized and may be without asymmetry.

Viscerosomatic reflex dysfunction and mechanical spinal somatic dysfunction, however, are often clinically encountered in a chicken-egg relationship at the same vertebral level,[21] making the differentiation between the two difficult or impossible. When the patient has established visceral pathology and concomitant mechanical dysfunction, it is impossible (and unnecessary) to discern whether primary spinal dysfunction resulted in the development of visceral pathology through somatovisceral effects or longstanding visceral pathology produced mechanical spinal dysfunction.

Paraspinal viscerosomatic reflexes, when identified, may be further confirmed by searching for Chapman's points. As stated earlier, these are found paired, anteriorly and posteriorly. They are in specifically mapped locations (Figs. 5.1 and 5.2) and are palpable as discrete gangliform masses that are firm but not hard. They are quite small, 2 to 3 mm in diameter, and very tender, and they lie upon deep fascia or periosteum. They will move slightly with palpatory pressure but remain attached to the deep tissues. They may be found alone or in groups, and when they are the result of chronic disease processes, they are of greater magnitude and tend to coalesce.

Somatic dysfunction that is the result of a viscerosomatic reflex is primarily of diagnostic value. It is definitively treated by treating the causative visceral pathology. The inseparable relationship between viscerosomatic reflexes and somatovisceral

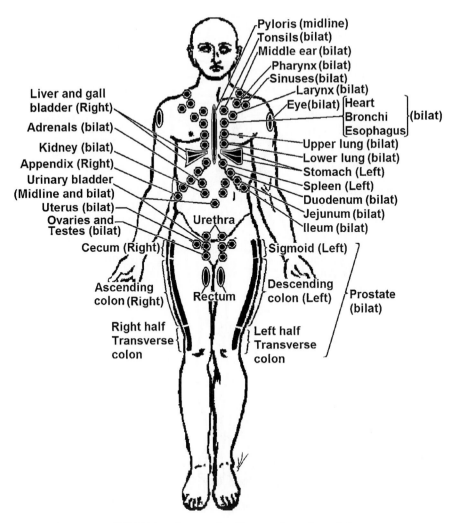

FIGURE 5.1   The anterior Chapman's tender points.

reactions that are the result of spinal facilitation, however, means that for every somatic dysfunction due to visceral pathology there is a segmentally related response that will in turn affect segmentally related viscera. As such, although therapies should be employed that are specifically directed at the visceral pathology, as discussed later, OMT may be used as adjunctive treatment through its effect upon somatovisceral physiology.

The Location of Viscerosomatic Reflexes

As Burns[8] suggested, viscerosomatic reflexes offer a significant contribution to the physical diagnosis of visceral pathology. For physical findings to have diagnostic value, however, they must be consistently reliable. Head[4] extensively mapped referred pain based in part upon increased tenderness to palpation. Following the earlier works on referred pain, Pottenger[7] provided one of the first thorough descriptions of the somatic manifestations of visceral disease. Much of the early osteopathic literature on viscerosomatic reflexes consists of anecdotal case studies.

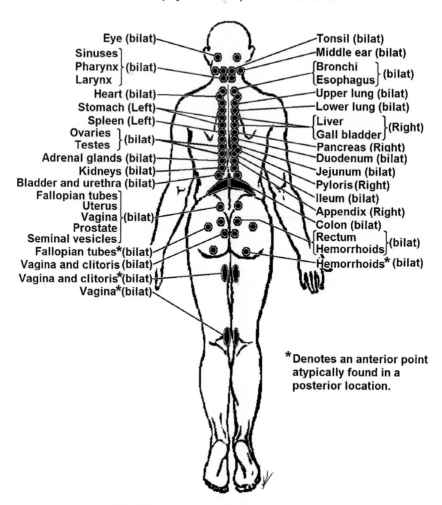

Eye (bilat)
Sinuses
Pharynx }(bilat)
Larynx
Heart (bilat)
Stomach (Left)
Spleen (Left)
Ovaries }(bilat)
Testes
Adrenal glands (bilat)
Kidneys (bilat)
Bladder and urethra (bilat)
Fallopian tubes
Uterus
Vagina }(bilat)
Prostate
Seminal vesicles
Fallopian tubes*(bilat)
Vagina and clitoris (bilat)
Vagina and clitoris*(bilat)
Vagina*(bilat)

Tonsil (bilat)
Middle ear (bilat)
Bronchi }(bilat)
Esophagus
Upper lung (bilat)
Lower lung (bilat)
Liver }(Right)
Gall bladder
Pancreas (Right)
Duodenum (bilat)
Jejunum (bilat)
Pyloris (Right)
Ileum (bilat)
Appendix (Right)
Colon (bilat)
Rectum }(bilat)
Hemorrhoids
Hemorrhoids* (bilat)

*Denotes an anterior point atypically found in a posterior location.

FIGURE 5.2   The posterior Chapman's tender points.

Consequently, the exact location of reported reflex findings varies slightly from author to author. Beal[20] reviewed this literature and provided probably the most thorough overview of the recorded locations of viscerosomatic reflexes to date.

Because viscerosomatic reflexes are mediated through general visceral afferent neurons traveling with the autonomic nerves that supply the target area or organ they represent, they are classified as sympathetic and parasympathetic. Viscerosomatic reflexes classified as sympathetic are found from the first thoracic segment through the mid lumbar region. As a rule, organs above the thoracoabdominal diaphragm manifest their sympathetic viscerosomatic reflexes in the paravertebral soft tissues at or above the level of T5, while organs below the diaphragm manifest their sympathetic viscerosomatic reflexes at or below the level of T5. The parasympathetic viscerosomatic reflexes are found in association with the vagus, cranial nerve X, with manifestation in the high cervical region. Parasympathetic viscerosomatic reflexes are also found in association with the pelvic splanchnic nerves, the second, third, and fourth sacral segments, with manifestation in the pelvic region. Certain exceptions are discussed as they are described later in the chapter.

Tissue texture changes of viscerosomatic reflex origin are predictably bilateral or asymmetrical, as well as being predictable as to the spinal segmental level where they are found. Midline organs, such as the pancreas, produce bilateral tissue texture change. Paired organs, such as the lungs, produce bilateral reflex findings when a generalized disease process, such as pulmonary fibrosis, affects both sides, while an asymmetrical disease process will produce an ipsilateral reflex response. Right lower lobe pneumonia therefore would be expected to result in a right-sided paravertebral reflex. Asymmetrically placed organs result in asymmetrical ipsilateral reflexes. Consequently, the myocardial reflex tends to be left-sided, while the reflex from liver disease will be right-sided.

The following listing of viscerosomatic reflex locations (Table 5.1) is compiled from sites listed by multiple sources.[4,7,17,20,22–24]

TABLE 5.1

Paravertebral Viscerosomatic Reflexes

System or Organ	Sympathetic	Parasympathetic
Head and neck	T1–T5	
Upper respiratory tract	T1–T5	
	Trigeminal: final common pathway, temporalis muscles, occiput, C1, C2.	
Cardiac		
Myocardial	T1–T5 left	Occiput, C1, C2
Coronary artery	C3–C5 (sympathetic?)	
Pulmonary		
Lung	T1–T4	Occiput, C1, C2
Bronchomotor reflex	T1–T3	Occiput, C1, C2
Asthma reflex	T2 left	Occiput, C1, C2
Bronchial mucosa reflex lung	T2–T3	Occiput, C1, C2
Parenchyma reflex	T3–T4	Occiput, C1, C2
Parietal pleura	T1–T12	Occiput, C1, C2
Upper GI		
Esophagus	T3–T6 right	Occiput, C1, C2
Stomach	T5–T10 left	Occiput, C1, C2
Duodenum	T6–T8 right	Occiput, C1, C2
Lower GI		
Small intestine	T8–T10 bilateral	Occiput, C1, C2
Appendix and cecum	T9–T12 right	Occiput, C1, C2
Ascending colon	T11–L1 right	Occiput, C1, C2
Descending colon, rectum	L1–L3 left	S2–S4
Pancreas	T5–T9 right or bilateral	Occiput, C1, C2
Liver, gallbladder	T5–T10 right	Occiput, C1, C2
Phrenic nerve somatosomatic reflex	C3–C5 right	
Spleen	T7–T9 left	

(Continued)

TABLE 5.1 (Cont.)

Paravertebral Viscerosomatic Reflexes

System or Organ	Sympathetic	Parasympathetic
Urinary tract		
Kidney	T9–L1 ipsilateral	Occiput, C1, C2
Proximal ureter	T11–L3 ipsilateral	Occiput, C1, C2
Distal ureter	T11–L3 ipsilateral	S2–S4
Bladder	T11–L3 bilateral	S2–S4
Urethra	T11–L2 bilateral	
Genital tract		
Fallopian tubes	T10–L2 bilateral	S2–S4
Seminal vesicles		
External genitalia	T12 bilateral	
Prostate	T10–L2 bilateral	S2–S4
Ovaries and testes	T10–T11 ipsilateral	
Uterus	T9–L2 bilateral	S2–S4
Adrenal glands	T8–T10 ipsilateral	

GI, gastrointestinal.

Viscerosomatic Reflexes from the Head, Eyes, Ears, Nose, and Throat

The sympathetic innervation of the head and neck emanates from the upper thoracic spine. Thus, T1–T5 dysfunction can be found in response to pathology of the structures of the head and neck.[22]

Upper Respiratory Tract

The final common pathway for sympathetic and parasympathetic innervation of the upper respiratory tract is the trigeminal nerve. Innervated by the trigeminal nerve, the muscles of mastication, particularly the temporalis muscles, serve as a somatic component for an upper respiratory tract viscerosomatic reflex that may be considered both sympathetic and parasympathetic. An additional upper respiratory tract viscerosomatic reflex site is occiput to C2. This represents a reflex between the trigeminal nerve and upper cervical nerves that innervate the posterior neck muscles.[25]

The Chapman points[17] associated with the upper respiratory tract are found bilaterally. They include the following:

Nasal sinuses. The anterior points lie 7 to 9 cm lateral to the sternum on the upper edge of the second ribs.

Pharynx. The anterior points lie upon the first ribs 3 to 4 cm medial to where the ribs emerge from beneath the clavicles.

Larynx. The anterior points lie upon the second ribs, 5 to 7 cm lateral to the sternocostal junction. The posterior points are found in the same location for the

nasal sinuses, pharynx, and larynx, upon C2 midway between the spinous
process and the tip of the transverse process.

Tonsils. The anterior points are between the first and second ribs adjacent to the
sternum, and the posterior points lie upon C1 midway between the spinous
process and the tip of the transverse process.

Middle ear. The anterior points lie upon the superior anterior aspect of the clavicles just lateral to where they cross the first ribs, and the posterior points lie
upon the posterior aspect of tips of transverse processes of C1.

Eye. The anterior points lie upon the anterior aspect of the humerus at the level of
the surgical neck, and the posterior points lie upon the squamous portion of
the occipital bone below the superior nuchal line.

Viscerosomatic Reflexes from the Heart

There is general agreement that the myocardial sympathetic viscerosomatic reflexes
are found from T1 to T5, with greater left-sided than right-sided incidence.[7,17,20,22–24] Larson[26] subdivided this region, noting a higher incidence of associated cardiac arrhythmia when the viscerosomatic reflex was observed at the T2
level. Reflex findings at the T5 level, he suggested, were more likely associated
with posterior wall myocardial infarctions.

Luciani,[6] reviewing the early literature on referred pain in association with
heart disease, described an area of cutaneous hypersensitivity in dermatomes C3
to C4. Larson identified reflex paravertebral tissue texture change at C3 to C5 that
was attributed to coronary artery disease and myocardial ischemia.[26]

The parasympathetic viscerosomatic reflex from the heart is the vagal reflex,
occiput, C1, C2.[23,24] These high cervical findings are, however, nonspecific for the
heart because the vagus innervates so many visceral structures, and the upper respiratory trigeminal reflex described earlier is also found at this level.

The Chapman points[17] associated with the heart are bilateral. The anterior
myocardial points are in the intercostal space between the second and third ribs at
the sternocostal junction. The posterior points are found in the space between the
transverse processes of T2 and T3 midway between the spinous process and the
tip of the transverse process.

Viscerosomatic Reflexes from the Lower Respiratory Tract

The viscerosomatic reflex from lung is generally agreed upon as being bilateral from
T1 to T4,[7,17,22–24] although Beal's review identified a broader area of involvement
from T2 to T8.[20] The upper thoracic pulmonary reflex has been further subdivided
into a bronchomotor reflex area, T1 to T3 (with T2 left referred to as the asthma
reflex), a bronchial mucosa reflex area, T2 to T3, and a lung parenchyma reflex area,
T3 to T4.[23] Because the parietal pleura receive somatic innervation, inflammation
involving the pleura may be found anywhere between T1 and T12, left- or right-
sided depending upon the location and extent of pleural invlovement.[7]

As stated earlier, general pulmonary involvement will result in bilateral paravertebral reflex findings, while lateralized pathology produces ipsilateral tissue texture change.

One would anticipate that the parasympathetic viscerosomatic reflex from the
lungs would manifest as the vagal reflex, occiput, C1, C2.[24]

The bilateral Chapman points[17] associated with the lungs include the following:

Bronchi. The anterior points are in the intercostal space between the second and
third ribs at the sternocostal junction, and the posterior points are on T2 midway between the spinous process and the tip of the transverse process.

Upper lung. The anterior points are in the intercostal space between the third and
fourth ribs at the sternocostal junction, and the posterior points are found in
the space between the transverse processes of T3 and T4, midway between the
spinous process and the tip of the transverse process.

Lower lung. The anterior points are in the intercostal space between the fourth and
fifth ribs at the sternocostal junction, and the posterior points are found in the
space between the transverse processes of T4 and T5, midway between the
spinous process and the tip of the transverse process.

Viscerosomatic Reflexes from the Gastrointestinal Tract

Because the gut develops as a midline structure that extends along the entire
length of the embryo, the gastrointestinal tract receives sympathetic innervation
from almost the entire length of the thoracolumbar spinal cord. The rostral-
to-caudal gastrointestinal sympathetic viscerosomatic reflexes progress sequentially along the thoracolumbar paravertebral soft tissues. Although it should be
expected that a midline structure would manifest bilateral paravertebral reflexes,
the rotation that occurs as the embryologic gut develops causes certain reflexes
to be predominantly left-sided (stomach), while others (cecum and appendix) are
right-sided.

The vagus provides the parasympathetic innervation of the gastrointestinal
tract proximal to the mid transverse colon, and consequently, most of the gut
demonstrates a parasympathetic viscerosomatic reflex at the level of the occiput,
C1, C2. The distal half of the transverse colon to the rectum receives its parasympathetic supply from the pelvic splanchnic nerves, S2 to S4, and consequently
demonstrates sacropelvic viscerosomatic reflex activity.[23,24]

Upper Gastrointestinal Viscerosomatic Reflexes

The esophagus has very little sympathetic innervation. Its reported reflexes are
variable: T3 right,[23] T5 to T6 right.[22] The stomach has been generally agreed upon
to manifest as a left-sided reflex from T5 to as low as T10.[7,20,22,23] The duodenum
reflex tends to be right-sided from T6 to T8.[23] A distinctive alternating pattern of
paravertebral findings emerges. It can be considered indicative of upper gastrointestinal pathology: high cervical vagal reflex accompanied by T3 right, T5 to T7
left, and T6 to T8 right. This offers assistance with differentiating an upper gastrointestinal disorder from possible cardiac or pulmonary etiology.

The Chapman points[17] associated with the upper gastrointestinal tract include
the following:

Esophagus. The anterior points are in the space between the second and third ribs
at the sternocostal junction, and the posterior points are found upon T2, midway between the spinous process and the tip of the transverse process.

Stomach. The anterior points are in the spaces between the fifth to seventh ribs, from
the midmammillary line on the left to the sternum. The posterior points are found
in the spaces between the transverse processes of T5 to T7, midway between the
spinous processes and the tips of the transverse processes on the left.

Pyloris. The anterior points are on the front of the sternum from the ster-
nomanubrial junction inferiorly to the xiphoid process. The posterior point is
found on the tenth rib at the costotransverse junction on the right.

Duodenum. The anterior points lie bilaterally in the spaces between the eighth and
ninth ribs near the costochondral junctions, and the posterior points are found
bilaterally in the space between the transverse processes of T8 and T9 midway
between the spinous processes and the tips of the transverse processes.

Lower Gastrointestinal Viscerosomatic Reflexes

The parasympathetic reflex as far as the mid transverse colon continues to be the vagal reflex, occiput, C1, C2. The sympathetic viscerosomatic reflex from the small intestine is T8 to T10, bilateral[22] (possibly right greater than left[23]).

The bilateral Chapman points[17] associated with the small intestine include the following:

Jejunum. The anterior points are in the space between the ninth and tenth ribs near the costochondral junctions, and the posterior points are found in the space between the transverse processes of T9 and T10, midway between the spinous processes and the tips of the transverse processes.

Ileum. The anterior points are in the space between the tenth and eleventh ribs near the costochondral junctions, and the posterior points are found in the space between the transverse processes of T10 and T11, midway between the spinous processes and the tips of the transverse processes.

Viscerosomatic Reflexes for the Remainder of the Gastrointestinal Tract

The vermiform appendix and cecum result in reflex tissue texture change from T9 to T12 on the right.[20,23,24] The ascending colon results in reflex tissue texture change from T11 to L1 on the right.[20,22–24]

At the level of the mid transverse colon, the parasympathetic viscerosomatic reflex shifts from vagal to pelvic splanchnic, S2 to S4, resulting in sacropelvic tissue texture change and tenderness. Pathology affecting the descending colon to the rectum results in reflex tissue texture changes from L1 to L3 on the left.[22–24]

The Chapman points[17] for the appendix are right-sided. The anterior point is near the tip of the twelfth rib on the right upon its superior edge, and the posterior point is found in the space between the tips of the transverse processes of T11 and T12 on the right.

The bilateral Chapman points[17] associated with the large intestine include the colon. Chapman's description of the reflex points associated with the colon necessitates further discussion. The posterior points representing the entire colon are found bilaterally in a triangular area, from the transverse process of L2 to the transverse process of L4 and extending laterally to the iliac crest. The anterior points of the colon lie bilaterally on the lateral aspects of the thighs in the tensor fascia lata and the anterior portion of the iliotibial tract. The colonic subdivisions, cecum to sigmoid, however, are individually represented within the anterior points, beginning with the cecum over the right greater trochanter and progressing to the right half of the transverse colon, proximal to the right knee. The anterior points for the left half of the transverse colon are found upon the left iliotibial tract distally, beginning proximal to the left knee and ascending the lateral thigh to the left greater trochanter, where the anterior points for the sigmoid colon are found.

The anterior colonic points are as follows:

Cecum. The anterior points are located laterally upon the upper fifth of the right thigh, anteriorly on the tensor fascia lata.

Ascending colon. The anterior points are located laterally upon the middle three-fifths of the right thigh, on the anterior aspect of the iliotibial tract.

Right half of the transverse colon. The anterior points are proximal to the right knee, laterally upon the anterior aspect of the iliotibial tract.

Left half of the transverse colon. The anterior points are proximal to the left knee, laterally upon the anterior aspect of the iliotibial tract.

Descending colon. The anterior points are located laterally upon the middle three-fifths of the left thigh, on the anterior aspect of the iliotibial tract.

Sigmoid colon. The anterior points are located laterally upon the upper fifth of the left thigh, anteriorly on the tensor fascia lata.

Additional lower gastrointestinal bilateral Chapman's points that have been described:

Rectum. The anterior points are located on the proximal inner thighs over the lesser trochanters bilaterally, and the posterior points are found on the sacrum, close to the ilium at the lower end of the sacroiliac articulation.

Hemorrhoids. The anterior points are located immediately above ischial tuberosities, and the posterior points are found on the sacrum, close to the ilium at the lower end of the sacroiliac articulation.

Viscerosomatic Reflexes from the Pancreas, Liver, Gallbladder, and Spleen

Pancreas

The sympathetic reflex is a multisegmental reaction from T5 to T9.[7,22,23] The tissue texture findings have been described as left-sided [7,22] and as bilateral.[23] In chronic pancreatitis, the area tends to become fixed in extension. This may occur as a direct somatic effect of the retroperitoneal location of the pancreas and the effect of inflammation and the liberation of pancreatic digestive enzymes upon the surrounding tissues.

The parasympathetic reflex is vagal, occiput, C1, C2. The intensity of this reflex may be monitored from day to day, as it tends to mirror the severity of acute pancreatitis.

The Chapman points[17] associated with the pancreas are right-sided. The anterior point is located in the space between the costal cartilages of the seventh and eighth ribs, and the posterior point lies between the transverse processes of T7 and T8, midway between the tips of the spinous processes and the transverse processes.

Liver and Gallbladder

The sympathetic reflex is a right-sided reaction, palpable from as high as the level of T5 to T10.[7,20,22,23] The parasympathetic reflex for the liver is vagal, occiput, C1, C2. Additionally, a somatosomatic reflex, mediated through the phrenic nerve, C3 to C5, is responsible for referred pain to the right shoulder and midcervical paravertebral tissue texture change.[7,24]

The Chapman points[17] associated with the liver and gallbladder are right-sided. The anterior points are in the spaces between the fifth and seventh ribs, from the midmammillary line to the sternum, and the posterior points are between the transverse processes of T5 to T7, midway between the tips of the spinous processes and the transverse processes.

Spleen

The sympathetic reflex is a left-sided reaction, palpable from the level of T7 to T9.[22]

The Chapman points associated with the spleen are left-sided. The anterior points are in the spaces between the seventh and eighth ribs near the costochondral junction, and the posterior points are located between the transverse processes of T7 and T8, midway between the tips of the spinous processes and the transverse processes.

Viscerosomatic Reflexes from the Urinary Tract

Kidney

The sympathetic reflex is ipsilateral with the side of the urinary tract of involvement; a palpable reaction may be present from T9 to L1.[7,22–24] The parasympathetic reflex for the kidneys is vagal, occiput, C1, C2.

The Chapman points[17] associated with the kidneys are found ipsilateral to the side of urinary tract involvement. The anterior points lie 1 inch above the umbilicus, laterally on either side of the midline, and the posterior points are between the transverse processes of T12 and L1, midway between the tips of the spinous processes and the transverse processes.

Ureter
The sympathetic reflex is ipsilateral with the side of the urinary tract of involvement; a palpable reaction may be present from T11 to L3.[7,22–24] As a kidney stone traverses the ureter, a corresponding viscerosomatic reflex will descend along the thoracolumbar paravertebral soft tissues.[24]

The parasympathetic reflex for the proximal ureters is vagal, occiput, C1, C2, and for the distal ureters, pelvic splanchnic, S2 to S4.

Bladder
The sympathetic reflex is bilateral T11 to L3.[22,24] The parasympathetic reflex is pelvic splanchnic, S2 to S4.

The Chapman points[17] associated with the urinary bladder are bilateral. The anterior points are located immediately surrounding the umbilicus and on the pubic symphysis, just lateral to the midline midway between the superior and inferior edges of the pubic bones. The posterior points are located upon the superior edge of the transverse process of L2.

Urethra
The sympathetic reflex is bilateral T11 to L2.[22]

The Chapman points[17] associated with the urethra are bilateral. The anterior points are on the superior aspect of the pubic symphysis, and the posterior points are on the superior edge of the transverse process of L2.

Viscerosomatic Reflexes from the Reproductive Organs

Fallopian Tubes (and Seminal Vesicles)
The sympathetic reflex from the fallopian tubes is ipsilateral to the side of pathology from T10 to L2.[23,24] The parasympathetic reflex is pelvic splanchnic, S2–S4.[23,24]

The Chapman points[17] associated with the fallopian tubes and seminal vesicles are bilateral. The anterior points are paradoxically located posteriorly, midway between the acetabulum and sciatic notch, and the posterior points are between the posterior superior iliac spine of the ilium and the transverse process of L5 on the iliolumbar ligament. (Owens' text reads "spinous process," not transverse process, but the illustration is most consistent with the description given here.)

Genital Organs
The sympathetic reflex is bilateral at T12.[22]

Chapman points[17] are identified bilaterally for the female genitalia (clitoris and vagina). The anterior points are located bilaterally on the distal medial thigh, 7 to 15 cm on the upper inner aspect of the posterior thigh, and the posterior points are located bilaterally between the posterior superior iliac spine of the ilium and the transverse process of L5 on the iliolumbar ligament. (Owens' text reads "spinous process," not transverse process, but the illustration is most consistent with the description given here.)

Prostate
The sympathetic reflex is bilateral from T10 to L2.[7,22,23] The parasympathetic reflex is from the pelvic splanchnic nerves, S2–S4.[7,22,23]

Bilateral Chapman points[17] are identified for the prostate. The anterior points are located bilaterally on the lateral aspect of the thighs in a similar distribution to that of the colon, from the trochanter downward on the outer aspect of the femur to within 2 inches of the knee joint laterally, and the posterior points are located bilaterally between the posterior superior iliac spine of the ilium and the transverse process of L5 on the iliolumbar ligament. (Owens' text reads "spinous process," not transverse process, but the illustration is most consistent with the description given here.)

Ovaries (and Testes)
The sympathetic reflex is ipsilateral with the side of gonadal involvement from T10 to T11.[22,24]

The Chapman points[17] identified for the ovaries are bilateral. The anterior points are located upon the anterior surface of the pubic bone, from the pubic tubercle inferiorly to the origin of the adductor muscles. The posterior points are located in the spaces between T9 and T11.

Uterus
The sympathetic reflex is bilateral from T9 to L2.[20,22–24] The parasympathetic reflex is from the pelvic splanchnic nerves, S2-S4.[23,24]

The Chapman points[17] identified for the uterus are bilateral. The anterior points are on the medial margins of the obturator foramina, and the posterior points are located bilaterally between the posterior superior iliac spine of the ilium and the transverse process of L5 on the iliolumbar ligament. (Owens' text reads "spinous process," not transverse process, but the illustration is most consistent with the description given here.)

Viscerosomatic Reflexes from Endocrine Glands

Pancreas
See page 44.

Adrenal Glands
The sympathetic reflex is ipsilateral with the side of the adrenal involvement from T8 to T10.[22]

The Chapman points[17] identified for the adrenal glands are bilateral. The anterior points are located 5 to 7 cm above and 2 to 3 cm on either side of the umbilicus, and the posterior points are located bilaterally in the intertransverse spaces between T11 and T12, midway between the tips of the spinous processes and transverse processes.

TREATMENT CONSIDERATIONS

Somatic dysfunction that is the reflex result of primary visceral pathology, a viscerosomatic reflex, is treated by employing the medical treatment specifically indicated for the underlying pathology responsible for the reflex. This is not debatable. The spinal segmental facilitation that is the result of the viscerosomatic reflex can, however, produce a somatovisceral reflex demonstrating lowered thresholds for autonomic neuronal firing. Sustained hyperactivity of sympathetic pathways has been demonstrated to be deleterious to target tissues, resulting in such clinical conditions as peptic ulcer disease, pancreatitis, neurogenic pulmonary edema, and fatal arrhythmias following myocardial infarction.[14] Sustained parasympathetic activity will result in bradycardia and gastrointestinal hyperactivity. If pancreatitis, as an example, results in a viscerosomatic reflex with segmental facilitation from T5 to T9, the facilitation will in turn expose the pancreas to sustained sympathetic hyperactivity. Thus, it has been argued that manipulative treatment may be directed at the somatic dysfunction to decrease the facilitated state, even if it is of viscerosomatic reflex origin, with resultant beneficial effect upon the site of pathology.[12,14,20]

Early osteopathic research differentiated between stimulatory and inhibitory manipulative treatment and its somatovisceral impact.[8] When treating the somatic component of a viscerosomatic reflex to induce a somatovisceral effect, inhibitory pressure procedures, as described at the end of this chapter, are most often the treatment of choice. Chapman's points are treated by applying inhibitory pressure in a slow circular fashion for 10 to 30 seconds until any associated tissue texture change resolves.

Stimulatory procedures utilizing articulatory range of motion and soft-tissue stretching are appropriate when treating congested states, such as pneumonia, or hypoactive conditions, such as constipation. Somatosensory input, with resultant stimulation of internuncial neurons that synapse in the intermediolateral cell column of the thoracic and upper lumbar cord, will produce a segmentally related sympathetic response. Similarly, high-cervical or sacral stimulation will result in a parasympathetic response.

The anatomic areas of consideration, when using manipulation to effect a somatovisceral response, are essentially the same as those noted earlier as loci for viscerosomatic reflexes. As Burns noted, however, they are "less circumscribed and less direct than are viscerosomatic reflexes."[8] As such, the areas listed hereafter are the places to begin looking for the source of somatovisceral impact. Also, particular sympathetic reflexes may emanate from a much broader area than the viscerosomatic reflexes described herein.

Viscerosomatic reflexes are often identified in spinal segments that also demonstrate mechanical somatic dysfunction. The same neurophysiology that is responsible for the paravertebral response to visceral pathology in the viscerosomatic reflex explains the effect of somatic dysfunction upon a segmentally related viscus through a somatovisceral reflex. The level of spinal mechanical somatic dysfunction is maintained in a facilitated state by the mechanical dysfunction and can affect segmentally related viscera as a somatovisceral reflex.

The treatment of somatic dysfunction as it relates to systemic visceral disease can be appreciated once it is decided what effect the somatic dysfunction has upon the status of the patient. The effect of somatic dysfunction may be mechanical and/or the result of somatovisceral reflex activity.

Consideration of the somatovisceral effect of somatic dysfunction should prompt the physician to ask the following questions:

- Is there facilitation of sympathetic (thoracolumbar) or parasympathetic (high cervical or sacral) components of the spinal cord? If so, how does it affect the patient?
- What sympathetic somatovisceral mechanisms are present? Spinal facilitation, with resultant increased sympathetic tone, increases vascular tone, which decreases tissue perfusion and nutrient and oxygen supply to tissues and thereby increases any need for anaerobic glycolysis. It relaxes the gallbladder and biliary ducts and decreases the glandular secretions and peristalsis, producing constipation or ileus. Sympathetic stimulation of the gastrointestinal tract decreases peristalsis, which predisposes the patient to constipation or the development of an ileus.
- What parasympathetic somatovisceral mechanisms are present? Spinal facilitation, with resultant increased parasympathetic tone, increases the secretion of the digestive enzymes amylase and lipase. It causes contraction of the gallbladder

and biliary ducts and increased glandular secretions and peristalsis, producing diarrhea and colic.

The consideration of somatovisceral mechanisms as they relate to the individual organ systems and specific disease processes are discussed in later chapters.

The Mechanical Effect of Somatic Dysfunction

Consideration of the mechanical effect of somatic dysfunction should cause the physician to seek answers to the following questions:

- Does the patient have a pain complaint that is the result of, or is compounded by, somatic dysfunction? Physicians often become so focused upon the patient's primary illness that they overlook simple problems that contribute greatly to the patient's discomfort.
- How is musculoskeletal dysfunction affecting the patient's ability to respond to the disease process? For example, restriction of the thoracic cage and diaphragm, while detrimental to anyone, is particularly deleterious to a patient with pulmonary disease.
- Does the mechanical component of the somatic dysfunction result in venous and/or lymphatic stasis? Efficient movement of the thoracic inlet, thoracic cage, abdominal diaphragm, mesenteries, and pelvic diaphragm is necessary for optimal low-pressure fluid (lymphatic and venous) dynamics and tissue perfusion. Inefficiency of this mechanism further adds to the tendency to develop tissue congestion.

DISCUSSION

When considering the care of a patient with significant visceral pathology, it is easy to become focused upon the precise therapeutic protocol for the specific disease process and lose sight of the individual patient. The urgency of many disease processes causes us to focus only upon the intervention that offers the greatest immediate therapeutic effect. Treatment of peripheral, seemingly unrelated and trivial conditions may be considered ineffective and inappropriate.

If one considers somatic dysfunction only in the context of the musculoskeletal system, it could arguably be seen as trivial in the presence of such disease processes as myocardial infarction, pyelonephritis, or Crohn's disease. From a distinctively osteopathic perspective, however, somatic dysfunction in the presence of significant visceral pathology becomes highly significant.

Viscerosomatic reflexes are a useful part of the physical diagnosis of visceral pathology because they are somatic dysfunction that develops specifically in response to visceral pathology. They offer diagnostic clues to the location and severity of the etiologic pathology. Viscerosomatic reflexes are identifiable as tissue texture abnormality and tenderness in the dermatomes and myotomes that share innervation with the etiologic pathology. They are most easily palpable in the paravertebral soft tissues and in the specific areas represented as Chapman's reflexes.

Viscerosomatic reflexes offer valuable diagnostic information, particularly in the absence of overt visceral complaints. The recognition of a potential viscerosomatic reflex assists in the differential diagnosis of somatic pain, offering the clinician insights that might otherwise go unrecognized. Objective palpatory findings of a viscerosomatic reflex without associated disease should lead to a more focused review of the patient's history. Somatic dysfunction that resists manipulative treatment should raise the question of viscerosomatic origin.

Viscerosomatic reflexes are definitively treated first by treating the causative visceral pathology. Somatic dysfunction, however, affects visceral physiology through its mechanical effect as well as through somatovisceral reflexes. OMT of viscerosomatic reflexes has been advocated to reduce somatic dysfunction and interrupt the reflex arc, thereby influencing the viscus through stimulation of somatovisceral effects.

Additionally, the linkage between the musculoskeletal system and specific viscera through the segmental arrangement of the central nervous system allows the physician to associate seemingly unrelated areas into an integrated holistic approach to patient care. Anatomic systems are a convenient way of studying human physiology and pathology, and although not entirely arbitrary, the division of the human body into such systems is artificial. There are advantages to being able to recognize the connections between the different systems of the body through viscerosomatic, somatovisceral, somatosomatic and viscerovisceral connections. To approach the patient in this context means that the physician must consider the interrelationship of otherwise seemingly unrelated structures and systems; it fosters the holistic clinical approach for which osteopathic medicine is known.

Procedures

The following are examples of procedures that are valuable for diagnosing somatic dysfunction of visceral reflex origin and of OMT procedures that may be employed for their somatovisceral effect. Please note: The procedures that follow are examples of manipulative treatment that you may wish to employ. The actual choice of procedures used should be determined by the unique circumstances of each individual patient.

Diagnosis

Palpation for Tissue Texture Abnormality, Layer Palpation

This procedure is employed to identify tissue texture change that may be found in association with viscerosomatic reflexes. The patient may be in any position that lends itself to the examination and the requirements of the health status of the patient. The physician's position depends upon the patient's position. This procedure is described in Chapter 3.

Red Reflex

This procedure is employed to assess for vasomotor irritability as an indicator of spinal segmental facilitation commonly found in association with acute somatic dysfunction, including viscerosomatic reflexes.

Patient position: seated or prone. Physician position: standing behind the seated patient or to the side of the prone patient.

Procedure

1. Stroke the paravertebral skin. (The standard palpatory examination of the paravertebral soft tissues is also sufficient to produce a red reflex.)
2. Observe for areas that become hyperemic. Facilitated segments demonstrate vasomotor instability and become hyperemic sooner, demonstrate a greater degree of hyperemia, and remain hyperemic longer than adjacent segments.

Skin Drag

This procedure is employed to assess for sudomotor hyperactivity as an indicator of spinal segmental somatic dysfunction facilitation, including viscerosomatic reflexes.

Patient position: seated or prone. Physician position: standing behind the seated patient or to the side of the prone patient.

Procedure

1. With the pads of the fingers, lightly stroke the paravertebral skin.
2. Areas of sudomotor hyperactivity indicative of acute dysfunction will be moist and provide greater friction (skin drag) than adjacent tissues when stroked with the pads of the fingers. Areas of chronic dysfunction will be dry and provide less friction.

Beal's Compression Test

This procedure, employed to diagnose somatic dysfunction, is particularly valuable for assessing the patient who is confined to a hospital bed.

Patient position: supine. Physician position: seated at the side of the bed facing the patient.

Procedure

1. Slide the hands, palms up, beneath the patient.
2. Place the pads of the fingers in contact with the paravertebral soft tissue on the side of the spine closest to the examiner and to the area of maximal tissue texture abnormality and muscle contraction. Palpate the paravertebral soft tissues.
3. Apply gentle pressure in an anterior direction relative to the supine patient, thus compressing the paravertebral soft tissues.
4. Using the principles of layer palpation, compare the soft tissues at each vertebral level with those of the segment above and below. Look for the spinal level of maximum tissue texture change in the context of subcutaneous turgidity, fascial tension and deep paravertebral muscle tension.
5. This procedure can be repeated up and down the paravertebral soft tissues of the thoracic and lumbar regions on the side nearer the physician.
6. To examine the opposite side, it is necessary to move to the other side of the bed and repeat the process.

As an alternative method in which both sides are examined simultaneously, the physician can sit at the head of the bed and slide the hands, palms up, beneath the supine patient on either side of the spine. From this position, the physician can evaluate and compare left side with right side and segments above and below. This approach is limited, however, to evaluation of the cervical region and upper thoracic spine.

Treatment

Inhibitory Pressure

This procedure is employed to treat any dysfunction severe enough to discourage more aggressive intervention. It is intended to reduce tissue texture abnormality and muscle spasm. It is particularly valuable for addressing the somatovisceral component of an acute viscerosomatic reflex.

The patient may be treated in any position that lends itself to the area being addressed and to the health status requirements of the patient. The position of the physician depends upon the position in which the patient is treated. For purposes of this discussion, the patient is supine because this is the position typically required when treating severely ill individuals. The physician in this instance should therefore be seated or standing at the side of the bed or treatment table facing the patient.

Procedure

1. Slide the hands, palms up, beneath the patient and palpate the paravertebral soft tissues.
2. Place the pads of the fingers in contact with the area of maximal tissue texture abnormality and muscle contraction.
3. Apply gentle pressure to the tight muscles.
4. Gradually increase pressure as the muscles relax.
5. When maximum pressure has been applied, hold it for 1 to 2 minutes and then very slowly release it.

Stop the intervention, slowly releasing, if you detect spasticity. At no time should the treated tissue be rapidly released. Such action will result in immediate reestablishment of muscle spasm.

Treatment of Chapman's Reflexes (Figs. 5.1 and 5.2)

This procedure is employed to treat viscerosomatic Chapman's reflexes. Such reflexes exhibit the following traits: Small (2–3 mm) nodular masses that are palpable in soft tissue and that demonstrate sharp pinpoint nonradiating tenderness. They exert a therapeutic somatovisceral effect when treated.

In the past, the anterior points have been designated as diagnostic and the posterior points as treatment points.[17] Many clinicians today who employ Chapman's reflexes therapeutically treat either or both the anterior and posterior points. The patient may be treated in any position that lends itself to the area being addressed and the health status requirements of the patient. The position of the physician depends upon the position in which the patient is treated. It has also been recommended that the specific treatment of the reflex points should not be initiated until the pelvis has been thoroughly treated for somatic dysfunction.[17–19]

Procedure

1. Place the palmar distal pad of the index finger in contact with the palpable nodular mass of the Chapman's point to be treated.
2. Apply pressure to the point. The amount of pressure necessary will be "somewhat heavy and uncomfortable"[18] for the patient.
3. Apply the therapeutic pressure in a circular fashion, massaging the point in an attempt to gradually dissipate it. This treatment usually requires 10 to 30 seconds.
4. The treatment ceases when the palpable point resolves or when the physician fatigues.

Soft Tissue/Range of Motion, Patient on Side, a Stimulatory Procedure (e.g., Thoracic [Fig. 5.3] and Lumbar [Fig. 5.4] Regions)

For a description of the cervical soft tissue and range-of-motion procedure, see Chapter 16.

This procedure is employed to decrease muscle spasm and soft tissue tension in a manner that is sufficiently aggressive to result in somatovisceral stimulation. The description is directed at treating the right paravertebral region.

Patient position: lying on the left side, with one or two pillows under the head and the knees bent. Physician position: standing at the side of the table facing the patient.

Procedure

1. Position the patient's bottom arm under the head and the top arm wherever it is comfortable and out of the way. Flex the patient's hips for stability.

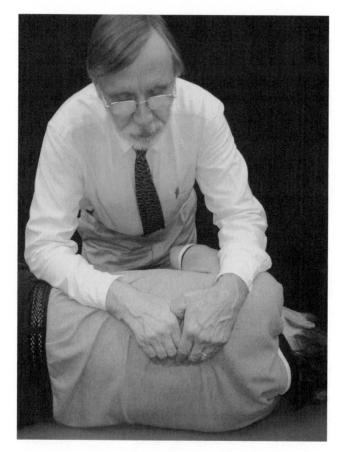

FIGURE 5.3 Stimulatory procedure for the thoracic region.

2. Hook the fingers over the paraspinal musculature of the side facing up at the level of the thoracolumbar junction. Wrap the hands over the patient's flank.
3. Apply a controlled force through both hands that is directed anterolaterally, cephalad, and caudad. Keep your back straight. Place one foot in front of the other. Lean back and use your full body weight.
4. Release the force in a controlled fashion. Work up the thoracic spine and down the lumbar spine as necessary.

Soft Tissue/Range of Motion, Patient Prone (Fig. 5.5)

This procedure is employed to decrease muscle spasm and soft tissue tension in a manner that is aggressive enough to result in somatovisceral stimulation. The description is directed at treating the right paravertebral region. The patient should be lying prone and the physician standing

Patient position: prone on the bed or treatment table. Physician position: standing at the left side facing the patient.

Procedure

1. Place the thenar eminence and hypothenar eminence of the treating hand between the spinous processes and the paraspinal muscle group on the patient's right side. Place the other hand over the opposite paraspinal muscles.

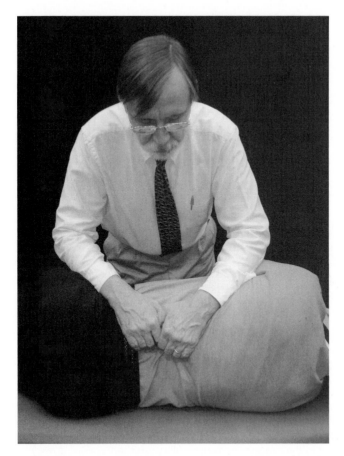

FIGURE 5.4   Stimulatory procedure for the lumbar region.

2. Use the treating hand to apply a controlled force in the anterolateral direction. The depth and rate of the applied force determines whether you are primarily treating the soft tissues (soft tissue procedure) or articulating the vertebrae (deep articulation procedure).
3. Stop advancing the force when the barrier is reached (limit of tissue stretching or patient's tolerance).
4. Release the forces in a controlled fashion. Work up and down the thoracic lumbar spine as necessary. Continue until the paravertebral soft tissues are relaxed.

Rib Raising to Stimulate Sympathetic Activity (Fig. 5.6)

Treatment by rib raising reduces constriction of larger lymphatic vessels. Rib raising that raises the rib heads also stimulates the thoracic sympathetic chain ganglia. This treatment initially stimulates regional sympathetic efferent activity to organs related to that spinal level of sympathetic innervation, but in the long run, rib raising results in a prolonged reduction in sympathetic outflow from the area treated. Freeing rib motion also frees the excursion of the rib cage during respiration. Freeing the rib heads increases the excursion of the chest during breathing and improves lymphatic flow.

Patient position: supine. Physician position: standing or seated at the patient's side.

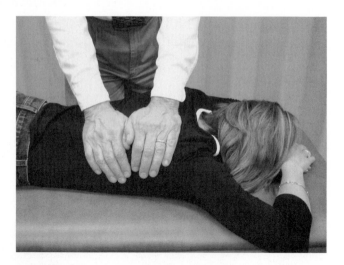

FIGURE 5.5   Soft tissue and range of motion, patient prone.

Procedure

1. Place the hands (palms) under the patient's thorax, contacting the rib angles with the pads of the fingers.
2. Flex the fingers to achieve contact with the rib angle and the patient's posterior thorax.
3. Apply traction on the rib angle.
4. While maintaining traction, bend your knees and lower your trunk, which raises the ribs when your hands move up. This is a fulcrum/lever action; the wrists are not bent. (Particularly if the patient is in a hospital bed, it is easier to move the hands upward if in the process you reciprocally push the forearms down.)
5. Move the hands to subsequent rib angles until all ribs are treated.
6. Treat the opposite side of the rib cage in the same manner.

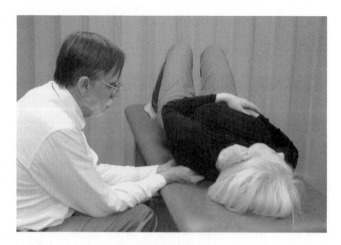

FIGURE 5.6   Rib raising.

References

1. Hazzard C. Principles of Osteopathy. 3rd ed. Kirksville, MO: Author, 1899;8–11.
2. Tasker DL. Principles of Osteopathy. 2nd ed. Los Angeles: Baumgardt, 1905;211–256.
3. Bernard C. Leçons de physiologie, expérimentale appliquée à la médicine. Paris: Baillière, 1855–1856.
4. Head H. On disturbances of sensation with especial reference to the pain of visceral disease. Brain 1893;16:1–133.
5. MacKenzie J. Some points bearing on the association of sensory disorders and visceral disease. Brain 1893;16:321–354.
6. Luciani L. Human Physiology. Vol 4. London: Macmillan, 1917:68.
7. Pottenger FM. Symptoms of Visceral Disease. 5th ed. St. Louis: Mosby, 1938.
8. Burns L. Viscero-somatic and somato-visceral spinal reflexes. J Am Osteopath Assoc 1907;7(2):51–60.
9. Burns L. Symposium on the A. T. Still Research Institute. J Am Osteopath Assoc 1930;29: 433–437.
10. Burns L. Certain cardiac complications and vertebral lesions. J Am Osteopath Assoc 1947; 47:199–200.
11. Denslow JS. An analysis of the variability of spinal reflex thresholds. J Neurophysiol 1944; 7:207–215.
12. Korr IM. The neural basis of the osteopathic lesion. J Am Osteopath Assoc 1947;47: 191–198.
13. Korr IM. Skin resistance patterns associated with visceral disease. Fed Proc 1949;8:87.
14. Korr IM, ed. The Neurobiologic Mechanisms in Manipulative Therapy. New York: Plenum, 1978.
15. Van Buskirk RL. Nociceptive reflexes and the somatic dysfunction: A model. J Am Osteopath Assoc 1990;90:792–809 [review].
16. ICD-9CM International Classification of Diseases. 9th revision. Clinical Modification. 5th ed. Salt Lake City: Medicode, 1999.
17. Owens C. An Endocrine Interpretation of Chapman's Reflexes. 2nd ed. Indianapolis: Academy of Applied Osteopathy (American Academy of Osteopathy), 1963.
18. Patriquin DA. Viscerosomatic reflexes. In: Patterson MM, Howel JN, eds. The Central Connection: Somatovisceral Viscerosomatic Interactions. Athens, OH: University Classics, 1992;4–12.
19. Patriquin DA. Chapman's reflexes. In: Ward RC, ed. Foundations for Osteopathic Medicine. 2nd ed. Philadelphia: Lippincott Williams & Wilkins, 2002;1051–1055.
20. Beal MC. Viscerosomatic reflexes: A review. J Am Osteopath Assoc. 1985;85:786–801.
21. Cole WV. The body economy. In: Hoag JM, ed. Osteopathic Medicine. New York: McGraw Hill, 1969;68–100.
22. Dowling DJ. Neurophysiologic mechanisms related to osteopathic diagnosis and treatment. In: DiGiovanna EL, Schiowitz S, eds. An Osteopathic Approach to Diagnosis and Treatment. 2nd ed. Philadelphia: Lippincott, 1997;29.
23. Van Buskirk RL, Nelson KE. Osteopathic family practice: An application of the primary care model. In: Ward RC, ed. Foundations for Osteopathic Medicine. 2nd ed. Philadelphia: Lippincott Williams & Wilkins, 2002;289–297.
24. Kuchera ML, Kuchera WA. Osteopathic Considerations in Systemic Dysfunctions. 2nd ed. Columbus, OH: Greyden, 1994.
25. Sumino R, Nozaki S, Kato M. Central pathway of trigemino-neck reflex. In: Oral-facial sensory and motor functions. International Symposium. Rappongi, Tokyo. Oral Physiol 1980;28 [abstract].
26. Larson NJ. Summary of site and occurrence of paraspinal soft tissue changes of patients in the intensive care unit. J Am Osteopath Assoc 1976;75:840–842.

CHAPTER 6

Psychoneuroimmunology

Jan Lei Iwata

"First, there is the material body; second, the spiritual being; third, a being of mind which is far superior to all vital motions and material forms, whose duty is to wisely manage this great engine of life. To obtain good results, we must blend ourselves with and travel in harmony with Nature's truths."

A. T. Still[1]

INTRODUCTION

The biopsychosocial model is one of the tenets of family medicine.[2] A good starting place, therefore, is to consider history while examining the role that psychoneuroimmunology (PNI) has played in bringing together the best in basic scientific research as it applies to the holistic framework of total patient care. Psychoneuroimmunology and osteopathic medicine should be synonymous when one is talking about the role of osteopathic manipulative medicine in primary care. Osteopathic family physicians care for the whole patient, providing a strong doctor–patient interface and psychological support in the form of listening, empathy, and compassion. Therefore, their excellent medical diagnostic skills and osteopathic manipulative treatment (OMT) position them as unique and distinctive health care providers and help to distinguish osteopathic medicine from other forms of health care.[3]

The holistic integrated view of patient care and how stress can affect one's health should be the starting point in care management and focus. Osteopathic manipulation for chronic spinal pain results in greater short-term improvement than acupuncture or medication,[4] and it has been shown to lessen the use of pain medications compared to standard care in subacute low back pain[5] and to require less physical therapy.[6] Since there is a close association between the spinal vertebrae and the autonomic nervous system via the sympathetic nervous system and the sympathetic trunk and ganglia, the neuromuscular system is considered to play a vital role in maintaining homeostasis. Any changes in the musculoskeletal system can affect other organs (somatovisceral reflex) or allow visceral pathology to manifest as musculoskeletal tissue texture and intervertebral joint motion (viscerosomatic reflex) changes, hence somatic dysfunction.[7]

Historically, in osteopathic medicine, Andrew Taylor Still is credited with stating that the best way to fight disease was by naturally stimulating the body's immune system. He also believed that the solution to disease was to find out what was creating the bodily disturbance and remove that interference, so that the body could return to its normal state of homeostasis. Still believed that we possessed all of the "elements and principles of remedy in the divine chemical laboratory within the body."[8] He also believed that the body and mind were inseparable. Future neuropharmacologic and neuroscience research eventually proved his premise to be true, that the "chemical factory" included various peptides that communicated with and regulated many systems, including pain perception and early inflammatory events, when an injury occurred. In perhaps the first publication addressing the "psychic origin of disease," Hoover[9] summarized these concepts and proposed a theoretical construct that was remarkably insightful.

A primary goal of PNI research is to translate basic research into clinically relevant health applications. In this context, PNI's premier position in evidence-based health care in the twenty-first century is increasingly recognized and is poised to be the gold standard in the next decades.[10] PNI is a relatively new scientific field that defines and describes the concept of a vast unified psychosomatic communication network of neuropeptides in brain and other nonneural tissues and their corresponding receptors in the immune, endocrine, and central nervous systems, linking body to mind.[11] They do not exist independently, as was once believed, but are in constant communication with one another via neuropeptide ligands and their identical target receptor molecules.[12] This has been strengthened by animal and human research demonstrating relationships between behavior and neuropeptide-mediated regulation of immune function. To understand its application to clinical medicine, it is important to review the research behind psychosomatic illness and how it applies to wellness models. Robert Ader,[13] who demonstrated that immunosuppression could be behaviorally conditioned in rats, coined the term "psychoneuroimmunology" in 1981.

HISTORY

Much credit goes to the pioneering work led by Candace Pert at Johns Hopkins University in the 1970s. Pert, as a neuropharmacologist and neuroscientist, discovered and identified the first brain receptor, the opioid receptor. This receptor bound exogenous opioid drugs and analogs and endogenous opioid neuropeptides (endorphins) with powerful pain- and mood-modifying properties.[14,15] Through brain mapping, Pert found that the highest concentrations of these receptors resided in the limbic, amygdala, and hippocampus system, implying that neuropeptides and their receptors join the brain, glands, and immune system in a network of communication between brain and body. Later on, as section chief of the brain chemistry and clinical neuroscience branch at the National Institute for Mental Health (NIMH), she demonstrated how endogenously produced neuropeptide ligands bind to their cell surface receptors. This communication system operates outside the hardwired linear channels of neurotransmissions via a parallel extracellular parasynaptic system. The extracellular system allows neuropeptides to flow throughout the brain and body and act at distances without linear connections to their cellular targets, thereby effecting their change through receptor signal specificity.[16,17] This new paradigm explained how peptides could act as neurotransmitters and hormones. This led to brain mapping of other endogenous neuropeptides and study of the actions of molecules, such as morphine, phencyclidine, benzodiazepine, substance P, bombesin, corticotropin (ACTH), cholecystokinin, vasoactive intestinal polypeptide (VIP), neurotensin, transferrin, and insulin receptors. She believed that the 70 to 80 neuropeptides identified to date are the "biochemical correlate or substrate of emotion." Most, if not all, alter behavior and mood states. Also, many of these ligands influence immune cell function and immune system trafficking, influencing the intensity and duration of immune response to foreign entities.[11]

Specific "nodal points" of neuropeptide receptor distribution, identified by Pert and colleagues,[16] include emotion-mediated brain areas, the mobile cells of the immune system, and the dorsal horn of the spinal cord, where information from glands, skin, and other peripheral organs first make their contact with the central nervous system (CNS). Other receptor-rich loci include the periaqueductal gray region of the brainstem, which is hard-wired to limbic and emotional brain structures by neuronal pathways and has been shown to modulate pain thresholds. Additional nodal points include the gastrointestinal tract from the esophagus to the large intestines, which is lined with neuropeptides and receptors, including serotonin. The kidney, testes, and pancreas are other such sites. Other nodal points lie along the spinal cord (with a distribution similar to that of autonomic nervous system ganglia), internal organs, and skin. Since "informational substances" reside in all systems, Pert suggested that the neuromusculoskeletal system stores information in the form of "tissue memory" of injury, trauma, or disease. Nerve cells secreting immune products, such as interleukins, tumor necrosis factor, and cytokines, communicate directly with the brain via the vagus nerve or through the blood-brain barrier and cerebrospinal fluid.[18] Malfunction of the operation of cell receptors can cause disease, which suggests that perhaps emotional states can alter the course and outcome of biological illnesses.[14]

Pert also discovered peptide T (DAPTA). This peptide is the first viral entry inhibitor proving hopeful in the treatment of neuro-AIDS. It blocks the chemokine receptor–mediated chemotaxis receptor (CCR5) to reduce the HIV viral load to undetectable levels. This action permits a safe reversal of the devastating mental and neurological damage and cognitive impairment commonly seen in neuro-AIDS patients[19–22] and again demonstrates how the behavioral effects seen with endogenously produced neuropeptides can affect emotion and immune disease states.

Receptors for thyroid-stimulating hormone, pheromones, leuteinizing hormone–releasing hormone–like peptides, thyrotropin-releasing hormone–like peptides, endorphin-related peptides, and interferon-related peptides are found in higher plants and unicellular microorganisms (bacteria, protozoa) that bind to these substrates, resembling receptors. The manner of binding is analogous to that of the hormone receptors found in higher animals, which leads to the assumption that the molecules of intercellular communication are highly conserved and probably arose much earlier in evolution than the endocrine, nervous, and immune systems in mammals and other vertebrates.[23]

In 1981, J. Edwin Blalock, an immunologist at The University of Texas, was the first to study this aspect of the immune system. He reported the presence of endorphins and ACTH receptors bound to lymphocytes.[24] Other papers confirmed that ACTH and endorphin receptors and ligands found on lymphocytes were identical to those produced by the pituitary.[18] In fact, the immune system was capable not only of sending information to the brain via immunopeptides but also of receiving information from the brain via neuropeptides.[25] Immunocytes, monocytes, macrophages, and T lymphocytes also were found to produce many other neurohormones: VIP, somatostatin, substance P, oxytocin, neurophysin, gonadotropin, growth hormone, and throtropin.[26]

The Vagus Nerve and Substance P

The vagus nerve was identified as one of several routes through which cytokines signal the brain that the immune system has been activated. The vagus is thus an important conduit for neuroimmunomodulation.[18] Blalock viewed the immune system as a sense organ that alerted the brain to the presence of detected pathogens and infectious agents via the neuroendocrine system.[25] The paraganglia of the vagus nerve possess proinflammatory immune-associated cytokines to do just this. Also, it has been postulated that cytokines released within the brain itself, by accessory lymphoid cells and/or glial cells, could activate neural structures.[27] Substance P also is highly concentrated in the spleen at the site of antigen uptake and processing, which suggests that it is involved as well in the control of sensory functions of the immune system. In the intestinal tract, it evokes potent excitatory action. In sensory nerves supplying local sites of chronic inflammation, elevated levels of substance P have been detected, indicating a role for substance P in mediating allergic reactions while modulating the severity of joint injury in experimental arthritis.[28,29]

It is well known that in the CNS the vagus nerve is involved with pain neurotransmission from its activity in the dorsal horn of the spinal cord, because it is capable of directly irritating peripheral afferent nociceptors (PANs). These peripheral nociceptors are the small-caliber pain fibers that are activated by the high mechanical, thermal, and chemical stimuli that are highly damaging or that are involved in local tissue injury. This rapid firing of projections communicates to the limbic system as pain, causing the neuroendocrine and emotional responses known as "sickness behavior," or acute phase response (decreased locomotion, decreased libido, decreased exploration and aggression, decreased food and water intake, and hormonal changes). Local signaling of the PAN to the spinal cord at the level of the dorsal horn therefore is critical to the formation of spinal facilitation and its effect on the body. The output of the glial cytokine response is enhanced pain perception (hyperalgesia) and activation of the arousal system.[30]

Locally, substance P release from the PAN fibers causes mast cells to release histamine and vascular endothelial cells to release prostaglandins, producing swelling, while bradykinin is released from the numerous cell types in fascia. White blood cells migrate to the area and release cytokines. These proinflammatory neuropeptides trigger increased sensitization of the stimulated nerves, leading to further secretion of substance P to activate sympathetic catecholamines in the damaged tissue. Other neuropeptides released are calcitonin gene–related polypeptide and somatostatin, vasodilators that release more histamine in the area, causing further swelling and inflammation. Tissue acidosis ensues, which activates PAN in the skin, contributing to tissue texture changes that indicate somatic dysfunction. If this spinal facilitation continues, producing excitatory toxicity (further production of dynorphin) leading to interneuron (pain inhibitory fiber) death, the dorsal horn neurons compensate by undergoing membrane molecular changes. "In this mode, dorsal horn neurons have altered their membrane properties such that they over-respond to very minimum input, and in some cases, to no input at all."[30] This creates an ongoing spinal facilitation that links the complex network of information shared between the endocrine, brain, and immune systems during painful events.[30] Hence, somatic dysfunction increases cytokine and PAN activity in hyperalgesia.

Visceral afferent fibers in the vagus signal dysfunction to the solitary nucleus in the brainstem, releasing proinflammatory cytokines by macrophages, dendritic cells, and other immune cells at the nerve endings, thereby stimulating the primary afferent fibers. This signal ascends through the brainstem to the thalamus and the limbic forebrain, initiating behavioral changes, such as activation of the sympathetic nervous system and of the hypothalamic-pituitary-adrenal axis (HPA), to arrive at a general adaptive and protective response. The amygdala is associated with fear or negative memory and has descending projections to the locus coeruleus, known as the sympathetic nervous system of the brain, in the brainstem. The arousal system of the brainstem therefore receives sensory stimuli (somatic, visceral, visual, and acoustic) and emotional stimuli and channels this warning information into a wide-ranging output circuitry that significantly alters activity in the nervous, endocrine, and immune systems. From the locus coeruleus, projections go to the hypothalamus to coordinate the release of corticotropin-releasing hormone and the secondary release of ACTH, cortisol, and norepinephrine.[30] This phenomenon is known as the locus coeruleus–norepinephrine axis, which is activated in hyperalgesia.

Vasoactive Intestinal Polypeptide Implications

In sensory areas of the brain (the olfactory bulb, thalamic nuclei, several cranial nuclei, the area postrema), and the inner walls of the blood vessels of the brain and spleen, VIP receptors are abundant. VIP itself is a potent vasodilator and smooth muscle relaxant (esophageal sphincter, stomach, and gallbladder), inhibits gastric acid secretion and absorption in the intestinal lumen, and stimulates secretion of water into bile and pancreatic juice. VIP-secreting cells and receptors line the entire gastrointestinal tract, which suggests that they are possible mediators of so-called *gut feelings*. VIP, substance P, and calcitonin gene–related peptide were proved to be potent lymphocyte and monocyte chemoattractants, verifying the role of these peptides in immune system trafficking.[11] The distribution patterns in brain and lymphoid tissues indicate interrelatedness of the two organ systems and may serve as one biochemical rationale for a biopsychosocial view of health and disease since the gut is known as the *ancient brain* of the body and is rich with serotonin receptors.

Other Local Events Seen with OMT (Nitric Oxide, Endocannabinoids)

Nitric oxide (NO), operating as a neurotransmitter and locally acting hormone, recently has been implicated in osteopathic manipulation by restricting the development of inflammation and down-regulating the process.[31] Physical manipulation induces NO synthase (NOS) release of NO. Other beneficial effects include peripheral vasodilation and warming of the skin, decrease in heart rate, and an overwhelming sense of well-being, referred to as the relaxation response, along with salutary anti–lipid peroxidation, antibacterial, and antiviral effects. It does so by modulating neurotransmitter release, neurosecretion, and behavioral activities.[32] NO is a major signaling molecule in the immune, cardiovascular, and nervous systems. The presence of an endothelial mu opioid receptor further substantiates the role of opioids in vascular coupling in NO release.[33] Diabetic endothelium is known to have fewer mu opioid receptors present, and it has diminished constitutive basal and morphine-stimulated NO release.[34]

Other signaling molecules also in the blood notably include the endocannabinoids (anandamide [arachidonylethanolamine] and 2-arachidonylglycerol, interleukin (IL) 10, and 17–beta estradiol. These are naturally occurring constitutive NOS–derived, NO-stimulating signaling molecules that are expressed by nerve tissue and diffused into the blood. These signaling molecules can further initiate profound physiological effects when osteopathically stimulated (through the physical mechanotransduction mechanism).[31] Anandamide, as part of the ubiquitous arachidonate and eicosaid signaling cascade, as well as estrogen, through NO release, can down-regulate immunocyte and vascular function in women and may provide an additional mechanism whereby osteopathic treatment may aid in the relief of female-associated dysfunction (i.e., those occurring post-partum).[31] Similarly, 2-arachidonylglycerol can cause reduction in cytokines and adhesion molecules, an immunosuppressive response similar to that of anandamide[35] (Fig. 6.1).

"Furthermore, naturally occurring signaling molecules such as morphine, anandamide, interleukin-10, and 17-beta-estradiol appear to exert, in part, their beneficial physiological actions, i.e., immune and endothelial down regulation by the stimulation of cNOS."[33] Morphine, given its long latency before increases in its levels are detected in human tissue and blood, arises after high-impact motion. It and the other signaling molecules, through an NO mechanism, down-regulate the activities within neural and immune tissues, thus providing a possible mechanism for the analgesic effects attributed to high-impact manipulation.

"The capacity of the cannabinoids to regulate immune function is well established."[36] Cannabinoids have been reported to have anti-inflammatory effects and reduce joint damage in animal models of arthritis. Anandamide has been shown to prevent cartilage resorption by inhibiting cytokine-induced NO production by chondrocytes and also by inhibiting proteoglycan degradation.[37] John McPartland[38] demonstrated in a randomized, blinded, controlled clinical trial that in contrast to controls, cannabimimetic effects (i.e., the relaxation response) were seen post-OMT in patients receiving manipulation. Also, serum anandamide levels doubled post-OMT compared to pretreatment levels, using chemical ionization gas chromatography and mass spectrometry measures. During pain modulation, when nociceptors are firing in the dorsal horn of the spinal cord, cannabinoid receptors can dampen the efficacy of activators and sensitizers and prevent the nociceptors from firing, preventing peripheral sensitization and hyperalgesia,

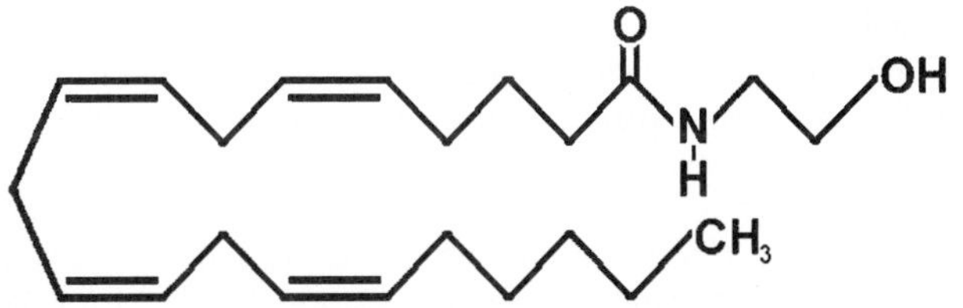

FIGURE 6.1   Chemical structure of the endocannabinoid anandamide.

especially in neuropathic and inflammatory pain. OMT can restore axoplasmic flow and restore the receptors to their active sites.[38] This restoration is critical to reestablishing homeostasis and restoring function after a painful or traumatic event that produces somatic dysfunction.

Thermal changes, in which temperature reduction occurs within 30 minutes following manipulative treatment, have been shown to occur in chronic somatic dysfunction areas of known musculoligamentous strain. Spontaneous localized motor activity that was seen on electromyography in patients who had chronic midthoracic back pain had an immediate reduction or cessation of spontaneous potentials, indicating that a change in the electromyographic pattern also occurred after osteopathic manipulation that correlated with palpatory changes.[39,40] This may be due to local NO effects.

The piezoelectric transducer model has been proposed to be operating in improved nerve conduction as well as in the functioning of tissue enzymes.[41] According to Bassett, piezoelectric properties are present in many biological systems and may theoretically control cell nutrition, local pH (skin tissue acidosis), enzyme activation and inhibition, orientation of intracellular and extracellular macromolecules, migratory and proliferative activity of cells, contractility and permeability of cell membranes, and energy transfer, including biomechanical deformation and physiological activity.[41,42] In fact, experimental acidosis in skin is due to nonadapting nociceptor excitation in a spatially restricted volume of tissue and appears to be a dominant factor in inflammatory pain.[43,44] Bassett proposed that the crystalline properties of bone and tendons produce electrical potentials when the collagen matrix is deformed (organic constituent). This was also found to be true in dentin and cartilage.[42] Manipulation therefore may be helpful in restoring proper tissue pH and in reducing nociceptor excitation, reducing pain through local NO-mediated events.

Travell trigger points have been implicated to produce somatic dysfunction and to be evoked from abnormal depolarization of motor endplates, producing the presynaptic, synaptic, and postsynaptic mechanisms of abnormal depolarization of acetylcholine, defects of acetylcholinesterase, and up-regulation of postsynaptic nicotinic receptors. When a person is under physical, chemical, or psychological stress, the hyperexcitability evokes trigger points in muscles. Since impaired circulation increases metabolic demands of muscle cells, resulting in an adenosine triphosphate (ATP) crisis, this further triggers presynaptic and postsynaptic decompensation. When circulation is impaired, increased contractile activity ensues; then all the local factors contributing to edema and inflammation are activated.[45]

Cranial Osteopathic Implications

In cranial osteopathy, it is believed that if there are imbalances in the circulation within the skull, neurological (nervous) and endocrine (hormonal) disturbances can follow. The pituitary lies cradled in the sphenoid, and distortions of the sphenoid bone are fairly common. Theoretically, therefore, pituitary dysfunction can result.[46] Many children with birth injuries have been treated successfully using cranial osteopathy. The primary respiratory mechanism, coined by William Sutherland,[47] is related to the fluctuation of the cerebrospinal fluid that occurs within the ventricles of the brain and the cisterns of the subarachnoid space, the meninges, the CNS, the articular mobility of the cranial bones, and the sacrum between the ilia.[48] Radiographic evidence has shown that 96.1% of patients treated using the cranial vault procedure exhibited measurement differences at three or more sites.[49] More recent findings are that cranial manipulation affects the blood flow velocity oscillation in its low-frequency Traube-Hering-Meyer components, believed to be mediated through parasympathetic and sympathetic activity and affecting the autonomic nervous system.[50] Since it is known that the periaqueductal gray region surrounding the cerebral aqueduct is contiguous with the fourth ventricle and rich with cannabinoid receptors that are activated by hydrostatic pressure, theoretically, a CV-4 (compression of the fourth ventricle) treatment can activate these receptors in the limbic system and cerebral cortex, causing cannabimimetic effects and resulting in an effective relaxation response.[38]

Pain Behavior and Allostasis

Frank Willard, a neuroanatomist, states that allostasis and its unhealthy effects on the body can lead to inflammatory and degenerative injury of the body and mind. He believes that somatic dysfunction activates related spinal cord circuits and releases humoral factors summating at the level of the brainstem and that these factors initiate general arousal and associated protective endocrine and neural reflexes, known as "sickness behavior."[27,30,51]

Willard concludes that the osteopathic approach to patient care is aimed at helping the patient restore a more natural homeostatic condition. Long-term allostasis has been correlated with increased sympathetic tone in the body that affects the cardiovascular system, hypertension, chronic pain, and insulin resistance. Any of these long-term effects can lead to other devastating diseases or mortality. Memory loss and depression are two manifestations of the effect of allostasis on the central nervous system. Long-term elevated levels of cortisol have been associated with significant damage to the hippocampal formation from dysregulation of the corticotropin-releasing hormone feedback control from the hippocampus to the hypothalamus. This also affects the renal and gastrointestinal systems, leading to increased water retention, sodium retention, hypervolemia, hypertension, and increased gastrointestinal and skin delayed-type hypersensitivity. Many inflammatory, neoplastic, and degenerative disease processes that we accept as common aging phenomena may be the result of accelerated compensation of dysregulated homeostatic processes.[31] The impact of psychoneuroimmunology on osteopathic medicine and primary care is, therefore, huge.

Application to Primary Care and Osteopathic Manipulative Medicine

From the perspective of psychoneuroimmunology, the body and mind are inseparably connected through the emotions via the peptide ligand network. In reality, this system is holographic and protective in its response to outside stimuli. More important, when the communication system breaks down on any level, the system becomes dysregulated and sets the course for disease and/or pain to occur and be maintained. As might be expected, chronic stress can contribute to this, as can emotional states (depression, anxiety, worry, hostility, fear) and diseases and disorders (e.g., cancer, diabetes, hypertension, asthma, sinusitis, allergies, dermatitis, irritable bowel syndrome).

The concepts of psychoneuroimmunology have application and profound implications for the primary care physician confronting disease prevention and health maintenance. Since the neuromuscular system is closely linked to the CNS and therefore the PNI pathways inherent in the body, many of the disorders and diseases presented by patients to the primary care doctor have a PNI component. In fact, when a person gets sick, the related feelings, or "sickness behavior' (fever,[27] fatigue, malaise, loss of interest in usual things, social isolation, loss of appetite, and altered sleep), are associated with an increase in proinflammatory cytokines similar to depression (IL-1, IL-6, and/or tumor necrosis factor). Psychomotor sickness behavior and sleep are related to IL-1; IL-1-beta also influences food intake, body temperature, and pain sensitivity in the hypothalamus and thalamus.[52] Disturbances of memory and cognitive impairment are related to IL-2 and in part to ATNF-alpha. Furthermore, since cytokines and their receptors are ubiquitously distributed in the brain, they have been shown to activate astrocytes and microglia in the CNS to produce even more cytokines locally.[53] Hypersecretion of cytokines has been implicated in schizophrenia and depressive disorders (IL-2, IL-6, respectively).[52]

The effects are far-ranging since lymphatic and neuroendocrine tissues are ubiquitous in the body, and the effects that are produced locally can simultaneously produce effects centrally, via the limbic-amygdala-hippocampus system (the emotional centers of the brain), affecting the whole body. These tissues also are in direct communication with the HPA, which is activated when stress and emotional responses influence the level of corticosteroid hormones released. In turn, these hormones modulate the immune cell function through an inflammatory response. Also, a hypothalamic-pituitary-gonadal feedback loop is regulated by thymosins.[54] Initially, acute stress up-regulates the immune system, increasing natural killer cells; however, chronic inescapable stress produces an opioid-like state that eventually down-regulates the immune system toward disease.[55] It is the HPA and locus coeruleus–norepinephrine axes together that constitute the major stress system of the body, providing the quick release of cortisol and norepinephrine into the system.

Somatic dysfunction relays an excitatory drive on the locus caeruleus–norepinephrine and HPA axes of the midbrain and hypothalamus. The release of cytokines from inflammatory tissues stimulates the HPA through humoral routes. The first phase is mediated by the peripheral nervous system (less than 1 hour), and the second phase develops more slowly (more than 3 hours), paralleling the rise of the inflammatory event. Overall, this sequence of events sets up the potential for cumulative catecholamine stress to continue the sympathetic nervous system–HPA coupling, leading to a long-term allostatic load and eventually damaging end organs. Immunosuppression and this loss of feedback autoregulatory control result in organ systems damaging one another.[30]

In the context of family practice, this implies that any treatment done medically and osteopathically can directly influence the PNI state of the body. The three aims of OMT are restoration to normal of the supporting tissues (bone, muscle, ligament, and fascia), normalization of movement and articulation, and normalization of the reflexes and/or the mechanical influences on the body as a whole.[46] Additionally, the aim is for the neurological integration, including central, peripheral, autonomic, neuroendocrine, neurocirculatory, and somatic elements, to be integrated with general patient care.[56] Any form of hands-on therapy, such as OMT, therefore, can improve local blood flow while reducing pain signals to the spinal cord and mitigating the concurrent effects on pain behavior. Cutaneous vascular changes in the region of the segmental spinal disorder have been demonstrated,[57] and the relationship of blood supply to the level of an organ function is important. There has been speculation that vital organ system function may be influenced by spinal segmental disorders, as seen in the facilitated segment. It has been shown that under conditions of strong emotion, organs innervated from levels of skeletal disturbance in areas with already altered autonomic outflow are especially vulnerable to facilitation-induced changes in vascular supply. Any attention given to correcting somatic dysfunction therefore may benefit the patient both in the local dysfunctional area and for general body reactions by reducing excessive cerebral excitation.[58] Additionally, OMT has been shown to provide immune enhancement.[7]

OMT can effect a change by stimulating the cannabinoid receptors peripherally at nociceptor sites and in the dorsal horn, down-regulating proinflammatory changes and central sensitization through the retrograde signaling of NO-induced anandamide postsynaptically. This retrograde signal acts on the cannabinoid receptors presynaptically by closing the excitatory calcium channels and stopping the release of substance P and glutamate, restoring axoplasmic flow to the receptors.[38] The reduction of somatic dysfunction using OMT could theoretically restore homeostatic mechanisms by disrupting the pain feedback loops that are locally and centrally mediated.

One of the known barriers—or shall we say challenges—facing family practice residents today is the lack of time available to perform manipulation. Time for OMT is further reduced in a managed care setting. Thus, very few osteopathic physicians use OMT in their daily practice once they graduate from osteopathic medical internships or residencies,[59-63] even though many of these physicians regarded holistic medicine as being the most distinguishing characteristic of their profession.[62] Many believe that OMT is efficacious and that the osteopathic approach to treatment is a primary distinguishing feature of their profession, incorporating, as it does, a caring doctor–patient relationship and a hands-on style of caring in the practice of medicine.[64] A recent study showed that family physicians were more apt to use HVLA thrust, or lymphatic or muscle energy procedures than non–primary care specialists and OMT specialists.[65] A focused treatment plan can provide an immediate option in regard to using OMT in a busy practice setting. Also, since some patients seeing osteopathic physicians for specialized OMT care may have poorer quality of life than the general population, early detection and treatment of musculoskeletal conditions may be important factors in preventing chronicity and its interference with one's quality of life.[66]

Conditions in the osteopathic literature that have shown positive responses on use of manipulative procedures include the following:

- Acute otitis media[67]
- Cardiac disease, coronary heart disease[68,69]
- Chronic tension headache[70] and neck pain, migraines,[71-77] cervical compressive myelopathy with herniated disc,[78] intraocular pressure[79]
- Fibromyalgia,[80] rheumatic disease[81,82]
- Sinusitis[83,84]
- Upper and low back pain[5,58,85-95]
- Shoulder pain[96,97]
- Upper respiratory conditions: acute respiratory failure,[98] asthma,[99,100] colds,[101] pneumonia[102-105]
- Temporomandibular joint dysfunction,[106] malocclusion[107]
- Cerebral palsy,[108] multiple sclerosis,[109] idiopathic parkinsonism[110,111]
- Mild osteoarthritic pain, thoracic outlet syndrome[112]
- Scoliosis[113]
- Post surgery,[114] post pulmonary resection,[115] post knee and hip arthroplasty[116,117]
- Carpel tunnel,[111,118] lateral epicondylitis,[119] bursitis, Achilles tendonitis, plantar fasciitis[120]
- Prenatal care,[121] birth trauma[48,122]
- Chronic musculoskeletal pain[4,5,95]
- Hospitalization,[3] traumatic brain injury[123]
- Hypertension[124,125]

Other effective manipulative therapies include myofascial release, positional release, soft tissue deep articulation, cranial, counterstrain, torque unwinding, and muscle energy procedures. HVLA of the cervical spine, however, has fostered controversy and is contraindicated in cases of severe osteoporosis under any condition. There have been reports in the literature of iatrogenic cervical fractures[126] and of vertebral basilar artery and carotid artery dissection involving chiropractic,[127-132] less so with physical therapy,[133] and rarely OMT.[134] Currently the American Academy of Osteopathy recommends that information regarding the risks be provided to trainees and that all physicians continue to offer this form of treatment along with other modalities to treat the cervical spine.[135] Soft tissue myofascial release includes various procedures: effleurage, pétrissage, friction, and tapotement. Manipulative procedures have been shown to improve flexibility, decrease the perception of pain, and decrease the levels of stress hormones.[136]

Since 60% of the body is bone, tendon, and ligaments, with 206 bones in the human structure, it is important for wellness therapies[46] to consider treating the musculoskeletal system. Poor postural mechanics, strain, repetitive stress, and injuries can benefit from OMT procedures, since any structural or mechanical abnormality can affect the body's natural homeostasis. The relationship between structure and function not only is relevant to the treatment of disease; it provides a framework in which the body may begin the process of resuming its natural order.

For example, in asthma, a focused treatment plan for manipulation would include using the lymphatic pump procedure to stimulate the immune system to reduce inflammation and would also include using any appropriate form of manipulation to treat the corresponding viscerosomatic dysfunctions found in the upper thoracic and cervical areas. In low back pain, the standard of care necessitates a focused treatment plan that includes treatment of the lumbosacral region with manipulation.[94] It is also important to administer the initial manipulation in conjunction with an exercise program for the first 2 weeks of treatment. A patient home care and treatment plan at a frequency of up to two to three times a week may incorporate an active exercise program during the first month as part of a strengthening program. Clear-cut therapeutic goals should be established at the onset of treatment. Lack of improvement after three to four treatment sessions should result in a discontinuation of the current treatment plan and a reassessment of the problem.[95]

Other adjunctive care that contributes to relaxing the patient, that provides support in bringing the body back into homeostasis and balance, and that has been advocated and used with success in primary care includes massage, acupuncture, mindfulness meditation, guided imagery, relaxation training, low-frequency pulsed electromagnetic field, essential oils, and herbal remedies.[137-144] Therefore, comprehensive holistic care aimed at addressing the cause of disease, combined with individually tailored treatment and preventative measures, examining the environmental, social, mental and behavioral aspects of disease, is paramount for understanding how PNI and OMT are related. Additionally, any positive action, such as treating a somatic dysfunction that results in a change in the psychoneuroimmunologic milieu of the mind and brings about an effective change in outcomes warrants further consideration by the family practice physician.

References

1. Still AT. The Philosophy and Mechanical Principles of Osteopathy. Kirksville, MO: American School of Osteopathy, 1892.
2. Trilling JS. Selections from current literature. Psychoneuroimmunology: validation of the biopsychosocial model. Fam Pract 2000;17:90–93.
3. Shubrook JH, Dooley J. Effects of a structured curriculum in osteopathic manipulative treatment (OMT) on osteopathic structural examinations and use of OMT for hospitalized patients. J Am Osteopath Assoc 2000;100:554–558.
4. Giles LG, Muller R. Chronic spinal pain: A randomized clinical trial comparing medication, acupuncture, and spinal manipulation. Spine 2003;28:1490–1502; discussion 1502–1503.

5. Andersson GB, Lucente T, Davis AM, et al. A comparison of osteopathic spinal manipulation standard care for patients with low back pain. N Engl J Med 1999;341:1426–1431.

6. Assendelft WJ, Morton SC, Yu EI, et al. Spinal manipulative therapy for low back pain. A meta-analysis of effectiveness relative to other therapies. Ann Intern Med 2003;138: 871–881.

7. Lesho EP. An overview of osteopathic medicine. Arch Fam Med 1999;8:477–484.

8. Still AT. American manual therapy. In: The Autobiography of A. T. Still. Kirksville, MO: Author, 1908.

9. Hoover HV. Selected osteopathic papers: Place of psychosomatics in osteopathy. In: Northup TL. Academy of Applied Osteopathy 1950 Yearbook. Morristown, NJ: American Osteopathic Association, 1950:85–86. (Now available through the American Academy of Osteopathy, Indianapolis.)

10. Prolo P, Chiappelli F, Fiorucci A, et al. Psychoneuroimmunology. New avenues of research for the twenty-first century. Ann NY Acad Sci 2002;966:400–408.

11. Pert CB, Dreher HE, Ruff MR. The psychosomatic network: Foundations of mind-body medicine. Altern Ther Health Med 1998;4:30–41.

12. Pert CB. The wisdom of the receptors: Neuropeptides, the emotions, and bodymind. Advances 1986;3(3):8–16.

13. Ader R, Cohen N. Behaviorally conditioned immunosuppression. Psychosom Med 1975; 37:333–340.

14. Pert CB, Snyder SH. Opiate receptor: Demonstration in nervous tissue. Science 1973;179:1011–1014.

15. Pert CB, Pasternak G, Snyder SH. Opiate agonists and antagonists discriminated by receptor binding to brain. Science 1973;182:1359–1361.

16. Pert CB, Ruff MR, Weber RJ, Herkenham M. Neuropeptides and their receptors: A psychosomatic network. J Immunol 1985;135(2 suppl):820S–826S.

17. Schmitt FO. Molecular regulation of brain function: A new view. Neuroscience 1984; 13:991–1001.

18. Pert CB. Molecules of Emotion: Why You Feel the Way You Feel. London: Simon & Schuster, 1997;143.

19. Polianova MT, Ruscetti FW, Pert CB, et al. Antiviral and immunological benefits in HIV patients receiving intranasal peptide T (DAPTA). Peptides 2003;24:1093–1098.

20. Pert CB, Hill JM, Ruff MR, et al. Apeptides deduced from the neuropeptide receptor-like pattern of antigen T4 in brain potently inhibit human immunodeficiency virus receptor binding and T-cell infectivity. Proc Natl Acad Sci USA 1986;83:9254–9258.

21. Redwine LS, Pert CB, Rone JD, et al. Peptide T blocks GP120/CCR5 chemokine receptor-mediated chemotaxis. Clin Immunol 1999;93:124–131.

22. Heseltine PN, Goodkin K, Atkinson JH, et al. Randomized double-blind placebo-controlled trial of peptide T in HIV-associated cognitive impairment. Arch Neurol 1998;55:41–51.

23. Roth J, Leroith DL, Collier ES, et al. Evolutionary origins of neuropeptides, hormones and receptors: Possible applications to immunology. J Immunol 1985;13(2 suppl):816S–819S.

24. Smith EM, Blalock JE. Human lymphocyte production of corticotropin and endorphin-like substances: Association with leukocyte interferon. Proc Natl Acad Sci USA 1981; 78:7530–7534.

25. Blalock JE. A molecular basis for bidirectional communication between the immune and neuroendocrine systems. Physiol Rev 1989;69:1–32.

26. Blalock JE. The syntax of immune-neuroendocrine communication. Immunol Today 1994; 15:504–511.

27. Fleshner M, Laudenslager ML. Psychoneuroimmunology: Then and now. Behav Cogn Neurosci Rev 2004;3:114–130.

28. Wiedermann CJ, Sertl K, Pert CB. Substance P receptors in rat spleen: Characterization and autoradiographic distribution. Blood 1986;68:1398–1401.

29. Wiedermann CJ, Sertl K, Zipser B, et al. Vasoactive intestinal peptide receptors in rat spleen and brain: Shared communication network. Peptides 1988;9(suppl 1):21–28.

30. Willard FH. Nociception, the neuroendocrine immune system, and osteopathic medicine. In: Ward RC, ed. Foundations for Osteopathic Medicine. Philadelphia: Lippincott Williams & Wilkins, 2002:137–156.

31. Salamon E, Zhu W, Stefano GB. Nitric oxide as a possible mechanism for understanding the therapeutic effects of osteopathic manipulative medicine. Int J Mol Med 2004;14(3): 443–449 [review].

32. Stefano GB, Ottaviani E. The biochemical substrate of nitric oxide signaling is present in primitive non-cognitive organisms. Brain Res 2002;924:82–89.

33. Stefano GB, Goumon Y, Bilfinger TV, et al. Basal nitric oxide limits immune, nervous and cardiovascular excitation: Human endothelia express a mu opiate receptor. Prog Neurobiol 2000;60:13–30.

34. Bilfinger TV, Vosswinkel JA, Cadet P, et al. Direct assessment and diminished production of morphine stimulated NO by diabetic endothelium from saphenous vein. Acta Pharmacol Sin 2002;23:97–102.

35. Stefano GB, Bilfinger TV, Rialas CM, Deutsch DG. 2-Arachidonyl-glycerol stimulates nitric oxide release from human immune and vascular tissues and invertebrate immunocytes by cannabinoid receptor 1. Pharmacol Res 2000;42:317–322.

36. Roth MD. Pharmacology: Marijuana and your heart. Nature 2005;434:708–709.

37. Mbvundula EC, Bunning RA, Rainsford KD. Effects of cannabinoids on nitric oxide production by chondrocytes and proteoglycan degradation in cartilage. Biochem Pharmacol 2005;69:635–640.

38. McPartland JM. The endocannabinoid system and OMT. Lecture notes. American Academy of Osteopathy New Ideas Forum. Colorado Springs, CO, March 19, 2005.

39. Deibert PW, England RW. Crystallographic study: Thermal changes and the osteopathic lesion. J Am Osteopath Assoc 1972;72:223–226.

40. England RW, Deibert PW. Electromyographic studies: Part I. Consideration in the evaluation of osteopathic therapy. J Am Osteopath Assoc 1972;72:221–223.

41. Boguslaw L. Biological significance of piezoelectricity in relation to acupuncture, hatha yoga, osteopathic medicine and actions of air ions. Med Hypotheses 1977;3:9–12.

42. Bassett CA. Biological significance of piezoelectricity. Calcif Tissue Res 1968;1:252–272.

43. Steen KH, Issberner U, Reeh PW. Pain due to experimental acidosis in human skin: Evidence for non-adapting nociceptor excitation. Neurosci Lett 1995;199:29–32.

44. Steen KH, Steen AE, Kreysel HW, Reeh PW. Inflammatory mediators potentiate pain induced by experimental tissue acidosis. Pain 1996;66:163–170.

45. McPartland JM. Travell trigger points: molecular and osteopathic perspectives. J Am Osteopath Assoc 2004;104:244–249.

46. Chaitow L. Osteopathy: Head-to-Toe Health Through Manipulation. Wellingborough, UK: Thorsons, 1974;23, 72.

47. Sutherland WG. The Cranial Bowl. Mankato, MN: Free Press, 1939.

48. Kimberly PE. Osteopathic cranial lesions. J Am Osteopath Assoc 1948;47:261–263.

49. Oleski SL, Smith GH, Crow WT. Radiographic evidence of cranial bone mobility. Cranio 2002;20(1):34–38.

50. Sergueef N, Nelson KE, Glonek T. The effect of cranial manipulation on the Traube-Hering-Mayer oscillation as measured by laser-Doppler flowmetry. Altern Ther Health Med 2002; 8(6):74–76.

51. Hart BL. Biological basis of the behavior of sick animals. Neuroscience Biobehav Rev 1988;12:123–137.

52. Muller N, Ackenheil M. Psychoneuroimmunology and the cytokine action in the CNS: Implications for psychiatric disorders. Prog Neuropsychopharmacol Bio Psychiatry 1998; 22(1):1–33.

53. Haas HS, Schauenstein K. Neuroimmunomodulation via limbic structures: The neuroanatomy of psychoimmunology. Prog Neurobiol 1997;51:195–222.

54. Wiedermann CJ. Shared recognition molecules in the brain and lymphoid tissues: The polypeptide mediator network of psychoneuroimmunology. Immunol Lett 1987;16: 371–378.

55. Shavit Y, Depaulis A, Martin FC, et al. Involvement of brain opiate receptors in the immune-suppressive effect of morphine. Proc Natl Acad Sci USA 1986;83:7114–7117.

56. Seffinger, MA, King HH, Ward RC, et al. Section 1. Osteopathic philosophy and history. In: Ward RC, ed. Foundations for Osteopathic Medicine. Philadelphia: Lippincott Williams & Wilkins, 2002;4–18.

57. Korr IM, Thomas PE, Wright HM. Symposium on the functional implications of segmental facilitation. J Am Osteopath Assoc 1955;54:265–268.
58. Bradford SG. Role of osteopathic manipulative therapy in emotional disorders: A physiologic hypothesis. J Am Osteopath Assoc 1965;64:484–493.
59. Gamber RG, Gish EE, Herron KM. Student perceptions of osteopathic manipulative treatment after completing a manipulative medicine rotation. J Am Osteopath Assoc 2001; 101:395–400.
60. Fry LJ. Preliminary findings on the use of osteopathic manipulative treatment by osteopathic physicians. J Am Osteopath Assoc 1996;96:91–96.
61. Johnson SM, Kurtz ME, Kurtz JC. Variables influencing the use of osteopathic manipulative treatment in family practice. J Am Osteopath Assoc 1997;97:80–87.
62. Johnson SM, Kurtz ME. Diminished use of osteopathic manipulative treatment and its impact on the uniqueness of the osteopathic profession. Acad Med 2001;76:821–828.
63. Mann DD, Eland DC, Patriquin DA, Johnson DF. Increasing osteopathic manipulative treatment skills and confidence through mastery learning. J Am Osteopath Assoc 2000;100: 301–304, 309.
64. Johnson SM, Kurtz ME. Perceptions of philosophic and practice differences between US osteopathic physicians and their allopathic counterparts. Soc Sci Med 2002;55(12): 2141–2148.
65. Johnson SM, Kurtz ME. Osteopathic manipulative treatment techniques preferred by contemporary osteopathic physicians. J Am Osteopath Assoc 2003;103:219–224.
66. Licciardone JC, Gamber RG, Russo DP. Quality of life in referred patients presenting to a specialty clinic for osteopathic manipulative treatment. J Am Osteopath Assoc 2002;102:151–155.
67. Zaphiris A, Mills MV, Jewell NP, Boyce WT. Osteopathic manipulative treatment and otitis media: Does improving somatic dysfunction improve clinical outcome? J Am Osteopath Assoc 2004;104:11–EOA.
68. Johnson FE. Some observations on the use of osteopathic therapy in the care of patients with cardiac disease. J Am Osteopath Assoc 1972;71:799–804.
69. Rogers JT, Rogers JC. The role of osteopathic manipulative therapy in the treatment of coronary heart disease. J Am Osteopath Assoc 1976;76:21–31.
70. Bronfort G, Assendelft WJ, Evans R, et al. Efficacy of spinal manipulation for chronic headache: A systematic review. J Manipulative Physiol Ther 2001;24:457–466.
71. Sloop PR, Smith DS, Goldenberg E, Dore C. Manipulation for chronic neck pain: A double-blind controlled study. Spine 1982;7:532–535.
72. Bronfort G, Evans R, Nelson B, et al. A randomized clinical trial of exercise and spinal manipulation for patients with chronic neck pain. Spine 2001;26:788–797; discussion 798–799.
73. Swenson RS. Therapeutic modalities in the management of nonspecific neck pain. Phys Med Rehabil Clin North Am 2003;14:605–627.
74. Boyce RH, Wang JC. Evaluation of neck pain, radiculopathy, and myelopathy: Imaging, conservative treatment, and surgical indications. Instr Course Lect 2003;52:489–495.
75. Hardin J Jr. Pain and the cervical spine. Bull Rheum Dis 2001;50(10):1–4.
76. Kriss TC, Kriss VM. Neck pain: Primary care work-up of acute and chronic symptoms. Geriatrics 2000;55(1):47–48, 51–54, 57.
77. Cassidy JD, Lopes AA, Yong-Hing K. The immediate effect of manipulation vs. mobilization on pain and range of motion in the cervical spine: A randomized controlled trial. J Manip Physiol Ther 1992;15:570–575.
78. Browder DA, Erhard RE, Piva SR. Intermittent cervical traction and thoracic manipulation for management of mild cervical compressive myelopathy attribute to cervical herniated disc: A case series. J Orthop Sports Phys Ther 2004;34:701–712.
79. Iwata JL, Multack RF, Kappler R, Glonek T. Effectiveness of using osteopathic manipulation in treating ocular tension headache patients in an ambulatory setting with corresponding reduction in intraocular pressure. J Osteopath Coll Ophthalm Otolaryngol 2000;12:15–19.
80. Gamber RG, Shores JH, Russo DP, et al. Osteopathic manipulative treatment in conjunction with medication relieves pain associated with fibromyalgia syndrome: Results of a randomized clinical pilot project. J Am Osteopath Assoc 2002;102:321–325.

81. Fiechtner JJ, Brodeur RR. Manual and manipulation techniques for rheumatic disease. Rheum Dis Clin North Am 2000;26(1):83–96, ix.

82. Ernst E. Complementary and alternative medicine in rheumatology. Baillieres Best Pract Res Clin Rheumatol 2000;14:731–749.

83. Dudley G. Sinusitis: Supplement missing osteopathic component. J Am Osteopath Assoc 1998;98:539–540.

84. Hopp RJ. Revisiting the role of osteopathic manipulation in primary care. J Am Osteopath Assoc 1999;99:88.

85. Lee H, Nicholson LL, Adams RD. Cervical range of motion associations with subclinical neck pain. Spine 2004;29:33–40.

86. Coughlin P, Kriebel R, Fogel R. New England Journal of Medicine article may be misleading about OMT. J Am Osteopath Assoc 1999;99:561–565.

87. Jermyn RT. A nonsurgical approach to low back pain. J Am Osteopath Assoc 2001; 101(4 suppl pt 2):S6–S11.

88. Bronfort G, Haas M, Evans RL, Bouter LM. Efficacy of spinal manipulation and mobilization for low back pain and neck pain: A systematic review and best evidence synthesis. Spine 2004;4:335–356.

89. Danto JB. Review of integrated neuromuscular release and the novel application of a segmental anterior/posterior approach in the thoracic, lumbar, and sacral regions. J Am Osteopath Assoc 2003;103:583–596.

90. Raftis KL, Warfield CA. Spinal manipulation for back pain. Hosp Pract (Off Ed) 1989;24(3): 89–90, 95–96, 102 passim.

91. Abend DS. Osteopathic manipulation for low back pain. Postgrad Med 1997;101:56, 58.

92. Connelly C. Patients with low back pain: How to identify the few who need extra attention. Postgrad Med 1996;100:143–146, 149, 150, 155–156.

93. Williams NH, Wilkinson C, Russell I, et al. Randomized osteopathic manipulation study (ROMANS): Pragmatic trial for spinal pain in primary care. Fam Pract 2003;20: 662–669.

94. Evidence-Based Medicine Guidelines. Cochrane Back Review Resources. Helsinki: Duodecim Medical, 2005.

95. Mior S. Manipulation and mobilization in the treatment of chronic pain. Clin J Pain 2001;17(4 suppl): S70–S76.

96. Knebl JA, Shores JH, Gamber RG, et al. Improving functional ability in the elderly via the Spencer technique, an osteopathic manipulative treatment: A randomized controlled trial. J Am Osteopath Assoc 2002;102:387–396.

97. Jacobson EC, Lockwood MD, Hoefner VC Jr, et al. Shoulder pain and repetition strain injury to the supraspinatus muscle: Etiology and manipulative treatment. J Am Osteopath Assoc 1989;89:1037–1040, 1043–1045.

98. Stretfanski MF, Kaiser G. Osteopathic philosophy and emergent treatment in acute respiratory failure. J Am Osteopath Aug 2001;101:447–449.

99. Bockenhauer SE, Julliard KN, Lo KS, et al. Quantifiable effects of osteopathic manipulative techniques on patients with chronic asthma. J Am Osteopath Assoc 2002;102:371–375.

100. Rowane WA, Rowane MP. An osteopathic approach to asthma. J Am Osteopath Assoc 1999;99:259–264.

101. Magoun HI. More about the use of OMT during influenza epidemics. J Am Osteopath Assoc 2004;104:406–407.

102. Northrup TL. Pneumonia under osteopathic manipulative therapy. In: Northrup TL, ed. Academy of Applied Osteopathy 1945 Yearbook. Manipulative Therapy Demonstrations. Ann Arbor, MI: Edwards Brothers, 1945:101–105. (Now available through the American Academy of Osteopathy, Indianapolis.)

103. Noll DR, Shores J, Gamber RG, et al. Benefits of osteopathic manipulative treatment for hospitalized elderly patients with pneumonia. J Am Osteopath Assoc 2000;100:776–782.

104. Facto LL. The osteopathic treatment of lobar pneumonia. J Am Osteopath Assoc 1947;46:385–392.

105. Chila AG. Pneumonia: Helping our bodies help themselves. Consultant 1982:174–188.

106. Knutson GA, Jacob M. Possible manifestation of temporomandibular joint dysfunction chiropractic cervical X-ray studies. J Manip Physiol Ther 1999;22:32–37.

107. Jecmen JM. A cranial osteopathic approach to correcting malocclusions employing Kernott and fixed labial appliance therapy. J Am Acad Gnathol Orthop 1988;5(1):10–15, 17.

108. Duncan B, Barton L, Edmonds D, Blashill BM. Parental perceptions of the therapeutic effect from osteopathic manipulation or acupuncture in children with spastic cerebral palsy. Clin Pediatr (Phila) 2004;43:349–353.

109. Yates HA, Vardy TC, Kuchera ML, et al. Effects of osteopathic manipulative treatment and concentric and eccentric maximal-effort exercise on women with multiple sclerosis: A pilot study. J Am Osteopath Assoc 2002;102:267–275.

110. Rivera-Martinez S, Wells MR, Capobianco JD. A retrospective study of cranial strain patterns in patients with idiopathic Parkinson's disease. J Am Osteopath Assoc 2002;102: 417–422.

111. Wells MR, Giantinoto S, D'Agate D, et al. Standard osteopathic manipulative treatment acutely improves gait performance in patients with Parkinson's disease. J Am Osteopath Assoc 1999;99:92–98.

112. Sucher BM. Palpatory diagnosis and manipulative management of carpal tunnel syndrome: II. "Double crush" and thoracic outlet syndrome. J Am Osteopath Assoc 1995;95:471–479.

113. College of Osteopathic Physicians and Surgeons. Handbook of Osteopathic Technique. Los Angeles: Haynes Printers, 1941:96–101.

114. Nicholas AS, Oleski SL. Osteopathic manipulative treatment for postoperative pain. J Am Osteopath Assoc 2002;102(9 suppl 3):S5–S8.

115. Hirayama F, Kageyama Y, Urabe N, Senjyu H. The effects of postoperative ataralgesia by manual therapy after pulmonary resection. Man Ther 2003;8(1):42–45.

116. Licciardone JC, Stoll ST, Cardarelli KM, et al. A randomized controlled trial of osteopathic manipulative treatment following knee or hip arthroplasty. J Am Osteopath Assoc 2004;104:193–202.

117. Millett PJ, Johnson B, Carlson J, et al. Rehabilitation of the arthrofibrotic knee. Am J Orthop 2003;32:531–538.

118. Sucher BM, Hinrichs RN. Manipulative treatment of carpal tunnel syndrome: Biomechanical and osteopathic intervention to increase the length of the transverse carpal ligament. J Am Osteopath Assoc 1998;98:679–686.

119. Struijs PA, Damen PJ, Bakker EW, et al. Manipulation of the wrist for the management of lateral epicondylitis: A randomized pilot study. Phys Ther 2003;83:608–616.

120. Huang HH, Qureshi AA, Biundo JJ Jr. Sports and other soft tissue injuries, tendinitis, bursitis, and occupation-related syndromes. Curr Opin Rheumatol 2000;12:150–154.

121. King HH, Tettambel MA, Lockwood MD, et al. Osteopathic manipulative treatment in prenatal care: A retrospective case control design study. J Am Osteopath Assoc 2003;103: 577–582.

122. Turney J. Tackling birth trauma with cranio-sacral therapy. Pract Midwife 2002;5(3):17–19.

123. Greenman PE, McPartland JM. Cranial findings and iatrogenesis from craniosacral manipulation in patients with traumatic brain syndrome. J Am Osteopath Assoc 1995;95:182–188, 191–192.

124. Morgan JP, Dickey JL, Hunt HH, Hudgins PM. A controlled trial of spinal manipulation in the management of hypertension. J Am Osteopath Assoc 1985;85:308–313.

125. Spiegel AJ, Capobianco JD, Kruger A, Spinner WD. Osteopathic manipulative medicine in the treatment of hypertension: An alternative, conventional approach. Heart Dis 2003;5:272–278.

126. Ea HK, Weber AJ, Yon F, Liote F. Osteoporotic fracture of the dens revealed by cervical manipulation. Joint Bone Spine 2004;71:246–250.

127. Parenti G, Orlandi G, Bianchi M, et al. Vertebral and carotid artery dissection following chiropractic cervical manipulation. Neurosurg Rev 1999;22(2-3):127–129.

128. Hurwitz EL, Morgenstern H, Vassilaki M, Chiang LM. Adverse reactions to chiropractic treatment and their effects on satisfaction and clinical outcomes among patients enrolled in the UCLA Neck Pain Study. J Manipulative Physiol Ther 2004;27(1):16–25.

129. Haldeman S, Kohlbeck FJ, McGregor M. Stroke, cerebral artery dissection, and cervical spine manipulative therapy. J Neurol 2002;249:1098–1104.

130. Cote P, Cassidy JD, Haldeman S. Spinal manipulative therapy is an independent risk factor for vertebral artery dissection. Neurology 2003;61:1314–1315.

131. Haldeman S, Carey P, Townsend M, Papadopoulou C. Clinical perceptions of the risk of vertebral artery dissection after cervical manipulation: the effect of referral bias. Spine 2002;2:334–342.

132. Haldeman S, Carey P, Townsend M, Papadopoulou C. Arterial dissections following cervical manipulation: the chiropractic experience. CMAJ 2001;165:905–906.

133. Di Fabio RP. Manipulation of the cervical spine: Risks and benefits. Phys Ther 1999;79:50–65.

134. Vick DA, McKay C, Zengerle CR. The safety of manipulative treatment: Review of the literature from 1925 to 1993. J Am Osteopath Assoc 1996;96:113–115.

135. AOA Position Papers. American Osteopathic Association House of Delegates Meeting. Chicago: American Osteopathic Association, August 2004.

136. Nadler SF. Nonpharmacologic management of pain. J Am Osteopath Assoc 2004;104(11 suppl 8):S6–S12.

137. Furlan AD, Brosseau L, Imamura M, Irvin E. Evidence-based medicine guidelines: Massage for low back pain. Cochrane Database Syst Rev 2004;(2):CD1929.

138. Astin JA. Mind-body therapies for the management of pain. Clin J Pain 2004;20:27–32.

139. Sherman KJ, Cherkin DC, Connelly MT, et al. Complementary and alternative medical therapies for chronic low back pain: What treatments are patients willing to try? BMC Complement Altern Med 2004;4(1):9–16.

140. Astin JA, Shapiro SL, Eisenberg DM, Forys KL. Mind-body medicine: State of the science, implications for practice. J Am Board Fam Pract 2003;16:131–147.

141. Lazar JS. Mind-body medicine in primary care: Implications and applications. Prim Care 1996;23:169–182.

142. Jacobs GD. Clinical application of the relaxation response and mind-body interventions. J Altern Complement Med 2001;7(suppl 1):S93–S101.

143. Bassett CAL. Bioelectromagnetics in the service of medicine. In: Blank M, ed. Electromagnetic Fields: Biological Interactions and Mechanisms. Advances in Chemistry Series No 250. Washington: American Chemical Society, 1995;261–277.

144. Price S, Price L. Aromatherapy for Health Professionals. 2nd ed. London: Harcourt, 2000.

Patient Populations

CHAPTER 7

The Psychiatric Patient

Andrew Lovy

INTRODUCTION

The fundamentals of osteopathic medicine are applicable not only to the practice of family medicine but also to the diagnosis and treatment of the psychiatric patient. Since its inception osteopathic medicine has approached the patient as an indivisible unit. This concept goes beyond a holistic approach to the body to include the mind and spirit as the triune nature of humanity.[1] Thus, mental function and dysfunction have always been part of the osteopathic approach to patient care. J. Martin Littlejohn, an early student of osteopathic medicine, founder of the Chicago College of Osteopathic Medicine, and later of the British School of Osteopathy in England, summarized this holism in his description of psychiatry as follows:

"Mind, however, is not in the brain, but in the body. In the psychology of the mind the entire nervous system is included, and this includes, in addition to the nervous system proper, the entire terminal system, that is, muscle, mucous membrane, etc. To understand the mind and the mental diseases, we must have (a) a knowledge of the structure, functions and relations of every part of the body to the nervous system, and (b) the clinical facts brought out by those cases in which the mind is in an abnormal state. Hence our knowledge of the mind is based on anatomy, physiology, psychology and psychopathology."[2]

Because of this approach there has always been the possibility of considering the impact of somatic dysfunction and its effective treatment upon mental health.[3] Throughout the first half of the twentieth century, the Still-Hildreth Sanatorium, an osteopathic institution in Macon, Missouri, was dedicated exclusively to the study and treatment of mental and nervous diseases.[4-7] Attempts to correlate specific manifestations of somatic dysfunction with various forms of mental illness met with only limited success.[6-8] Anecdotal reports describe efficacy with the use of osteopathic manipulative treatment (OMT) in the treatment of schizophrenia, but there are insufficient substantial data to verify this statistically.[4-6,9] Recently, however, a small pilot study (treatment N = 8; control N = 9) has statistically demonstrated positive effects for hospitalized depressed patients treated with OMT.[10]

Whether or not one wishes to accept Littlejohn's global interpretation of the mind, the presence of the nervous system throughout the body and recent information supporting the concepts of psychoneuroimmunology (see Chapter 6) make a holistic understanding of physical and mental wellbeing readily appreciable.[11] Thus, the interaction between dysfunction in the periphery and the neural and endocrine effects of the central nervous system on the periphery makes the reduction of peripheral nociception with OMT a potentially viable contribution to psychotherapeutics.

CONTEMPORARY PRACTICE

The family physician is by definition a primary health care provider and as such assumes responsibility for all manner of patients. It has been estimated that as many as 50% of all primary care visits involve chief complaints with strong psychologic undercurrents.[12] Patients with obvious psychiatric problems are, however, in a minority. All too often the presenting complaint is an elusive physical symptom. Actually, nearly every physical complaint has a psychic component. A list of common physical complaints that may be psychologically motivated or at least linked includes low back pain, chronic pelvic pain, tinnitus, headache, dizziness, atypical chest pain, dyspnea, temporomandibular joint pain, generalized musculoskeletal pain, fatigue, irritable bowel syndrome, hypoglycemia, and multiple chemical sensitivity.[13] Many of these complaints are obviously referable to the musculoskeletal system and consequently are particularly likely to appear before a practitioner who uses OMT. These patients have been said to be somatizing. Thus, these symptoms may appropriately lend consideration to psychiatric diagnoses and the need for treatment. Certain psychiatric diagnoses are more likely than others to involve somatization focused upon the musculoskeletal system. Personality disorders, those of cluster B in the DSM-IV-TR (antisocial, histrionic, narcissistic, and borderline) are likely to somatize. Additionally, affective disorders, including major depressive disorder, dysthymia, and minor depression, can cause somatic complaints, as can the paranoid type of schizophrenia and anxiety disorders, such as panic disorder, generalized anxiety disorder, and obsessive-compulsive disorder.[14,15]

The irony of these situations is that when the somatizing patient with a musculoskeletal or visceral complaint is subjected to a thorough osteopathic structural examination, somatic dysfunction consistent with the complaint is often identified. This is because the patient is not necessarily fabricating the complaint but rather is intensely focused upon it. The association between somatic dysfunction and psychosomatic symptoms has been recognized in the osteopathic literature for decades.[16-18]

The term *psychosomatic* refers to the inseparable interaction between the psyche (mind) and the soma (body). More properly referred to as psychophysiologic disorders, this group of illnesses presents primarily as physical conditions that are affected by emotional factors. They typically involve a single organ system and are usually associated with increased activity of the autonomic nervous system. Symptoms result from physiologic changes that normally accompany certain emotional states, but these changes are more intense and sustained than normal.[14]

It is not difficult to understand the neurophysiology of viscerosomatic and somatovisceral reflexes.[19] (See Chapter 5.) The psychophysiologic relationship is acknowledged, so why should there not be similar psychosomatic and somatopsychologic pathways? The psychosomatic pathway can be explained neurophysiologically by the ability of the segmental facilitation, found in association with spinal somatic dysfunction, to focus descending neurologic impulses from increased cortical activity, as might be found in many psychiatric conditions.[20–22] This produces segmental hypersensitivity to nociceptive stimuli, which in turn results in increased cortical awareness of structures, somatic and/or visceral, innervated by the facilitated segment.[21] It also explains how emotional distress, acting through descending pathways, can be directed by the facilitated segment to result in gastrointestinal hypermotility or bronchospasm, depending upon the anatomic level of the spinal cord facilitated.

A somatopsychologic pathway is equally plausible. It is generally acknowledged that when an individual has discomfort, there is commonly an accompanying psychologic response. Painful discomfort is transmitted to the central nervous system by nociceptive neurons. This results in segmental facilitation, and impulses continue up the spinal cord and through the limbic system, where emotional associations can be made, eventually reaching cortical awareness.

Osteopathic medicine has always considered the integration of psyche and soma, just as it has soma and viscera, as part of its theory and practice. Physicians who incorporate manipulative therapy into their practice will inevitably use the integrative concepts to treat some patients who present with psychopathology. Conversely, they treat many individuals with physical symptoms who have psychologic issues affecting the soma and viscera. In a holistic model, somatic dysfunction and psychologic dysfunction are inseparably linked.

Manipulation has been recommended to reduce stress-related musculoskeletal tension and sympathetic hyperactivity found in association with a multiplicity of psychiatric illnesses, including schizophrenia,[5,17] depression,[10] anxiety,[17,23,24] and somatoform disorders.[16–18,23,24] OMT has been recommended as an appropriate procedure for all age groups, including children[5] and the elderly.[18]

The family physician must learn to recognize psychiatric issues. Among these are somatic presentations that originate in psychologic and emotional issues. The questions, then, are these: How does one integrate the diagnosis and treatment of somatic dysfunction into the treatment of the patient whose musculoskeletal dysfunction is significantly linked with psychologic dysfunction? Under what circumstances is OMT indicated? What forms of OMT are appropriate, and when is OMT contraindicated?

The Somatizing Patient

Somatization is a defense mechanism, an automatic psychologic process that protects the individual from anxiety and the awareness of internal or external stressors or dangers. It mediates the individual's reaction to external stressors and emotional conflicts. Somatization as a defense mechanism is characterized by physical complaints not fully explained by an existent medical condition but severe enough to result in medical treatment or alteration in lifestyle. Symptoms can include pain in various anatomic areas, often suggest neurologic involvement, and often involve the gastrointestinal and reproductive systems.[14]

To be classified as having somatization disorder, a complex of symptoms known in the past as hysteria or Briquet's syndrome, the patient must demonstrate a constellation of pain and gastrointestinal, sexual, and pseudoneurologic symptoms before age 30, and the condition must have been present for years. This is one of the somatoform disorders, the others being undifferentiated somatoform disorder, conversion disorder, pain disorder, psychogenic pain disorder, hypochondriasis, neurasthenia, and pseudocyesis.[14]

Patients with many types of mental disorders employ somatization as a defense. Affective disorders, including major depressive disorder, dysthymia, and minor depression, can cause somatic complaints, as can anxiety disorders, such as panic disorder, generalized anxiety disorder, and obsessive-compulsive disorder.[15] An anxiety disorder of childhood and adolescence, overanxious disorder, considered by some to be equivalent to the adult diagnosis of generalized anxiety disorder, may present as general tension and an inability to relax, with recurrent somatic complaints for which no organic cause can be found. Personality disorders, particularly those comprising Cluster B in DSM-IV-TR (histrionic, antisocial, narcissistic, and borderline) are likely to somatize.[14] Among psychotic patients, schizophrenics may demonstrate somatic concerns that can reach delusional proportions.

Posttraumatic Stress Disorder

Another group of individuals likely to seek treatment for a somatic complaint that is intimately linked to psychologic issues are patients with posttraumatic stress disorder (PTSD). This is a specific form of anxiety disorder involving exposure to an exceptional mental or physical stressor, such as experiencing, witnessing, or confronting an event involving actual or threatened death or injury of oneself or another. The immediate reaction is intense fear, helplessness, or horror. It is followed by recurrent reliving of the event, avoidance of stimuli associated with the event or numbing of general responsiveness and by manifestations of fear and increased arousal. This can occur immediately or may not appear for months or much longer after the trauma. Reliving of the event can occur as recurrent, intrusive, and distressing recollections of it, as images, thoughts, or perceptions. PTSD also can manifest as recurrent distressing dreams of the event or a sudden feeling as if the event were recurring. In these patients some aspect of the body can be literally or symbolically linked to the past trauma. Patients can experience powerful psychologic distress or physiologic reactivity if they are exposed to internal or external cues that symbolize or resemble some part of the original event. The affected person will consequently try to avoid thoughts or feelings associated with the event or anything that might arouse recollection of it. There can be amnesia of an important aspect of the event, or it may be entirely repressed, as is often the case with PTSD from sexual abuse. Such patients may lose interest in significant activities. They may feel detached or estranged from others, have a sense of a foreshortened future, have difficulty sleeping, be irritable, be prone to angry outbursts, have difficulty in concentrating, or demonstrate an exaggerated startle response.

According to Hans Selye in his key work on general adaptive syndrome, once there is a stress, tissues react in their characteristic way.[25] Factors that influence the effect of trauma include genetic predisposition, plasticity of the individual brain (as the brain develops, the significance of a stressor or its permanence may change), the chemical matrix, past experiences including formative tutorials (what one is taught early in life about oneself, one's abilities, and how safe or unsafe the world is), and the duration, intensity, and frequency of the traumatic event. These factors determine how one defends oneself.

A further determinant is the individual's perception of the viability of defense. A person who feels that defense is viable may defend or attack. If the individual does not feel it is viable, flight is the alternative. If defense is perceived as unviable and no escape is possible, the response is freezing. Experiments using *executive* animal models (rats,[26] monkeys[27]) demonstrate that learned helplessness over time can result in integrated altered chemistries, altered structure, altered brain pathways, and altered posture. We are all familiar with the difference between the gait and station of an individual who is profoundly depressed or anxious and the same person's mobility when he or she is feeling well.

Character defenses are traits of the individual's personality that serve unconscious protective purposes. Wilhelm Reich, a student of Freud's, described a link between suppressed or repressed aspects of an individual's personality and the body, and he developed the concept of body language. He concluded that people form a kind of armor to protect themselves from the blows of the outside world and from their own desires and instincts. The mechanism of PTSD is a form of character defense in which in part unconscious positioning that stems from previous physical or psychologic trauma provides the patient with a symbolic or real postural defense against further attack. Thus, the soma comes to symbolize an aspect of the unconscious psyche. Reich went on to develop techniques to interpret patients' defensive body language and to help them deal with it by understanding how it came about in the first place.[28]

The main defense mechanism active here is repression. When something is so painful, so unacceptable, that one cannot deal with it and continue to survive, the memory is shut out of awareness. It is still present, but it has been moved into the unconscious. It still has power, shown by the way people act, sometimes in ways that are not necessarily driven by what is happening at the time. The treatment from the psychiatric perspective often is to make the person aware of the original trauma, to bring it back into consciousness and deal with it in the present. When a traumatic memory is suppressed and eventually repressed, it is not only the thought that is blocked but possibly also the associated action or need for action, because the two are intimately linked. For example, if a boy must repeatedly raise his right hand to protect himself from being struck, he may not only repress the fact that he has been struck but also the reason he raised his hand. When this occurs, the muscles employed in defense are frequently tense.

In this circumstance, the psychologic issues that the trauma created accompany physical issues. Muscles tighten or become slack; internal organs respond by either shutting down or becoming hyperactive. The individual survived the initial trauma and pushed it into the unconscious, where it is taken out of awareness. The person can function but must expend energy to keep the original hurt from conscious awareness. Occasionally such a defense fails. If a thought, feeling, body posture, or some other reminder occurs, the body again reacts for an instant or longer, not to what is occurring now, but to what occurred in the past.

Osteopathic physicians are sensitive to the medical problems the patient faces and their effect upon the musculoskeletal system as viscerosomatic reflexes. Consequently, the osteopathic physician can diagnose visceral malfunction through palpatory skills and the ability to integrate this information into the musculoskeletal findings. In the same sense, the osteopathic physician should address psychologic issues. The term *somatoemotional* has been used to describe the relationship between the soma and the psyche, but the relationship goes far beyond this. This relationship may be viewed as a mind-body-mind feedback loop or syndrome. As with the interrelationship between viscerosomatic and somatovisceral reflexes, there is a reverberating relationship between mental action and reaction and the soma.

Clinical experience demonstrates that muscles are frequently tense, and somatic dysfunction produces troublesome imbalance. This is often not because the origin was physical or mechanical but rather because the origin was emotional. The resultant somatic response is an attempt at physical resolution. Just as emotional blocking occurs at an unconscious level, musculoskeletal dysfunction may result from unconscious mechanisms. If the patient is observed carefully, the links between emotional issues and physically defensive positions, such as arm, leg, or head position, can be identified. The patient does not separate the experience into its elements, although many elements of an experience are stored in different areas of the brain and can be triggered by differing stimuli. It is possible for some of the elements to be suppressed while others are fully active. Frequently individuals pick up only portions of a memory, while other parts require more triggering or cueing before they are recalled.

Occasionally, any nonspecific stimulus triggers recollection of the entire experience or perhaps only the anxiety and fear that the original experience caused. The osteopathic physician can palpate the effects of this recollection in the musculoskeletal system. Certain issues are more likely to cause suppression than repression.

It is not a quantum leap to see that some unpleasant incidents involve the patient's emotions, body, and total life and survival. These incidents are aversive, painful, and unacceptable, and the patient moves them, or at least the dangerous portions, out of consciousness. The patient can now continue to function without being preoccupied by defending against trauma. This defense, however, extorts a price; psychologic effort expends mental energy. Many events that may trigger a partial recall of the original painful incident can occur during the rest of life. The patient responds partially to the triggering event in the present situation but also partially as a defense against the former, now unconscious, insult. Much uncovering psychotherapy is based upon this return to consciousness of what was repressed and dealing with the situation in the present.

Trauma to the individual can cause temporary or permanent changes in structure, function, and ability to integrate the total body mechanism. When the trauma is emotional, the influence can be felt not only at the time of the trauma but long afterward. If the trauma is sufficient to overload the person's defenses, the actual incident may be pushed deep into the unconscious so that the person can continue to function. It does, however, take its toll. The individual may reflect the effect of the trauma in unconscious ways. It may result in partial memories or fear, even when there seems to be no connection to the original situation in the present. These fears can lead to partial and even total immobilization of the individual, who then cannot function in most areas of life. Whether the diagnosis is PTSD, somatoform disorder, or any other of the anxiety disorders, the effect is devastating.

The Psychodynamics of Somatic Dysfunction

Somatic dysfunction, be it the result of postural imbalance, sprain, strain, or viscerosomatic reflexes, can be present without psychologic implications. In somatic dysfunction with psychologic implications, however, there is literal or symbolic significance to associated muscle tension, a position that may have been held as a means of expression or defense, such as tilting of the head or moving an arm into a certain position, as if to defend oneself. Sometimes a muscle will tense although there is no actual motion, and the alerting mechanism is called into play; the defense is mobilized, but the muscle does not move for any of several possible reasons.

Sometimes the symptom manifests during conversation; the person takes a particular position when discussing a certain topic. This is different from a habit, which causes the person to assume a particular body position. Sometimes the voice or demeanor changes regardless of the topic—although that, too, can be a result of unconscious feelings. Consider an individual trying to move a particular body part but not being able to, as when being forcibly held. Muscular tension can be identified in those body parts even though the muscle did not actually contract. Neurolinguistic phenomena occasionally manifest as an image, a sound, a smell, or a tactile sensation rather than verbal output. The comment "This makes my skin crawl," for example, illustrates the somatic equivalent of a psychic feeling.

It is as if every memory, every trauma, and every pleasant as well as unpleasant experience is stored in the brain. When recalled, the entire picture may reappear: sights, sounds, smells, body positions, emotions, and so forth. The experience may be stored in a hidden place, the unconscious, for diverse reasons. This usually is the result of a happening so unpleasant that it had to be blocked out of awareness and hidden from consciousness. Sometimes a partial memory comes back; this can be triggered deliberately or by accident and result in inexplicable symptoms.

So some people assume certain body postures. The osteopathic physician may not know exactly why a patient does so or why it occurs at specific times in the patient's life, but understanding how the person came to assume the posture can help the physician understand the patient. Without understanding, it is difficult to explain why a particular muscle or group of muscles is tense. Sometimes it is possible to gain understanding while working with the patient. From a psychiatric perspective, talking to patients and listening to what they say lets the clinician pick up themes and build upon those themes. Similarly, patients respond to the physical examination and treatment with OMT. Often treatment successfully alleviates the somatic dysfunction. Occasionally, though, those problem areas return in spite of expert treatment. In that case it is necessary to reevaluate. Has treatment addressed only the symptom of a more pervasive underlying problem? Is there postural imbalance, a leg length difference, an overuse syndrome, or viscerosomatic influence? Sometimes the somatic dysfunctions do not stay corrected. Possibly an emotional conflict causes a physical response, and sometimes a physical situation has emotions attached to it. The cycle continues until it becomes difficult to tell which came first.

Although the fund of osteopathic literature dedicated to the treatment of psychiatric patients is limited, it is significant in terms of the recognition of the mind-body interface and actions and is worthy of study. Many of the writings are single case studies or small samplings, but they point out not only a need for further research but also a need for practitioners to address these phenomena. Review of old psychiatric literature reveals that concepts and models of behavior rarely change, and so they are worth examining for an understanding of the thinking of the times. What changes as science progresses is neurologic, neuropharmacologic, and psychologic knowledge. Based upon this advancing knowledge, treatment modalities change, but they seldom negate the value of the original hypothetical constructs and the theoretical models.

The Role of OMT

Patients' patterns of somatic dysfunction are as unique as the individual. If somatic dysfunction is diagnosed and appropriately treated with OMT, it should resolve.

Manipulative procedures may be classified according to how aggressive they are as physical intervention. (See Chapter 4.) It is thought that psychiatric patients are probably most appropriately treated with procedures from the least aggressive end of this continuum. Certainly, high-velocity, low-amplitude treatment should be avoided under most circumstances.[18,24] It is recommended that treatment begin in the least painful areas, starting with soft tissue and avoiding forceful procedures. If vertebral mobilization is attempted, it is best accomplished by rhythmic articular rocking or springing procedures.[16]

Touch is a primal form of communication, and because of the possibility of misinterpretation, it must be employed with the greatest caution in treatment of a patient with psychopathology. OMT is contraindicated if the patient does not wish to be touched or feels that the intervention is too uncomfortable.[24]

OMT is the definitive treatment for somatic dysfunction only. Just as the recognition of a viscerosomatic reflex offers diagnostic information that can lead to the specific treatment of visceral pathology, recognition of the linkage between somatic dysfunction and psychologic dysfunction can provide entrée for effective psychotherapy.

Recognizing a Connection

After the structural evaluation and treatment with OMT, an unanticipated response may occur. Something happens to the patient, who reports a smell, a sound, a tune in the head, or a change in muscle tension that is not explained entirely by the manipulation or by the reduction of somatic dysfunction. This should alert the physician that there is something more, an unidentified emotional component. The treatment of the somatic dysfunction has not corrected the entire problem. It is no different from using the musculoskeletal component as an indicator of a visceral phenomenon, a viscerosomatic reflex. In that case, the visceral pathology must be addressed, whether it is the gallbladder, stomach, heart, or lungs, before the reflex-associated somatic dysfunction will respond to treatment.

The converse also is true. Through somatovisceral action OMT can affect cholangitis, gastroenteritis, or any internal organic problem with musculoskeletal manipulation. Although it is appropriate also to treat the visceral component specifically, the task is not complete until both visceral and somatic components of the reflex relationship, that is, all of the components responsible for maintaining a state of dysfunction, have been treated. This relationship also applies between the somatic and emotional components. Changing position or relieving muscular tension with OMT may alleviate the emotional component. If the patient then is able to link that response to the present, the defensive position may no longer be necessary. The symptomatic relief may drive the repressed memory from the unconscious into the conscious, allowing it to dissipate.

Once traumatized, the patient reacts, and treatment is directed toward repairing the damage, regardless of the etiology. Finding the etiology may help explain the presence of the trauma and assist in prevention of further trauma. Etiology is important in understanding the cause of the reaction, but it does not necessarily direct one to the most effective course of treatment.

Which came first, the chicken or the egg? The somatic dysfunction or the emotional issue? The complex interaction between the soma and the psyche often makes this a difficult question. In the case of PTSD, the trauma, if it was emotional, most probably preceded the somatic response; if the original trauma was physical, the somatic and emotional components may have occurred almost simultaneously. The somatizing patient, whose physical complaint is focused upon an area of somatic dysfunction, on the other hand, may well have become focused upon a prior musculoskeletal discomfort. In any case, because the family physician deals with the here and now, the clinical questions are these: How much of this can or should the primary care physician attempt to treat? When does it become necessary to consult a psychiatrist to address the emotional component? The family physician can diagnose and treat many emotional conditions. But more complex issues, individuals who demonstrate extensive or persistent disability, should be referred to the specialist for concomitant psychotherapy while the family physician may continue, if appropriate, to address the somatic component.

Anxiety and Tension

Does reduction of anxiety reduce tension? Is reduction of tension enough? Not all psychopathology is a result of tension, but tension can make it worse. The physician can make the perfect correction, use the appropriate procedures, but uncover an unexpected somatoemotional component. On occasion a clinician who uses OMT becomes aware of something happening that appears to go beyond the physical touch or the positioning of the patient, something that defies intervention. As the physician moves the patient during treatment, the purpose is to relieve tension, reduce muscle spasm, enhance available range of motion, and correct positional imbalance.

It is fairly common for the emotional component to become troublesome again. The clinician makes a physical diagnosis, identifies a therapeutic plan, and implements it, only to find that the patient received little or no relief and that the original dysfunction, possibly along with others, is still troublesome. Another try fails to produce the desired therapeutic response. Possibly the OMT or even the diagnostic evaluation appears to have greater significance for the patient than warranted.

The Emotional Release

Many patients are shy. They have problems with looking at others, exposing themselves, or having their bodies palpated, but this reaction can go beyond simple modesty. Otherwise neutral areas of the body may be defended vigorously, or significant areas may not be defended at all. The patient may become frightened, tense up, even begin to cry uncontrollably. The patient has an emotional response or a brief recollection of a forgotten past event. It is seldom a total recall experience, but it can be. Some body areas, some movements, some positions, and some therapists are particularly likely to trigger these emotions that seem unrelated to the stimulus. When this occurs, notice whether there is muscular tension or total relaxation and try to link the person's position at the moment to a similar or identical traumatic position in the past. The response may be surrender, as the muscles go flaccid, or it may be rigidity, particularly if the defensive behavior was useful at the time of the original trauma. Putting the person in the position of the original injury frequently exposes but not necessarily releases the emotional components. Physical, emotional, or sexual abuse, either at key times in development or over a protracted period, with the person not able to launch an effective defense, is frequently the culprit. The patient had to tolerate the abuse to survive or survived in spite of the abuse. The person was able to defend in some way by blocking out what was happening or what could not be controlled. The person either did not or could not physically defend against the abuse. Once one reaches this point in the treatment session, the real work begins: the process of integrating the patient's emotions with the body. Although it may not make sense to the physician at the time, this procedure is very similar to performing a myofascial release. One works through the tension of the various fascial planes. One cannot guide the process, or force it; one can merely try to follow it.

At this point, one needs to ask oneself and the patient: Has this ever happened before? Has it happened before under similar circumstances? Does this remind the patient of something? Sometimes the patient has avoided the particular position because it was so well defended. Other times the patient may have accidentally assumed the position, had a reaction, did not understand it, did not link it with anything, and so did not see a physician to explore it. Many have had full neurologic evaluations because the problem seemed more neurologic than somatoemotional. A strange smell, a partial paralysis or weakness, or seeing bright flashing lights can lead one in that direction, and of course, it is appropriate to go there. When looking at an organic component as the problem, it is also necessary to consider the organic finding as part of a full somatoemotional constellation.

By now, the physician should realize that a repressed memory may have been triggered, and until this aspect of the patient's problem is dealt with, alleviation of the somatic symptom is impossible. Moreover, the depth, nature, and severity of the emotional trauma is not always mirrored by the severity of the associated somatic dysfunction. Some dysfunctions are very resistant to treatment without fully exploring the original incident, while others are not. An original incident that was terribly significant at the time may in the broad scope of things turn out not to be all that important and may be shrugged off. At other times, what appears to be a minor tic or annoyance may in fact have a representation from childhood of something very traumatic and important to the development of the person's personality. Thus, the physician must consider defense mechanisms from a psychologic perspective as well as from a biomechanical one.

OMT: Releasing the Emotional Component

Bearing in mind that a patient's anatomically neutral (the physical midpoint), functionally neutral (balanced muscular tension), and emotionally balanced (comfortable, at equilibrium) states may not all necessarily reflect the same position, the physician attempts to put the patient into a neutral position where opposing tensions are balanced. Tissue tension must direct the physician, not vice versa. While moving the patient into position, it is useful to visualize the muscle groups that might have been involved in the original trauma and attempt to place them in the least physically stressful position. It may require trial and error to identify the position of maximum relaxation. This is a dynamic process. Each time the physician successfully positions the patient, the patient readjusts and new tensions emerge. As the patient shifts into each new neutral position, the physician develops new concepts and thoughts about the origin of the patient's problem. Through this process, new hypotheses arise as old ones fade. Any sensory stimulus—sounds, sights, smells—may originally have been involved. Although the physician is dealing with body position in terms of intervention, a new defensive position may be assumed as a result of the presence of another hidden memory associated with a sound, a smell, or a thought or when the patient is under stress or tired. As the physician proceeds with the intervention, the emotional component will eventually be released, and the patient may suddenly feel sad, angry, or frightened or begin to cry, bringing repressed emotions into the present moment where they can be dealt with.

As defenses are removed, the release can be so pronounced that an emotional crisis may be precipitated, and the physician must be prepared to make an appropriate response. The physician may find a raw, exposed psyche suddenly revealed, and it must be dealt with. Usually one cannot leave the patient in that position physically or emotionally in order to call the specialist and say, "Here's where we are. Here's what we have. So what do I do now?" Sometimes that may be the only option, and one must say, "Hang on there and let me see if I can get a psychiatrist on the phone." But it is better to have basic psychiatric knowledge, a conceptual model to work with, and procedures that will alleviate the emotional distress and seal it back up—while making it available again for treatment by a specialist.

Pitfalls, Pratfalls, and Precautions

A number of patients with psychiatric conditions have somatic complaints. The challenge for the primary care physician is how to identify these patients and address their physical complaints as well as their psychologic issues. These patients have somatic dysfunction. Therefore, when they are examined and somatic dysfunction is diagnosed, their somatization is corroborated. OMT, if it furthers this corroboration or fulfills needs for attention, can create dependence.[18]

Somatizing patients who are not manifesting overt psychiatric symptoms before treatment can develop them when their somatic dysfunction is effectively resolved with OMT. This may be the result of the use of somatic symptoms as a defense mechanism that the treatment has disabled, so that somatization is no longer effective. At this point the patient's underlying psychiatric issues rise to the surface. The question is not whether OMT is inappropriate. The questions are when the proper time is, what the proper procedures for maximum benefit to the patient are, what psychotherapy is appropriate, and when it should be employed.

Defenses, like somatization and repression, serve protective purposes, and disruption of them leaves the patient vulnerable. The simplest recourse for the patient is to cling tenaciously to the disrupted defense in an attempt to restore it. This is why, when the somatic component of the somatizing patient is effectively treated with OMT, the patient may demonstrate a paradoxical response. Even though the objective findings associated with the dysfunction are decreased, the patient may report that the subjective complaint is worse. Identifying the somatic dysfunction corroborates the patient's defensive position. Treating the dysfunction removes or significantly weakens the defense, impelling the patient to try desperately to maintain it. If that particular defense cannot be maintained, the focal point of the somatization may be shifted to a new area of the body, or there may be a switch to an entirely different defense.[18] If the patient's defenses have been systematically stripped away without providing alternative methods of coping, the patient may be left with no alternative but suicide. Consequently, when a defense is eliminated, an effective alternative must be provided. Failure here can result in serious problems for the patient.

The physician–patient relationship is ideally based upon reciprocal, honest communication with mutual respect and understanding. Patients with delusions and misinterpretations are honest in their presentation of the phenomenon as they perceive it. The misinterpretations and delusions can be worked out as the physician–patient relationship solidifies and the patient's trust in the physician increases.

The psychiatric patient, however, presents a complex clinical problem. It is impossible to treat somatic dysfunction with the physical intervention of OMT without exerting a psychologic effect. Transference in psychiatric terms is the unconscious assignment to others of feelings and attitudes that were originally associated with important figures (e.g., parents, siblings) in early life. The transference relationship follows the pattern of its prototype. In the patient–physician relationship, the transference may be negative (hostile) or positive (affectionate).

In classical psychoanalysis, the physician avoids all physical contact with the patient to prevent transference from interfering with the pure psychotherapeutic relationship. Psychotherapists from other schools of thought may use this phenomenon as a therapeutic tool to help the patient understand emotional problems and their origins. If simply shaking hands can foster transference, one can imagine what can result from physical contact that entails the diagnosis of somatic dysfunction and its treatment with OMT. The simplest transference between the patient and physician is the recognition that the physician is a person of authority. In the medically focused relationship that most commonly occurs between a physician and patient, this can be very beneficial; however, because touch is such a primal form of communication, it is open to misinterpretation.

One of Freud's concepts was that it is not what happened but the fear and concern that something bad could have happened that creates the problem. One does not always accurately remember incidents because they were emotionally charged. Suggestibility is heightened, and memories of just who did what, and how, and when may be false. The body, however, is not fooled; it responds with a defense that may have been used to ward off the original negative stimulus. It is incumbent upon the physician, therefore, to explore all of the links—the somatovisceral, the somatopsychologic, the musculoskeletal and the rest—and to keep an open mind regarding all etiologic possibilities.

The patient who has been abused frequently comes into therapy, whether general medical, musculoskeletal specialty, or psychiatric specialty, with concerns and fears of authority figures. The patient can be very suggestible, wanting badly to please so as to undo the pain. It is essential that the physician understand this and be trained in the presentation and interpretation of data without judgment prior to the initiation of treatment.

With the individual's desire to get well and the authority of the physician, sometimes the patient's need to please and the physician's desire for a quick and reasonable answer can lead to problems. Memories have been known to be manufactured when a therapist guides a patient to see issues of abuse in childhood that either never occurred or did not occur as anticipated. I recall one patient who came to me for psychiatric help and who had clear evidence of emotional and physical abuse. There was no doubt that her father did actually abuse the patient in her early years. However, I did not plant any suggestions; I merely followed her where she wanted to go, with comments, suggestions, and positions that gave her either relief or more discomfort. As therapy developed, she clearly recalled a key incident hidden from her consciousness in which she was indeed sexually assaulted, not by her father but by an uncle. This fact was later verified by family members who thought that she had forgotten the incident.

If we treat the somatic dysfunction, are we treating the core problem or the consequences of emotion? It is in the feedback from the patient that we gain our greatest clues regarding this. If it was a core issue, the somatic dysfunction will more than likely respond and clear up. If, on the other hand, it is a somatoemotional consequence, the somatic dysfunction may move to another part of the body in a process similar to unwinding as each defense is analyzed and worked through until the core issue or defense is revealed.

CONCLUSION

Because the practice of family medicine necessitates that the practitioner address all of the health issues of the patient from all aspects of medicine and surgery and because of the inseparability of physical and mental health, osteopathic medicine, with its recognition of the triune nature of the patient, offers an effective model for the understanding of these complex issues. The diagnosis and treatment of somatic dysfunction provide the practitioner with a system of clinical problem solving that provides an opportunity to approach the patient holistically. At every level of the central nervous system along the spine, the neurophysiology of somatic dysfunction inseparably links viscera, soma, and psyche through complex viscerosomatic, somatovisceral, somatopsychologic and psychosomatic feedback interrelationships.[20–22] One component of these complex relations cannot become problematic without affecting the other two, and treatment of no one aspect is complete without consideration of the others.

Preexisting organic pathology and functional complaints, whether visceral or somatic, may be augmented by personality traits. Visceral or somatic conditions can provide defenses against psychologic stress. These conditions in themselves may prove more debilitating than the originating stressors would have been if they had been more effectively dealt with. Ambiguous physical complaints may represent occult organic pathology, or they may be manifestations of repressed psychologic issues. Thus, in daily clinical practice the family physician must possess a thorough knowledge of psychopathology, and the osteopathic family physician is in a unique position to integrate that knowledge thoroughly into a highly organized holistic approach to the patient.

References

1. Still AT. Philosophy of Osteopathy. Kirksville, MO: Author, 1899. Reprinted by the American Academy of Osteopathy, Indianapolis, 1971;26.
2. Littlejohn JM. Psychiatry. Bound monograph in the personal library of K. E. Nelson. Publisher and date unknown; pp 1–2.
3. Still AT. Osteopathy, Research and Practice. Kirksville, MO: Author, 1910. Reprinted by Eastland Press, Seattle, WA, 1992;136–139.
4. Gerdine LVH. Osteopathy and insanity. J Am Osteopath Assoc June 1917;1199–1200.
5. Hildreth AG, Still FM. Schizophrenia. J Am Osteopath Assoc 1939;38:422–426.
6. Still FM. Dementia praecox. J Osteopathy 1940;33:534–536.
7. Woods JM, Woods RH. A physical finding related to psychiatric disorders. J Am Osteopath Assoc 1961;60:988–993.
8. Iwata JL, Rodos JJ, Glonek T, Habenicht A. Comparing psychotic and affective disorders by musculoskeletal structural examination. J Am Osteopath Assoc 1997;97:715–721.
9. Magoun HI Sr. The cranial concept in general practice. Osteopath Ann 1976;4:206–212.
10. Plotkin BJ, Rodos JJ, Kappler R, et al. Adjunctive osteopathic manipulative treatment in women with depression: A pilot study. J Am Osteopath Assoc 2001;101:517–523.
11. Kropiunigg U. Basics in psychoneuroimmunology. Ann Med 1993;25:473–479.
12. Kroenke K, Mangelsdorff D. Common symptoms in ambulatory care: Incidence, evaluation, therapy and outcome. Am J Med 1989;86:262–266.
13. Walker EA. Medically unexplained physical symptoms. Clin Obstet Gynecol 1997;40:589–600 [review].
14. Diagnostic and Statistical Manual of Mental Disorders: DSM-IV-TR Text Revision. 4th ed. Washington: American Psychiatric Association, 2000.
15. Barsky AJ. A comprehensive approach to the chronically somatizing patient. J Psychosom Res 1998;45:301–306.
16. Dunn FE. The osteopathic management of psychosomatic problems. J Am Osteopath Assoc 1948;48:196–199.
17. Dunn FE. Osteopathic concepts in psychiatry. J Am Osteopath Assoc 1950;49:354–357.
18. Bradford SG. Osteopathic considerations in psychiatric disorders of the elderly. Osteopath Ann 1974;2:26–27, 29–31.
19. Patterson MM, Howell JN, eds. The Central Connection: Somatovisceral/Viscerosomatic Interaction. Proceedings of the 1989 American Academy of Osteopathy International Symposium. Athens, OH: University Classics, 1992.

20. Korr IM. The neural basis of the osteopathic lesion. J Am Osteopath Assoc 1947;47:191–198.
21. Korr IM. The emerging concept of the osteopathic lesion. J Am Osteopath Assoc 1948;48:127–138.
22. Korr IM. IV. Clinical significance of the facilitated state. J Am Osteopath Assoc 1955;54:277–282.
23. Mark BT. Psychologic stress and muscle tension. Osteopath Ann 1977;5:212–217.
24. Osborn GG. Manual medicine and its role in psychiatry. AAO J 1994;4(1):16–21.
25. Selye H. The general adaptive syndrome and the disease of adaptation. J Clin Endocrinol 1946;6:117–230.
26. Weiss J. Psychological factors in stress and disease. Sci Am 1972;226(6):104–113.
27. Brady JV. Ulcers in executive monkeys. Sci Am 1958;199(4):95–98 passim.
28. Reich W. Charakteranalyse: Technik und Grundlagen. Vienna: Zelbstverlag (Manzsche, Vienna), 1933.

CHAPTER 8

The Pediatric Patient

Nicette Sergueef and Kenneth E. Nelson

INTRODUCTION

Pediatric anatomy, physiology, and specific disease processes encountered in clinical practice can be relatively predictable. Specific disease processes, once diagnosed, have well-defined therapeutic protocols. However, clinical practice is not quite that simple; every patient is unique. All patients have their own individual history, anatomic variations, and consequently functional (and dysfunctional) differences. As well as treating disease processes, the osteopathic clinician must optimize function wherever possible. Effective diagnosis and treatment of somatic dysfunction enhances the self-healing ability of human physiology, which should enhance the efficacy of all other appropriate therapeutic protocols in the treatment of disease processes.

Yet all too often, clinicians, even those skilled in the use of osteopathic manipulative treatment (OMT) for their adult patients, hesitate to use manipulation upon their younger patients. The preverbal patient will not provide a specific complaint, so the diagnostician must think to look for contributory somatic dysfunction. And even if somatic dysfunction is suspected, the clinician may be hesitant to employ OMT for fear of injuring a delicate infant or child. This concern is unjustified if the somatic dysfunction is specifically diagnosed and the treatment modality is judiciously selected. The purpose of this chapter is to provide the clinician a logical approach to the diagnosis and treatment of somatic dysfunction in the neonatal and pediatric population.

PEDIATRIC SOMATIC DYSFUNCTION

It has been said that infants and children do not demonstrate somatic dysfunction. This is not true. It is true that the pediatric patient almost never has the musculoskeletal complaints commonly associated with adult somatic dysfunction. Dysfunctional mechanics of the neuromusculoskeletal system do, however, exert significant influence upon the health status of these patients.

Primary somatic dysfunction in the adult is frequently the result of trauma (macro or micro) associated with the individual's neutral postural mechanical pattern. Compensatory postural mechanics, as encountered in accommodation for minor inequities of leg length, is recognized in adult patients. Similarly, neonatal or pediatric somatic dysfunction is often caused by birth trauma and/or childhood injuries upon the mechanical pattern of intrauterine posture and environment. Neonates may have asymmetric musculoskeletal mechanics that are the result of asymmetric intrauterine positioning preferentially assumed during the prenatal period. These asymmetries, confounded by the physical stress of birth, produce somatic dysfunction. As the infant or child matures, this pattern is further affected by the evolution of developmental milestones and weight-bearing mechanics and possibly by trauma.

A thorough understanding of anatomy offers particular insight into the role of somatic dysfunction in the development of functional complaints and in specific disease processes. We know that structure and function are intimately related, that form follows function in both the intrauterine and extrauterine environments. Malposition of the bones of the pelvis can produce the positional dysfunctions of the lower extremities and gait errors encountered in pediatric practice. It is obvious that the ulnohumeral articulation of the elbow acts as a hinge joint. So too, potential patterns for motion between the bones of the skull may be extrapolated by closely observing the anatomy of their articulations. Knowledge of the anatomy of the skull and face is extremely important. Malpositional molding of the bones of the skull and face can contribute to functional ear, nose, and throat problems, such as poor feeding, strabismus, and recurrent otitis media. Such cranial dysfunction can also result in symptoms of cranial nerve entrapment.

We know that movement of the unossified articulations of the human skull is possible. The molding that occurs in an infant's skull during birth makes this readily apparent. At birth, the sutures of the cranial vault provide sufficient mobility that overlapping of adjacent bones frequently occurs during delivery.

The cranial base consists of several synchondroses, where the tissue connecting the osseous components is cartilage that turns into bone before adult life. A significant synchondrosis, the spheno-occipital or sphenobasilar synchondrosis (SBS), exists between the occipital bone and the sphenoid. Synchondroses are also found between the component parts of the sphenoid bone and between the petrous and squamous portions of the temporal bones. The occipital bone at birth consists of four parts, each separated by a synchondrosis. The anterior intraoccipital synchondroses, between the basiocciput and the bilateral exocciputs, have clinical significance because when they fuse, they form the occipital condyles and the hypoglossal canals (Fig. 8.1).

The synchondroses function as hinges during birth and are sometimes stressed. Persistent dysfunctional patterns between different bones are interosseous, while persistent dysfunctional patterns between the component parts of a bone are intraosseous.

In most individuals, these synchondroses ossify before adulthood. Ossification of the intraosseous synchondroses of the sphenoid and temporal bones is usually

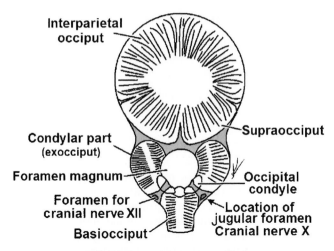

FIGURE 8.1 The occiput at birth.

complete in the first 2 years of life and in the occipital bone at 7 to 9 years. The SBS is ossified in most individuals between 8 and 18 years.[1-5] Thus, the greatest therapeutic effect of OMT upon these areas is expected before the synchondroses ossify.

Somatic dysfunction throughout the body is often described as impairment of articular mechanics, while cranial dysfunctions have been described as membranous articular strains.[6,7] This designation is made because of the significance of the dural membranes in the embryologic development of the skull and consequently in cranial somatic dysfunction (ICD-9CM 739.0[8]).

Embryologically the outer layer of the dura mater and the future skull are of the same origin. They are both derived from the ectomeninx. The ectomeninx divides into an inner layer that becomes the dura mater and an outer layer that forms the bony structures. "The relationship between the developing skull and the underlying dura mater continues during postnatal life when the bones of the calvaria are still growing."[9] It is very difficult to separate the bone from the dura in the skull of an infant. The dura membranes play a mechanical role in the transmission of intracranial forces. The dura is a template for the growing bones, and any imbalance in the tension of its fibers will give rise to disturbance in the bone growth processes.

Also, the venous sinuses lie between layers of dura, and the cranial nerves go through or are surrounded by dural fibers. Dural strain can therefore result in venous stasis and cranial nerve entrapment. Using functional OMT to balance the dural fibers is a fundamental aspect of the treatment of the infant or child.

The palpable phenomenon of the cranial rhythmic impulse (CRI) has been demonstrated to correspond to low-frequency fluctuations in blood flow velocity.[10] These fluctuations are a manifestation of rhythmicity in the autonomic nervous system.[11] It has further been demonstrated that cranial manipulation increased the amplitude of these fluctuations and the fluctuations of similar frequency in intracranial fluid content.[12-14] Although the therapeutic implications of these observations are not yet clearly identified, for maximum efficacy manipulative treatment should be applied in association with these fundamental body rhythms.

DIAGNOSIS AND TREATMENT OF THE PEDIATRIC PATIENT

An osteopathic physician begins the diagnosis of an infant or child in the same fashion as the adult patient, approaching pediatric care with these things in mind and answering the following questions:

1. How does dysfunction of the musculoskeletal system mechanically affect the patient?
2. What effect does the sympathetic nervous system have upon the patient?
3. What effect does the parasympathetic nervous system have upon the patient?
4. How does circulatory stasis affect the patient?

OMT may be employed to decrease physical discomfort, to improve function, and ultimately to affect structure. The malleability of very young tissue makes the application of functional and cranial procedures more effective in youngsters than in older individuals, in whom ossification has more rigidly fixed dysfunctional patterns. Treatment of dysfunction may augment the effectiveness of specifically indicated treatment protocols. It may also offer a specific therapeutic approach for conditions otherwise treated only by symptom suppression or watchful waiting. Because of the rapid growth rates of infants and small children, recognizing and treating reversible dysfunctional asymmetries, as opposed to watchful waiting, fosters symmetric musculoskeletal development. While manipulative treatment for adult patients is often directed at alleviating discomfort and improving function, the effect of functional balance upon structure is much greater for the infant or child.

Dysfunction of the musculoskeletal system will affect functional and eventually structural development. The physical discomfort associated with somatic dysfunction of upper thoracic, cervical, suboccipital, or cranial mechanism may affect infant latching, sucking, and swallowing, and may result in gastroesophageal reflux. Similarly, dysfunction of the lumbar or pelvic region and/or the lower extremity may inhibit the infant from sitting or crawling according to the normal developmental schedule. Pain and discomfort may manifest as irritability, failure to meet developmental milestones, and/or the asymmetric use of muscles. Continued asymmetric use of muscles will hypertrophy the overused side and further weaken the underused side. Forces transmitted through muscles and fascia, including the dura, may contribute to asymmetric skeletal growth, delay in the developmental milestones, and structural dysfunction in adulthood.

The clinician must consider how somatic dysfunction can affect specific systems, such as upper respiratory and gastrointestinal tracts, along with their affects upon the general growth and development of the patient. Somatic dysfunction can predispose the patient to the development and/or recurrence of disease processes, such as otitis media, and reduce the ability to respond to any such disease process. Somatic dysfunction can also present as functional symptoms, such as gastrointestinal irritability or sleep disturbance.

An osteopathic examination should be performed upon every infant and child, particularly those at high risk for the development of somatic dysfunction: prolonged labor and complicated prenatal courses, cephalopelvic disproportion, breech deliveries, deliveries using vacuum extraction or forceps, cesarean sections, and multiple births. At birth the infant should be able to assume all positions. Persistent asymmetry with or without discomfort in certain positions may be a sign of dysfunction requiring further intervention.

The physician should not feel intimidated by pediatric somatic dysfunction; the same principles apply as for diagnosing and treating adults. Infants and small children are apt not to cooperate with this process. The diagnosis and treatment of somatic dysfunction necessitate that the diagnostician physically invade the patient's space. Obviously this is more easily accomplished when the clinician is able to explain the process and its intent to the patient. For infants and children, who do not understand the verbal communication, physical communication and sincerity of approach are more important as the clinician addresses the child's total environment.

Infants and children require great delicacy of touch and sensitivity to asymmetric tension for the effective diagnosis of somatic dysfunction. The best results are obtained when the diagnosis and treatment are done without causing distress. The patient should not cry. Preverbal infants and children may not be able to tell you specifically when something feels good or not, but they will express themselves by cooperating when the procedure is properly applied and resisting when it is not. It is not possible to persuade an infant or child that what feels bad is ultimately going to be good for them. Because you are attempting to place the patient in the position of comfort, these patients offer you the ultimate feedback as to the proper application of your approach.

OMT is categorized as direct or indirect according to how the manipulative procedure is applied in relation to diagnosed motion restriction. By definition, indirect OMT takes the area of somatic dysfunction away from the dysfunctional restrictive barrier. Often it is said that the patient is placed in a position of ease. The etiologies of pediatric somatic dysfunction and the pliability of the pediatric musculoskeletal system make indirect procedures the treatment modalities of choice. Physiologically these patients are typically hyperreactors. As such, they tend to respond rapidly to low doses of OMT. Therefore, constant monitoring of their response to treatment is essential.

Inexperienced clinicians are often hesitant to use OMT on infants and children because they are concerned about injuring them. It is almost impossible to injure any patient with indirect OMT. It is necessary to be very careful if the patient cannot react, as perhaps with an infant who is extremely premature or small for gestational age. During application of indirect OMT, the dysfunctional barrier is disengaged and the patient is gently moved to a position of ease. This approach is ideal when treating the preverbal patient because when properly done the patient will experience comfort and cooperate with the process.

The principles of indirect functional OMT apply here.[15,16] The examination of the pediatric musculoskeletal system is directed at identifying the patterns of dysfunctional imbalance. Imbalance necessitates compensation, which is less efficient than unencumbered functional balance. The infant should be observed at rest. The infant will assume a posture that most approximates its position of comfort. Infants usually assume their intrauterine position. When dysfunctional mechanics are identified, adjacent anatomic areas should be evaluated for contributory dysfunction. Dysfunctional patterns following intrauterine posture very often involve several regions, for instance occipital, cervical, and thoracic.

CLINICAL CONDITIONS

The following is a list of problems frequently encountered in pediatric patients along with the dysfunctional mechanics that can produce them. The use of OMT is specifically indicated to treat the somatic dysfunction that results in a myriad of functional conditions. It *should not* substitute for a thorough history and physical examination to rule out organic pathologies.

Dysfunction of the Skull and Axial Skeleton

Plagiocephaly

Plagiocephaly[17] is distorted shape of the infant's skull, typically recognized in the first year of life. Functional plagiocephaly must be differentiated from synostotic plagiocephaly, a condition brought on by premature fusion of the cranial sutures. Synostotic plagiocephaly is demonstrable radiographically and treated surgically. In functional plagiocephaly, the cranial sutures are unfused and there is dysfunctional molding of the infant's skull. Etiologies proposed for functional plagiocephaly include intrauterine position, trauma during birth, and feeding and sleeping positions.[18]

Dysfunctional patterns between the occiput and the atlas (C1) and lateral strain of the SBS have been reported in correlation with plagiocephalies.[19] In 1992, the American Academy of Pediatrics suggested that to prevent sudden infant death syndrome (SIDS), infants be placed supine to sleep. Since then the incidence of posterior plagiocephaly has increased dramatically.[20] Asymmetric sleeping and/or feeding posture is a likely contributing factor for this condition. A baby should be able to rest comfortably. If only one side or position is chronically chosen, the head will become asymmetric. The infant with posterior plagiocephaly has asymmetric flattening of the occipitotemporal region and commonly contralateral flattening of the frontal region. Rotational dysfunction of occiput upon the atlas (C1) will predispose the infant to sleep with a preferential asymmetric head position, fostering the development of unilateral occipitotemporal flattening (Fig. 8.2). This results in a parallelogram deformity of the head viewed from above that is consistent with SBS lateral strain.[21] The effects upon the cervical and thoracic spine may also be grossly evident.

Torticollis

Torticollis, or wryneck, a malposition of the head and neck upon the torso, is the result of muscular imbalance involving the sternocleidomastoid, trapezius, and/or

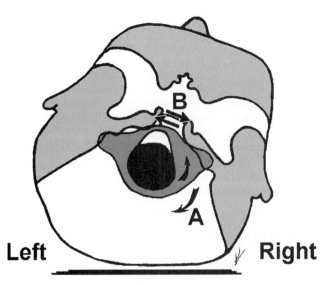

FIGURE 8.2   Viewed from above, the parallelogram shape of posterior plagiocephaly on the right, illustrating the relationship between occipital flattening (right), occipitoatlantal rotation (A) to the right and spheno-occipital synchondrosis right lateral strain pattern (B).

scalenes. In infants, "congenital torticollis" most commonly appears as cervical side bending and rotation in opposite directions. Various etiologies have been suggested: intrauterine position, impairment of the vascularization of the sternocleidomastoid, compartment syndrome,[22] and dysfunction between the first cervical and the occipital bone.[23]

The two components, side bending and rotation, may manifest to different degrees. Where side-bending mechanics are dominant, significant dysfunctional lateral translation of the occiput may be found. Torticollis may also be associated with dysfunction of the upper thoracic and cervical regions. Cranial dysfunction often involves the occiput and temporal bones, both acting upon cranial nerve XI.[24]

Infantile Scoliosis

Infantile scoliosis manifests between birth and age 3. It is often a non–weight-bearing spinal curvature. Intrauterine compressive forces were suggested as an etiology as early as Hippocrates.[25] Somatic dysfunction of the upper thoracic vertebrae is a straightforward cause of scoliosis in early life. The spinal curvature can also be the result of compensation from cranial somatic dysfunction. Infantile scoliosis is found in association with asymmetric developmental deformation of the occiput. Intraosseous dysfunction of the occiput can produce asymmetry of the occipital condylar parts, resulting in compensatory mechanics in the spine below. Somatic dysfunctions of the SBS, torsion, side bending, rotation, and lateral strains will also produce asymmetric head position that affects spinal mechanics. Additionally, compensatory spinal curves can occur as the result of somatic dysfunction caudal to the scoliosis. Intraosseous dysfunction of the sacrum with resultant asymmetry of the sacral base should be considered.

OMT is effective for infantile scoliosis that is the result of somatic dysfunction. Incomplete resolution should lead to a search for more significant etiologies, such as genetic disorder or congenital malformation.

Kyphosis

Similar to the side-bending deformity of infantile scoliosis, increased anteroposterior curvature of the thoracic spine can occur as the result of primary thoracic somatic dysfunction or compensatory mechanics. Dysfunctional mechanics should be sought in the upper thoracic vertebrae, ribs, or pectoral girdle. As a compensatory etiology, dysfunctional extension of the occiput upon the atlas (C1) can position the head upon the cervical spine such that increased cervical lordosis and thoracic kyphosis result.

Pectus Excavatum and Pectus Carinatum

Posterior deformation (pectus excavatum) of the sternum can result from direct derangement of the internal fascial structure of the thoracic cage and intraosseous dysfunction of the sternum. This can be associated with internal rotation of the paired structures, specifically the pectoral girdle. In pectus carinatum, similar mechanisms exist but with a tendency for external rotation of the paired structures.

Disorders of Weight-Bearing Mechanics

Disorders of the Hip

Hip disorders have varying degrees of severity. Congenital dislocation of the hip is an orthopedic condition. Subluxation, however, may respond well to OMT. Ortolani's sign indicates the need for further radiographic or ultrasonic diagnosis.

Location of the femoral capital epiphysis within the acetabular space is indication for conservative treatment.

Insufficient depth of the acetabulum without dislocation of the femoral head can be associated with pelvic somatic dysfunction. Intraosseous dysfunction at the conjunction of the ilium, ischium, and pubes results in a shallow acetabulum. There may also be associated dysfunction between the sacrum and homolateral innominate. This disorder demonstrates the importance of function on structure.

Patellar Disorders

Recurrent dislocation of the patella associated with improper tracking can result from inappropriate myofascial tension in the quadriceps. If the condition is unilateral tibial internal rotation, external rotation or glide dysfunction upon the femur should be considered. Bilateral conditions are more likely to have significant somatic dysfunction affecting the pelvis or even upper thoracic or craniocervical junction.

Valgus and Varus Patterns of the Lower Extremity

Varus problems of the knees and ankles are very often associated with flexion and external rotation patterns on the same side at the level of the lower extremity, the pelvis, the temporal bone, or the occipital bone. Similarly, valgus problems are associated with extension and internal rotation patterns of these same areas.

Flat and Hollow Feet

It is necessary to differentiate total flatfoot or hollow foot from partially flat foot or hollow foot. In the latter, only the posterior portion of the longitudinal arch is involved, resulting from dysfunction of the talocalcaneal junction.

Total flat foot is usually associated with a pattern of extension and internal rotation. Total hollow foot is associated with a pattern of flexion and external rotation. Dysfunctional mechanics may be found at the level of the feet as well as elsewhere in the lower extremity. Or the problem may be the result of weight bearing associated with dysfunction of the midline bones. Extension of the sacrum, increased anteroposterior curvatures of the spine, extension of the occiput upon the atlas (C1), and extension of the SBS can be associated with flat feet. In contrast, flexion of the sacrum, decreased anteroposterior curvatures of the spine, flexion of the occiput upon the atlas (C1), and flexion of the SBS are associated with hollow feet.

Disorders of the Digestive Tract

Suckling Dysfunction

Suckling is a reflex-mediated activity. When difficulty with suckling is encountered, a common solution is to provide a nipple with a larger opening or a softer consistency to reduce the effort necessary for successful nursing. Although this solution may be effective, it reduces the amount of muscular effort required. Adequate muscular action contributes to the growth of orofacial structures and may prevent malocclusion.

Treatment of cranial somatic dysfunction offers an additional approach when addressing suckling difficulties. Somatic dysfunction between the occipital and the temporal bones affects cranial nerve IX, the glossopharyngeal nerve, as it passes through the jugular foramen. Intraosseous dysfunction of the occipital bone can result in entrapment of cranial nerve XII, the hypoglossal nerve (Fig. 8.1).

Gastroesophageal Reflux

Infants normally bring up small amounts after feeding. Excessive vomiting may be associated with overfeeding or with the consumption of formula that is irritating to the infant. Often, however, in spite of carefully controlled feedings and multiple attempts to identify an acceptable formula, the infant continues to vomit excessively. OMT can be used to treat somatic dysfunction of the base of the skull to improve upper gastrointestinal irritability. Somatic dysfunction between the occipital and the temporal bones affects cranial nerve X, the vagus nerve, as it passes through the jugular foramen. Additionally, somatic dysfunction of the thoracoabdominal diaphragm should be treated to address the relationship between the esophagus and the diaphragm.

Colic and Constipation

The colicky infant is often irritated and crying. The constipated child may stay several days with incomplete or no bowel movements. Organic causes, such as congenital megacolon, hypothyroidism, cystic fibrosis, or Hirschsprung's disease, must be ruled out. Treatment of somatic dysfunction of the lumbar and pelvic regions commonly relieves the functional conditions of the gastrointestinal tract.

Ear, Nose, and Throat

Treatment of ear, nose, and throat problems should first address somatic dysfunction of the upper thoracic region, origin of the sympathetic supply to the head and neck. The suboccipital region is also important, possibly because of the reflex relationship with the trigeminal nerve, the final common pathway of both sympathetic and parasympathetic upper respiratory innervation.[26] Cranial somatic dysfunction may be specifically identified in relationship to various ear, nose, and throat dysfunctions.

Conditions of the ear, such as recurrent otitis media, have been demonstrated to respond to the treatment of somatic dysfunction.[27] After considering upper thoracic and cervico-occipital dysfunction, attention can be directed at the mechanics of the base of the skull. The occiput, sphenoid, and temporal bones provide attachment for muscles of the oropharynx. The tensor veli palatini and levator veli palatini affect the efficient opening and closing of the auditory tube and drainage of the middle ear. Also, the cartilaginous portion of the auditory tube that lies beneath at the petrosphenoid articulation is directly affected by dysfunctional mechanics between the sphenoid and temporal bones.

Nasal dysfunction may result from compression of the frontal bone with the ethmoid, lachrymal, maxillary, and nasal bones. This often arises from stresses placed upon the frontal bone by the maternal pelvis in the last trimester of pregnancy and during vertex delivery. Dysfunctional mechanics may result in nasal obstruction, noisy nasal respiration, and a predisposition to rhinitis and mouth breathing.

Recurrent pharyngitis in toddlers can be associated with cervical somatic dysfunction. Somatic dysfunction may contribute to impaired lymphatic drainage of the area with resulting edema and pain.

Dental Disorders

Oral respiration disrupts muscular forces exerted by the tongue, cheeks, and lips upon the maxillary arch. Oral respiration can be associated with malocclusion, gingivitis, and dental caries. Malocclusion and temporomandibular joint dysfunction can be produced by temporal, maxillary, and mandibular asymmetries. Bruxism may be associated with temporal dysfunction, temporomandibular dysfunction, and malocclusion.

Eyes

Myopia, hyperopia, certain types of strabismus, and lachrymal duct obstruction can be the result of craniofacial somatic dysfunction. The sagittal diameter of the orbital cavity is decreased with flexion and external rotation of the cranial bones and increased with extension and internal rotation. Myopia is associated with an increased anteroposterior diameter of the eyeball, hyperopia with a decreased diameter.

Because the extraocular muscles originate from the sphenoid and frontal bones and the maxillae, disorders involving asymmetric muscle pull mechanics, such as strabismus, can be addressed by checking for dysfunctions in this area. Dysfunction of cranial nerve VI, the abducens nerve, can occur because of mechanical stresses upon it as it passes beneath the petrosphenoid ligament. Altered mechanics between the temporal bones and sphenoid can produce this.

In mechanics similar to those described in the discussion of the nasal dysfunction, the frontal bone is compressed downward during the delivery. Compression of the lachrymal canal will result from dysfunction between the frontal, lachrymal, and maxillary bones. This condition should be addressed as soon as possible to prevent infection. Patients often respond dramatically to a single treatment.

Pulmonary Disorders

Bronchitis and asthma can be improved following the treatment of somatic dysfunction of the upper thoracic and cervical areas. In asthma, experience shows that T2 is frequently involved. The upper thoracic dysfunction is commonly encountered and is possibly the consequence of stress put upon the thoracic region when the shoulders are delivered during the birth process.

Psychomotor Development Dysfunctions

Delayed prone to supine position (average 3 to 6 months), supine to prone (average 4 to 7 months), or tripod sit (average 4 to 6 months) may be the consequence of cervical or thoracic dysfunction. Delayed sit position (average 4 to 6 months), creeping (average 4 to 8 months), and crawling (average 9 months) may result from pelvic dysfunctions.

Sleep Disorders

Somatic dysfunction anywhere in the body will disturb the infant and can result in irritability and sleep disorders. Somatic dysfunction of the skull is encountered in sleep disorders. A statistical correlation has been demonstrated between cranial dysfunction, specifically lateral strain of the SBS, and sleep disorder.[19] The SBS dysfunction can be treated with specific procedure described later in the chapter. Membranous articular dysfunction of the vault should also be addressed.

DIAGNOSING AND TREATING THE PEDIATRIC PATIENT

The palpatory diagnosis of somatic dysfunction is discussed at length in Chapter 3. However, a discussion of the most basic mechanics of cranial osteopathy is warranted here. Midline bones, including the ethmoid, vomer, sphenoid, occiput, and all of the vertebral segments, including the sacrum and coccyx, demonstrate flexion and extension as their primary motions. The paired bones of the skull, ribs, pelvic, and upper and lower extremities demonstrate external rotation, normally coupled with midline flexion. Internal rotation is normally coupled with midline extension. A detailed description of the specific motions of individual bones is available from the textbooks on the subject.[6,28-30]

The following protocol is intended to provide the clinical diagnostic information and the therapeutic sequence needed to initiate an intervention. In all of the clinical conditions described in this chapter, the examination and treatment can proceed as the following series of steps. They are described here, but the exact sequence in which they are performed should be dictated by the preference of the individual patient. There should be no separation between the diagnostic examination and treatment. As dysfunctional asymmetries are identified, they are treated using indirect principles. Allowing the patient to dictate the preferential sequence for the examination and treatment applies the concept of indirectness to the entire intervention. The connection with the child is essential. No harm should be done if one pays close attention to the reaction of the child. A child will not let anything uncomfortable happen; he or she will respond to any discomfort. Treating infants and children with OMT is a good school. The patient is the teacher and will provide feedback on how well the treatment is progressing.

Connect with the child. The first and possibly most important step is to establish nonverbal contact with the patient. All of the action to follow in the examination and treatment must be performed respectfully and with the full consent of the child. In the case of the preverbal infant, this will manifest as overt acceptance.

Observation is very important. Observe the child's preferential resting posture, position and movements of the feet, the legs, the pelvis, the torso, the arms, and the neck (side bending and rotation). Observe the shape of the head and the face. Children almost always position in the dysfunctional pattern. They will lie asymmetrically and prefer to move away from the dysfunctional barrier. Astute observation will allow one to recognize the areas of dysfunctional motion restriction.

Establish physical contact with the child. Older children can be instructed to lie on the examination table in the same manner as the adult patient. The physical examination of the infant often presents difficulties that require accommodation on the part of the physician. The best position for examination and treatment is lying on the examination table. The infant, however, may not willingly assume this position, and therefore, alternative positions should be considered. The infant can be examined while being held on the physician's lap or in the parent's arms.

The palpatory examination can begin with the pelvis. Place one warm hand under the sacrum palm up, with the index and little fingers each contacting one of the posterior superior iliac spines. Assess symmetry and motion restriction of the innominates to one another and the sacrum between the innominates. Maintaining sacral contact, place the other hand beneath the patient so that the fingertips are palpating the lumbar spinous processes. Assess the sacrum and the lumbar spine. Correct any dysfunctional pattern with indirect principles of treatment.

Next, examine the torso with attention to the thoracic cage. With one hand still in contact with the sacrum, place the other hand on the sternum. Assess for abnormalities in the shape of the torso. Assess the inherent rhythm of the child's body, CRI, and costal respiration. Determine whether the sacrum and sternum move in harmony. Any lack of freedom in the sternal area should lead to consideration of somatic dysfunction of the thoracic spine. Again, correct any dysfunctional pattern.

Leave one hand under the pelvis in contact with the sacrum and place the other hand on the top of the head, assessing the shape of the skull, palpating the vault, the forehead, and the temporal and the occipital parts. Leave this hand on the vault or on any area more comfortable for the child. Determine whether the sacrum and skull move in harmony. Palpate for asymmetry in the inherent motion, correct any dysfunctional pattern.

Now place both hands upon the skull and assess the SBS and any other cranial area and correct any dysfunctional pattern.

Description of Basic Procedures

Please note: The procedures that follow are examples of manipulative treatment that you may wish to employ. The actual choice of procedures used should be determined by the unique circumstances of each individual patient.

Lumbopelvic Release (Fig. 8.3)

This procedure is used to treat somatic dysfunction of the lumbar spine and pelvis.

Patient position: supine. Physician position: standing or seated facing in the direction of the patient's head and to the side of the patient such that the physician's dominant hand is closest to the patient.

Procedure

1. Place your dominant hand under the sacrum palm up, with the index and little fingers each contacting one of the posterior superior iliac spines.
2. Assess symmetry and motion restriction of the innominates to one another and the sacrum between the innominates.
3. Place the other hand beneath the patient so that your fingertips are palpating the lumbar spinous processes.
4. Assess the sacrum and the lumbar spine and palpate the motion associated with myofascial tensions and the inherent motion of the CRI.
5. Using indirect principles, correct any dysfunctional pattern.
6. When the procedure is complete, reassess the dysfunctional area.

Thoracic Release (Fig. 8.4)

This procedure is used to treat somatic dysfunction of the thoracic cage.

Patient position: seated or supine. Physician position: standing or seated to the side.

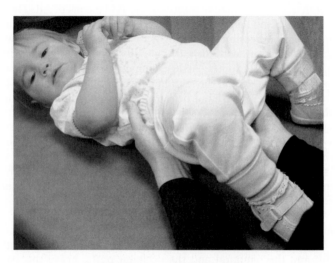

FIGURE 8.3   Lumbopelvic release.

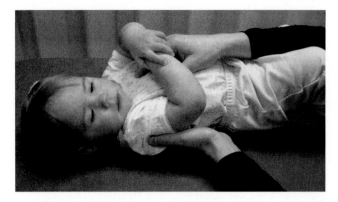

FIGURE 8.4   Thoracic release.

Procedure

1. Place one hand under the thorax palm up, with the tips of the fingers contacting the spinous processes of the thoracic spine.
2. Place the other hand on the sternum, paying attention to the sternocostal joints.
3. Palpate the motion associated with myofascial tensions, pulmonary respiration, and the inherent motion of the CRI.
4. Identify asymmetric tensions and motion restriction.
5. Using indirect principles, correct any dysfunctional pattern.
6. When the procedure is complete, reassess the dysfunctional area.

Cranial Membranous Release (Fig. 8.5)

This is a general procedure used to balance membranous tension in the skull and beyond. It can be employed as a first step to treat cranial dysfunction. The patient is preferably supine (but may be seated as in Fig. 8.5), and the physician is seated at the head of the table.

Procedure

1. Place one hand under the occiput.
2. Place the other in contact with the frontal bone.
3. Palpate the motion associated with membranous tensions between the frontal and occipital bones.
4. Palpate the rate and amplitude of the inherent motion of the CRI.
5. Identify asymmetric tensions and motion restriction.
6. Using indirect principles, correct any dysfunctional pattern.
7. When the procedure is complete, reassess the dysfunctional area.

Sphenobasilar Release (Fig. 8.6)

This procedure is used to treat somatic dysfunction between the occiput and the sphenoid at the SBS. The patient is preferably supine, and the physician is seated at the head or to the side of the table.

Procedure

1. Place your nondominant hand transversely in contact with the occiput so as to avoid contact with the occipitomastoid sutures.
2. Place your dominant hand with the palm resting gently across the frontal bone with the tip of the thumb in contact with the lateral aspect of the greater wing of the

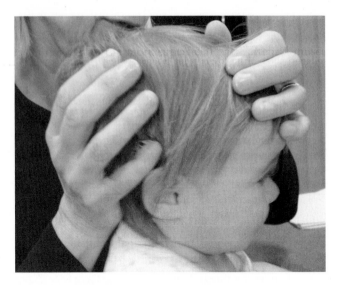

FIGURE 8.5 Cranial membranous release.

sphenoid on one side and with the tip of the middle finger in contact with the lateral aspect of the greater wing of the sphenoid on the other side.
3. Palpate the rate and amplitude of the inherent motion of the CRI.
4. Palpate the motion between the sphenoid and occipital bones, thus evaluating the SBS. Assess for flexion, extension, torsion, side-bending rotation, lateral and vertical strains, and compression.
5. Identify asymmetric tensions and motion restriction.
6. Using indirect principles, correct any dysfunctional pattern.
7. When the procedure is complete, reassess the dysfunctional area.

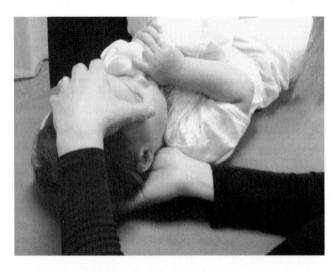

FIGURE 8.6 Sphenobasilar release.

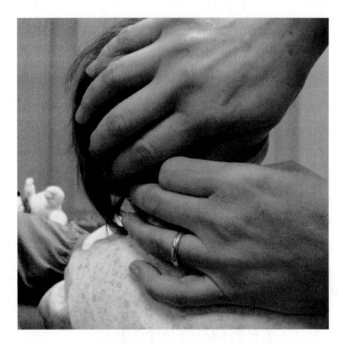

FIGURE 8.7   Occipital release.

Occipital Release (Fig. 8.7)

This procedure is used to treat dysfunction of the craniocervical junction. The patient is supine (but may be seated as in Fig. 8.7), and the physician is seated at the head of the table.

Procedure

1. Place your dominant hand palm up beneath the patient's head, contacting the occiput but not the occipitomastoid sutures.
2. Place the tip of the index or middle finger of the other hand at the level of the spinous process of the atlas (C1).
3. Palpate the motion between the occipital bone and the atlas (C1). Assess for flexion, extension, side bending, and rotation.
4. Identify asymmetric tensions and motion restriction.
5. Using indirect principles, correct any dysfunctional pattern.
6. When the procedure is complete, reassess the dysfunctional area.

Occipitomastoid Release (Fig. 8.8)

This procedure is used to treat dysfunction of the occipitomastoid suture. In this example, the right occipitomastoid suture will be treated.

Patient position: supine or seated as in Fig. 8.8. Physician position: seated at the head of the table.

Procedure

1. Place your left hand transversely palm up beneath the patient's head, contacting the occiput such that the tip of the fingers are medial to the right occipitomastoid suture.
2. Place the right hand such that the tips of the index and middle fingers are in contact with the mastoid portion of the temporal bone.

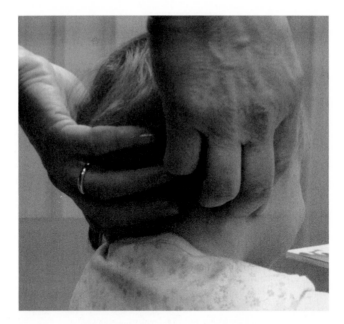

FIGURE 8.8 Occipitomastoid release.

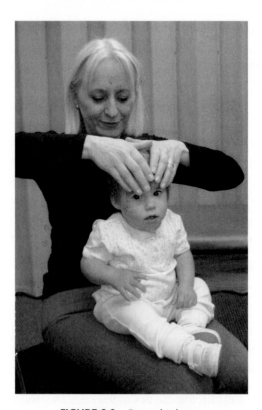

FIGURE 8.9 Frontal release.

3. Palpate the motion between the occipital and temporal bones.
4. Identify motion restriction.
5. Using indirect principles, correct any dysfunctional pattern.
6. When the procedure is complete, reassess the dysfunctional area.

Frontal Release (Fig. 8.9)

This procedure is used to treat somatic dysfunction of the frontal bone. It is particularly important to treat somatic dysfunction of the frontal bone before any attempt to treat specific problems involving the face.

Patient position: supine or seated as in Fig. 8.9. Physician position: seated at the head of the table.

Procedure

1. Place both hands in contact with the frontal bone, such that the index fingers are aligned on either side of the metopic suture and the other fingertips contact the brow ridges bilaterally.
2. Palpate the motion between the left and right halves of the frontal bone and the rate and amplitude of the inherent motion of the CRI.
3. Identify motion restriction.
4. Using indirect principles, correct any dysfunctional pattern.
5. When the procedure is complete, reassess the dysfunctional area.

References

1. Irwin GL. Roentgen determination of the time of closure of the spheno-occipital synchondrosis. Radiology 1960;75:450–453.
2. Madeline LA, Elster AD. Suture closure in the human chondrocranium: CT assessment. Radiology 1995;196:747–56.
3. Mann SS, Naidich TP, Towbin RB, Doundoulakis SH. Imaging of postnatal maturation of the skull base. Neuroimaging Clin North Am 2000;10:1–21, vii.
4. Melsen B. Time of closure of the spheno-occipital synchondrosis determined on dry skulls: A radiographic craniometric study. Acta Odontol Scand 1969;27:73–90.
5. Okamoto K, Ito J, Tokiguchi S, Furusawa T. High-resolution CT findings in the development of sphenooccipital synchondrosis. Am J Neuroradiol 1996;17:117–120.
6. Magoun HI. Osteopathy in the Cranial Field. 2nd ed. Kirksville, MO: Journal, 1966.
7. Sutherland WG. The Cranial Bowl. Mankato, MN: Free Press, 1939:45.
8. ICD-9CM International Classification of Diseases, 9th Revision: Clinical Modification. 5th ed. Salt Lake City: Medicode, 1999.
9. Collins P. Embryology and development. In: Williams PL, ed. Gray's Anatomy. 38th ed. Edinburgh: Churchill Livingstone, 1995:257.
10. Nelson KE, Sergueef N, Lipinski CM, et al. Cranial rhythmic impulse related to the Traube-Hering-Mayer oscillation: Comparing laser-Doppler flowmetry and palpation. J Am Osteopath Assoc 2001;101:163–173.
11. Akselrod S, Gordon D, Madwed JB, et al. Hemodynamic regulation: Investigation by spectral analysis. Am J Physiol 1985;249(4 pt 2):H867–H875.
12. Sergueef N, Nelson KE, Glonek T. The effect of cranial manipulation upon the Traube-Hering-Mayer oscillation as measured by laser-Doppler flowmetry. Altern Ther Health Med 2002;8:74–76.
13. Moskalenko YE, Kravchenko TI. Wave phenomena in movements of intracranial liquid media and the primary respiratory mechanism. AAO J 2004;14(2):29–40.
14. Nelson KE, Sergueef N, Glonek T. Cranial manipulation induces sequential changes in blood flow velocity on demand. AAO J 2004;14(3):15–17.

15. Bowles CH. A functional orientation for technic. 1955 Yearbook. Indianapolis: American Academy of Osteopathy, 1955;177–191.

16. Johnston WL, Friedman HD. Functional Methods: A Manual for Palpatory Skill Development in Osteopathic Examination and Manipulation of Motor Function. Indianapolis: American Academy of Osteopathy, 1994.

17. Sergueef N. Approche ostéopathique des plagiocéphalies avec ou sans torticolis. Paris: Spek, 2004.

18. Peitsch WK, Keefer CH, LaBrie RA, Mulliken JB. Incidence of cranial asymmetry in healthy newborns. Pediatrics. Dec 2002;110(6):e72.

19. Sergueef N, Nelson KE, Glonek T. Palpatory diagnosis of plagiocephaly. Complement Ther Clin Pract 2006;12:101–110.

20. Kane AA, Mitchell LE, Craven KP, Marsh JL. Observations on a recent increase in plagio-cephaly without synostosis. Pediatrics 1996;97(6 Pt 1):877–885.

21. Sergueef N, Nelson KE, Glonek T. Palpatory diagnosis of plagiocephaly. J Am Osteopath Assoc 2004;104:339.

22. Davids JR, Wenger DR, Mubarak SJ. Congenital muscular torticollis: Sequela of intrauterine or perinatal compartment syndrome. J Pediatr Orthop 1993;13:141–147.

23. Jacquemart M, Piedallu P. Le torticolis "congénital" est-il simplement un torticolis obstétri-cal? Concours Méd 1964;36:4867–4870.

24. Sergueef N. La thérapie cranio-sacrée chez l'enfant. Paris: Spek, 1988.

25. Dunn PM. Congenital postural deformities. Br Med Bull 1976;32:71–76.

26. Sumino R, Nozaki S, Kato M. Central pathway of trigemino-neck reflex. In: Oral-facial sensory and motor functions. International Symposium. Rappongi, Tokyo; Oral Physiol. 1980:28 [abstract].

27. Mills MV, Henley CE, Barnes LL, et al. The use of osteopathic manipulative treatment as adjuvant therapy in children with recurrent acute otitis media. Arch Pediatr Adolesc Med 2003;157:861–866.

28. Sutherland WG. The Cranial Bowl. Mankato, MN: Free Press, 1939; reprinted 1986.

29. Upledger JE, Vredevoogd JD. Craniosacral Therapy. Chicago: Eastland, 1983.

30. King HH, Lay E. Osteopathy in the cranial field. In: Ward RC, ed. Foundations for Osteopathic Medicine. 2nd ed. Philadelphia: Lippincott Williams & Wilkins, 2002; 985–1001.

CHAPTER 9

The Female Patient

Kenneth E. Nelson and Joey Rottman

INTRODUCTION

The practice of osteopathic medicine stresses the importance of dysfunction of the neuromusculoskeletal system in all aspects of patient care. Somatic dysfunction may be primarily responsible for the patient's complaints. It may contribute to a greater or lesser extent to concomitant illness. Or it may be a reflection (viscerosomatic reflex) of existent visceral pathology. Application of this understanding to the diagnosis and treatment of gynecologic and obstetric patients affords a distinctive approach to care.

The skills necessary to diagnose somatic dysfunction and the effects of its treatment offer multiple advantages in the practice of obstetrics and gynecology. The identification of viscerosomatic reflexes augments physical diagnosis. The ability of clinicians skilled in the diagnosis of somatic dysfunction to palpate lightly and appreciate subtle tissue texture abnormalities is also useful for diagnosis of gynecologic and obstetric conditions other than somatic dysfunction. Emphasis upon dysfunction of the neuromusculoskeletal system, with its resultant pain, neural facilitation (somatovisceral effects), and circulatory compromise, gives the osteopathic approach to medical practice an advantage in the treatment of the conditions unique to female patients. The ability to employ specifically controlled forces as applied in osteopathic manipulative treatment (OMT) can be beneficial in obstetric procedures.

It is not the purpose of this chapter to review the practice of gynecology and obstetrics. That information is readily available elsewhere. Rather this chapter addresses the diagnostic and therapeutic approach to the care of the female patient that is unique to osteopathic medicine.

GYNECOLOGY

A significant number of gynecologic patients present with pelvic pain as a chief complaint. The pain may be deep within the pelvis, in the perineum, in the lower abdomen, or in the low back. Many gynecologic problems, such as endometriosis, adenomyosis, mittelschmerz, and various pelvic infections, present as pelvic pain. These conditions result in viscerosomatic reflexes involving the spinal segments innervating the site of pathology.

Viscerosomatic Reflexes

Viscerosomatic reflexes offer diagnostic clues. They are mediated through general visceral afferent neurons in either the sympathetic or parasympathetic nerves. The resultant reflex manifests as palpable tissue texture abnormality and tenderness in the dermatomes and myotomes of the spinal cord level from which the primary cell bodies of respective sympathetic and parasympathetic efferent neurons originate. The intensity of the palpable tissue texture abnormality of a viscerosomatic reflex offers an indication of the severity of the visceral pathology responsible for the reflex.

The locations of viscerosomatic reflexes may demonstrate slight variation among individuals. Yet they are reliable because of the overall consistency of the anatomy of the nervous system. The sympathetic gynecologic viscerosomatic reflexes are as follows: ovaries T10 to T11 lateralized, uterus T9 to L2 bilateral, fallopian tubes T10 to L2 lateralized. The preponderance of parasympathetic innervation of the female genitourinary tract emanates from the pelvic splanchnic nerves, S2 to S4. The lateral half of the fallopian tubes, however, receives parasympathetic innervation from the vagus nerve. Thus, the high cervical vagal viscerosomatic reflex may explain the occurrence of some headaches in association with various gynecologic problems.

If visceral inflammation involves the parietal peritoneum because it is innervated by somatosensory nerves, a somatosomatic reflex will be present at the spinal level innervating the inflamed peritoneum.

The identification of tissue texture abnormality and tenderness resulting from viscerosomatic and somatosomatic reflexes in any of these paraspinal regions should lead the physician to consider the possibility of segmentally related visceral pathology as part of the differential diagnosis. Treatment of these somatic findings results in transient pain relief at best and more often has no effect. The definitive treatment of the underlying visceral pathology is the only effective treatment.

Somatovisceral Reflexes

The segmental spinal facilitation associated with a viscerosomatic reflex also results in increased efferent stimulation (sympathetic or parasympathetic depending upon the spinal level) to the site of visceral pathology. OMT can be employed adjunctively to affect these somatovisceral reflexes. OMT may also be employed to treat residual somatic dysfunction after the primary visceral pathology has been treated.

Primary spinal somatic dysfunction results in facilitation that can affect segmentally related organs through increased sympathetic or parasympathetic activity. Functional visceral symptoms that are the result of somatovisceral reflexes may be alleviated by treating the underlying somatic dysfunction and when appropriate, postural imbalance that predisposes the individual to that somatic dysfunction. It has been suggested that correction of inequality of leg length, which is responsible for chronic sacral somatic dysfunction, may be a prime factor in the treatment of pathophysiologic changes affecting the pelvic organs.[1]

Dysmenorrhea is cramping pelvic pain associated with menstruation. Although this is an oversimplification, sympathetic activity results in uterine contraction, and parasympathetic activity results in uterine relaxation. Treatment of thoracolumbar somatic dysfunction will reduce sympathetic input to the uterus. Clinical experience has demonstrated that pressure applied over the sacrum of a prone patient frequently reduces the severity of menstrual cramps. If effective, the procedure can be taught to a family member.

Somatic Dysfunction

It is fairly common for a specific organic cause for pelvic pain to fail to be identified and for the patient to be described as having chronic pelvic pain, that is, pelvic pain of unidentified etiology of more than 6 months' duration. More than one-third of 60 women in a random series of outpatient gynecologic visits presented with pain as the primary symptom. Of these individuals, 75% had no identifiable organic cause.[2] Commonly, the somatic dysfunction responsible for persistent pelvic pain first develops during or just after pregnancy because of the stresses placed upon the low back and pelvis.

Somatic dysfunction must not be overlooked as an etiology for pain resembling gynecologic pathology. Because visceral pain is often dull and vague as to location, it is often mimicked by musculoskeletal pain of somatic dysfunction. Spinal and sacropelvic somatic dysfunction can result in low back, lower abdominal, and perineal pain. Recognizing this may save many a patient from unnecessary diagnostic procedures.

Spasm of psoas major often produces lumbosacral pain. There may also be pain in the inguinal region and in the upper inner thigh, where the iliopsoas tendon crosses over the pubic ramus and where it inserts upon the lesser trochanter of the femur respectively. The primary dysfunction in this instance is often Fryette's type II flexion mechanics in the upper lumbar spine. Such dysfunctional mechanics may also result in inguinal pain because of segmental facilitation with resultant hypersensitivity in the L1, L2 dermatomes.

Sacropelvic somatic dysfunction produces pelvic pain. Sacroiliac somatic dysfunction is complex. A complete discussion of these mechanics is beyond the scope of this chapter. Many sources are available to the individual who wishes to review this subject in depth.[3–8]

Within the pelvis are three articulations, the pubic symphysis and the two sacroiliac joints, that can become dysfunctional. When there is dysfunctional motion restriction in one of these articulations, compensatory stresses are placed on the other two, and the pelvis often twists in accommodation.[9] The patient's pain complaint may therefore be in the region of the primary dysfunction or in an adjacent area that is under compensatory stress.

Sacroiliac articular somatic dysfunction results in restricted motion of the involved joint. Sacroiliac dysfunction often results in pain directly referable to the involved joint. It is often accompanied by pain in the buttocks and—in response to involvement of the ilium—inguinal region.

Pubic symphysis dysfunction results in symphyseal suprapubic pain and perineal pain. It is often encountered as a result of the stress of walking with a change in the center of gravity caused by the ever-expanding uterus. Or it may be encountered post partum as a result of the stresses placed upon the pelvis by labor and delivery. Pubic symphysis dysfunction typically occurs as a superior or inferior shearing stress. The pelvic bone on the side of the superiorly displaced pubis will be displaced slightly superiorly and posteriorly. This will tend to produce pain in the superior aspect of the sacroiliac joint and the inguinal ligament on that side. The pelvic bone on the side of the inferiorly displaced pubis will be displaced slightly inferiorly and anteriorly. This will tend to produce pain in the inferior aspect of the sacroiliac joint on that side.

Twisting of the pelvis, whether from sacroiliac dysfunction, pubic symphysis dysfunction or from mechanics above (psoas spasm, scoliosis) or below (unequal leg length) the pelvis, will result in asymmetric stresses upon the soft tissues within the pelvis. Pain in the musculature of the pelvic floor and the sacrospinous and sacrotuberous ligaments may be confused with pain from pathology of the pelvic organs. Tenderness of these structures produces dyspareunia. Asymmetric spasm of the levator ani muscle (levator ani syndrome or proctalgia fugax) confuses clinicians who do not understand pelvic somatic dysfunction.

Central Facilitation

Chronic pelvic pain patients are commonly incapacitated by the pain. The pain is frequently exacerbated by emotional factors. The fact that no etiology has been identified may lead the patient to question her own perceptions. Further, because no etiology has been identified, no definitive treatment is available other than symptom suppression.

In a significant number of cases, chronic pelvic pain is associated with childhood sexual abuse and as with other forms of chronic pain, with current or past physical abuse, which necessitates a thorough psychosocial history to elucidate somatoemotional and somatoform mechanisms that may be active in pelvic pain. (See Chapter 7.)

The frustration, anger, and anxiety of patients with chronic pelvic pain results in a state of facilitation within the central nervous system. This central facilitation may lower thresholds for nociception, making even normal sensory input painful.[10]

OBSTETRICS

The practice of obstetrics has been an integral part of osteopathic medicine since its inception.[11] Osteopathic principles and the diagnosis and treatment of somatic dysfunction in the obstetric patient are the same as for any other patient.

The obstetric patient, however, is subject to altered musculoskeletal mechanics as the gravid uterus expands. The patient's weight increases, and her center of gravity shifts anteriorly. This affects the lumbar lordosis. The area of T8 to T11 generally becomes the area of transition between the lumbar lordosis and thoracic kyphosis due to the anterior shift of the center of gravity and the exaggeration of the thoracic and lumbar curves that progresses during pregnancy. (See Chapter 27.) These alterations also cause a progressively widening gait.[12]

Most people have inequality of leg length.[13] (See Chapter 26.) The weight-bearing stresses of pregnancy introduce new or aggravate preexisting compensated dysfunctional mechanics and make low back pain one of the most frequently encountered complaints during pregnancy. Although these conditions are unavoidable, the effective treatment of somatic dysfunction alleviates discomfort without the use of unnecessary medications and makes pregnancy significantly more tolerable.

Total body water increases progressively during pregnancy, reaching 6 to 8 L, most of which is distributed in the extracellular space.[14] Fluid exchange between the intravascular and interstitial spaces, as described by Starling's equilibrium, is such that more than 10% of the water that leaves the intravascular space must be returned to the general circulation via the lymphatic system. Swelling of the extremities is a common complaint during pregnancy. Interstitial edema can be sufficient to compromise structures within confined spaces. Carpal tunnel syndrome during pregnancy is extremely common. The diagnosis and treatment of myofascial dysfunction of the extremities may be used to enhance the efficiency of the muscular pump's ability to decongest the interstitial space. Direct stretching of the transverse carpal ligament,[15] active articulation of the carpal bones, and treatment of pectoral girdle and upper thoracic (sympathetic supply to the upper extremity) somatic dysfunction[16] have been shown to reduce median nerve compression within the carpal tunnel.

As the uterus expands, it displaces the abdominal contents upward, limiting excursion of the diaphragm and consequently the mechanical efficiency of the respiratory effort. Pulmonary respiratory efficiency actually increases during pregnancy in compensation for the mechanical compromise of respiration. Alternating positive and negative intrathoracic pressure as the result of inspiratory and expiratory mechanics is also responsible for returning venous blood and lymph to the heart. It is therefore appropriate to address somatic dysfunction of the thoracic spine, ribs, and diaphragm to optimize the function of the thoracic cage as a central lymphatic pump.

DIAGNOSIS AND TREATMENT

The diagnosis and treatment of somatic dysfunction in obstetric and gynecologic patients is no different from that of any other adult. There are, however, some issues that are particularly commonly encountered in this patient population. Low back pain is a common complaint of obstetric patients. Chronic and acute pelvic pain is a frequently perplexing gynecologic diagnosis that may simply indicate undiagnosed somatic dysfunction. Dyspareunia may have its origin in somatic dysfunction.

The osteopathic approach to the female patient provides unique diagnostic methods and treatment modalities to support the patient with obstetric and gynecological needs. It is an obligation that OMT be one of the tools at the osteopathic practitioner's disposal. No pregnant patient who complains of low back pain should leave the office with only a prescription for acetaminophen. No nonpregnant patient with pelvic pain should be scheduled for an imaging study or an invasive surgical procedure without a thorough evaluation for somatic dysfunction, including an internal pelvic structural examination.

Therefore, this chapter focuses upon the diagnosis and treatment of pelvic somatic dysfunction. The diagnosis of pelvic somatic dysfunction must include consideration of structures above and below the pelvis. That a patient's complaint identifies a specific anatomic structure or area does not necessarily mean that is the primary site of somatic dysfunction responsible for the complaint.

The diagnosis of somatic dysfunction necessitates a thorough knowledge of anatomy. If one knows the structure of an area, one can understand its function and recognize how the functional limitation of somatic dysfunction can produce the patient's complaint. One of the problems encountered when attempting to diagnose nonvisceral pelvic pain is the failure to identify the specific painful structures. When performing the gynecologic bimanual examination, it is standard procedure to palpate the uterine cervix, fundus, and adnexa. Rarely does anyone consider the sacrospinous and sacrotuberous ligaments, the iliopsoas tendon, the levator ani muscles, or the small muscles of the perineum.

When a patient complains of chronic pelvic pain or dyspareunia, such an internal pelvic structural examination is imperative. Notice asymmetric tension (tissue texture change) when the muscles and ligaments are palpated and on which side a painful response (tenderness) is elicited. Correlate these findings with the findings of the remainder of the structural musculoskeletal examination. Once treatment is initiated, recheck the muscles and ligaments internally for change and note the difference.

The anatomy of the female neuromusculoskeletal system, with the exception of the fine anatomy of the perineum, is not unique. The ordinary mechanics of somatic dysfunction apply for diagnosis and treatment here. The obstetric patient, however, does present some difficulty, particularly in the later months of pregnancy, when it is not possible for her to comfortably lie prone. For this reason, descriptions of diagnostic methods in the following section focus upon an approach suitable for diagnosis of a patient in the third trimester of pregnancy. With one exception, these procedures are done with the patient supine or laterally recumbent.

Many authors[3–8] have described somatic dysfunction of the sacrum and pelvis. Although initially these descriptions may appear incongruous, one who thoroughly understands pelvic anatomy can appreciate the commonality and differences of the various descriptions. Somatic dysfunction typically involves restrictions of musculoskeletal physiologic motion. These are the mechanics reviewed in this chapter. However, the potentially traumatic forces of the birth process upon the pelvis result in a multitude of shearing stresses that can result in aberrant dysfunctional patterns.

Sacropelvic Somatic Dysfunction

The Physiologic Motion of the Sacrum

Sacral mechanics can be considered relative to the ilia (anterior and posterior sacrum) or relative to the lumbar spine (forward and backward torsion). Under both circumstances, sacral rotation occurs about either the right or left oblique axis. Sacroiliac dysfunctions typically demonstrate the pattern of rotation and side bending in opposite directions.

The Sacrum and the Ilium

Anterior and Posterior

An anterior sacrum by definition is anterior to the ipsilateral ilium. Therefore, if the ilium is described relative to the sacrum, it is posterior to the sacrum. This does not necessarily mean it is a "posterior ilium." The terms *anterior ilium* and *posterior ilium* refer to the position of one ilium relative to the other. This may result from asymmetric soft tissue tensions, dysfunctional sacroiliac articulation, pubic symphysis, or lumbosacral mechanics. A similar relationship exists between the sacrum and ipsilateral ilium on the side of the posterior sacrum.

As the sacrum moves, so goes the ilium: When rotational forces are applied to the sacrum from above and the sacrum rotates, the sacroiliac ligaments are placed on tension and the ilia move with the sacrum but to a lesser degree.[9]

Sacroiliac somatic dysfunction is associated with spasm and pain of pelvic musculature. A posterior sacrum is often accompanied by spasm in the piriformis muscle. As the sacrum rotates posteriorly, its ventral surface moves away from the greater trochanter, placing the ipsilateral piriformis muscle on tension. This initiates a stretch reflex, which results in spasm.

A similar relationship between an anterior sacrum and gluteus medius tension is less immediately obvious. The anterior sacrum is anterior to the ipsilateral ilium. Posterior movement of the sacrum relative to the ilium on the dysfunctional side is restricted. With normal weight bearing, forces acting upon the anterior sacrum from above through the lumbar spine tend to pull it posteriorly (toward a neutral position). Because of the sacroiliac restriction, the ilium is also pulled posterior relative to the femur. This places tension upon the gluteus medius (and gluteus minimus), which originates on the ilium between the iliac crest and the posterior gluteal line above and the anterior gluteal line below and inserts upon the lateral aspect of the greater trochanter. The increased tension on the muscle results in spasm.

Lumbosacral Mechanics, Sacral Torsions

Side bending of the lumbar spine upon the sacrum engages the sacral oblique axis on the side of the bending. That is, side bending right engages the right oblique axis, and side bending left engages the left oblique axis. With neutral weight bearing (absence of significant forward or backward bending), the sacrum relative to L5 moves forward on the side opposite the engaged oblique axis. This forward torsion is further identified by the sacral mechanics on the involved oblique axis, that is, right on right or left on left.

In the presence of significant forward or backward bending, the sacrum relative to L5 will move backward on the side opposite the engaged oblique axis. This backward torsion is further identified by the sacral mechanics on the involved oblique axis, that is, left on right or right on left.

The Symphysis Pubis

Superior and inferior shearing mechanics are most commonly seen in association with pubic dysfunction. This dysfunction is seen both ante and post partum and following strenuous use of the adductor muscles of the thighs.

Iliopsoas Mechanics

Psoas spasm occurs bilaterally; however, one side frequently exerts more force. This asymmetry of muscle pull produces an active pelvic side shift in the direction away from the side of the predominantly tight psoas. Psoas spasm may be classified as primary or secondary.

Primary

Somatic dysfunction in the upper half of the lumbar spine produces psoas spasm. Type II mechanics of L1 on L2 or L2 on L3, typically in flexion with rotation and side bending toward the side of the predominant psoas muscle, are the most commonly encountered dysfunctional etiology.

Secondary

In the presence of lumbosacral inflammation (discitis) or instability (herniated nucleus pulposis, spondylolisthesis), physiologic splinting of the surrounding musculature results in psoas spasm. The forward displacement of the patient's center of gravity as the gravid uterus grows results in increased stress upon the lumbosacral junction, with resultant psoas spasm a common occurrence.

Forces Acting Upward (See Chapter 26)

Short leg mechanics result in sacral unleveling, producing lumbosacral and sacropelvic somatic dysfunction. (See Chapter 6.) Errors in locomotion, another cause of lumbosacral and sacropelvic dysfunction, affect the pelvis from below.

Forces Acting Downward (See Chapters 26, 27, and 28)

Psoas spasm and idiopathic scoliosis are two examples of conditions above the pelvis that produce sacropelvic dysfunction. (See Chapters 26 and 28.)

Cranial Considerations

The sacrum and pelvis are thought to be linked to the cranial mechanics through the reciprocal tension membrane.

Viscerosomatic Considerations (See Chapter 5)

Hyperactivity in visceral afferent nerves due to visceral disease or dysfunction will produce segmentally related reflex somatic dysfunction. Genitourinary and lower gastrointestinal pathology produce reflexes referable to the lower spine.

Structural Examination of the Obstetric Patient (See Also Chapter 3)

Because of the shift in center of gravity that results from fetal growth and uterine enlargement, examination of the obstetric patient for somatic dysfunction may seem difficult. In particular, during the latter stages of pregnancy, the patient cannot comfortably lie prone. In fact, with minimal modification the structural examination of the pregnant patient is relatively simple. The following sequence may be employed.

Patient Standing

1. Monitor gait. Is the gait symmetric from side to side? How wide is the patient's gait? Evaluate spinal anteroposterior curves. As the pregnancy progresses, the transition between the thoracic kyphosis and the lumbar lordosis tends to shift upward to between T11 and T8.
2. Evaluate for asymmetry of bilateral landmarks: mastoid processes, acromion processes, inferior angles of the scapulae, iliac crests, sacral sulcae, and greater trochanters. Do a pelvic side shift to test for iliopsoas mechanics.
3. Instruct the patient to bend forward, and do a standing flexion test to assess iliosacral mechanics.
4. While the patient is bent over, observe for asymmetric paravertebral prominence indicative of the spinal rotation associated with type I spinal curves.

Patient Seated on an OMT Table

1. Stand behind the patient and perform a seated flexion test to assess for sacroiliac restriction.
2. To evaluate the sacroiliac motion restriction more specifically, with the patient again sitting up straight, palpate the right sacral sulcus and rotate the patient's upper torso to the left. This will introduce rotation down through the sacroiliac joints. The sacrum should rotate with the trunk to the left and side bend to the right. The right sacral sulcus should become deeper.
3. Repeat the process for the left sacroiliac joint by rotating the patient's torso to the right and palpating the left sacral sulcus.

4. Palpate the superior and inferior poles of the sacroiliac joints for tissue texture abnormality and tenderness. Compare tissue reactivity of the superior pole to that of the inferior pole. This information, in association with findings of asymmetric motion restriction, will allow you to diagnose articular sacroiliac somatic dysfunction. Tissue reactivity greater at the inferior pole is consistent with a posterior sacrum on that side. Tissue reactivity at the superior pole is consistent with an anterior sacrum.
5. Assess the lumbar and thoracic spine for TART (**t**enderness to palpation, **a**symmetry of position, **r**estriction of motion, and **t**issue texture change) findings.

Patient Supine

1. Evaluate the rest of the musculoskeletal system with the patient supine. This portion of the examination may be less efficiently performed in the lateral recumbent position if the uterus compresses the inferior vena cava when the patient lies supine. Include the occipitoatlantal, thoracolumbar, and lumbosacral transition areas. These areas are the most stressed as the pregnancy progresses.
2. Palpate the sacrum by placing your hand palm up beneath the patient and rock it to assess restriction of articular motion. Assess the inherent sacral motion of the cranial rhythmic impulse (CRI).
3. Check anterior counterstrain points and innominate and pubic bone dysfunction.

Procedures

Please note: The procedures that follow are examples of manipulative treatment that you may wish to employ. The actual choice of procedures used should be determined by the unique circumstances of each individual patient.

Sacrum, Inhibitory Pressure (Fig. 9.1)

This procedure is employed to decrease the severity of dysmenorrhea. It is simple and effective and may appropriately be taught to the patient's family members. (For diagnosis, see Chapter 3.)

Patient position: prone. Physician position: standing to one side at the level of the patient's pelvis.

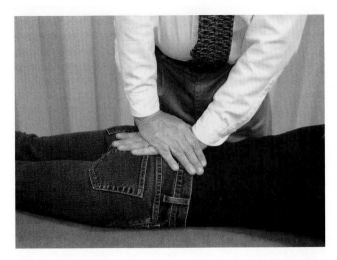

FIGURE 9.1 Inhibitory pressure applied over the sacrum for dysmenorrhea.

Procedure

1. Place one hand palm down along the patient's vertical axis upon the sacrum (the direction, cephalad or caudad, of the fingers should be determined by personal comfort) and place your other hand palm down over the first hand.
2. Fully extend your elbows and lock them.
3. Apply pressure slowly to the sacrum through your arms by gradually lowering the weight of your torso onto the patient's pelvis.
4. When you have applied as much weight as is tolerable to the patient, hold this pressure steadily for at least 1 or 2 minutes.
5. Release the pressure very slowly by gradually lifting your torso.
6. Repeat as necessary.

Lumbar Paravertebral Muscles (Soft Tissue) (Fig. 9.2)

This procedure is employed to relax hypertonic lumbar paravertebral muscles. It is useful in the third trimester and during labor, as it reduces the low back discomfort of this time. It is described here with the patient on her side. It can be modified, since during labor position changes become inappropriate or difficult. Under these circumstances allow the patient to remain supine and slide your hands palm up beneath her low back and perform the soft tissue stretch in a fashion similar to that employed for rib raising. (See Chapter 5.) These procedures are simple and effective and may appropriately be taught to the patient's family members.

The patient lies on either side with her hips and knees comfortably flexed to provide stability for her torso. The lower arm may be placed under her head and the other arm, wherever it is comfortable and out of the way. The physician stands facing the patient at the level of the lumbar spine.

Procedure

1. Wrap your hands over the patient's flank and grasp the upper paraspinal musculature at the level of the thoracolumbar junction.
2. Place one of your feet in front of the other for stability.

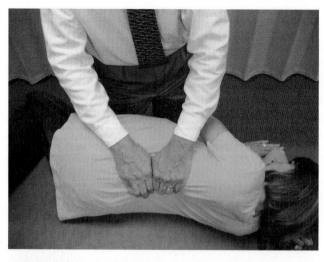

FIGURE 9.2 Lumbar paravertebral muscles soft tissue stretching.

3. Keeping your back straight, lean back and use your body weight to apply antero-lateral traction slowly through both hands.
4. Hold this position until the muscles relax.
5. Release the force slowly and work up and down the lumbar spine, treating tight areas.
6. When the procedure is complete, reassess the dysfunctional area.
7. Have the patient roll to the other side and repeat the procedure.

Psoas Release (Indirect) (Fig. 9.3)

This procedure is employed to reflexively reduce hypertonicity of the psoas major muscle. (See Chapter 26.)

Patient position: supine. Physician position: standing on the side of the tight psoas muscle at the level of the pelvis, facing the patient's head.

Procedure (Example: Right Psoas Muscle)

1. Stand on the patient's right side.
2. Place your left hand under the right upper lumbar paraspinal musculature and palpate for areas of tension. The paraspinal musculature that is antagonistic to the tight right psoas muscle will be palpably tight.
3. Monitor the area of palpable paravertebral tension with your left hand throughout the remainder of the procedure.
4. Grasp the patient's right leg in the region of the tibial tuberosity with your right hand and flex the knee and hip.
5. When you have flexed the patient's hip to approximately 90 degrees, begin to apply very small amounts of additional flexion and extension, external and internal rotation, and abduction and adduction.
6. Adjust these fine-tuning motions until the paravertebral tension that your left hand is monitoring begins to dissipate.
7. Hold the hip in this position and allow the paravertebral and psoas muscles to relax.

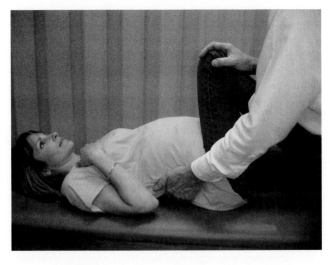

FIGURE 9.3   Indirect release for psoas spasm.

8. Maintaining your monitoring hand in place, slowly lower the patient's right leg to the table. As you perform this part of the procedure, move no faster than the paravertebral tension will allow. If the monitored muscles begin to tighten, use fine tuning motions as described in step 5 to find the most effective route to return the patient's leg to the table and yet maintain paravertebral relaxation.
9. When the procedure is complete, reassess the dysfunctional area.

Psoas (Muscle Energy) (Fig. 9.4)

This procedure is employed to relax a spastically contracted psoas major muscle and thereby reduce low back pain and improve extension of the ipsilateral hip. (See Chapter 26.)

Patient position: supine. Physician position: standing beside the table on the side of the tight psoas muscle.

Procedure (Example: Tight Right Psoas Muscle)

1. The patient's right hip is toward the edge of the right side of the table.
2. Standing next to the patient's right side, lower the right leg off the side of the table.
3. Place your left hand upon the patient's anterior thigh proximal to the patella.
4. Stabilize the patient's pelvis upon the table by applying a holding force with your right hand over the left anterior superior iliac spine.
5. Extend the patient's right hip by gently pushing the thigh downward until the barrier is reached.
6. While maintaining a holding force against the patient's thigh, instruct her to lift it into your hand for 3 seconds and then to relax.
7. It is important to allow the patient to relax briefly (2 seconds) before engaging the new barrier.
8. Extend the patient's hip further until the new barrier is reached.
9. Repeat the entire sequence as necessary to stretch the tight muscle.
10. When the procedure is complete, reassess the dysfunctional area.

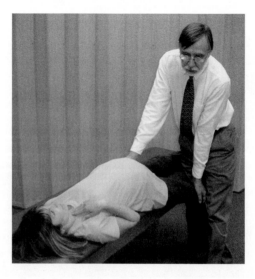

FIGURE 9.4 This same muscle energy procedure may be used to treat both psoas spasm and ipsilateral posterior innominate.

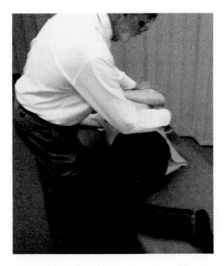

FIGURE 9.5   Anterior sacrum, muscle energy.

Anterior Sacrum (Muscle Energy) (Fig. 9.5)

This procedure is employed to introduce motion to a dysfunctional sacroiliac articulation. (See Chapter 3.)

Patient position: on the side on the treatment table with hips and knees flexed. Physician position: standing at the patient's hips.

Procedure (Example: Left Anterior Sacrum, Sacral Rotation Right on the Right Oblique Axis, with Motion Restriction of the Superior Pole of the Left Sacroiliac Articulation)

Patient position: on the right side.

1. Using your left hand, place the pads of your index and middle fingers over the patient's left sacral sulcus to monitor the dysfunctional sacroiliac articulation.
2. With your right hand, grasp both of the patient's legs just above the ankles.
3. Flex the hips until you palpate motion between the sacrum and ilium in the left sacroiliac articulation.
4. Further flex the patient's left hip and allow the left leg to drop off the side of the treatment table. This produces external rotation of the left hip and introduces side bending of the sacrum to the right. It also rotates the sacrum to the left between the ilia.
5. Brace the patient's left leg with your right thigh to stabilize her on the table and to maintain the introduced side bending and rotation.
6. Switch your monitoring hand and palpate the patient's left sacral sulcus with your right hand.
7. Grasp the patient's right arm above the elbow with your left hand and pull toward you until you palpate left rotational force in the left sacroiliac joint.
8. Maintain the left rotational forces applied to the sacrum by releasing the patient's right arm and contacting the left anterior shoulder with your left forearm.
9. Keep your left forearm in contact with the patient's left shoulder, and again, switch hands so that you are monitoring the patient's left sacral sulcus with your left hand.
10. Contact the patient's left iliac crest with your right forearm and rotate the pelvis toward you, rotating the pelvis to the right with your right forearm while maintaining sacral rotation to the left from above with your left forearm.

11. Tell the patient to push the pelvis back against the holding force of your right forearm and/or to push the left shoulder against your left forearm for 3 to 5 seconds.
12. Maintain your holding force during the patient's contraction.
13. Instruct the patient to relax for 2 to 3 seconds.
14. Increase pressure through your right forearm to rotate the patient's pelvis farther to the right while maintaining sacral rotation to the left by holding the upper torso with your left forearm as in step 10 to reengage the barrier, and repeat steps 11 through 14 as many times as necessary to establish the desired sacroiliac range of motion.
15. When the procedure is complete, reassess the dysfunctional area.

Anterior Sacrum Leg Pull (HVLA) (Fig. 9.6)

This procedure is employed to treat sacroiliac articular dysfunction found in association with sacral forward torsion. With an anterior sacrum, the innominate is posterior to the sacrum. During this procedure the leg does not have to be extended to load the quadriceps group, because the acetabulum lies anterior to the sacrum. (See Chapter 3.) Please note: This procedure should not be used if the patient has potential instability of the knee or hip on the side being treated.

Patient position: supine. Physician position: standing at the foot of the treatment table.

Procedure (Example: Right Anterior Sacrum, Sacrum Rotated Left on the Left Oblique Axis, Restriction of the Right Sacroiliac Joint, Superior Pole)

1. Grasp the patient's right ankle just above the malleoli with both hands.
2. Instruct the patient to relax all of the muscles in the low back and leg.
3. Internally rotate the leg to accumulate forces at the right sacroiliac joint. This pulls the ilium away from the sacrum, thereby gapping the sacroiliac joint.

    The patient's leg and thigh should *not* be lifted from the treatment table, so tension is maintained upon the anterior thigh.

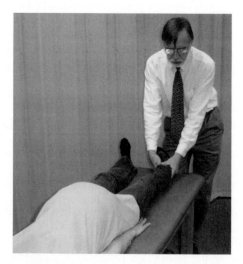

FIGURE 9.6   HVLA leg pull for anterior sacrum.

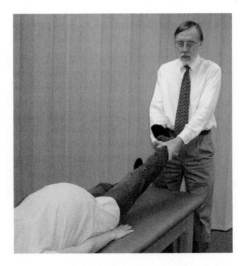

FIGURE 9.7   HVLA leg pull for a posterior sacrum.

4. Apply the final corrective force with a quick pull on the patient's leg, carrying the right innominate anteriorly to meet the sacrum.
5. When the procedure is complete, reassess the dysfunctional area.

Posterior Sacrum Leg Pull (HVLA) (Fig. 9.7)

This procedure is employed to treat specific sacroiliac articular dysfunction in association with sacral forward torsion. Considering a posterior sacrum, the innominate will be relatively anterior to the sacrum. When employing this procedure, the hip must be flexed to load the hamstring muscular group. Please note: This procedure should not be used if the patient has potential instability of the knee or hip on the side being treated.

Patient position: supine. Physician position: standing at the foot of the treatment table.

Procedure (Example: Right Posterior Sacrum, Sacrum Rotated Right on the Right Oblique Axis, Restriction of the Right Sacroiliac Joint, Inferior Pole)

1. Grasp the patient's right ankle just above the malleoli with both hands.
2. Instruct the patient to relax all of the muscles in the low back and leg.
3. Internally rotate the leg to accumulate forces at the right sacroiliac joint. This pulls the ilium away from the sacrum, thereby gapping the sacroiliac joint.
4. While keeping the knee extended, flex the hip until tension is placed on the hamstrings.
5. Apply the final corrective force with a quick pull on the patient's leg, carrying the right innominate posteriorly to meet the sacrum.
6. When the procedure is complete, reassess the dysfunctional area.

Piriformis Muscle (Muscle Energy) (Fig. 9.8)

This procedure is employed to increase restricted internal rotation of the hip. This dysfunction is often seen as a result of spasm of the piriformis muscle.

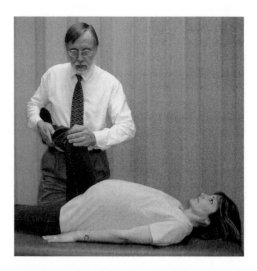

FIGURE 9.8   Muscle energy for piriformis spasm.

Patient position: supine. Physician position: standing at the side of the table on the side of the dysfunctional hip, facing the patient.

Procedure (Example: Restriction of the External Rotators of the Right Hip)

1. Grasp the patient's right knee with your left hand and the right leg with your right hand.
2. Flex the right hip and knee each to 90 degrees.
3. Cradle the patient's right calf in your right hand so that the ankle is firmly held between your right arm and side.
4. Place your left palm upon the lateral aspect of the patient's right knee.
5. Internally rotate the patient's right thigh by abducting the leg from the midline while maintaining the knee in a fixed position until the barrier is engaged.
6. Instruct the patient to externally rotate the thigh by contracting the hip muscles and attempting to move the foot back to midline for 3 to 5 seconds.
7. Maintain your holding force during the patient's contraction.
8. Instruct the patient to relax for 2 to 3 seconds.
9. Further internally rotate the patient's right thigh as in step 5 to reengage the barrier. Repeat steps 6 to 8 as many times as necessary to establish the desired range of motion.
10. When the procedure is complete, reassess the dysfunctional area.

Anterior and Posterior Innominate (Muscle Energy)

This procedure is employed to improve motion of the dysfunctional innominate. Dysfunctional restriction of motion between the two pelvic bones can occur such that one innominate bone is anterior (anterior innominate dysfunction) or posterior (posterior innominate dysfunction) to the other.

Patient position: supine. Physician position: standing at the side of the table on the side of the innominate, facing the patient.

Posterior Innominate Dysfunction (Muscle Energy) (Fig. 9.4)

Procedure

1. Draw the patient's pelvis toward the edge of table on the side of the dysfunctional innominate sufficient to permit the lower extremity on that side to hang off the table.
2. Reach across the table and place one hand upon the opposite innominate to stabilize the patient's pelvis upon the table.
3. Place your other hand above the knee of the lower extremity that has been allowed to hang off the side of the table.
4. Apply a downward force to the thigh, extending the hip to engage the barrier.
5. Instruct the patient to push the knee upward against your holding force for 3 to 5 seconds.
6. Maintain your holding force during the patient's contraction.
7. Instruct the patient to relax for 2 to 3 seconds.
8. Further extend the patient's hip as in step 4 to reengage the barrier. Repeat steps 6 to 8 as many times as necessary to establish the desired motion of the innominate.
9. When the procedure is complete, reassess the dysfunctional area.

Anterior Innominate Dysfunction (Muscle Energy) (Fig. 9.9)

Procedure

1. Place one hand beneath the patient's pelvis on the side of the dysfunctional innominate so that your finger tips are contacting the posterior superior iliac spine and sacroiliac joint.
2. With your other hand flex the patient's knee and hip on the dysfunctional side until the barrier is engaged.
3. Instruct the patient to lace the fingers together, reach down, and grasp the flexed knee, and hold it in the flexed position.
4. Place the hand flexing the patient's hip over the hands upon the knee.
5. Instruct the patient to extend the hip by pushing the knee against the holding force for 3 to 5 seconds.

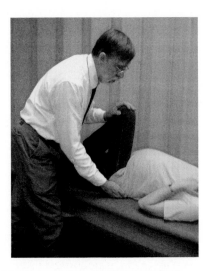

FIGURE 9.9 Muscle energy for anterior innominate.

6. Maintain the holding force during the patient's contraction.
7. Instruct the patient to relax for 2 to 3 seconds.
8. Further flex patient's hip as in step 2 to reengage the barrier and repeat steps 5 to 8 as many times as necessary to establish the desired motion of the innominate.
9. When the procedure is complete, reassess the dysfunctional area.

Symphysis Pubis Superior or Inferior Shear (Muscle Energy) (Fig. 9.10)

This procedure is employed to improve motion between the two pelvic bones at the pubic symphysis. Dysfunctional restriction of motion between the two pelvic bones can occur at the pubic symphysis such that one pubic bone is held in a superior (superior pubic dysfunction) or inferior (inferior pubic dysfunction) position relative to the other. Since the relationship between these two bones involves a single articulation, the symphysis, this nomenclature is somewhat arbitrary.

Patient position: supine. Physician position: standing beside the table and facing the patient.

Procedure

1. Tell the patient to flex the hips and knees and to keep the feet flat on the table.
2. The patient's foot on the side of the superiorly displaced pubic bone may be slightly farther from the buttocks than the other foot. This asymmetric foot placement flexes the hip on the side of the superiorly displaced pubic bone slightly less than the other hip. It is thought that when the patient performs the therapeutic isometric contraction, this results in a more inferiorly directed force applied through the adductor magnus on the side of the superiorly displaced pubic bone.
3. Abduct the patient's thighs and place your forearm between them such that your palm is in contact with one of the patient's knees and your elbow is in contact with the other.
4. With your other hand palpate the patient's pubic symphysis.
5. Instruct the patient to adduct the knees for 3 to 5 seconds against the holding force of your forearm between the knees.
6. Once gapping is felt at the symphysis pubis, instruct patient to relax for 2 to 3 seconds.

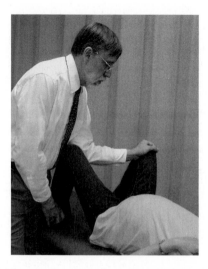

FIGURE 9.10   Muscle energy for pubic symphysis dysfunction.

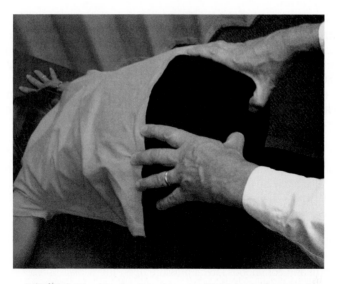

FIGURE 9.11   Myofascial release, ischial tuberosity spread.

7. Further abduct the patient's thighs as in step 2 to reengage the barrier, and repeat steps 4 to 6 as many times as necessary to establish the desired motion of the of the pubic symphysis.
8. When the procedure is complete, reassess the dysfunctional area.

Ischial Tuberosity Spread (Myofascial Release) (Figs. 9.11 and 9.12)

This procedure is employed to separate the ischial tuberosities and consequently to promote motion between the sacrum and the innominates. It may be employed as a general articular procedure to reduce sacral torsion and flexion dysfunctions.

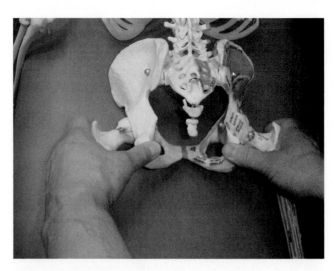

FIGURE 9.12   Thumb placement, medial to the ischial tuberosities, for myofascial release of ischial tuberosity spread.

It is also intended to facilitate pelvic diaphragm relaxation during respiratory exhalation. It may thus be employed as a soft tissue myofascial procedure to improve the function of the urogenital and pelvic diaphragms as part of the management of such conditions as dyspareunia, chronic pelvic pain, cystitis, prostatitis, proctitis, hemorrhoids, and constipation.

Patient position: prone, or in the knees to chest position if pregnant, with the pelvis as close to the foot of the table as comfort and positioning stability permit. Physician position: standing at the foot of the table.

Procedure

1. If the patient is prone, flex the knees to 90 degrees. In the knee chest position, the knees will already be flexed.
2. Internally rotate the patient's thighs by keeping the knees fixed upon the table and abducting the legs. This tends to draw the pelvic bones away from the sacrum and places tension upon the perineum.
3. Place the pads of your thumbs bilaterally upon the medial aspects of the patient's ischial tuberosities.
4. Apply firm and continuous lateral pressure upon the ischial tuberosities.
5. Instruct the patient to cough.
6. As the perineum is felt to relax, with sensitivity for patient discomfort, apply increased cephalad pressure upon the pelvic diaphragm and lateral pressure against the ischial tuberosities.
7. Repeat steps 5 and 6 as many times as necessary to establish the desired relaxation of the pelvic diaphragm and/or sacral motion.
8. When the procedure is complete, reassess the dysfunctional area.

Sacrum Diagnosis and Treatment (Cranial) (Fig. 9.13)

The CRI may be palpated throughout the body. Cranial osteopathic theory places great significance upon harmonious motion of the sacropelvic region with cranial motion. This reciprocal relationship means that treating the sacrum and pelvis can have broad influence upon the whole body's cranial mechanism. This procedure is

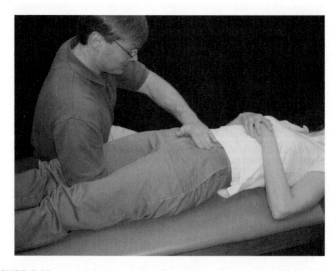

FIGURE 9.13   Cranial osteopathy diagnosis and treatment of the sacrum.

employed to enhance symmetric motion of the sacrum and consequently of the entire cranial mechanism.

The patient lies supine, and the physician sits beside the table, facing the head of the table and with the dominant hand to be employed for palpation and treatment closest to the table.

Procedure for Diagnosis and Treatment

1. Place your palpating hand and forearm between the patient's thighs palm up upon the table, with your fingers pointed toward the patient's head.
2. Instruct the patient to flex the knee farther from you, put the foot flat upon the table, and lift the pelvis off the table.
3. Slide your hand beneath the patient's sacrum such that your fingertips contact the base of the sacrum and the sacral sulci bilaterally. The apex of the sacrum should lie in the palm of your hand.
4. Instruct the patient to lower the pelvis onto your hand and to straighten out the leg.
5. Lean your weight on your elbow.
6. Palpate the CRI. During cranial flexion, the base of the sacrum moves into your fingertips, and during cranial extension, the apex of the sacrum moves into the palm of your hand.
7. Assess the quality, quantity, and symmetry of this subtle motion and identify asymmetric motion, propensity for flexion or extension, and diminished amplitude of the CRI.
8. Maintaining your hand in the same position, use indirect treatment methods and apply gentle force to move the sacrum toward the freedom of motion, or use direct treatment methods and apply gentle force to move the sacrum toward the restriction of motion.
9. Hold the selected indirect or direct position and await a release of the sacrum.
10. When the procedure is complete, reassess the dysfunctional area.

References

1. Burrows EA. Disorders of the female reproductive system. In: Hoag JM, ed. Osteopathic Medicine. New York: McGraw Hill, 1969;676–684.
2. Morris N, O'Neill D. Out-patient gynaecology. Br Med J 1958;14:1038–1039.
3. Heinking KP, Kappler RE. Pelvis and sacrum. In: Ward RC, ed. Foundations for Osteopathic Medicine. 2nd ed. Philadelphia: Lippincott Williams & Wilkins, 2002;601–622.
4. DiGiovanna EL, Schiowitz S. Evaluation of the pelvis and sacrum. In: An Osteopathic Approach to Diagnosis and Treatment. Philadelphia: Lippincott, 1991;189–212.
5. Fryette HH. Principles of Osteopathic Technic. Indianapolis: American Academy of Osteopathy, 1954, 1980;67–107.
6. Greenman PE. Pelvic girdle dysfunction. In: Principles of Manual Medicine. 2nd ed. Philadelphia: Williams & Wilkins, 1996;305–367.
7. Kuchera WA, Kuchera ML. Diagnosis and manipulative treatment of the lumbopelvic region. In: Osteopathic Principles in Practice. 2nd ed. Columbus, OH: Greyden, 1994;393–512.
8. Nelson KE. The sacrum: A bone of contention. AAO J 1997;7(4):17–24.
9. Strachan WF, Beckwith CG, Larson NJ, Grant JH. A study of the mechanics of the sacroiliac joint. J Am Osteopath Assoc 1938;37:576–578.
10. Pearce S. A Psychological Investigation of Chronic Pelvic Pain in Women. University of London, 1986 [PhD thesis].
11. Still AT. Philosophy of Osteopathy. Kirksville, MO: Author, 1899. Reprinted by the American Academy of Osteopathy, Indianapolis, 1971:234–249.

12. Tettambel M. Obstetrics. In: Ward RC, ed. Foundations for Osteopathic Medicine. 2nd ed. Philadelphia: Lippincott Williams & Wilkins, 2002;450–461.
13. Nelson KE. The management of low back pain. AAO J 1999;9(1):33–39.
14. Physiology of pregnancy. In: West JB, ed. Best and Taylor's Physiological Basis of Medical Practice. Philadelphia: Williams & Wilkins, 1990;892–934.
15. Sucher BM. Palpatory diagnosis and manipulative management of carpal tunnel syndrome. J Am Osteopath Assoc 1994;94:647–663.
16. Ramey KA et al. MRI assessment of changes in swelling of wrist structures following OMT in patients with carpal tunnel syndrome. AAO J 1999;9(2):25–31.

CHAPTER 10

The Surgical Patient

Janet M. Krettek

INTRODUCTION

The art of surgery is significantly enhanced when the osteopathic model is used to manage a patient's care. Surgery can be used as a diagnostic test and/or as a measure to provide a cure. The osteopathic model assists in diagnosis and treatment perioperatively. There are various aspects of the patient's care to consider, depending on when the patient is encountered. These aspects of patient management fall into three phases: preoperative, intraoperative, and postoperative. Though we artificially dissect the patient into separate systems to reveal the physiological processes, it is important to treat the patient as a whole, integrated person.

PREOPERATIVE

For minor surgical procedures, little or no other treatment is necessary. The removal of a skin lesion, for example, is minimally stressful to the patient. However, if the patient is undergoing a more extensive procedure, such as arthroscopy or breast biopsy, preoperative considerations include checking the patient for overall state of health, nutrition, and hydration. Optimize the patient's circulation, arterial, venous, and lymphatic, to the proposed surgical area. Check for local or viscerosomatic areas of somatic dysfunction. If the patient will be undergoing general anesthesia, ensure optimal pulmonary function, including the musculoskeletal component of respiration.

For major surgery, it is desirable to optimize patients' health status prior to surgery. However, surgery is often required on an urgent or emergency basis, which makes this impossible. Patients should be prepared mentally, emotionally, and spiritually to optimize recovery. Patients should understand the procedure, benefits, risks, possible complications, and likelihood that these will occur in their situation. Patients should be confident in the skills and compassion of all personnel involved in their care. Thus, every caregiver must be kind and attentive to patients' needs.

All affected systems, including pulmonary, renal, cardiac, gastrointestinal, neuromusculoskeletal, and circulatory (arterial, venous, lymphatic, and primary respiratory) should be checked. Age and nutrition should be considered as well. Smoking cessation ideally begins 2 weeks prior to surgery.[1] All systems should be functioning as well as possible preoperatively. Preparation may include osteopathic manipulative treatment (OMT), medications, nutrition, and education.

The use of OMT varies according to the individual needs and the areas of somatic dysfunction. Ensure that the thoracic cage, the diaphragm, and the cervical spine all have good motion and are free of significant somatic dysfunction. Midcervical (C3–C5) somatic dysfunction is associated with increased postoperative pulmonary complications. This has been described as a somatovisceral mechanism. In reality, it most likely represents a somatosomatic reflex in which the cervical somatic dysfunction affects the thoracoabdominal diaphragm through the phrenic nerve, and the resultant dysfunction predisposes the patient to develop pulmonary complications. The use of OMT preoperatively to reduce midcervical somatic dysfunction has been shown to significantly decrease postoperative pulmonary complications.[2] Further, specifically treating somatic dysfunction reduces postoperative complications and discomfort.[3–5]

Diagnosis

Diagnosis of acute abdominal pain is often perplexing. Heightened palpatory skills of the astute examiner offer insight into abdominal processes. Viscerosomatic reflexes in particular can be helpful in diagnosis. (See Chapter 5.)

Viscerosomatic reflexes are segmentally predictable dermatomal and myotomal responses to inflammatory visceral pathology. The location of the reaction identifies the involved organ, and the intensity of the tissue texture abnormality indicates the degree of visceral inflammation. Neoplastic lesions that are not specifically innervated may not produce a viscerosomatic response commensurate with the severity of the disease process unless a significant inflammatory reaction is produced in the tissues surrounding the neoplasm.

The tissue texture change of the viscerosomatic reflex is most readily palpated in the paravertebral soft tissues of the spinal level, sympathetic or parasympathetic, that innervates the structure responsible for the reflex. General visceral afferent nociceptive neurons return to the spinal cord in the same nerves that carry the efferent autonomic fibers. The reflexes lateralize to the paravertebral soft tissues on the same side of the body as the viscus. Midline organs produce bilateral reflex reactions. The location of these palpatory findings is often at the spinal level, where the patient may report referred pain. Consequently, cholecystitis results in a right-sided response in the area of T5 to T10; appendicitis produces tissue texture abnormality at T12 on the right, the dermatomal level of McBurney's point; and pancreatitis produces a bilateral reaction in the mid thoracic region, T5 to T9.

Although the somatovisceral impact of a viscerosomatic reflex may be treated preoperatively, the definitive treatment of the underlying pathology is the specific surgical procedure. These areas of tissue texture change, and tenderness to palpation resulting from viscerosomatic reflexes are manifestations of visceral pathology, not primary somatic dysfunction.

INTRAOPERATIVE

Intraoperatively, the osteopathic physician must demonstrate extreme respect for the patient. The patient is in a vulnerable position, and great care to prevent unintended visceral, somatic, or emotional injury is necessary. Warm, gentle speech should be used in the operating room. The patient must be placed in a position that is both comfortable for the patient and convenient for the surgeon. For example, when positioning a patient in stirrups for a pelvic or rectal procedure, ensure symmetry of position. Asymmetric placement of the lower extremities may result in sacropelvic somatic dysfunction postoperatively.

When operating, the surgeon must take care to respect the tissue. The tissue should be retracted gently and smoothly and only as needed. Students must be taught how to touch the various tissues to avoid injury.

Before incising the skin, the area of incision can be injected with local anesthetic, even if the patient is undergoing general anesthesia. This prevents the pain reflex by blocking the C fibers, thereby reducing postoperative pain and somatosomatic reflexes.

POSTOPERATIVE

During the first 1 to 3 postoperative days, the systems approach should be taken to regain or develop health overall. The systems to be concentrated upon first are those that are central to life, the pulmonary and circulatory systems. It is appropriate to use procedures to facilitate lymphatic flow and improve the mobility of the thoracic diaphragm and the cranial mechanism. Ensure that gentle care is given with attention to the patient's level of pain and tolerance to your treatment as well as consideration of the surgical site. Goals at this time are prevention of atelectasis and maintaining adequate circulation. The most common reason for postoperative fever is atelectasis. General anesthesia causes some alveolar collapse, which can be easily corrected if the patient is alert, active, and able to resume full, normal respiration postoperatively. However, chest or abdominal surgery will inhibit the patient's respirations as a result of splinting secondary to pain. Prolonged bed rest, such as post hip pinning, will also decrease full diaphragmatic excursion. Manipulative procedures to consider include lymphatic pump, rib raising, pedal pump, compression of the fourth ventricle (CV-4), and diaphragm and soft tissue procedures.

Pain control is very important. The most obvious reason is to decrease suffering, but there are other reasons. Treating the patient's pain early breaks the pain cycle and interrupts the viscerosomatic and somatosomatic reflexes. If it is left unchecked, pain can be much harder to manage the second or third postoperative day as the patient's pain tolerance falls in response to hyperactivity of the sympathetic nervous system. When the pain is lessened or obliterated, the patient can take deeper breaths and increase activity, thus improving the pulmonary, lymphatic, gastrointestinal, and cranial systems. This has a spiraling effect to a better recovery. Opioids and their derivatives are most useful early and in combination with pain relievers using other mechanisms of actions, such as a nonsteroidal anti-inflammatory drug or acetaminophen. Diminished gastrointestinal motility is less important than pain control. Do not be concerned at this time with the possibility of starting an addiction. Addiction will not result from adequate treatment of postoperative pain.

Additional treatment modalities may be added at day 2 to 4, depending on the type of surgery. Remember to have the patient participate in the healing by breathing deeply to improve pulmonary function and walking as soon as possible to improve circulation and gastrointestinal motility. Today, with the use of minimal-access procedures, more about the effects of early activity on recuperation from surgical trauma is revealed. Patients can have less pain and less ileus, leading to more physical activity, earlier discharge times, and more rapid resumption of normal activities.

Patients are often discharged from the hospital so early that the physician does not get a chance to provide any further extensive postoperative care in the hospital setting. For patients who remain hospitalized, however, the gastrointestinal tract and renal and autonomic nervous systems may now be approached. Though patients are discharged earlier, this does not change the body's reaction to the stress and injury of surgery. The first phase of healing, the inflammatory stage, takes place over the first 3 postoperative days. One can change the intensity of this phase with ice, rest, elevation, anti-inflammatory medications, and OMT, but it still takes place. On postoperative day 4, the diuresis phase begins, in which the patient loses the retained fluids from the intracellular and extracellular spaces, including the surgical site. This is the time to ensure that renal and circulatory functions are at their peak. The lymphatic system picks up 8 to 12 L of fluid daily, of which 2 to 4 L returns to the venous circulation via the thoracic duct. The remainder returns via capillary exchange in the lymph nodes.[6] During the diuretic phase, the fluid load increases. Thoracic cage mobility is imperative, not only for efficient respiration but also for returning lymph to the general circulation. The thoracic duct terminates into the left subclavian vein; therefore, mobility of the thoracic outlet is critical to prevent obstruction to the flow of lymph.

Rib raising is of great value in reducing postoperative atelectasis and consequent pneumonia.[4] Motion of the thoracoabdominal diaphragm, which may be decreased by abdominal splinting, should be enhanced. Cephalic traction on the anterior axillary folds of the supine patient pulls the thoracic cage into the position of inhalation. This transiently reduces thoracic cage excursion, necessitating that the patient breathe by using the diaphragm, thereby stimulating diaphragmatic motion. Various modifications of thoracic lymphatic pump may be employed if the patient (and the surgical site) can tolerate them.

The motion of the diaphragm results in alternating negative and positive intrathoracic pressure coupled with alternating positive and negative intraabdominal pressure. This two-chambered pump mechanism and the unidirectional flow that results from the presence of valves in the lymphatic vasculature pulls the lymph centrally into the venous circulation. Enhancing thoracic cage mobility preoperatively is directed at postoperatively reducing lymphatic congestion and the likelihood of pulmonary stasis.

Lymphatic flow occurs as the result of lymphatic vasomotion augmented by movement of structures surrounding the lymphatic vasculature.[7] The cranial rhythmic impulse (CRI) has been demonstrated to be synchronous with the Traube-Hering (baroreflex) fluctuation in blood flow velocity and pressure.[8] This fluctuation in sympathetic tone may also be a driving force behind lymphatic vasomotion and is a possible explanation for how cranial manipulative procedures, such as CV-4, affect the patient.[9-11]

Preexistent spinal (and to a lesser extent appendicular) somatic dysfunction should be identified and treated. Spinal somatic dysfunction results in spinal cord–level segmental facilitation with somatovisceral effects. High cervical and sacropelvic dysfunction results in parasympathetic somatovisceral reflexes. Thoracolumbar dysfunction results in sympathetic somatovisceral reflexes. Check for temporal bone dysfunction and upper cervical dysfunction when considering the function of the vagus nerve. The patient may need some assistance in stimulating the gastrointestinal tract via stimulation of the underactive parasympathetic nervous system and inhibiting the overactive sympathetic nervous system. Increased sympathetic tone contributes to postoperative ileus and results in vasospasm that decreases tissue perfusion. The supply of arterial blood will decrease, and diminished lymphatic and venous capacity will increase passive congestion. The sympathetic ganglia lie between T1 and L2. Combining the two procedures, inhibitory pressure and rib raising, when treating the thoracic and lumbar spinal regions, can inhibit sympathetic tone. The parasympathetic nervous system is divided into cranial and sacral portions. The vagus nerve innervates the pulmonary, gastrointestinal, and cardiac systems. The parasympathetic nervous system should be stimulated with manipulation, therefore, to resolve an ileus.

Somatic dysfunctions occur just from inactivity, lying in a hospital bed for a few days. Be sure to ask the patient about any back, neck, or appendicular discomfort. The treatment of these somatic dysfunctions may be a bit difficult, particularly without an OMT table, but procedures can be modified for application in a hospital bed, and the benefits are great. The patient's comfort will be much improved. This will allow the patient to recuperate more quickly.

LATE POSTOPERATIVE

A few weeks after surgery is the time to work more on the somatic dysfunctions of the fascia and other layers of tissue involved at the time of the surgery. If there were complications of the surgical site, such as infection, the timing of the OMT should be further delayed. The residual somatic component from preoperative viscerosomatic reflexes is best treated at this time. The area has had time to settle down from the trauma of the disease process and that of the surgery. If somatic dysfunction is still present at the area of a viscerosomatic reflex, it now should be treated. The condition postcholecystectomy syndrome is an example of a viscerosomatic reflex that persists postoperatively. The postcholecystectomy patient has the symptoms of cholecystitis even though the gallbladder is no longer present. Treatment of the residual gallbladder viscerosomatic reflex effectively treats this condition.

Determining OMT Dosage

Dosage and tolerance are important to the treatment of the surgical patient. (See Chapter 4.) Tolerance is determined by age, by severity of illness, and postoperatively, by the circumstances of the surgical site. How much OMT is enough? One should choose a procedure the patient will tolerate and treat the patient until a response occurs.

What kind of response should the clinician look for? Relaxation of the soft tissues in the area being treated is a good response, often referred to as a *release*. Vasodilation resulting in increased skin temperature or redness and increased sudomotor activity indicates it is time to stop treatment. Increased heart or respiratory rate also indicates that the patient has reached the level of tolerance. If the patient feels that the intervention is too uncomfortable, the clinician should stop and choose another approach or return later and try again. It is often best to apply small doses of OMT daily or even several times daily.

CONCLUSION

Every patient should be examined and treated using the osteopathic model. As long as the clinician respects the patient's tolerance and the integrity of the surgical site, employing OMT preoperatively and postoperatively should increase the patient's comfort, decrease postoperative complications, and reduce the potential for late postoperative somatic dysfunction.

Procedures

The diagnosis and treatment of somatic dysfunction offers the osteopathic surgeon a valuable tool. Viscerosomatic reflexes add to the armamentarium of physical diagnosis. Somatic dysfunction should be treated preoperatively whenever possible. The selection and application of a procedure are determined by the somatic dysfunction and the physical status of the patient.

Treatment of the postoperative patient is determined by the same principles as the treatment of the preoperative patient. The postoperative period, however, does consist of the relatively predictable series of events of the recuperative process. The following procedures are examples of OMT that can be employed to treat the postoperative surgical patient. Please note: The procedures that follow are examples of manipulative treatment that you may wish to employ. The actual choice of procedures used should be determined by the unique circumstances of each individual patient.

Inhibitory Pressure

This procedure is employed to affect reflex activity by suppressing the somatic component of a somatovisceral reflex. (See Chapter 5.)

Compression of the Fourth Ventricle, CV-4 (Cranial) (Fig. 10.1)

This procedure is employed to stimulate the body's inherent recuperative ability by promoting fluid interchange; it is thought especially to influence lymphatic and cerebrospinal fluid circulation.

Patient position: supine. Physician position: seated at the patient's head.

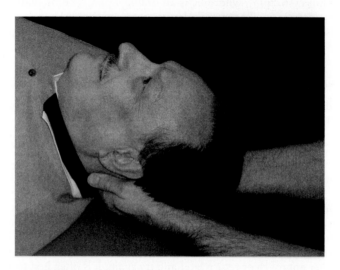

FIGURE 10.1 Compression of the fourth ventricle, CV-4.

Procedure

1. Place your hands, palms up with one resting in the palm of the other so that the thenar eminences are parallel, beneath the patient's head in contact with the lateral angles of the occiput. It is very important that your thenar eminences, the points of contact with the patient's head, are medial to the occipitomastoid suture.
2. The weight of the patient's head should be resting upon your thenar eminences, placing medially directed pressure upon the lateral angles of the occiput.
3. Palpate the occiput for the flexion and extension phases of the CRI for a few cycles. As the occiput moves into flexion, you will perceive a sense of lateral and caudal displacement of your thenar eminences. As the occiput moves into extension, you will perceive a sense of medial and cephalad displacement of your thenar eminences.
4. Begin treatment by following the occiput into extension and gently increasing the medial pressure from your thenar eminences upon the lateral angles of the occiput.
5. After the occiput reaches full flexion, you will feel it reverse direction and enter the extension phase of the cycle. Gently resist this and maintain the occiput in flexion.
6. Repeat this process of following the occiput into extension and resisting flexion. The amplitude of the palpable CRI will become smaller with each cycle until a still point is reached, the moment when the CRI seems to stop.
7. After the still point, wait for the motion of the CRI to return and move with it into flexion and extension.
8. When the procedure is complete, reassess the amplitude of the CRI.

Cervical (Soft Tissue/Articulation) (Fig. 10.2)

This procedure is employed to decrease cervical tissue tension and enhance the symmetric range of motion of the cervical spine.

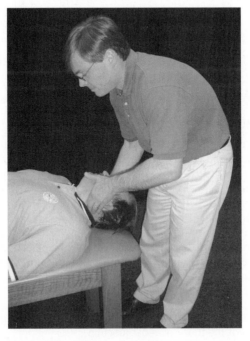

FIGURE 10.2   Soft tissue and articulation of the cervical spine.

Patient position: supine. Physician position: seated at the head of the treatment table.

Procedure

1. With both hands, place the pads of your fingers bilaterally over the cervical paraspinal tissues at the level of maximal palpable paravertebral tension.
2. Symmetrically apply bilateral anterior and cephalad pressure until you sense the stretch of the cervical paraspinal soft tissues. Applying more pressure will produce articular motion.
3. Hold with this degree of applied force position until the tissues relax.
4. Slowly release the holding force, exerting care not to unload the muscles too rapidly.
5. Repeat this sequence several times, working up and down the cervical spine, until the desired decrease in paraspinal tension is achieved. As you become proficient with this procedure, you will learn to focus specifically upon asymmetric areas of paraspinal tension.
6. When the procedure is complete, reassess the dysfunctional area.

Thoracic, Patient on Side (Soft Tissue) (See Fig. 5.3)

This procedure is employed to decrease paravertebral muscle spasm and soft tissue tension of the thoracic spine.

Patient position: lying on one side with a pillow beneath the head and the knees bent to stabilize the torso. Physician position: standing at the side of the table or bed facing the patient.

Procedure

1. Curl your fingers over the paraspinal musculature beginning at the thoracolumbar junction.
2. Place one foot in front of the other for stability.
3. Keeping your back straight, lean back and use your body weight to apply anterolateral traction slowly through both hands.
4. Hold this position until the muscles relax.
5. Release the force slowly and work up and down the thoracic spine, treating tight areas.
6. Have the patient roll to the other side and repeat the procedure.
7. When the procedure is complete, reassess the dysfunctional area.

Lumbar Paravertebral Muscles (Soft Tissue) (See Fig. 5.4)

This procedure is employed to relax hypertonic lumbar paravertebral muscles. It is described here with the patient on the side. It can be modified to accommodate the postoperative patient since position changes may be inappropriate or difficult for the patient. Under these circumstances, allow the patient to remain supine and slide your hands, palm up, beneath the low back and perform the soft tissue stretch in a fashion similar to that employed for rib raising. (See Fig. 5.6.)

Patient position: lying on one side with hips and knees comfortably flexed to provide stability for the torso. The bottom arm may be placed under the head and the other arm placed wherever it is comfortable and out of the way. Physician position: standing facing the patient at the level of the lumbar spine.

Procedure

1. Wrap your hands over the patient's flank and grasp the upper paraspinal musculature at the level of the thoracolumbar junction.
2. Place one of your feet in front of the other for stability.

3. Keeping your back straight, lean back and use your body weight to apply antero-lateral traction slowly through both hands.
4. Hold this position until the muscles relax.
5. Release the force slowly and work up and down the lumbar spine, treating tight areas.
6. Have the patient roll to the other side and repeat the procedure.
7. When the procedure is complete, reassess the dysfunctional area.

Rib Raising (See Fig. 5.6)

Rib raising reduces constriction of larger lymphatic vessels. Raising the rib heads also stimulates the thoracic sympathetic chain ganglia. This treatment initially stimulates regional sympathetic efferent activity to organs related to that spinal level of sympathetic innervation, but in the long run, rib raising results in a prolonged reduction in sympathetic outflow from the area treated. Freeing rib motion also frees the excursion of the rib cage during respiration. Freeing the rib heads increases the excursion of the chest during breathing and improves lymphatic flow.

Patient position: supine. Physician position: standing or seated at the patient's side.

Procedure

1. Place your palms under the patient's thorax, contacting the rib angles with the pads of your fingers.
2. Flex your fingers to achieve contact with the rib angle and the patient's posterior thorax.
3. Apply traction on the rib angle.
4. While maintaining traction, bend your knees and lower your trunk, which raises the ribs when your hands move upward. This is a fulcrum and lever action; do not bend your wrists. (Particularly if the patient is in a hospital bed, it is easier to move the hands upward if you reciprocally push your forearms down.)
5. Move your hands to subsequent rib angles until all ribs are treated.
6. Treat the opposite side of the rib cage in the same manner.
7. When the procedure is complete, reassess excursion of the thoracic cage.

Rib Balancing

This procedure gently balances the right and the left sides of the thoracic cage, promoting ease of respiratory excursion.

Patient position: supine. Physician position: standing at the side of the table or bed facing the patient.

Procedure

1. Place the palmar surfaces of your hands on the right and left side of the lower rib cage of the patient with your fingers pointing toward the surface of the table or bed and your thumbs pointed toward each other.
2. Move both halves of the thoracic cage cephalad and caudad, rotate left and right, and laterally translate left and right, and determine the directions of restriction and freedom of motion.
3. Move the thoracic cage in the direction of ease of each of these motions, individually or in combination, and hold.
4. Wait for a release, the perception of relaxation of tension, to occur.
5. At this point, if the patient tolerates the procedure, you can move the thoracic cage back in the direction of the previously observed restrictions to enhance the release.
6. When the procedure is complete, reassess the dysfunctional area.

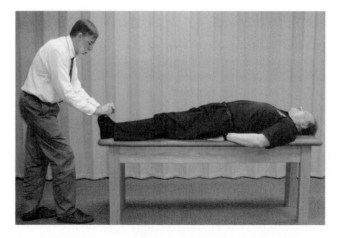

FIGURE 10.3 Dalrymple's pedal lymphatic pump.

Pedal Pump (Dalrymple's Pump) (Fig. 10.3)

This procedure is employed to enhance low-pressure venous and lymphatic return to the heart and thereby reduce passive congestion of the lower extremities, abdominal contents and lungs.

Patient position: supine. Physician position: standing at the patient's feet.

Procedure

1. Grasp the patient's toes with both hands.
2. Abruptly push cephalad, dorsiflexing the patient's ankles, and then quickly return them to the neutral position. This action should send a wave of motion cephalad, followed by a rebound wave.
3. As the rebound wave returns to the feet, reapply the dorsiflexion force, creating an oscillatory pump.
4. The oscillating motion moves the lower extremities in approximation of the muscular pump. It also moves the abdominal contents intermittently up against the thoracoabdominal diaphragm, facilitating alternating positive and negative intra-abdominal and intrathoracic pressure and decongesting the liver and spleen.

Pectoral Traction to Enhance Motion of the Diaphragm (Fig. 10.4)

This procedure enhances thoracoabdominal diaphragmatic excursion. It can be used with relative ease for postsurgical patients and for patients in the intensive care unit, where multiple lines, tubes, and monitoring devices may be in place.

Patient position: supine. Physician position: standing at the patient's head.

Procedure

1. Curl your fingertips bilaterally over the inferior border of the pectoral muscles of the anterior axillary folds, taking care not to gouge or tickle the patient. Alternatively, apply traction through the arms, as in Fig. 10.4.
2. Lean back, using your body to produce cephalad traction on the anterior thoracic cage.

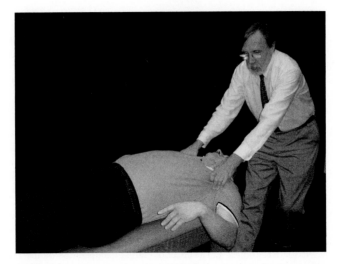

FIGURE 10.4   Pectoral traction to enhance motion of the diaphragm.

3. While maintaining the traction, instruct the patient to breathe deeply.
4. Because the pectoral traction tends to pull the anterior thoracic cage into the position of inhalation, to breathe deeply the patient must employ the motion of the thoracoabdominal diaphragm.
5. When the procedure is complete, reassess motion of the thoracoabdominal diaphragm.

Wound or Scar Release (Indirect)

This procedure may be employed to reduce asymmetric tension and restore functional balance to stresses transmitted through a surgical wound or scar.

The position of the patient and physician depend upon the site of the wound being treated. In this example, an abdominal wound may be treated with the patient supine and the physician standing or seated beside the patient at the level of the pelvis.

Procedure

1. Place the palms of your hands parallel to and on either side of the wound. You may spread your fingers, depending upon the surface of the abdomen it is appropriate to cover.
2. Approximate your hands gently, reducing tension on the wound.
3. Move the tissues on either side of the wound gently in different directions (cephalic, caudal, left, right) to determine the tension pattern in the surrounding tissues.
4. Gently move your hands and the tissues on either side of the wound in the direction that most reduces tension until you perceive a sense of balance.
5. Hold both sides of the wound in this balanced position until you perceive a release (further relaxation of tension).
6. Having the patient exhale and hold the breath, if feasible, during step 5 may be employed to enhance the balance of tension.
7. When the procedure is complete, reassess tension of the soft tissue surrounding the wound or scar.

References

1. Townsend CM, Beauchamp RD, Evers BM, Mattox K, eds. Sabiston Textbook of Surgery: The Biological Basis of Modern Surgical Practice. 17th ed. Philadelphia: Saunders, 2004;1769.
2. Henshaw RE. Manipulation and postoperative pulmonary complications. DO 1963;4(1): 132–133.
3. Stiles EG. Osteopathic treatment of surgical patients. Osteopath Med 1976;1(3):21–23.
4. Larson NJ. Manipulative care before and after surgery. Osteopath Med 1977;2(1):41–49.
5. Sleszynski SL, Kelso AF. Comparison of thoracic manipulation with incentive spirometry in preventing postoperative atelectasis. J Am Osteopath Assoc 1993;93:834–838, 843–845.
6. Townsend CM, Beauchamp RD, Evers BM, Mattox K, eds. Sabiston Textbook of Surgery: The Biological Basis of Modern Surgical Practice. 17th ed. Philadelphia: Saunders, 2004;93.
7. Johnston MG, ed. Experimental Biology of Lymphatic Circulation. Vol 9. Research Monographs in Cell and Tissue Physiology. Amsterdam: Elsevier, 1985;8–9.
8. Nelson KE, Sergueef N, Lipinski CM, et al. Cranial rhythmic impulse related to the Traube-Hering-Mayer oscillation: Comparing laser-Doppler flowmetry and palpation. J Am Osteopath Assoc 2001;101:163–173.
9. Sergueef N, Nelson KE, Glonek T. The effect of cranial manipulation on the Traube-Hering-Meyer oscillation as measured by laser-Doppler flowmetry. Altern Ther Health Med 2002;8(6):74–76.
10. Nelson KE, Sergueef N, Glonek T. Cranial manipulation induces sequential changes in blood flow velocity on demand. AAO J 2004;14(3):15–17.
11. Nelson KE, Sergueef N, Glonek T. The effect of an alternative medical procedure (CV-4) upon low-frequency oscillations in cutaneous blood flow velocity. J Manip Physiology Ther 2006, in press.

CHAPTER 11

The Athlete

Kurt P. Heinking

INTRODUCTION

Osteopathic physicians are uniquely suited to care for athletes. Andrew Taylor Still saw athletic patients. Still also encouraged students, both men and women, to join the athletic association at the American School of Osteopathy.[1] Still was a pioneer in treating professional athletes and patients in collegiate sports.[2] The American School of Osteopathy had numerous sports teams and a very good reputation for producing many famous athletes and coaches. Osteopathic primary care sports medicine focuses on treating injuries and improving athletic performance while enhancing the function of the musculoskeletal system.

Sports injuries account for a large portion of visits to the primary care physician's office. Approximately 20% of the American public regularly participates in exercise programs, and this health-conscious attitude about physical fitness is encouraging.[3] This increase in athletic participation also means an increase in injuries seen by the primary care practitioner, not only in adults but in children and geriatric patients as well. It is estimated that every year more than 17 million Americans seek medical care because of athletic and recreational issues.[4] More than 55 million women participate in recreational sports annually, and by 2030, 20% of our population will be more than 65 years old.[5] This large number of geriatric athletes, especially those older than 85, are the most rapidly growing segment of the population.[6]

Patients exercise for a number of reasons. Some have specific reasons based on published guidelines. Some of these include protection against an initial cardiac episode, reducing the risk of recurring cardiac events, obtaining a more favorable lipid profile, controlling obesity, decreasing blood pressure, improving glucose tolerance, increasing bone density, improving self-image, and reducing stress and tension.[5] Others exercise as part of a social routine, and still others for general health.

Athletes exercise because they love to participate and compete. They compete against themselves and others. They are proud of their abilities and define who they are through their athletic prowess. It is because of this that athletes seek medical care for many unusual reasons. Athletes hold off seeking the physician for pain, but they do consult when they see poor performance or inability to do what they like. Athletes also tend to procrastinate and ignore "little" aches and pains. Sometimes they consult only because they were pulled from a game by a coach or a trainer.

On the field, the management of injured athletes is primarily focused on eliminating urgent conditions and determining whether they can go back into the game. Sometimes it is necessary to confiscate the helmet or to move the patient to the training room for protection; otherwise the injured athlete will go back into the game. Primary care physicians are an integral part of athletes' health care team, along with orthopedic surgeons, physical therapists, certified athletic trainers, physiatrists, neurologists, pediatricians, geriatricians, rheumatologists, and cardiologists. It is this team that provides the best care for injured athletes. Physicians not only are gatekeepers; they also must motivate discouraged players and reduce risks to players. Primary care physicians must also make medical decisions based upon specialists' recommendations and help guide patients down the appropriate medical pathway.

THE HISTORY

A complete history is essential. Many athletes have multiple complaints. Each should be delineated and fully prioritized at the initial visit. Why is the patient presenting now? Is the patient getting better, staying the same, or worsening? What has been done so far? Determining the specifics regarding pain is important, but equally important is determining the specifics of any functional limitations. Was there only one specific injury (macrotrauma) or is a repetitive overuse syndrome (microtrauma) present? If microtrauma has occurred over time, are abnormal stresses applied to normal tissues, or are normal stresses applied to abnormal tissues?

Clinical investigation of these questions is of paramount importance when obtaining a history. Taking a history from athletes includes the who, what, where, why, and how of the chief complaint; however, it also has some unique components, such as patients' level of play or activity. Do they participate in more than one sport? Do they play other sports, or are they participating in club activities? Where are they in the season? How long is the season? How is the team doing? Do they use specific gear or protective equipment? Do they take ergogenic aids to maintain their performance? These types of questions assist in clinical problem solving by elucidating the causes of their problems.

Young athletes may not give a reliable history, and older athletes may be stoic and not provide all of the necessary information. Dealing with the parents of an injured athletic child or the family member may be difficult. The history leads to a differential diagnosis. The physical examination can be performed in a problem-focused fashion. The clinician uses osteopathic palpatory skills, the physical examination, and other studies to narrow the differential diagnosis. An adequate history and physical, including a thorough structural examination, will provide the diagnosis in 90% of cases. Do not rely heavily on diagnostic tests; on the contrary, diagnostic tests should complement a thorough history and physical.

THE PHYSICAL EXAMINATION

An efficient physical examination includes the palpatory diagnosis of somatic dysfunction throughout the examination. Specific orthopedic tests should be selected and integrated according to the patient's specific complaint. The examination should start with gait and balance. Then evaluate the patient seated, supine, and prone (if tolerated). It is critical to examine not only the injured region but also distant regions that may be related. Palpating for tissue texture abnormality is fundamental to the evaluation of the injured athlete.[7]

Evaluation of Gait

When observing gait, look at the patient's stance for the initial foot position. Evaluate the arches, overpronation, supination, and hind foot position. Evaluate the heel strike, midstance, swing-through and push-off phases. Always evaluate for a limp, and look to see if the patient is favoring one extremity or the other.

Look for leg rotation or hip hiking. Evaluate the shoes for wear; inquire about use of orthotics, and examine the feet for calluses. Mitchell[8] described a cycle of walking that described motion of the pelvic bones, sacroiliac joints, and postural compensations during gait. Understanding this turns the evaluation of the patient's gait into a whole-body assessment.

The Standing Structural Examination

The standing structural examination of the athlete focuses on asymmetry, with evaluation of anatomic landmarks for levelness and anterior, posterior, and lateral curvature of the spine. Perform a standing flexion test and evaluate for pelvic side shift. Athletes may develop unique postures brought on by their particular sport, especially if they are using one arm or one leg repeatedly. Runners may have a variety of lower extremity problems. For example, structural examination may reveal that a patient with an asymmetric dropped arch has a short leg syndrome. Always look at levelness of the iliac crests, the greater trochanters, and pelvic side shift, as these findings may indicate unequal leg length. (See Chapters 3 and 26.)

It is fairly common to find significant paravertebral muscle development on the side of the patient's dominant hand. This must be differentiated from a scoliotic curve. Flattened thoracic kyphosis may indicate an extended Fryette's type II somatic dysfunction. These are clinically painful and produce many symptoms in the upper back, neck, and upper extremity.[9]

The Seated Examination

The seated examination includes an examination of the following regions:

- Head, eyes, ears, nose, throat
- Neurologic examination
- Cardiac examination

- Pulmonary examination
- Musculoskeletal examination (See Chapter 3)
  - Thoracic spine
  - Ribs
  - Neck (active range of motion, passive range of motion, Spurling's sign)
  - Knee, ankle, and foot
  - Seated flexion test for sacral dysfunction

Supine Examination

The supine examination includes examination of the following regions:

- Abdomen
- Pelvis (ilium motion tender points, pubic symphysis)
- Hip, knee
- Lower extremity
- Pulses, sensations
- Straight leg raising sign
- Ankle and foot
- Cervical spine
- Cranial strain pattern assessment

Prone Examination

The prone examination includes the following examination of each of the following regions:

- Lumbar spine
- Hip extension
- Sacral motion
- Quadriceps muscle tension
- Hamstring muscle tenderness and tone
- Soft tissue diagnosis of somatic dysfunction

Palpation and motion testing in the clinical examination are integrated. It is very important that the osteopathic examination not be a separate examination. The integration of the diagnosis of somatic dysfunction with the standard physical examination helps the clinician make the link between somatic dysfunction and abnormalities in the general physical examination or orthopedic examination.

The Functional (Dynamic) Examination

Many times it is beneficial to examine an athlete performing a certain movement or exercise. A physician can palpate various tissues or muscles for activation, weakness, or tightness. This approach also evaluates motions used in the swing, throw, block shot, or tackle. Digital video recording also can be very useful, because motion, gait, and speed when they throw or swing can be analyzed. This also can be sped up or slowed down to evaluate the various component parts of the motion in the search for faults or defects. It is important to differentiate orthopedic pathology from functional conditions: Remember, every patient has certain musculoskeletal compensations that allow them to adapt to their injury. Sometimes compensations become abnormal and are themselves a problem.[7] In considering the dynamic examination, one must consider the ground reaction force, the patient's center of gravity, the muscle firing patterns, and the postural findings on the structural examination. Then these factors are evaluated and integrated into their treatment plan. When a clinician adds balance and proprioception to this list and when these factors are addressed in the treatment plan, the patient's entire kinetic system is evaluated.

CLINICAL PROBLEM SOLVING

Is there a somatic component to the patient's chief complaint, injury or illness? How do the palpatory findings relate to the condition? Is there a general postural pattern contributing to this situation? Are viscerosomatic reflexes causing facilitation of a specific spinal region? How does the patient respond to osteopathic manipulative treatment (OMT), and does OMT improve orthopedic testing? Keeping these issues in mind determines what is to be treated first. Acute injuries may not tolerate palpation, motion testing, or OMT. In this situation, begin by working in distant yet related anatomic areas until the tissue texture and sensitivity improves. Chronic conditions require chronic treatment. Look for the most significant area of tissue texture change and motion restriction, the key somatic dysfunction.

Use exercises not only to stabilize areas of the spine or extremity that are hypermobile but also to mobilize restricted tissues and joints. Tissue injury needs time to heal; sometimes rehabilitation and/or exercises are added too soon, before sufficient healing occurs. This is commonly seen in rotator cuff tendonitis. Rest and relative rest is important. Athletes need to participate actively in their healing and rehabilitation. Determine a timeline and treatment plan; discuss it with the patient, and stick to it. Support the host, especially with OMT, as it sets the stage for this healing to begin. OMT will improve tissue perfusion and facilitate lymphatic drainage from an area.

Another important aspect is deciding when to mobilize an injured area. If there is instability due to ligamentous sprain or fracture, obviously it is necessary to immobilize it with a splint or cast appropriately; also, sometimes casting is necessary to protect patients from themselves. Many athletes use an injured extremity against medical advice. In this situation, applying a cast may be the most appropriate thing to do. The primary care physician also must decide what aspects of physical therapy will benefit the patient. There is a right time and a wrong time to send a patient to physical therapy. Communicating with the physical therapist on a regular basis is critical for the patient's wellbeing. Also decide how much rest and how long. Be very specific with athletes about what they may and must not do.

Provide specific instructions on when to use ice or heat or contrasting baths, when to use compression or traction to the area, exactly when to take their medication. Such instruction will foster an improved treatment plan. Always consider what will be gained from a referral to another specialist and how this will fit into the patient's overall therapeutic scheme. Patients should always be an active participant in their health care as the primary care physician educates them and guides them down the path of wellness.

Allow patients to decide which way they would like to go with their healing process. Providing a patient with a graded return to activity is important. For example, with runners, determine the total number of miles they are to run per week; consider frequency and duration. It may be important to adjust their mileage and time, for example, by decreasing their mileage by 50% and slowing their pace. As the athlete heals and the injury improves, the guidelines can be altered according to their symptoms. Provide them with a timeline extending perhaps over 4 weeks that lists exactly how much they should run and at what pace. Each week increase their time and/or duration based as their symptoms allow. Recommend what to do if their symptoms recur or worsen as their mileage increases; this may be instructions to increase medication, use ice, adjust warm-up or cool-down activities, walking, or stretching. Also tell them that if they tolerate their graded progression back to exercise, it is not wise to increase activities over the recommendations that have been made.

While injured structures are healing, it is also important to maintain cardiac conditioning. Athletes may cross-train with bicycle, pool, or other modalities to maintain their cardiovascular fitness. Encouraging the athlete to do more of these activities instead of the activity in which they were injured usually is beneficial.

Commonly Seen Athletic Conditions in Family Medicine

The Patient with an Acute Ankle Sprain

Ankle sprains are the most common athletic injury seen by sports medicine practitioners. Inversion sprains make up of 75% of ankle sprains.[10] Most ankle injuries occur in plantar flexion, because plantar flexion decreases the stability of the ankle joint. In plantar flexion, the anterior aspect of the talus is no longer wedged between the malleoli, which increases the mobility of the joint.

Upon initial presentation after an acute inversion sprain, it is common to have bruising along the lower aspect of the lateral side of the foot and tenderness over the peroneal tendons. The injured structures are typically anterior talofibular, calcaneofibular, and posterior talofibular ligaments. Diffuse swelling typically surrounds the lateral malleolus, ankle, and dorsum of the foot. Bony point tenderness may indicate a fracture. Pain to vibration over any bony structure may also signify fracture. Radiographs with comparative views are generally taken in children due to the potential for growth plate injuries. The Ottawa Ankle Rules (Table 11.1) were developed to guide clinicians in deciding when to obtain a radiograph of an athlete who sustains an ankle sprain.[11]

Associated somatic dysfunction is common in ankle sprains and should be treated as soon as possible. An anterior lateral malleolus dysfunction is seen in typical ankle inversion. Muscle energy treatment of this dysfunction is quick and efficient. Myofascial restrictions due to muscle splinting and local swelling are common.

TABLE 11.1

Ottawa Ankle Rules: Decision Rule for Radiography in Acute Adult Ankle Injuries

Is the patient
    Unable to bear weight immediately and in the emergency department?
    Tender on the tip or posterior aspect of the lateral malleolus?
    Tender on the tip or posterior aspect of the medial malleolus?
Any affirmative answer indicates that a radiograph should be obtained.

Stiell IG, Greenberg GH, McNight RD, et al. Decision rules for the use of radiography in acute ankle injuries: Refinement and prospective validation. JAMA 1993;269:1127–1132.

Removal of myofascial restrictions can help with lymphatic drainage of a swollen, tender ankle. Changes in gait, the use of crutches, and limping contribute to dysfunction of the innominate, sacrum, and lumbar spine. Use OMT in these areas to produce a negative seated flexion test and equalize pelvic side shift.

Anterior Knee Pain

Anterior knee pain is a common finding in the athletic population, especially among females. Because many orthopedic terms are grouped into this category, there is a consensus that a detailed history and physical examination are critical in making the diagnosis.[12] The most common diagnosis is chondromalacia of the patella. Other terminology includes patellofemoral pain syndrome, miserable malalignment syndrome, and patellar tracking abnormality. It is a painful condition that usually starts as repetitive overuse and tends to occur in the patient who develops tight hamstrings and weakness in the medial aspect in the quadriceps muscle. As the process continues, malalignment of the patella causes abnormal tracking along the femoral groove. Over time this causes the cartilage of the patella to soften and roughen. Patients complain of pain around the patella, a variable amount of swelling, and difficulty negotiating stairs or hills. The patella may feel like it locks or catches if they sit with their knees crossed for long; this is the classic *movie goer's sign.*

The osteopathic examination includes palpation for restriction of patellar motion with an evaluation of the ability of the vastus medialis muscle to contract. Atrophy and/or flaccidity of this muscle is a common finding, as is tightness of the hamstring muscles and iliotibial band. Counterstrain and other indirect procedures for the hamstring and calf muscles are beneficial. It is also common to find fibular motion restrictions and dysfunction of the ipsilateral innominate. Tightness and tender points along the iliotibial band are common. OMT should be applied to the axial skeletal component in the lumbar spine and to any innominate sacroiliac dysfunction. Indirect myofascial release of the patella and anterior knee is beneficial for an acute condition. It is also important to improve fibular motion through an articulatory or muscle energy procedure. Following OMT, it is important to give the patient flexibility exercises for the hamstring and calf muscles and open- and closed-chain kinetic exercises for the vastus medialis oblique muscle.

Closed-chain exercises, such as mini-squats against a wall or extension of the knee against a resistance extension lockout, help facilitate a more functional return to activity. Always treat the lumbar and innominate dysfunction prior to giving the patient static or dynamic flexibility exercises for the hamstrings. If lumbar dysfunction is not treated, hamstring tension tends to recur. It is also important to control swelling of the knee. As little as 5 mL of effusion can stimulate the hamstring to tighten and the vastus medialis to weaken or become flaccid.

Hamstring Strain

Hamstring strains are common, unfortunate, and recurrent. They typically occur in sports that require sudden bursts of speed, like football, track, and rugby.[13] The predisposing factors include fatigue, cramping, improper warm-ups, and muscle tension. The athlete may have superficial bruising, a palpable defect or rent in the muscle, a local intramuscular hematoma, or an avulsion of the ischial tuberosity. In milder injuries, there is local tension with multiple tender points in the hamstring group of muscles.

Occasionally there is a tear (or epiphyseal injury) off the ischium rather than in the belly of the muscle. The mechanism of injury is typically simultaneous abrupt hip flexion and knee extension. Somatic dysfunction of the ilium (especially an anterior ilium dysfunction) can predispose the athlete to a hamstring strain. Spasms of the biceps femoris may be related to the dysfunction of the fibula as well. Treating dysfunction of the tibia and fibula and using the indirect procedures for the hamstrings facilitates muscle healing. Always look at the patient's feet, especially for signs of overpronation and malalignment of the patellar femoral joint. Hamstring strains are usually secondary to other biomechanical factors of the feet, knees, or ankles and can be avoided through proper warm-up and cool-down exercises and static or dynamic flexibility programs.

Following an acute injury on the playing field, move the patient to the sidelines or the training room for proper evaluation and treatment. Indirect manipulative procedures that place the injured part in a position of ease are the most appropriate. Subsequent treatment should address any segmental dysfunction in the upper lumbar and low thoracic region, as this would maintain sympathetic tone to the lower extremity, maintaining hamstring tightness. The next components addressed should be the ilium and the sacroiliac joint, as proper motion of this joint will also allow more normal motion of the pelvis during gait. Gentle seated dynamic range-of-motion exercises for the hamstring muscles also help facilitate moving lymphatic fluid from the area and improving range of motion. Always finish the manual treatment by applying the RICEM principle: rest, ice, compression, elevation, and medication for pain control.

Rotator Cuff Tendonitis: Impingement Syndrome

Rotator cuff tendonitis and subacromial bursitis typically occur together and are probably the most common sports medicine diagnoses of the shoulder. Patients have pain, weakness, and limited shoulder mobility overhead. With a complete tear, patients may develop pain near the deltoid insertion, which occurs at night, along with difficulty reaching the arm overhead. The rotator cuff is composed of four muscles: the supraspinatus, infraspinatus, teres minor, and subscapularis. The supraspinatus tendon is torn in approximately 90% of cases of rotator cuff tendonitis.

There are four proposed mechanisms of injury in repetitive overuse (microtrauma).[14] Primary impingement occurs with repetitive overhead motion as the supraspinatus tendon impinges under the inferior portion of the acromion. The shape and slope of the acromion are important. A congenitally hooked acromion or perhaps an arthritic spur can aggravate the supraspinatus tendon. Secondary impingement occurs with glenohumeral laxity and instability of the shoulder. In this situation, cephalad migration of the humeral head and undersurface tears may occur. Tensile failure during throwing may fatigue the cuff muscles and develop a tear with eccentric loading. Overhead throwing may also cause an internal (posterosuperior glenoid impingement). In this situation the inferior aspect of the supraspinatus is trapped between the greater tuberosity of the humerus and the posterior superior labrum. Patient apprehension resulting from external rotation of the shoulder (at 90 degrees of abduction) indicates glenohumeral instability and is another cause of tendonitis.

Physical examination reveals tenderness in the subacromial space; instability testing (e.g., apprehension and relocation tests, sulcus sign) may reveal laxity. Resistance testing of the supraspinatus is done with the arms internally rotated and abducted 90 degrees in the scapular plane. Inability to resist the examiner's downward force indicates supraspinatus weakness. The impingement sign of Neer involves injecting 10 mL of 1% lidocaine hydrochloride into the subacromial space and repeating the resistance test of the supraspinatus.[14] Pain relief confirms impingement. Occasionally cervical neuropathy, such as C5 to C6, C6 to C7, can cause rotator cuff muscle weakness and pain to the shoulder that would mimic rotator cuff tendonitis. This possibility always must be ruled out in a patient with rotator cuff tendinopathy.

There is usually significant structural somatic dysfunction of the upper thoracic spine and ribs. An extended (Fryette's type II) dysfunction is commonly found. Treatment of this dysfunction with an epigastric high-velocity, low-amplitude (HVLA) thrust is beneficial, because the procedure allows some upward traction as well as the right amount of spinal flexion. Rotator cuff patients tend to "hike" their shoulder causing scalene hypertonicity, upper trapezius muscle tender points, and segmental lower cervical dysfunction. It is fairly common to find an elevated first rib as well, partly due to dysfunction at the T1 segment as well as anterior scalene hypertonicity. Tenderness and tightness of the ipsilateral pectoralis minor muscle are common, as is ropy tissue texture change of the infraspinatus and posterior axillary fold. A Jones tender point[15] in the subscapularis muscle (in the axilla) is also an indicative finding.

Rotator cuff injuries may be associated with other orthopedic problems, depending on the type and duration of trauma. Plain radiographs may reveal a compression fracture of the humeral head (Hill-Sachs deformity), dislocations, arthritic changes, and calcific deposits. When these situations occur simultaneously with rotator cuff tear, orthopedic consultation is warranted.

Manipulative treatment of these areas should start with the upper thoracic spine and ribs and the cervical spine and then should move into the shoulder, elbow, wrist, and hand. Myofascial or muscle energy procedures that involve the shoulder should stay away from painful arcs of motion and work with tissues in an indirect position (position of ease) until range of motion improves. The cornerstone of improving rotator cuff tendinopathy and impingement syndrome is posture-based work. Patients must improve their core abdominal strength initially, then progress to scapular stabilization and retraction exercises. When patients have reeducated their lower rhomboids and lower trapezius muscles, more-specific strengthening of the rotator cuff muscles themselves can begin. Patients should not aggressively exercise the shoulder without first addressing core muscle strength imbalances and lower scapular muscle inhibitions.

Heel Pain and Plantar Fasciitis

Heel pain is problematic and persistent. Plantar fasciitis (heel spur syndrome) is one of the most common causes. It is a condition of repetitive impact loading and microtrauma. It produces local heel pain at the medial plantar insertion on the calcaneus. Runners, basketball players, and volleyball players are at the highest risk. The first few steps in the morning are painful, and there is tenderness near the medial plantar fascia insertion on the calcaneus. Tenderness along the sidewall of the calcaneus in the adult athlete may indicate a calcaneus stress fracture instead of plantar fasciitis. Radiographs may show a calcaneal heel spur. These are generally not clinically significant, as they may be seen in patients without fasciitis as well. The clinician should look for intrinsic and extrinsic causes. Always look at the six S's of running injuries: shoes, surface, speed, stretching, strength, and structure.[9]

From a biomechanical approach, one should look for tension in the iliopsoas, hamstring, gastrocnemius, and soleus muscles. Tender points along the plantar fascia may be treated with Jones counterstrain.[15] Moreover, muscular tension along the tender points may occur in the calves and hamstring muscle groups. Release procedures, such as counterstrain, are effective for these areas. OMT for the patient with heel pain should start with the axial component in the lumbar spine and then proceed to the sacrum, pelvis, and distally to the hamstrings, calf, and finally the foot. Always treat with the objective to obtain both a negative seated flexion test and a negative pelvic side-shift test. If there is a leg length inequality, use a heel lift to level the sacral base. (See Chapter 26.) Use of gel heel cups with activity modification and stretching of the calves and hamstrings may be beneficial as well.

Integration of OMT into Conservative and Surgical Management

Conservative Management

OMT provides beneficial support to the host through healing of a variety of athletic injuries. Recall that there are specific phases of healing. The patient's body must progress through these phases for proper healing to take place. It is fairly common to see patients start aggressive strengthening programs in physical therapy before the inflammatory phase of the process is complete. That is why it is important to have a proper amount of rest initially. Relative rest is considered to be resting the injured part while still maintaining activity with the rest of the body. For example, a patient with a leg fracture who is in a cast may sit on an exercise bike moving the arms back and forth. This allows the patient to receive a cardiovascular workout while the legs remain stationary. It is possible for a patient who has a wrist or elbow injury to use a stationary or recumbent bike or walk on a track or a treadmill for aerobic training. Relative rest is important for maintaining athletes' cardiovascular status as they heal. It is also important for the sports medicine practitioner to practice *aggressive conservatism,* making patient–athletes an active and integral part of their healing process. This may include cross-training with other activities to maintain cardiovascular function, contrasting baths, and the use of medications, OMT, static or dynamic flexibility exercises, relaxation techniques, and psychological techniques, such as mental imagery. The multifactorial approach is the preferred manner in which *aggressive conservatism* is used in treatment.

OMT sets the stage for exercises to work. For example, if significant lumbar somatic dysfunctions are not treated and a patient tries to strengthen core abdominal muscles doing a simple curl-up exercise, the spine will not move in a segmented fashion and will skip over the restricted areas. Some areas of the spine will be overworked while others are skipped over altogether. OMT tends to decrease local swelling and to improve pain tolerance. It supports the innate healing power of the patient and improves fluid transfer and medication distribution. OMT may also decrease dependence on medication in patients with chronic pain. A multidisciplinary approach also improves the ability to compensate for injury. Consider patients who have been using a cast and crutches. They transfer abnormal stresses to the lumbar spine and pelvis. OMT to those regions can decrease pain and improve function, especially when the athletes return to their sport.

Conservative treatment of athletic injury includes the **RICEM** and **PRICEM** principles. These acronyms, pad (or protection), along with rest, ice, compression, elevation, and medication, as mentioned earlier, are commonly used in sports medicine. Besides applying these principles, it is critical to determine whether an area should be immobilized. For an acute ligamentous sprain, immobilization with a cast or splint is indicated. OMT, however, may also be indicated for areas distant or related. Consider, for example, a patient with a lumbar sprain at the L5 to S1 region. Such an athlete may have some reactive muscle spasm of the erector spinae muscle mass and tightening of the iliopsoas. OMT applied to these regions, which are distant yet related sites, may unload these muscles and help the injured area heal. It is also critical to pay attention to the area of injury from a standpoint of what needs to be padded or protected when the patient returns to play. It is important sometimes to shift forces away from the injured area. This is commonly done with foot injuries. For example, for the patient who has a metatarsal sprain or sesamoiditis, specific metatarsal pads are placed in the shoes to reduce pressure on the injured areas and redirect forces from the painful sites to other structures.

Conservative management also includes use of ice, heat, contrasting baths, ultrasound, muscle stimulation, iontophoresis, and/or phonophoresis. Ice therapy, good for acute injuries and acute inflammations, is usually kept in place for 15 to 20 minutes. Ice massage is also useful for tendonitis and can be used for shorter times. Contrasting baths, alternating use of ice and heat (always end with ice), also helps exercise, and it pumps the lymphatic fluid from the injured area by stimulating vasoconstriction and vasodilation. For deep muscle spasm, ultrasound may be used. Ultrasound applies deep heat to a muscular area and causes vasodilation. This causes relaxation and improves regional blood flow. Muscle stimulation, most commonly interferential current, is useful for controlling and modulating pain and also promoting vasodilation and the movement of fluids from an area. Iontophoresis is use of interferential current with application of a steroid gel to the skin. The electric current helps the steroid permeate into the soft tissues. Phonophoresis is use of ultrasound with a steroid gel to help the steroid permeate into the soft tissues and decrease pain. Combinations of these numerous modalities are used on a daily basis by athletic trainers in the training room.

Throughout the conservative management of the athlete, physicians, physical therapists, and athletic trainers work to improve free range of motion, strength, posture, and proprioception while mitigating pain as the treatment proceeds. In conservative management, it is important to consider the dosage and sequence of rehabilitation. This includes the dosage and sequence of OMT to various regions and dosage of other modalities, such as electrical muscle stimulation, ultrasound, ice, and heat. Some athletes receive these treatments daily in hopes of accelerating healing. Sometimes the patient is overdosed—too much of a good thing. Overuse of these conservative measures can worsen the patient's condition. The physician must be mindful of this circumstance.

Surgical Management

An important part of surgical management of athletic injury is *prehab,* or rehabilitation prior to surgery. This is true especially for a patient with a knee injury who is going to have arthroscopy or anterior cruciate ligament reconstruction. In this example, it is critical that the patient undergo some rehabilitation before surgery to learn how to fire the vastus medialis oblique muscle, stretch and strengthen the hamstrings, and strengthen the core abdominal and pelvic muscles. Rehabilitation exercises can be done isometrically so as not to aggravate the injured area. This will foster a faster recovery from the surgery and a faster return to sport. Presurgical OMT is also useful, not only to control pain and decrease swelling but also to improve function and motion of restricted tissue and improve anatomic relationships. Postoperatively, OMT is directed at the removal or reduction of functional impediment, to assist patients' ability to mount a recuperative response. Specifically, treating somatic dysfunction reduces postoperative complications, such as atelectasis and ileus. It also makes the patient more comfortable. Enhancing the thoracic cage motion preoperatively is critical because most patients need general anesthetics. Even if a spinal anesthetic is used, the patient will be lying for long periods. Improving thoracic cage mobility with OMT helps reduce lymphatic congestion postoperatively, as well as decreasing the incidence of pulmonary atelectasis. OMT decreases sympathetic tone postoperatively, and this improves bowel function, decreasing postoperative ileus. Common manipulative procedures used postoperatively are paraspinal inhibition, lymphatic pump, and rib raising.

The surgical patient may also develop viscerosomatic reflexes as a result of surgery, injury, and prolonged medication use. Usually patients who elect to have surgery have a severe injury and are taking a significant amount of nonsteroidal anti-inflammatory drugs. Often they develop upper thoracic viscerosomatic reflexes, indicating subclinical gastrointestinal irritation from these medications. Such reflexes can be addressed with OMT. It is important to decrease these musculoskeletal responses to inflammatory visceral pathology as well as to make appropriate changes in prescribed medication.

Early range-of-motion exercises after surgery are usually recommended, depending on the anatomic structures treated. For most postoperative knee arthroscopies, the patient can go home the following day and attempt to bear weight. More extensive cases may necessitate use of a continuous passive motion machine. OMT helps to improve function as these patients heal and may permit decreased use of opioid pain medication. It improves function of their new anatomic relationships and new structure.

Return-to-Play Considerations

A physician must consider the level of the athlete and the participation guidelines that were determined initially. The duration of the patient's condition must be taken into account along with the severity. Athletes may have comorbid conditions, especially if they are older; these must be taken into account. How patients respond to rehabilitation, what prior injuries they have had, and how those prior injuries were rehabilitated will also help guide the physician in determining return-to-play considerations. There are specific return-to-play considerations for some conditions, such as concussion. Since these guidelines are controversial and tend to change frequently, it is important to consult the most recent medical literature.

Every athlete has a unique rehabilitation potential. Some of this is determined from prior injury history and some is found during the current rehabilitation. The physician may notice that an athlete will respond more quickly to one therapeutic modality than to others. Sometimes modalities have to be rotated to obtain maximum gain from each modality. The rehabilitation plan for each patient must take into account the timeline, the team's level of play, and pressures from coaches and the team to have the athlete return. Once a decision is made by a treating physician, it is recommended that the physician stick to the decision and not succumb to these external pressures. Always provide adequate communication and a release form for the athlete, especially a student athlete.

Prevention, Patient Education, and Performance Enhancement

Prevention is an integral part of caring for athletes. OMT plays a significant role in preventing athletic injury, as much as if not more than proper warm-up and cooling down. Patients who have a full pain-free active range of motion and know when they are developing a specific pain or problem tend to come to the office sooner and avoid exacerbating an injury. If somatic dysfunction goes undiagnosed or untreated, its severity can increase in such a way that a patient can develop an injury secondary to compensation from the somatic dysfunction. It is also important that athletes have proper gear for their activity and proper access to training services. Often a patient knows enough to rest an injured area or to cross-train to unload tissue stresses applied by repetitive overuse. In this situation, the patient may be able to prevent or reduce the severity of an injury.

Patient education is a critical aspect of athlete care. Handouts and demonstrations of stretches and exercises by the physician, therapist, or trainer are important.

It also is a good practice to have additional visual aids (still pictures, videotapes, DVDs) available for the patient. Occasionally it is necessary to film a patient's throwing or swinging mechanics. This film can be used to find biomechanical errors and to educate the patient. It is important to educate the coach and the relatives of the athlete as the athlete goes through the stages of rehabilitation. Education is not only an important part of the treatment of athletic injury; it is also an important part of prevention of the use of anabolic steroids, creatine, stimulants, and other over-the-counter drugs and banned substances.

Patients who have completed a rehabilitation program and have returned to their sport and athletes who have noticed a decline in their performance may need performance enhancement. OMT can help by removing hindrances to compensations from older injuries and by improving biomechanical function. Performance can also be enhanced by use of appropriate gear and work with specialized coaches, such as batting coaches, golf swing coaches, throwing coaches, and shooting coaches. Finding patients' functional deficits is important. There may be a deficit in their form that is not noticed initially. Sometimes this can be found if film footage is taken of an athlete's motion and then slowed down and evaluated.

Another critical component of performance enhancement is patients' state of mind and emotional factors regarding their own performance, their relationship with the coach and other players, and where they fit on the team. Many times an emotional issue is the primary problem or functional deficit in an athlete, and the musculoskeletal findings are only a distant effect. Psychotherapy, relaxation techniques, and mental imagery can be useful for working through a slump in athletic performance. Abrupt cessation of a sport because of athletic injury may lead to poor sleep and be the initiating event in the development of fibromyalgia. Osteopathic physicians believe the mind, body, and spirit are integrally linked. The emotional component of the athlete's injury should never be underestimated. Athletes can quickly become very depressed if their performance falls off. This situation often promotes a higher rate of medication usage and the use of nutritional supplements, recreational drugs, and ergogenic aids.

CONCLUSION

Osteopathic primary care physicians who use OMT and their structural medicine skills have a unique advantage in helping athletic patients who are injured. The treatment of somatic dysfunction with OMT sets the stage for proper healing to begin. It improves the function of therapeutic exercises, decreases pain, decreases complications after surgery, and improves function. Osteopathic physicians who use OMT in sports medicine are highly sought after for treatment of athletic injuries. They make significant differences in the lives and performance of the athletic patients.

Procedures

Please note: The procedures that follow are examples of manipulative treatment that you may wish to employ. The actual choice of procedures used should be determined by the unique circumstances of each individual patient.

Anterior Lateral Malleolus (Muscle Energy) (Fig. 11.1)

Consider the dysfunction of a left anterior lateral malleolus. The objective is to improve posterior movement of the lateral malleolus. An anterior lateral malleolus is associated with a posterior proximal fibula.

Patient position: supine. Physician position: standing at the foot of the table.

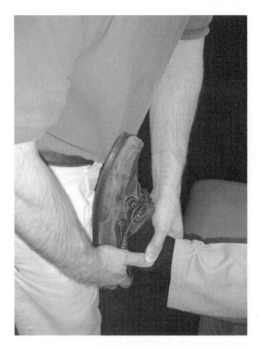

FIGURE 11.1 Muscle energy, anterior left lateral malleolus.

Procedure
1. Cup the patient's left heel in the palm of your right hand. Place your right thumb over the anterior aspect of the lateral malleolus, with the remaining fingers of your right hand projecting downward and around the posterior aspect of the calcaneus. Place your left thumb over your right thumb (reinforcement), with the remaining fingers of your left hand encircling the medial aspect of the ankle.
2. Contact the sole of the patient's foot with your abdomen, and while leaning forward, use your body to position the patient's foot in dorsiflexion. Maintain a posteriorly directed force over the anterior aspect of the lateral malleolus with your thumbs.
3. Corrective movement: Instruct the patient to gently push the foot into plantar flexion while restricting this motion with your body (maintain dorsiflexion). Maintain the posteriorly directed force with your thumbs. Have the patient hold the contraction for 3 to 5 seconds.
4. Instruct the patient to relax. Wait 2 seconds, then engage the new barrier by moving the patient's foot further into dorsiflexion while moving the lateral malleolus posteriorly with your thumbs.
5. Repeat two or three times or until motion improves.
6. When the procedure is complete, reassess posterior motion of the lateral malleolus.

Indirect Hamstring Release (Myofascial Release) (Fig. 11.2)

Consider the dysfunction of a hypertonic left hamstring. The objective is to decrease hamstring hypertonicity. The principles of counterstrain can be applied to treat dysfunction between agonist and antagonist muscle groups. A specific tender point is not necessarily present. The physician loads the antagonist and unloads the agonist. This may be considered a direct myofascial release to the antagonist or an indirect procedure to the agonist.[15]

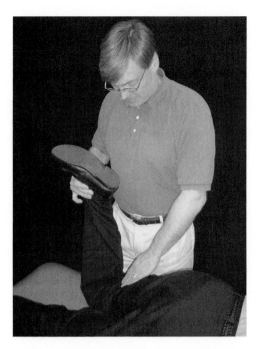

FIGURE 11.2   Indirect myofascial release of the left hamstring muscles.

Patient position: prone. Physician position: standing on the side of the dysfunctional hamstring.

Procedure

1. Palpate for an area of increased tension of the hamstring with both hands. Monitor this area with your left hand. A tender point is not necessary.
2. With your right hand, grasp the ankle and flex the knee slowly until the patient begins to feel tension in the quadriceps muscle. At this point tension of the hamstring should be minimal.
3. Unload the hamstring (agonist) and load the quadriceps (antagonist).
4. If the patient has pain in the low back with knee flexion, do not flex as far or choose another procedure.
5. Fine-tuning may be achieved by internally or externally rotating the tibia to achieve the least amount of tension in the hamstring.
6. Fine-tuning may also be achieved by translating the hamstring group medially or laterally with your left hand to achieve the least amount of tension in the hamstring.
7. After a several seconds, the hamstring will soften or release. Palpate for this release (or softening) of the hamstring group.
8. Slowly return the leg down to the table.
9. When the procedure is complete, reassess the dysfunctional muscle for tension.

Knee (Indirect Myofascial Release) (Fig. 11.3)

Consider the dysfunction of a myofascial restriction of the knee. The objective is to remove the fascial restriction and improve knee function.

Patient position: supine. Physician position: standing at the side of the patient.

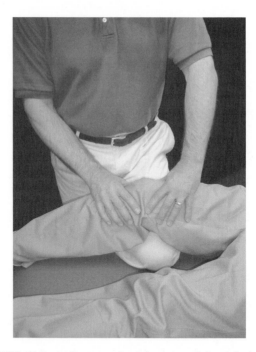

FIGURE 11.3 Indirect myofascial release of the right knee.

Procedure

1. Place your knee under the patient's knee to give a slight amount of flexion. Place your left hand above the patella on the distal thigh and your right hand below the patella on the tibia.
2. Conduct a motion test to find the direction of ease of the myofascial tissues. This will include a side-to-side (translatory) motion, an internal and external rotation, and a compression and distraction of the tissues.
3. For an indirect release, *unload and follow*. That is, move the tissues in the direction of freer motion, taking into account all aspects of translation, internal and external rotation, and either compression or distraction.
4. Hold this position and wait for an inherent release or softening of tissue tension.
5. When the procedure is complete, reassess the dysfunctional area.

Anterior Innominate Dysfunction (Muscle Energy) (See Fig. 9.9)

Consider the dysfunction of an anterior left innominate. The objective is to improve motion of the dysfunctional innominate into the restrictive barrier. In treating the anterior innominate, a modification includes grasping the ischium on the dysfunctional side to help augment posterior rotation of the innominate.

Patient position: supine. Physician position: standing at the side of the patient's dysfunctional innominate bone.

Procedure

1. Flex the patient's affected knee and hip until the restrictive barrier is engaged.
2. Apply your shoulder or axilla to the patient's knee, using both hands to grasp the sides of the table. Firmly hold the hip and knee in this flexed position.

3. Instruct the patient to press the knee into your shoulder area (extending the hip) against your holding force, starting with minimal force and increasing the amount of force only at your request. Instruct the patient to maintain the force for 3 to 5 seconds.
4. Have the patient rest and relax for a few seconds, then engage the new barrier and repeat the process; two or three efforts are usually sufficient.
5. When the procedure is complete, reassess the dysfunctional innominate.

Plantar Fasciitis (Counterstrain) (Fig. 11.4)

Consider point tenderness of the right plantar fascia insertion on the calcaneus. The objective is to reduce this tenderness. Jones[15] treats this condition in a prone position with the knee flexed and the heel pushed toward the front of the plantar-flexed foot.

Patient position: supine. Physician position: seated on the end of the table, facing the patient.

Procedure

1. Locate the region of the plantar fascia insertion on the inferior and anterior surface of the right calcaneus. Palpate for a significant tender point.
2. Monitor that tender point with one thumb, and with the other hand plantar-flex the ankle and flex the toes until tension or loading of the tibialis anterior muscle is achieved. Your right thumb acts as a fulcrum to flex around.
3. Supination or pronation of the foot may be required to fine-tune while obtaining a position of symptomatic relief (no tenderness).
4. The tibialis anterior is loaded; the gastrocnemius and soleus are unloaded.
5. Hold this position for 90 seconds or until a palpable softening of the tissues occurs.

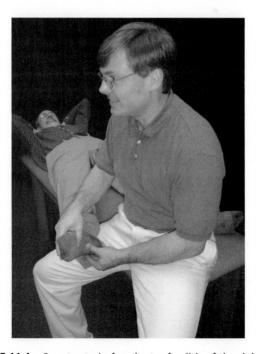

FIGURE 11.4 Counterstrain for plantar fasciitis of the right foot.

6. Slowly return the foot to its normal position. Your monitoring finger should not leave the point.
7. When the procedure is complete, reassess the dysfunctional plantar fascia for tenderness.

Epigastric Thrust (HVLA) (Fig. 11.5)

Consider the dysfunction T6 flexed, rotated right, side-bent right. The objective of this procedure is to restore motion in extension, left side bending, and left rotation. This procedure may be used on midthoracic dysfunctions. The barrier is primarily engaged with lateral translation. Keeping your knee on the table helps stabilize your forces so you do not hurt your own back.

Patient position: seated. Physician position: standing behind the patient with the right knee on the table on the side of the posterior component.

Procedure

1. Instruct the patient to sit comfortably on the table and clasp the hands behind the neck.
2. Fold a small pillow in half, place it in direct contact with the left transverse processes of T7 in a horizontal position, and hold it there firmly with your epigastrium.
3. Pass your left hand under the patient's left axilla and grasp the back of the patient's left forearm. Pass your right hand under the patient's right axilla and grasp the back of the patient's right forearm.
4. Extend the patient's upper thoracic area down to and including T6. Keep the patient's upper torso centered over the pelvis during this procedure.
5. Translate the patient's trunk to the right above T7 to introduce side bending to the left of T6 upon T7.

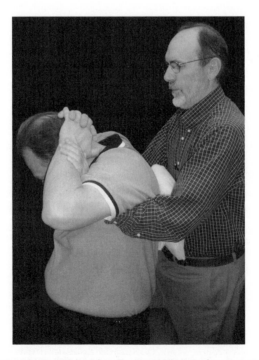

FIGURE 11.5 HVLA epigastric thrust for thoracic type II dysfunction, T6 flexed, rotated right, side bent right.

6. Rotate the upper thoracic area to the left, making sure you localize forces down to T6 upon T7.
7. The final corrective force is through the pillow and abdomen against the engaged barrier. It is an accentuation of the accumulated motions. Rotation is not a significant component.
8. When the procedure is complete, reassess the dysfunctional area.

CONSIDERATION

For extended dysfunctions, follow the previous procedure; however, have the patient flex forward by slumping while bringing the shoulders posterior in a translatory movement. The final corrective force is a quick thrust with short forward and lateral motion of the pillow and epigastrium coordinated with an increase in the amount of traction through the patient's axillae.

Biceps, Long Head (Counterstrain) (Fig. 11.6)

Consider a tender point in the tendon of the right long head of the biceps muscle near the bicipital groove. The objective is to alleviate the tender point by initiating a mild stretch to the antagonist muscle group (triceps).

   Patient position: standing. Physician position: standing behind the patient.

Procedure

1. Locate the biceps tender point near the distal tendon insertion.
2. Monitor the tender point with the middle or index finger of your left hand. (You will monitor the tender point for the whole procedure.)
3. Use your right hand to flex the elbow and shoulder. A mild stretch is placed on the triceps as the biceps is shortened. Try to achieve a position that maximally decreases

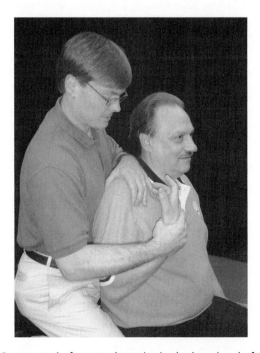

FIGURE 11.6   Counterstrain for a tender point in the long head of the right biceps.

tension under your monitoring finger. Supination of the forearm is usually necessary as well.

4. Hold the arm in this position for 90 seconds. As release occurs, you will feel a decrease in tension under your monitoring finger.
5. Slowly return the arm to the neutral position. (Do not let the patient assist you.)
6. When the procedure is complete, reassess the tender point.

Note: Counterstrain can be used for any tender point.

References

1. Walter GW. The First School of Osteopathic Medicine. Kirksville, MO: Thomas Jefferson University, 1924 (reprinted 1992):39–45.
2. Still CE Jr. Frontier Doctor—Medical Pioneer: The Life and Times of A. T. Still and His Family. Kirksville, MO: Thomas Jefferson University, 1907 (reprinted 1991, Truman State University):205–216.
3. Patrick K, Sallis JF, Long B, et al. A new tool for encouraging activity: Project PACE. Phys Sports Med 1994;22:45–52.
4. Scuderi GR, McCann PD, Bruno PJ, eds. Sports Medicine: Principles of Primary Care. St. Louis: Mosby, 1997.
5. Strauss RH. Cardiovascular benefits and risks of exercise: the scientific evidence. In: Wickland EH Jr, ed. Sports Medicine. 2nd ed. Philadelphia: Saunders, 1991;72–80.
6. Ward RC. Geriatrics. In: Ward RC, ed. Foundations for Osteopathic Medicine. 2nd ed. Philadelphia: Lippincott Williams & Wilkins, 2002;327–337.
7. Brolinson PG, Heinking KP, Kozar AJ. An osteopathic approach to sports medicine. In: Ward RC, ed. Foundations for Osteopathic Medicine. 2nd ed. Philadelphia: Lippincott Williams & Wilkins, 2002;534–550.
8. Mitchell FL. Structural pelvic function. In: 1958 Yearbook. Indianapolis: American Academy of Osteopathy, 1958:71–90.
9. Heinking KP. The geriatric athlete. In: Karageanes SJ, ed. Principles of Manual of Sports Medicine. Philadelphia: Lippincott Williams & Wilkins, 2005:629–640.
10. Brennanan FH Jr, Campagna K, Feldner W. Foot and ankle common conditions. In: Karageanes, SJ, ed. Principles of Manual Sports Medicine. Philadelphia: Lippincott Williams & Wilkins, 2005;424–441.
11. Stiell IG, Greenberg GH, McNight RD, et al. Decision rules for the use of radiography in acute ankle injuries: Refinement and prospective validation. JAMA 1993;269:1127–1132.
12. Cutbill JW, Ladly KO, Bray RC, et al. Anterior knee pain: A review. Clin J Sport Med 1997;7:40–45.
13. Best TM, Garrett WE. Hamstring strains: Expediting return to play. Physician Sports Med 1996;24(8):37–44.
14. Wolin PM, Tarbet JA. Rotator cuff injury: Addressing overhead overuse. Physician Sports Med 1997;25:54–74.
15. Jones LH. Strain and Counterstrain. Newark, OH: American Academy of Osteopathy, 1981.

CHAPTER 12

The Geriatric Patient

Kenneth E. Nelson, Ann L. Habenicht,
and Nicette Sergueef

INTRODUCTION

Osteopathic practitioners acknowledge that the body has the inherent ability to heal itself. If this is so, why isn't everyone healthy, and why don't we live forever? The answer to this question is obviously that this self-healing mechanism varies in efficacy from individual to individual and to a great extent is a manifestation of the individual's ability to compensate for stress. As the individual ages, the ability to compensate for stress decreases, while physiologic sources of stress increase. An individual's age can therefore be considered in the contexts of both physiology and time. A person may be old in years and yet remain young physiologically. Conversely, a much younger patient with a chronic illness will be physiologically aged. Eventually, however, every individual who is fortunate enough not to die young is subject to the cumulative effects of age.

This chapter focuses upon helping the patient to compensate for the inevitable decompensation brought on by aging. Preventive medicine is extremely important in this context; thus, nutrition and the function of the musculoskeletal system are two areas where preventive practices are readily applicable.

DIET AND NUTRITION

Nutrition is a subject unto itself and is beyond the scope of this chapter, but it should be part of the treatment of all patients. Dietetics for older patients must take into account several things. Cultural habits are formed. People learn their eating habits in early life, and these patients have had many years to establish bad dietetic habits that like everything else will have their greatest negative impact in the later years of life. Getting a patient to change a lifetime of eating habits can be difficult, particularly in old age, when gustatory pleasure may be one of the few enjoyments still available. Further, the patient may avoid eating even when adequate food is available, simply because meal preparation requires too much effort or they do not like to eat alone. Physical mobility may be impaired, further interfering with food buying and preparation. Energy expenditure is decreased, which decreases caloric requirements although the patient's requirements for micronutrients remain constant. The food the patient does eat is frequently poorly assimilated. Poor dental health, hyposecretion of the gastric mucosa, and senescent decrease in the production of enteric enzymes all interfere with the absorption of nutrients. As a person grows older, financial resources often diminish, and less money is available for food. Therefore, the physician must consider patients' dietary needs from all directions, a task that is by no means simple.

MUSCULOSKELETAL FUNCTION AND SOMATIC DYSFUNCTION

Aging brings with it distinct changes in the neuromusculoskeletal system. Somatic dysfunction is by definition an impediment of function of the musculoskeletal system that affects the patient mechanically and through its effect upon associated vascular and neurologic structures.[1] The individual must actively compensate for the resulting impairment. Somatic dysfunction is associated with irritability of the segmentally related nervous system that in itself may contribute to disease through direct somatovisceral and general systemic impact.[2] Somatic dysfunction can be found in patients of all ages. It is a reversible functional impairment that is readily amenable to osteopathic manipulative treatment (OMT).

As the individual ages and begins to lose muscle mass, strength and stamina diminish, with a resultant loss of functional capacity. The more efficiently patients function, the more they can compensate for the inevitable stresses of aging. As mentioned earlier, if the patient has an optimal diet, particularly as regarding calcium and vitamin D, augmented by an effective exercise program, this progression may be attenuated, if not arrested.

It is common knowledge that diet coupled with exercise may be employed to improve muscle tone and mass, prevent osteoporosis, reduce hyperlipidemia, maintain cardiovascular health, and enhance the efficacy of medical therapies for disease processes like diabetes. Thus, most older individuals have been told to exercise as part of their therapeutic regimen. These patients often work extremely hard to manage their diet and to increase their level of physical activity. Exercise programs like walking, low-impact aerobics, and tai chi are weight-bearing activities. Such activities, although highly desirable, paradoxically can contribute to postural decompensation. More than half of the general population demonstrate anatomic inequality of leg length of one-quarter inch or more.[3] This imbalance results in pelvic unleveling with compensatory type I group lateral curve spinal mechanics above the pelvis. Group spinal mechanics are not only associated with dysfunctional spinal side bending, they also increase the normal anteroposterior spinal curves. Thus, the patient is apt to decompensate due to weight-bearing stress in both the coronal and sagittal planes. The incidence of this decompensation increases with age as the patient loses the ability to accommodate for the asymmetric lateral and altered anteroposterior weight-bearing stresses. Most commonly this manifests as lumbosacral or sacro-pelvic pain.[3] Thus, the exercise prescribed to benefit the patient may result in postural decompensation and musculoskeletal pain. These issues may often be very simply addressed with lift therapy, core muscular strengthening, and if necessary, an antero-posterior orthotic (Levitor) device in association with appropriately applied OMT. (See Chapters 26 and 27.)

Postural imbalance and gait instability are particular issues with geriatric patients. Peripheral sensory input significantly provides for the maintenance of upright pos-ture. Aging is associated with a decrease in postural balance that increases the risk of falling.[4] When patients fall, they tend to fall to the side, commonly fracturing the hip. As the individual ages, visual, labyrinthine, and somatosensory input change their contribution to the dynamic maintenance of standing posture. Presbyopia, cataract formation, changes in the vitreous humor, and other ophthalmologic dis-eases of aging decrease visual acuity and consequently the individual's ability to rely upon vision for postural balance. Impaired visual acuity increases the chances of falling.[5] Thus, with loss of vision, the patient begins to rely more upon labyrinthine and somatosensory input.

Upper thoracic flexion and decreased cervico-occipital extension affect head position, lowering the visual field from the horizon and shifting the neutral posi-tion of the vestibular apparatus. The head-flexed position significantly increases postural instability.[6] When patients cannot rely upon visual cues for postural bal-ance, they tend to compensate by stiffening the muscles in their lower legs during upright standing.[4] The loss of muscle mass and strength impairs the efficacy of this compensation. Such patients can be treated by addressing somatic dysfunction of the upper thoracic, cervical, and cervico-occipital regions, particularly flexion dys-functions, and by providing exercises directed at strengthening the lower extremi-ties and enhancing freedom of ankle flexion and extension.

Evaluation of the Patient

Although the focus of this chapter is upon the diagnosis and treatment of somatic dysfunction, it is necessary to treat the entire individual, not just the musculoskele-tal system. An accurate diagnosis must obviously be predicated upon a thorough history and physical examination, inclusive of all systems and regions of the body. Viscerosomatic reflexes often provide clues to underlying occult visceral pathol-ogy. (See Chapter 5.) Treatment, be it OMT, pharmacotherapy, diet, or exercise is predicated upon proper diagnosis. The geriatric patient is subject to all of the mal-adies that affect younger patients. Therefore, the diagnosis and treatment of somatic dysfunction for geriatric patients with ear, nose, and throat (see Chapter 16); pulmonary (see Chapter 17); cardiovascular (see Chapters 18 and 19); and gas-trointestinal (see Chapter 20) problems are essentially the same as described else-where in this text. Geriatric patients are particularly likely to present with multiple chronic degenerative conditions that they may or may not be aware of. It is for these conditions in this population that the principles of osteopathic medicine, which focus upon diagnosing reversible somatic dysfunction and treating it with OMT to optimize function, possibly offer the greatest impact.

As individuals age, they become resigned to their diminished resilience and increased musculoskeletal discomfort. Chronic progressive conditions like hypertension, diabetes, and chronic renal failure can be present for extended periods without the patient knowing it. Physical symptoms that they might have found unacceptable in their younger days become normative, so they do not complain about them. Chronic lower urinary tract infections, low-grade upper respiratory infections, and dental sepsis can result in malaise that does not necessarily manifest as a specifically localized complaint. Occult hypothyroidism may be misinterpreted as normal loss of vitality with age. Benign conditions can present as perplexing complaints. Cerumen impaction, through irritation of the auricular branch of the vagus nerve, can present as a persistent nonproductive cough. Or simply because of diminished hearing, cerumen impaction may cause the patient to appear withdrawn and unresponsive.

Patients with an acute onset of musculoskeletal pain, no matter how vague or seemingly trivial, should have a thorough physical examination to rule out underlying medical and orthopedic disorders. Suboccipital headache may be caused by upper cervical somatic dysfunction, or it may be the result of eyestrain or a viscerosomatic reflex from the upper respiratory tract or from any of the viscera innervated by the vagus. OMT may be used to exert a positive effect upon segmentally related viscera through somatovisceral physiology, but the definitive treatment of a viscerosomatic reflex is the specific treatment of the underlying visceral pathology. Identification of spinal somatic dysfunction necessitates that pathology be ruled out in segmentally related viscera. Rib or thoracic spine pain that begins following an episode of coughing may well be the result of somatic dysfunction of the thoracic vertebrae or rib, but in an individual with osteoporosis, it may be a posttussive fracture. OMT is employed to treat somatic dysfunction, the functional reduction of motion, and as such is contraindicated if instability is a possibility.

The patient's chief complaint often dictates where to begin the musculoskeletal examination. If postural decompensation is suspected, a complete structural examination should be performed as for any other patient. From behind, with the patient standing, observe symmetrical anatomic landmarks that indicate the postural asymmetry of short leg mechanics. Compare the levels of the posterior superior iliac spines (PSIS), sacral dimples, the most lateral aspect of the iliac crests, and the tops of the greater trochanters. Typically, all of these are low on the side of the short leg. Next, check for compensatory spinal lateral curves. Have the patient bend forward and observe for asymmetrical paravertebral prominence, the result of the rotational component of type I mechanics. The typical accommodation to a short leg results in a compensatory curve that is convex on the side of the short leg. Further, observe for symmetry of anatomic landmarks above the pelvis (i.e., scapulae, acromion processes, and mastoid processes) and of anatomic landmarks of the lower extremity (i.e., popliteal creases and medial malleoli). Finally, check for pelvic side shift. Stabilize the upper torso by holding the shoulder with one hand and push medially over the lateral aspect of the opposite side of the pelvis with the other hand. The test is positive when the pelvis moves freely in one direction but resists movement in the opposite direction. A positive pelvic side shift is designated as either left or right as an indication of the direction of unrestricted pelvic motion. Inequality of leg length is associated with pelvic side shift toward the long leg, or the shift may be the result of asymmetric psoas major tension, with the resultant side shift away from the contracted muscle. The diagnosis of short leg syndrome is based upon a constellation of musculoskeletal and general body symptoms and upon physical findings that may be confirmed by radiography. (See Chapter 26.)

The musculoskeletal examination can be continued by systematically screening for regional and segmental somatic dysfunction. Palpation of an older person reveals readily observable tissue texture changes and motion restriction of somatic dysfunction. But the examination also reveals additional information to the discerning touch. Chronic disease states are accompanied by general subcutaneous tissue texture change. The myxedematous feel of chronic hypothyroidism is an obvious example. Diabetes has a similar feel that is the result of fluid shift from the intracellular to the extracellular compartment and as such is directly proportionate to the severity of hyperglycemia.[7,8] The degree of skin and muscle tone, the texture and amount of subcutaneous fat, the range and freedom of movement of joints, the presence or absence of crepitation are important indicators of physiologic age. Signs of aging are also noticeable in muscle power, circulation, coordination, and posture. This differentiation is significant because OMT is administered to patients as dictated by physiologic age to a far greater extent than chronological age. (See Chapter 4.)

Treating the Patient

The initial focus of any therapeutic regimen is dictated by the patient's problems. Once diagnoses have been made, appropriate treatments can be initiated. Specific therapies for the myriad of disorders, acute and chronic, that affect the geriatric patient are available in general medical texts. OMT should, of course, be employed as well. The treatment of somatic dysfunction as it relates to specific clinical conditions is covered elsewhere in this text. This approach is, however, disease oriented, while osteopathic medicine is said to be focused upon the patient, not the disease. So the clinician who is initiating disease-focused treatment, be it OMT or the use of medication, must approach the patient globally as well, considering not just a holistic approach to the body but also the mind and spirit. This aspect of treatment should be initiated at the same time as disease-focused therapies. It is here also that preventive interventions should begin. Consider the impact of somatic dysfunction upon the individual and apply the appropriate dose of OMT. Identify and address specific nutritional requirements. Define functional capacity and provide a realistic exercise program to enhance capabilities. Establish interpersonal communication, and patients will tell you in their own way what their feelings and needs are.

Somatic Dysfunction

In formulating a treatment plan and deciding for what purpose to employ OMT, it is useful to answer the following questions: How does dysfunction of the musculoskeletal system mechanically affect the patient? What are the effects of altered autonomic nervous activity (sympathetic and parasympathetic) resulting from somatic dysfunction? How does somatic dysfunction affect the patient's peripheral cardiovascular, arterial, venous, and lymphatic systems? Answers to these questions help the clinician to determine the desired therapeutic effect of OMT.

The clinician should also attempt to decide what component of the musculoskeletal system is predominantly responsible for the dysfunction. Is there articular restriction, muscle spasm, or dysfunctional fascial tension? Recognition of these conditions can help to determine the appropriate type of OMT. If the dysfunction results from articular restriction, a procedure that is directed at articular mechanics should be employed. Examples are high-velocity, low-amplitude (HVLA) technique and low-velocity, moderate- to high-amplitude articulation procedures. If the dysfunction results from soft tissue tension, a procedure that is intended to affect soft tissue (muscle energy, soft tissue stretching, myofascial release) is appropriate. If the dysfunction is best addressed by attempting to reduce neural reflex activity, counterstrain and facilitated positional release may prove to be the procedures of choice.

Somatic dysfunction resulting from viscerosomatic reflex activity should be addressed by treating the underlying visceral pathology; however, treatment of the pathology may be augmented but not replaced by manipulating the somatic component (somatovisceral reflex). The procedure or procedures chosen under these circumstances should result in somatic relaxation with minimal stimulation. Once the visceral component has been effectively treated, residual somatic dysfunction may be treated with appropriately selected OMT.

Patients may have a rebound reaction to OMT and should be cautioned about it. These reactions may range from a slight feeling of fatigue to an increase in pain at the site of the chief complaint or elsewhere. The elderly patient's response to OMT is slower than that of younger individuals. The typical rebound for these patients can last 12 to 48 hours. It is the result of the amount of soft tissue irritation present and the amount of OMT applied. Soft tissue procedures are particularly likely to produce such rebound reactions. Rebound responses occur most frequently after the first or second treatment. A reaction that lasts no more than 48 hours and that is followed by amelioration of symptoms is acceptable. If the patient has a more severe reaction, probably too much OMT has been administered at one time. The patient should be given 3 days to 2 weeks between interventions and the manipulation adjusted according to the response. A patient who remains unresponsive to intelligently applied manipulation after the second or third treatment should be reevaluated, and the possibility of an unrecognized viscerosomatic etiology should be considered.

The geriatric patient normally has a relatively strong response to relatively little stress and often with symptoms distant from the site of the chief complaint or therapy. Patients with chronic diseases, such as rheumatoid arthritis, may require the very gentlest of manipulative attention to prevent an acute exacerbation of symptoms. Osteoarthritis is often an indication of an attempt by the body to compensate for instability. As a consequence, adjacent areas of primary motion restriction should be sought out and treated to reduce stress upon the unstable osteoarthritic area. The patient with osteoporosis can benefit from manipulation, but this must be appropriately gentle. Procedures applying force downward upon the thoracic cage of the prone or supine patient put potentially traumatic force upon the costochondral, costovertebral, and mid shaft areas of the ribs and should be used only with the greatest caution. Stress caused by the psoas major muscle across the neck of the femur may be enough to cause spontaneous fracture, which is blamed upon the ensuing fall. The paravertebral muscles of the low back should have prophylactic attention to prevent chronic fibrocytic shortening and the consequent stresses upon the lumbar and sacral spines, the hip, and the femoral neck.

Patients must be comfortable during OMT if they are to give maximum cooperation. Indirect types of OMT may be considered initially because they are gentle and not threatening to the patient. The physician must be relaxed to avoid conveying a feeling of uncertainty to the patient. All movements should be slow, combining controlled force with skillful application. The therapeutic forces of direct procedures need not be brutal, and the proverbial *crack* following the application of the corrective force is not the sine qua non of therapy. Geriatric patients often do not demonstrate as full a range of articular motion as younger patients, and establishment of a full motion range is not always desired. Procedures may be modified to employ the patient's respiratory motion as a final corrective force, or if a forceful procedure is required, the corrective force is often most efficient when applied as the patient exhales. Direct manipulative procedures applied to the cervical spine should be slow and gentle, avoiding abrupt rotary forces. The dysfunctional barrier must be clearly diagnosed and specifically engaged before any corrective force is applied. Whenever possible, indirect procedures should be employed.

For treatment of lateral compensatory weight-bearing curves of the older patient with demonstrable inequality of leg length, specific OMT coupled with exercise directed at strengthening the core musculature should be employed before any attempt at lift therapy. These patients have had years to adapt to their balance pattern and may not require lift therapy. The objective is functional balance of the patient's sacral base to eliminate the propensity for chronic engagement of either the right or left oblique axis and to reduce the stress of asymmetric weight bearing in the spine above. If OMT and exercise alone do not accomplish this, lift therapy may be employed.[9] A heel pad typically no larger than one-eighth inch should be placed in the patient's shoe on the side of the short leg and adjusted upward, if necessary, in increments of one-eighth inch every 2 to 4 weeks. As long as the sacral oblique axis remains engaged on the side of the long leg (anterior sacrum on the side of the short leg or posterior sacrum on the side of the long leg), it is appropriate to increase the thickness of the heel pad. When the sacral mechanics reverse so that the oblique axis is engaged on the side that is being lifted, that is, the sacrum becomes anterior on the side opposite the anatomic short leg, you have created an artificial long leg and should reduce the size of the heel pad to the previous thickness. For older patients, an estimate of how much lift will probably be required may be calculated by dividing the inequality of leg length, as measured on the postural radiography, in half. When treating leg length inequality of recent onset (i.e., fracture or hip surgery), it is appropriate to attempt to correct most of the difference immediately and then determine the ultimate size of the heel pad using the principles described herein.

Placing a heel pad in a patient's shoe necessitates that the patient shift the pattern of accommodation accordingly. This shift in accommodation may be facilitated by specifically treating all existent somatic dysfunction before initiating lift therapy or when making changes in the size of the heel pad. During adjustment to the postural changes induced by heel pads, patients will have new areas of physical discomfort and should be informed of it, so that they realize it is part of the accommodation process.

Additional areas of the musculoskeletal system that it is appropriate to address prophylactically include the following: The craniocervical junction is important for postural balance. Mechanical perturbation, head flexed (tilted from the erect) position has been shown to increase postural instability.[5] Upper thoracic flexion contributes to the head-flexed position and necessitates low to mid cervical compensatory extension, placing stress on an area of the spine that is frequently unstable and osteoarthritic. The thoracic cage (thoracic inlet, ribs, vertebrae, and thoracoabdominal diaphragm) can be treated for efficiency of respiratory function and the return of venous blood and lymph to the heart. The lumbar pelvic and abdominal areas can be treated to promote lower gastrointestinal regulation.

Exercise

As individuals age, they undergo subtly progressive loss of function. From middle age on, there is a strong tendency for loss of muscle mass. By age 80 an active individual can be expected to have lost up to 20% of gastrocnemius mass.[10] Loss of muscle mass in turn affects functional capacity. Although these changes may be inevitable, preventive measures can retard the progression and maintain optimal functional status for as long as possible. Exercise can modify risk factors for disabling diseases.

It can alter the expression or consequences of diseases that are already present and indirectly affect other modifiers of disability, such as psychosocial functioning. Exercise may actually retard biologic aging.[11] Active and passive exercises may be prescribed to mobilize, stabilize, and strengthen the musculoskeletal system; to enhance balance; to develop and maintain physical fitness and increase endurance; and to improve body chemistry.

Therapeutic exercise should begin with identification of functional impediments that can prevent the patient from otherwise performing effectively. Problem areas of the musculoskeletal system should be identified and treated. Areas of hypermobility and instability are frequently found adjacent to and as compensation for areas of motion restriction. Therefore, motion impediment due to somatic dysfunction adjacent to areas of hypermobility should be sought out and treated before stabilization exercises begin. Short leg with pelvic unleveling and dysfunctional anteroposterior mechanics that will interfere with weight-bearing exercises must be addressed before the patient can take full advantage of these activities.

Exercise intended to mobilize, stabilize, and strengthen may be employed generally and may be expected to affect much, if not all, of the musculoskeletal system and to exert a positive cardiovascular effect. Swimming is an example of such an activity that has the added advantage of being non–weight bearing. Stretching exercises, such as yoga, may be employed to enhance range of motion but are probably most effective when performed under the supervision of an experienced teacher.

Progressive resistance and isometric exercises may be prescribed to provide stability and strength and to affect specific anatomic areas or in a total-body program. Free weights may be used only with caution. Compared to progressive resistance devices, free weights are hard to control and have the potential to exert traumatic stress if control is lost. If progressive resistance or free weights are used, low weights should be employed, and the focus of activity should be upon gradually increasing the number of repetitions. These exercises should be performed 2 or 3 times a week in 2 to 3 sets of 8 to 12 repetitions using 8 to10 major muscle groups. Each repetition should be performed slowly over about 10 seconds, and ballistic movements should be avoided. The patient should be encouraged to take at least one day of rest between exercise sessions.[11]

After addressing the motion restriction of upper thoracic somatic dysfunction, cervical isometric exercises (discussed later in the chapter) may be employed to stabilize and strengthen the mid to low cervical spine and to stretch contracted anterior muscles. Similarly, lumbosacral instability can be reduced by treating upper lumbar flexion dysfunction, stretching the prevertebral iliopsoas muscles, leveling the pelvis, addressing stressful anteroposterior pelvic mechanics, and strengthening core, abdominal, and lumbar paravertebral musculature (discussed later in the chapter).

To stabilize the sacroiliac joints, dysfunctional mechanics should be addressed as already described for the lumbosacral junction and exercise employed to strengthen the gluteal muscle group. A simple pelvic tilt (discussed later in the chapter) can be modified to strengthen the gluteal muscles if the patient tonically contracts the buttocks while tilting the pelvis. Slow squats are also effective for this purpose but must be employed with caution because they also stress the knees.

Exercises to enhance balance should stimulate the central neurologic control of equilibrium and posture by progressively narrowing the body's base of support, displacing its center of gravity to the limits of tolerance while removing visual, vestibular, and proprioceptive inputs.[11] Four independent fall-related predictors of hip fracture have been identified. They include slow gait, difficulty performing tandem (heel-to-toe) walk, reduced visual acuity, and small calf circumference.[12] The risk associated with three of these may be reduced by exercise.

As long as dysfunctional postural mechanics have been adequately addressed, the simplest exercise to enhance balance and reduce the risk of falling is walking. Patients can narrow the base of support and practice heel-to-toe walking. Unstable patients can employ a cane for security but should be encouraged to attempt the exercise while keeping the cane off the ground and using it only if they begin to lose balance.

To address diminished calf circumference, patients should strengthen the gastrocnemius muscles. While standing with their weight on both feet, they should shift their weight onto the balls of their feet and stand on their toes. Pelvic stabilization in the coronal plane is also important. Individuals who fall and sustain a hip fracture are likely to have fallen sideways.[13] Reinforcement of the gluteus medius muscles to encourage lateral pelvic strengthening should be addressed. The procedure is to stand, abduct one leg, and return to the initial position, then do the same thing with the other leg.

The intensity of these activities may be increased by narrowing the base of support. Patients should progress from standing on two feet while holding onto the back of a chair or the wall to standing on one foot with no hand support. While performing the exercises, if flexibility permits, they can challenge vestibular sensation by turning their head, neck, and upper torso to one side and then to the other. They can reduce sensory cues by closing their eyes or by standing upon a soft surface, such as a foam pillow. Shifting of the body's center of gravity adds challenge. This can be accomplished by having patients hold a heavy object out to one side while maintaining balance. They can stand upon one leg while lifting the other leg out behind the body, as with the standing psoas stretch, or they can lean forward as far as possible without falling or moving their feet. This exercise affects mainly the gluteus maximus.

Other examples of balance-enhancing activities include stepping over objects, climbing slowly up and down stairs, walking on a soft surface such as a foam mattress, tai chi, standing yoga, ballet exercises, and maintaining balance while standing on a moving vehicle, such as a bus.

Balance-enhancing exercise may be performed on a weekly to daily basis. Exercises should consist of 1 or 2 repetitions of 4 to 10 different exercises that emphasize dynamic rather than static posture. Patients should progress in difficulty as tolerated and should be cautioned not to progress too rapidly but rather to increase the difficulty of the exercise gradually as competence develops. The activities should be performed in a safe environment, and ideally someone else is available to monitor the activity.[11]

Total-body activities, including walking, bicycling, swimming, and dancing, can be employed to enhance cardiovascular status and to strengthen muscles and enhance balance among the elderly.[14] Regular physical activity reduces myocardial oxygen demand and increases exercise capacity, both of which are associated with lower levels of coronary risk.[15] In conjunction with other lifestyle considerations, such as smoking cessation and diet, regular exercise should be the first therapeutic modality employed in the treatment of hypertension.[16] As patients exercise, regardless of the type of activity, they will begin to develop and maintain physical fitness and increase endurance. They should be encouraged to select a form of activity that they find enjoyable. No matter what form of exercise they select, they should be encouraged to attempt to perform it to the optimum limits of their ability.

Regular exercise has been demonstrated to increase serum high-density lipoprotein concentrations and reduce low-density lipoproteins and triglycerides.[17] Also, exercise increases insulin sensitivity.[18]

These activities may be performed for 20 to 60 minutes 3 to 7 times a week. They should be low-impact weight-bearing activity if possible, and the workload should increase progressively to maintain the relative intensity of the exercise as determined by heart rate. Target heart rate is 45 to 80% of maximum heart rate for the individual.[11] Maximum heart rate can be calculated by subtracting the patient's age from 220.[19]

Even the gentlest of activities can prove beneficial if the patient is fragile. Deep-breathing exercises that actively move the thoracoabdominal diaphragm not only facilitate efficiency of respiration and maintain mobility of the thoracic cage; they also promote bowel activity and lymphatic drainage.[20] Deep-breathing exercises performed slowly, at 5 to 7 breaths per minute, have been demonstrated to affect the low-frequency Traube-Hering-Mayer fluctuations in autonomic tone.[21] Such respiratory activity has been shown to enhance heart rate variability and increase baroreflex sensitivity, both long-term indicators of favorable prognosis in cardiac patients.[22,23]

A gentle form of exercise based upon the principles of indirect OMT, autogenic functional balancing, has been demonstrated to affect baroreflex sensitivity similarly.[24] This activity also may be employed to improve musculoskeletal motion in a manner that is respectful of the tissues, presenting no risk of *overdoing it*. This type of activity can be adjusted to accommodate anybody, whatever the level of fitness.

Nutritional Considerations

Patients should be encouraged to follow a low-fat diet that provides fatty acids in a high ratio of unsaturated to saturated fats. They should avoid refined carbohydrates as much as possible and instead consume increased quantities of cereals, fruits, vegetables, and legumes. Protein consumption must be adequate to ensure maintenance of muscle mass. The ingestion of meats and dairy products, however, are also best limited to provide no more than 50% of daily protein consumption (total consumption: 0.8 g of protein per kilogram of body weight).[25]

Sodium intake should be limited. Although low-salt meals may initially be perceived as bland, the patient's appreciation for salty flavor is blunted by salt in the diet. After several weeks the individual's palate will accommodate, and previous levels of dietary sodium will seem to be excessive. Herbs and spices may be substituted as flavor enhancers. Wine used in cooking contains flavor-enhancing qualities and provides micronutrients, yet the cooking heat usually boils off the alcohol. If otherwise tolerated, the moderate (one to two drinks a day) consumption of alcohol, particularly in the form of red wine, is possibly beneficial to cardiovascular health.[26]

Patients should be encouraged to consume 1200 to 1500 mL (five to six 8-oz glasses) of water daily. Although they may prefer other beverages, adequate intake of water must be emphasized. It may prove advantageous to suggest that patients consider the water to be a medication and as such consume a full glass several times daily. The sense of thirst is often diminished with age, and dehydration can easily result. Also, many older individuals have xerostomia due to reduced saliva production that can result in decreased food intake.[27]

Other dietary supplements that should be provided include minerals and vitamins. A single multivitamin may prove sufficient, but it should include at least vitamin B complex, vitamin D, calcium, iron, zinc, and copper. Vitamin D and calcium are particularly important for musculoskeletal health. The significance of these nutrients for the prevention of osteoporosis is readily apparent, but they are also important in the maintenance of body muscle mass. During normal aging, there is a progressive loss of muscle mass that in the extreme progresses to sarcopenia, with a resultant loss of functional capacity.[28] This condition is associated with low levels of vitamin D and elevated parathyroid hormone levels.[29]

Another degenerative and functionally limiting process of aging, osteoarthritis, particularly of the weight-bearing joints, is properly addressed by weight reduction.[30] Additionally, glucosamine and chondroitin sulfate have been suggested as nutritional supplements for this condition. Although these compounds show efficacy in reducing symptoms, neither has been shown to arrest progression of the disease or regenerate damaged cartilage.[31]

Obesity has reached epidemic proportions in the United States. Body mass index (BMI), the ratio between weight and height, may be calculated as follows:

$$BMI = [(\text{weight in pounds})/(\text{height in inches})^2] \times 703.$$

The resulting indication of body fat content is classified in Table 12.1.

A quick and simple method for determining an individual's optimal body weight is to assume that a female who is 5 feet tall should weigh 100 pounds and then to add 5 pounds for each inch of height above 5 feet. Similarly, a male who is 5 feet tall should weigh 106 pounds, and 6 pounds should be added for each inch of height above 5 feet. Therefore, the optimal weight for a female who is 5 feet 6 inches tall is $[100 + (6 \times 5)] = 130$ lb (BMI = 21), and the optimal weight for a male of the same height would be $[106 + (6 \times 6)] = 142$ lb (BMI = 23). When calculating optimal weight for geriatric patients, it is appropriate to include an additional 10 to 15 pounds of reserve body fat to provide caloric support in the event of catastrophic illness.

Obesity is unquestionably detrimental, yet it is a reversible stressor. Exercise may be employed to augment weight reduction, but if patients do not restrict caloric intake as they exercise, they compensate by eating more. The individual whose weight causes physical distress may be unable to tolerate the stress of exercise. Thus, an effective weight reduction program must provide an effective admixture of caloric restriction and physical activity.

All too many patients feel powerless to address their weight problem. Providing patients with a highly structured program, if they are sufficiently motivated, can be empowering. There is a simple method that will allow patients to identify their own caloric requirements.

Before initiating any weight reduction program, baseline laboratory information should be obtained. This should include a complete blood count and a multichannel chemistry profile with serum glucose, renal and hepatic function parameters, lipid

TABLE 12.1

Body Mass Index

Weight Category	BMI Range
Underweight	<18.5
Normal weight	18.5–24.9
Overweight	25.0–29.9
Obese	>30.0

profile, and at least thyroid-stimulating hormone level. The incidence of occult hypothyroidism increases significantly with age, making this last test very important.

To begin the process, patients need one or more calorie counter reference books and a diary. If their weight is stable, they should begin by eating as they normally do for 2 weeks, recording in the diary the total caloric content of everything they eat. After 2 weeks, they should add up the daily caloric totals and divide by 14 to determine their average daily caloric intake for the period. The yield of 1 lb of body fat is approximately 3500 calories. Therefore, reduction of the average daily caloric intake by 500 to 1000 calories ($500 \times 7 = 3500$) results in a loss of 1 to 2 lb a week. This process is similar to what most individuals do to keep their checkbook balanced, and the analogy often works well as an explanation, except that to lose weight, patients must write *daily overdrafts* so that they are forced to withdraw from their adipose savings accounts.

Patients must compensate for the inevitable decrease in basal metabolic rate that accompanies caloric restriction with an exercise program as outlined earlier. Further, they should be cautioned not to attempt to lose more than 2 pounds weekly lest they place undue physiologic stress on their body and risk depletion of muscle mass.

Mind and Spirit

Existential anxiety at some point in life is almost universal. The very fact that one exists carries with it the unpleasant knowledge that sooner or later that existence as the individual knows it will cease and that cherished relationships will be severed. Only individuals with the very strongest spiritual belief systems do not find these thoughts troubling. In youth, life stretches before the individual with what often appears to be endless possibilities. In old age, the inevitable is undeniably near. Health often is a fragile and intermittent state, and pain and functional limitations are constant. Add to this that life's goals may have gone unmet and that cherished relationships have been lost, and it is a wonder the elderly are not all depressed. The physician–patient relationship in this environment is an extremely powerful one because the physician knows how to relieve suffering and even prolong life. Possibly the most important therapeutic agent in the treatment of many older patients is the personal interest of their physician. Often the mere attention of the physician activates the patient's mind and stimulates interest in life.

Here the fundamental principle of osteopathic philosophy, that the body possesses the inherent ability to heal itself, becomes not only promising to the patient but reassuring to the physician. Confronted by chronic illness that can only progress unto death and by pharmaceutical therapies with sequelae that are on occasion worse than what they treat, it is comforting to know that somatic dysfunction is not permanent, that it responds, often rapidly, to OMT and that OMT is virtually without untoward side effects. Andre V. Gibaldi once said that there are two procedures by which a physician can provide a patient with instant relief, I & D (incision and drainage) of an abscess and OMT. The fact that a headache may be eliminated with something as simple as suboccipital myofascial release, that dyspnea may be reduced by mobilization of the thoracic cage and diaphragm, that constipation may be relieved by stimulating the gastrointestinal tract through the abdominal wall, and that colic can be diminished by the appropriate application of inhibitory pressure to the paravertebral musculature is astounding.

On more than one occasion, a patient whose pain was relieved by OMT has become incensed because a physician seen previously said that there was *nothing wrong*. The irony of this is that that physician was in one sense correct. Somatic dysfunction is not disease; therefore, in the allopathic paradigm, nothing is wrong: Unfortunately, in that paradigm it follows that nothing can be done.

One of the obvious differences, therefore, between doctors of medicine and doctors of osteopathy is the use of OMT. It has been argued by individuals who do not use OMT and who consequently do not know what they are talking about that the benefit obtained through manual therapy is psychological. Even if that were the only way in which OMT affected the patient, what is wrong with that? It has been demonstrated that *healing touch* has a positive effect on both physiological and psychological variables.[33] Therapeutic touch has been suggested to promote comfort and reduce anxiety.[34] Are these not desirable treatment goals?

On the average, a patient visit in which somatic dysfunction is diagnosed and OMT is employed lasts longer than a regular medical visit. This extra time, combined with the healing touch, allows patients to speak about their life, to describe little bits of information that might be valuable for the physician. This physical contact builds a stronger physician–patient relationship. The physician becomes part of the patient's life in a very physical sense. This allows for truly holistic medicine, in which patients are cared for and that care becomes part of their global environment.

But the osteopathic approach is more than OMT. Patients are part of their treatment protocol. They are empowered and given the opportunity are encouraged to participate actively in self-healing. (See Chapter 1.) This inclusion alleviates the sense of powerlessness that so often accompanies the existential anxiety of the elderly.

CONCLUSION

The treatment of geriatric patients is one of the best examples of whole-body medicine. It offers significant opportunity to practice osteopathically distinctive health care. We must treat the patient's chief complaint. We must look at underlying illnesses. We must closely examine the patient's nutritional status. The recognition of somatic dysfunction as it links seemingly unrelated systems through viscerosomatic and somatovisceral mechanisms provides a uniquely holistic system of clinical problem solving. The diagnosis and treatment of reversible somatic dysfunction offers patients relief in a time in their life when most everything seems to be linked to unavoidable decline. But probably most important, we must stimulate patients' interest in living and empower them with methods by which they can participate in their own healing before we can ever begin to successfully treat them.

Procedures

Cervical Treatment (C2–C7), Patient Supine (Still Technique) (Fig. 12.1)

This procedure is employed to improve extension, right rotation, and right side bending at C3 to C4. The most common error in this procedure is failure to maintain compression or the distraction vector to the involved segment throughout the procedure. This procedure requires localization of motion to the affected segment.

Patient position: supine. Physician position: seated at the head of the table.

Procedure (Example: C3 on C4 Flexed [Forward Bent], Side Bent Left, Rotated Left [Tissue Texture Change, Motion Restriction, and Tenderness on the Left], Posterior C3 Left)

1. Place your right index finger on the posterior component of the dysfunction with your thumb on the other side.
2. Place your left hand on top of the patient's head.
3. With your left hand, apply gentle compression and introduce flexion down to the involved segment.

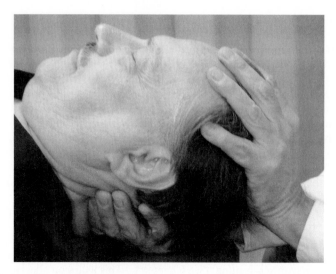

FIGURE 12.1   Still procedure for a type II cervical dysfunction, C3 on C4, flexed, side bent left and rotated left.

4. Position the dysfunctional segment in the direction of freer motion, involving all three planes of motion to a point of balance. Translation right will help left side bending.
5. While maintaining the vector force, quickly turn the segment in the opposite direction, toward and eventually through the restrictive barrier.
6. As you move the segment toward the restrictive barrier, you will note that the barrier no longer exits and the segment has free motion.
7. When the procedure is complete, reassess the dysfunctional area.

Cervical Treatment (C2–C7), Patient Seated (Still Technique) (Fig. 12.2)

This procedure is employed to improve flexion, right rotation, and right side bending at C3 to C4. The most common error in this procedure is failure to maintain compression or the distraction vector to the involved segment throughout the procedure. This procedure requires localization of motion to the affected segment.

Patient position: seated. Physician position: standing in front of the patient.

Procedure (Example: C3 on C4 Extended [Backward Bent], Side Bent Left, Rotated Left [Tissue Texture Change, Motion Restriction, and Tenderness on the Left], Posterior C3 Left)

1. Place your left index finger (sensing hand) on the posterior component of the dysfunction, with the remainder of the hand comfortably around the back of the neck as a support and fulcrum.
2. Place your operating (right) hand on the top of the patient's head.
3. Tilt the head back, extending the segment.
4. Side bend and rotate the head left until all tissue strains are removed from the affected segment. This position will be an exaggeration of the segment's rest position.

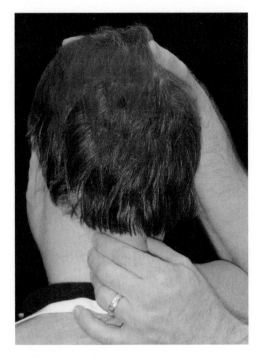

FIGURE 12.2   Still procedure for a type II cervical dysfunction C3 on C4, extended, side bent left and rotated left.

5. Introduce a gentle compression vector force down to the dysfunctional segment using the operating hand.
6. Rotate the head to the right through neutral into a right rotation with simultaneous flexion and side bending to the right toward the restrictive barrier.
7. As you take the head and neck through the range of motion, you may feel a release through the articular pillar.
8. Release the compression and return to neutral.
9. When the procedure is complete, reassess the dysfunctional area.

Thoracic Dysfunction (Still Technique) (Fig. 12.3)

This procedure is useful for thoracic somatic dysfunctions. It is employed to improve flexion, side bending left, and rotation left of T5 on T6. It is a gentle thoracic procedure that requires precise localization.

Patient position: seated. Physician position: standing behind the patient to the left.

Procedure (Example: T5 on T6, Extended, Side Bent Right and Rotated Right)

1. Place your left arm across the patient's anterior chest so that your left arm is draped over the patient's left shoulder and your left hand is on the patient's right shoulder.
2. Place your right sensing finger over the right transverse process of T5.
3. Gently introduce extension, right rotation, and right side bending until all three forces localize at T5 and the pathologic neutral is engaged (absence of tissue tension).

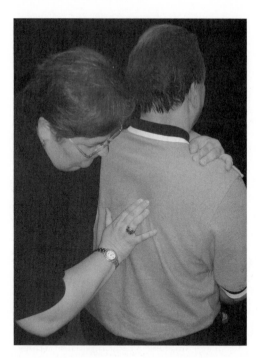

FIGURE 12.3   Still procedure for a type II thoracic dysfunction T5 on T6, extended, side bent right and rotated right.

4. Introduce a vector force in the shape of a V by pressure through the patient's shoulders with your left arm until the vector is localized at T5 right.
5. Maintaining the vector force, quickly flex, side bend left, and rotate left the T5 segment. As the segment T5 on T6 is about to reach the restrictive barrier, the barrier will melt away.
6. Return the segment to neutral.
7. When the procedure is complete, reassess the dysfunctional area.

Lumbar Dysfunction (Still Technique) (Fig. 12.4)

This procedure is useful for lumbar somatic dysfunctions. It is employed to improve flexion, side bending left, and rotation left of L2 on L3. It is a gentle lumbar procedure that requires precise localization.

Patient position: seated. Physician position: standing behind the patient to the left.

Procedure (Example: L2 on L3, Extended, Side Bent Right and Rotated Right)

1. Place your left arm across the patient's anterior chest (or shoulders as in Fig. 12.4) so that your left arm is draped over the patient's left shoulder and your left hand is on the patient's right shoulder.
2. Place your right sensing finger over the right transverse process of L2.
3. Gently introduce extension, right rotation, and right side bending until all three forces localize at L2 and the pathologic neutral is engaged (absence of tissue tension).
4. Introduce a vector force in the shape of a V by pressure through the patient's shoulders with your left arm until the vector is localized at L2 right.
5. Maintaining the vector force, with a moderate-speed flex, side bend left and rotate left the L2 segment. As the segment L2 on L3 is about to reach the restrictive barrier, the barrier will melt away.

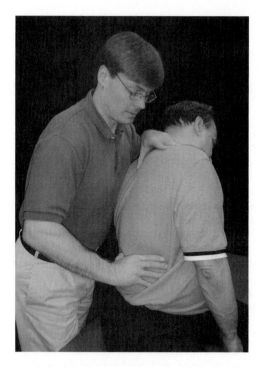

FIGURE 12.4   Still procedure for lumbar type II dysfunction L2 on L3, extended, side bent right and rotated right.

6. Return the segment to neutral.
7. When the procedure is complete, reassess the dysfunctional area.

Sacrum (Facilitated Positional Release)

Tender points are located along the sacroiliac joint, specifically upper pole L5 (UP5L) and lower pole L5 (LP5L). The UP5L point is medial to the PSIS at the upper pole of the sacrum, and the LP5L is approximately 2 cm caudal to UP5L (Fig. 12.5). This procedure is useful in relieving sacroiliac pain.

This procedure allows both tender points to be treated with the same start position with minimum modifications. The sacral base will move posteriorly when the sacrum is fully backward bent and when the pelvis is fully forward bent. Because of this finding, it is possible to treat these posterior tender points by placing the hip and subsequently the sacroiliac joint into flexion to allow the sacrum to extend. It is a gentle procedure that requires precise localization.

Patient position: supine. Physician position: standing on the affected side.

Procedure (Example: UPL5 Left Tender Point [Fig. 12.6])

1. Place your right hand on the UPL5 tender point to monitor.
2. With your left hand, gently flex the patient's knee and hip until motion is noted at the tender point.
3. Now gently externally rotate the hip until tenderness at the UP5L point is minimized to a level of 0 to 3 on a pain scale (10 = start position and most painful, 0 = no pain). If necessary, fine-tune the tender point position with adjustment of the leg position.

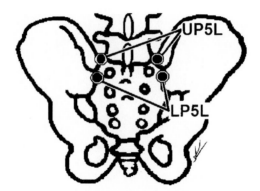

FIGURE 12.5   Tender points along the SI joint specifically, upper pole L5 (UP5L) and lower pole L5 (LP5L).

4. With your left hand, place a gentle vector force though the femur into the hip to facilitate the release.
5. A release will be perceived in 3 to 5 seconds.
6. Return the patient to the neutral position.
7. When the procedure is complete, reassess the dysfunctional area.

Simple Cervical Isometrics (Exercise)

This exercise is intended to strengthen cervicothoracic paravertebral musculature. Consequently, it may be employed to begin stabilizing mid to low cervical

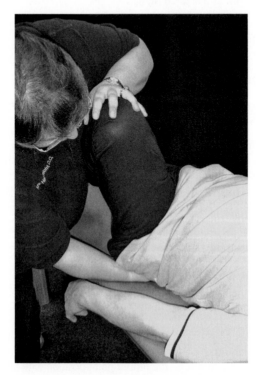

FIGURE 12.6   Facilitated positional release of a left sacroiliac dysfunction.

hypermobility and to reduce upper thoracic flexion. It should be performed at least once daily to tolerance and may be performed at night before the patient goes to sleep and in the morning upon awakening.

The patient lies supine in bed with the head on the pillow. For patients who cannot lie flat, this procedure can be modified to be performed seated. (See Cervical Isometrics below.)

Procedure

1. Palpate the posterior paravertebral musculature of the cervical spine with the pads of the fingers of both hands. This hand placement lets the patient monitor the intensity of the muscular contraction that follows.
2. Tuck the chin, inhale, and press the back of the head into the pillow for 3 to 5 seconds. The muscular contraction should be firm but should not result in cervical pain or other significant discomfort.
3. Exhale and relax.
4. This process may be repeated 5 to 10 times. The intensity with which the patient pushes the head into the pillow determines the level of the spine that is affected. Gentle pressure will strengthen the cervical region, while pushing with greater force will affect the upper thoracic spine.

Cervical Isometrics (Exercise) (Fig. 12.7)

This exercise is performed as 10 isometric contractions at each of 10 points of the head. The opposing arrows in Figure 12.7 indicate the contact points (with the exception of points 9 and 10, on the left and right cheeks respectively) and applied directions of the isometric contractions.

This exercise is employed to provide cervical stability by strengthening and balancing all of the cervical muscles. It may be used by patients with degenerative

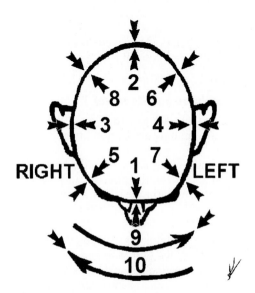

FIGURE 12.7   Cervical isometric exercise.

joint disease or herniated nucleus pulposus. It should be performed at least once daily to tolerance.

Patient position: seated.

Procedure

1. Place the tips of the index and middle fingers of one hand on the midline of the forehead just above the brow ridge (Fig. 12.7, position 1).
2. Simultaneously push the forehead into the fingertips while applying an equal amount of resistance with the hand. Hold this isometric contraction for 1 to 3 seconds, and then release the pressure.
3. Repeat this procedure 10 times for position 1.
4. Continue the exercise as above for positions 2 to 8 according to Figure 12.7. Although it does not matter which of the points of contact is first in the sequence of the exercise, it is important that the points of contact always alternate. That is, if the forehead is the first point of contact, the back of the head should be the second point of contact.
5. Points 9 and 10 differ slightly in their application (Fig. 12.7). Place one hand in contact with the side of the face and isometrically attempt to rotate the head in that direction, alternately contracting and relaxing, as in step 2, for 10 repetitions.
6. Repeat this rotational portion of the exercise in the opposite direction.

Simple Calf Strengthening to Stabilize Gait (Exercise)

This exercise is intended to increase gait stability. It should be employed by individuals whose gait is not stable enough to perform the standing exercise described later.

Patient position: seated on a chair. A straight-backed chair is preferable.

Procedure

1. Sit with the back straight and the feet about 12 inches apart flat upon the floor.
2. Place the hands upon the knees and lean the torso forward. The more you lean forward, the more weight you can place upon the knees.
3. Contract the gastrocnemius muscles, plantar flexing the ankles and raising slowly up onto the balls of the feet. Hold this position for 3 to 5 seconds.
4. Slowly return to the flatfooted position and rest for 3 to 5 seconds.
5. They now contract the pretibial muscles, dorsiflexing the ankles slowly until only the heels are contacting the floor. Hold this position for 3 to 5 seconds.
6. Slowly return to the flatfooted position and rest for 3 to 5 seconds. Repeat 5 to 10 times.

Calf Strengthening to Stabilize Gait (Exercise)

This exercise is intended to increase gait stability. It does so by strengthening the gastrocnemius muscles, maintaining ankle mobility and stimulating the vestibular apparatus.

Patient position: standing while holding onto the back of a chair or the wall for stability. With increasing adeptness, the patient can progress to doing them freehand but should always remain within reach of a support.

Procedure

1. Stand with the back straight and the feet flat on the floor, about 12 inches apart. Grasp the back of a chair or the wall to ensure stability. For any of the following variations of this exercise, releasing the hold on the chair or wall increases difficulty.
2. Contract the gastrocnemius muscles, plantar-flexing the ankles and rising slowly up onto the balls of the feet to stand on the toes. Hold this position for 3 to 5 seconds.

3. Slowly return to the flatfooted position and rest for 3 to 5 seconds. Repeat 5 to 10 times.
4. When comfortable performing this exercise, place the feet close together, narrowing the base of support, and repeat steps 1 to 3.
5. When comfortable performing this exercise, repeat steps 1 to 3 while standing upon one foot, further narrowing the base of support. Alternate standing on one leg and then on the other for 5 to 10 repetitions each.
6. Finally, if flexibility permits, challenge vestibular sensation while performing the exercises by turning the head, neck, and upper torso to one side and then to the other, and reduce sensory cues by closing the eyes or by standing upon a soft surface, such as a foam pillow.

Gluteal Strengthening to Stabilize Gait (Exercise)

Pelvic stability in the coronal plane is also important. Individuals who fall and sustain a hip fracture are likely to have fallen sideways. Reinforcement of the gluteus muscles to encourage lateral pelvic strengthening should be addressed.

Patient position: standing while holding onto the back of a chair or the wall for stability. With increasing adeptness, the patient can progress to doing them freehand but should always remain within reach of a support.

Procedure

1. Stand with the back straight and with the weight on one foot.
2. Slowly abduct the other leg; hold it in abduction for 3 to 5 seconds and then slowly return to the initial position.
3. Alternate standing on one leg and then on the other for 5 to 10 repetitions each.
4. While performing this exercise, if flexibility permits, challenge vestibular sensation by turning the head, neck, and upper torso to one side and then to the other. Reduce sensory cues by closing the eyes or by standing upon a soft surface, like a foam pillow.
5. Releasing the hold on the chair or wall adds difficulty.

References

1. Glossary of osteopathic terminology. In: Ward RC, ed. Foundations for Osteopathic Medicine. 2nd ed. Philadelphia: Lippincott Williams & Wilkins, 2002;1249.
2. Korr IM. Sustained sympathicotonia as a factor in disease. In: Korr IM, ed. The Neurobiologic Mechanisms in Manipulative Therapy. New York, London: Plenum, 1978;229–268.
3. Nelson KE. The management of low back pain. AAO J 1999;9(1):33–39.
4. Benjuya N, Melzer I, Kaplanski J. Aging-induced shifts from a reliance on sensory input to muscle cocontraction during balanced standing. J Gerontol A Biol Sci Med Sci 2004;59:166–171.
5. Lee HK, Scudds RJ. Comparison of balance in older people with and without visual impairment. Age Ageing 2003;32:643–649.
6. Buckley JG, Anand V, Scally A, Elliott DB. Does head extension and flexion increase postural instability in elderly subjects when visual information is kept constant? Gait Posture 2005;21:59–64.
7. Tarr R, Nelson KE, Vatt R, Richardson D. Palpatory findings associated with the diabetic state. AOA/NOF Research Conference Proceedings. J Am Osteopath Assoc 1985;85:604 [abstract].
8. Mnabhi A, Nelson KE, Glonek T. Quantifying the subjective assessment of tissue texture change: Comparison of osteopathic palpatory findings with random blood sugar in diabetic patients. J Am Osteopath Assoc 2001;101:472 [abstract].
9. Heilig D. Principles of lift therapy. J Am Osteopath Assoc 1978;77:466–472. Reprinted in Peterson B, ed. Postural Balance and Imbalance. Newark, OH: American Academy of Osteopathy, 1983;113–118.

10. Narici MV, Maganaris CN, Reeves ND, Capodaglio P. Effect of aging on human muscle architecture. J Appl Physiol 2003;95:2229–2234.
11. Singh MA. Exercise to prevent and treat functional disability. Clin Geriatr Med 2002;18:431–462, vi–vii.
12. Dargent-Molina P, Favier F, Grandjean H, et al. Fall-related factors and risk of hip fracture: The EPIDOS prospective study. Lancet 1996;348:145–149.
13. Greenspan SL, Myers ER, Kiel DP, et al. Fall direction, bone mineral density, and function: Risk factors for hip fracture in frail nursing home elderly. Am J Med 1998;104:539–545.
14. De Carvalho Bastone A, Filho WJ. Effect of an exercise program on functional performance of institutionalized elderly. J Rehabil Res Dev 2004;41:659–668.
15. Fletcher GF, Blair SN, Blumenthal J, et al. Statement on exercise: Benefits and recommendations for physical activity programs for all Americans. A statement for health professionals by the Committee on Exercise and Cardiac Rehabilitation of the Council on Clinical Cardiology, American Heart Association. Circulation 1992;86:340–344.
16. Kokkinos PF, Narayan P, Papademetriou V. Exercise as hypertension therapy. Cardiol Clin 2001;19:507–516.
17. Kreisberg RA, Oberman A. Medical management of hyperlipidemia/dyslipidemia. J Clin Endocrinol Metab 2003;88:2445–2461.
18. Mayer-Davis EJ, D'Agostino R Jr, Karter AJ, et al. Intensity and amount of physical activity in relation to insulin sensitivity: The Insulin Resistance Atherosclerosis Study. JAMA 1998;279:669–674.
19. Froelicher VF, Myers JN. Exercise and the Heart. 4th ed. Philadelphia: Saunders, 2000;100–112.
20. Abu-Hijleh MF, Habbal OA, Moqattash ST. The role of the diaphragm in lymphatic absorption from the peritoneal cavity. J Anat 1995;186(pt 3):453–467.
21. Ahmed AK, Harness JB, Mearns AJ. Respiratory control of heart rate. Eur J Appl Physiol Occup Physiol 1982;50:95–104.
22. Bernardi L, Sleight P, Bandinelli G, et al. Effect of rosary prayer and yoga mantras on autonomic cardiovascular rhythms: Comparative study. BMJ 2001;323:1446–1449.
23. Bernardi L, Spadacini G, Bellwon J, et al. Effect of breathing rate on oxygen saturation and exercise performance in chronic heart failure. Lancet 1998;351:1308–1311.
24. Sergueef N, Nelson KE, Glonek T. The effect of light exercise upon blood flow velocity determined by laser-Doppler flowmetry. J Med Eng Technol 2004;28(4):143–150.
25. Williams SR. Nutrition and Diet Therapy. 6th ed. St. Louis: Times Mirror/Mosby College, 1989;518–537.
26. Klatsky AL, Armstrong MA, Friedman GD. Red wine, white wine, liquor, beer, and risk for coronary artery disease hospitalization. Am J Cardiol 1997;80:416–420.
27. Sreebny LM, Valdini M. Xerostomia: A neglected symptom. Arch Intern Med 1987;147:1333–1337.
28. Visser M, Goodpaster BH, Kritchevsky SB, et al. Muscle mass, muscle strength, and muscle fat infiltration as predictors of incident mobility limitations in well-functioning older persons. J Gerontol A Biol Sci Med Sci 2005;60:324–333.
29. Visser M, Deeg DJ, Lips P. Low vitamin D and high parathyroid hormone levels as determinants of loss of muscle strength and muscle mass (sarcopenia): The Longitudinal Aging Study Amsterdam. J Clin Endocrinol Metab 2003;88:5766–5772.
30. Karlson EW, Mandl LA, Arweth GN, et al. Total hip replacement due to osteoarthritis: The importance of age, obesity, and other modifiable risk factors. Am J Med 2003;114:93–98.
31. Morelli V, Naquin C, Weaver V. Alternative therapies for traditional disease states: Osteoarthritis. Am Fam Physician 2003;67:339–344.
32. Calculate your body mass index. National Heart, Lung, and Blood Institute, National Institutes of Health. Available at http://nhlbisupport.com/bmi/bmicalc.htm. Accessed May 28, 2005.
33. Peters RM. The effectiveness of therapeutic touch: a meta-analytic review. Nurs Sci Q 1999;12:52–61.
34. Cox CL, Hayes JA. Reducing anxiety: The employment of therapeutic touch as a nursing intervention. Complement Ther Nurs Midwifery 1997;3(6):163–167.

CHAPTER 13

The Patient at the End of Life

Alice J. Zal

INTRODUCTION

In the not-too-distant past, people died, on average, much younger than today, often of infectious diseases. Contemporary medicine has greatly limited the toll that infections take upon the population. Chronic illnesses and malignancies are now the leading causes of death in the United States.[1] Advancing medical technology provides support to the terminally ill, but often with a dehumanizing effect. Physicians expend great efforts to assist patients to return to health. Yet, in spite of the greatest efforts, every patient eventually dies. Medical care can slow the course of the most devastating illnesses, but physicians must also protect and whenever possible improve the quality of life. Death is inevitable, and when the patient reaches the final phase of dying, osteopathic physicians must ask themselves what they can distinctively offer patients in the final days of life.

The holistic approach of the osteopathic philosophy of practice incorporates all systems of the human body into an integrated therapeutic protocol.[2] It addresses not just the disease process; rather, it embraces the patient and extended family. It is in this context that the osteopathic physician treats patients from birth to death. This approach empowers patients to *live until they die*. It also enables the family physician to play an integral part, as the leader of the patient's health care team, coordinating multiple consultants and conducting the symphony that concludes with a dignified death. Just as there is an art of living, there is an art of dying.

Thirty-five years ago at The University of Chicago School of Medicine, Elisabeth Kubler-Ross initiated open consideration of the need to support dying patients and to provide them with the means to live their final days to the fullest. She stressed the importance of the primary care physician stating: "We have long controversial discussions about whether patients should be told the truth. A question that rarely arises when the dying person is tended by the family physician who has known him from delivery to death and who knows the weaknesses and strengths of each member of the family."[3] She described the dying patient as being in a fluid state of five emotional stages. These stages are not stagnant, and the emotions of the patient and of their significant others can fluctuate from one stage to another and back again in a random sequence. Ideally, however, they should eventually progress to stage 5. The stages include (1) denial and isolation, (2) anger, (3) bargaining, (4) depression, and (5) acceptance. The recognition of this emotional sequence assists the attending physician to provide support to dying individuals although they may be belligerent and even accusatory.

The views expressed by Kubler-Ross incorporate a holistic approach that mirrors osteopathic physicians' approach to their patients. This system of support allows patients to die with dignity and with the health care team respecting their wishes. Her philosophy gives emotional support to dying patients, while we as osteopathic physicians give physical support and nurturing to patients and their circle of care. It is fundamental to osteopathic philosophy that the body possesses the inherent ability to heal itself. This holds true even as patients lie dying. Function can be optimized and discomfort reduced. The processes employed to treat terminally ill patients, including osteopathic manipulative treatment (OMT), are no different from those employed to treat patients at any other stage of life. The intensity of the intervention is, of course, variable and is dictated by the patient's level of physical tolerance.

It takes a team of health care providers to meet the needs of just one terminal patient. End-of-life issues pose a unique constellation of challenges to the physician. The terminally ill patient's physiology is stressed to its limits. Multiple dysfunctions affect the patient in a domino effect. Previously healthy systems become disrupted not because they are diseased but because they are incapable of continuing to function in the presence of the allostasis that is overwhelming the patient. These challenges demand that physicians use all of their knowledge of somatic dysfunction, disease entities, and systemic interactions—incorporate their osteopathic manipulative skills—and be the health facilitator for the patient. Physicians have to coordinate this care such that there is not an overlapping of care but rather a smooth concerted effort for the optimal level of support for patients. In this chaotic environment, osteopathic physicians' ability to identify dysfunction and to optimize function can provide relief and even comfort, possibly reducing patients' need for, and consequently the allostatic contribution of, analgesics, sedatives, laxatives, diuretics, and the like.

Some of the problems for end-of-life care that can be addressed and alleviated include the following:

- Pain
- Gastrointestinal dysfunction, including nausea, vomiting, ileus, and constipation
- Cardiopulmonary problems, including shortness of breath and central and peripheral edema

MUSCULOSKELETAL AND VISCERAL PAIN

Pain can come from numerous sources, including bone, muscles, fascia, or viscera. Visceral dysfunction and pathology can initially manifest as vaguely localized pain. Viscerosomatic and Chapman's reflexes[4] can be used to elucidate the source of pain during patients' final days of life. Often terminally ill patients demonstrate organ dysfunction in systems not immediately related to their primary disease process. Osteopathic physicians use the musculoskeletal system to offer diagnostic clues through viscerosomatic reflexes. The reflexes as described in Chapter 5 are mediated by general visceral afferent neurons that travel with either sympathetic or parasympathetic neurons from the dysfunctional or diseased viscera to the dermatomes and myotomes of the corresponding level of the spinal cord. Tissue texture abnormalities are palpable in the paravertebral tissue areas corresponding to the underlying visceral abnormality. These changes are located at the level from which the primary cell bodies of the respective sympathetic and parasympathetic efferent neurons originate. The intensity of the palpable tissue texture abnormality offers an indication of the severity and the source of the visceral pathology responsible for the reflex.

Viscerosomatic reflexes are segmentally predictable dermatomal and myotomal responses to inflammatory visceral pathology. The exact location of the reaction or increased tonicity of the overlying paravertebral muscles identifies the involved organ most of the time. General visceral afferent nociceptive neurons return to the spinal cord in the same nerve root bundles that carry the efferent autonomic fibers. The reflexes conducted by these neurons lateralize to the paravertebral soft tissues on the same side of the body as the viscus. Midline organs, hence, produce bilateral reflex reactions. Treatment of the somatic dysfunction is usually temporary, as the underlying organ must be treated to allay the discomfort in the soft tissues innervated by the viscerosomatic reflex. Tumors, whether benign or malignant, that do not in themselves have innervation consequently do not directly produce viscerosomatic reflexes. In this case, any response will result from direct irritation of adjacent innervated tissues exerted by the tumor.

Most patients as they enter their final phase of life equate death with the fear of pain. The main goal of the physician is to allow patients to live their last days fully. It is important that *one live until one dies*. The physician is the person who can make this possible through the use of appropriate OMT, medications, nerve blocks, neurostimulation, biofeedback, and physical therapy to alleviate discomfort. There are no upper limits to the dosage of pain medications, as long as the physician gradually increases the dose to match the increase in pain. Psychostimulants can be employed to antagonize the sedation produced by many opioids. With the use of psychostimulants, knocking out the pain does not mean knocking out the patient. In this arena, osteopathic physicians have an additional therapeutic modality to offer their patients to alleviate the pain of somatic dysfunction, which may in turn reduce patients' need for opioids. Along with medication, the use of OMT (soft tissue stretching, gentle articulatory procedures, rib raising, counterstrain, and lymphatic pump, to mention a few procedures) can be employed. Osteopathic physicians can help make pain more tolerable and enhance the homeostasis of the patient's body.

Osteopathic physicians have a unique armamentarium for diagnosis and treatment of these problems. Having taken an extensive history and physically examined the patient, including palpation for primary somatic dysfunction and viscerosomatic and Chapman's reflexes,[4] the physician can move on to choose the osteopathic procedure that is most appropriate for this patient.

Often, as patients become less mobile as a result of deteriorating physical health, they get multiple muscular contractions causing myofascial and bony articular dysfunction. These dysfunctional changes are often coupled with osteoporotic weakening of the skeletal structure. Osteoporosis can arise from lack of weight-bearing activities and poor dietary intake of calcium, vitamins, and other nutrients. Because of the fragile bone strength of these patients, one must be cautious when performing OMT. Physicians may have to adjust their manipulative procedures to accommodate the physical needs of the individual patient and do no harm to the already fragile individual.

The level of tolerance and the general health level of the patient dictate the level of aggressiveness of the procedure chosen. These procedures include the following:

- Articulation
- Soft tissue
- Direct fascial release
- Muscle energy
- Counterstrain
- Facilitated positional release
- Indirect fascial release
- Indirect cranial
- Lymphatic pump

High-velocity, low-amplitude (HVLA) procedures may be employed, but only with the utmost respect for the tolerance of the individual patient. When in doubt, it is best to err in the direction the less aggressive procedures.

GASTROINTESTINAL PROBLEMS

Nausea, vomiting, diminished peristalsis, constipation, and malabsorption of nutrients are all problems that patients face at the end of life. As A.T. Still put it, "The stomach is the mortar box for the retention and mixing for other workers."[5] The movement of the small intestine is a progressive wave of relaxations followed by constrictions from the pylorus to the ileocecal valve. According to Bayliss and Starling,[6] peristaltic movement is due to "intrinsic nerve activation contained in the Auerbach's plexus." This intrinsic gastrointestinal component of the autonomic nervous system provides a self-regulatory mechanism for the gut. Mechanical stimulation of the gut wall from distension or from the external effect of physical activity, as occurs with walking and other normal activities of daily living, results in a peristaltic response. The progressive loss of physical mobility, as occurs with chronic diseases and in the terminal stages of illness, results in decreased mechanical stimulation of the gastrointestinal tract. Therefore, direct mechanical stimulation of the gut with transabdominal OMT may be employed to stimulate peristalsis. These procedures should be applied frequently and can often be taught to the patient or to a family member. Including the patient and their family in the process not only provides regular application of the procedure but also empowers them by providing them with an opportunity to contribute, often dramatically, to their own well being.

Passive congestion of the abdominal organs may be addressed with OMT. The liver and spleen, large subdiaphragmatic organs, are capable of sequestering large volumes of blood and lymph. Mechanical stimulation of these organs may be employed to decrease passive abdominal congestion. The undersurface of the thoracoabdominal diaphragm is rich in lymphatic vasculature. The cisterna chyli is strategically located at the lower end of the thoracic duct in approximation with the abdominal aorta between the descending crura of the diaphragm. Not only does ensuring optimal thoracoabdominal diaphragmatic excursion enhance abdominal lymphatic drainage but the slow rhythmic motion of the diaphragm also massages the liver and spleen, augmenting venous return to the heart.

Optimal parasympathetic tone to the gastrointestinal tract may be facilitated by treating somatic dysfunction that affects the vagus and pelvic splanchnic nerves through somatovisceral mechanisms. The vagal reflex is the cervical parasympathetic viscerosomatic reflex. These vagal reflexes are located at the occiput, C1, and C2, with a greater tendency of a right-sided reaction from the pancreas, liver, gallbladder, small intestine, ascending colon, and right side of the transverse colon. The left-sided upper cervical reaction occurs with the esophagus, the stomach, and the duodenum. The sacral parasympathetic reflex (S2 to S4) is associated with conditions involving the left side of the transverse colon, the descending colon, the sigmoid colon, and the rectum.

Food that enters the colon has movement that is a combination of peristalsis and antiperistaltic motion. The forward and backward action slows down the food bolus to allow further digestion and absorption of the intestinal contents. It takes 2 hours for the bolus to move from the cecum to the hepatic flexure and 4 to 5 hours for it to move through the transverse colon. The slow movement of the colon comes from inhibitors in the spinal autonomic system (both in the upper and mid lumbar segments), whereas those supplying the rectum come from the hypogastric nerve, a plexus containing sympathetic (L1–L3) and parasympathetic (S2–S4) nerve fibers.

The neurologic supply to the digestive tract helps the osteopathic physician to locate the areas that require correction to normalize the digestive process. The correction of the somatic dysfunction causing the gastrointestinal dysfunction can normalize the nerve supply. The correction of the neuronal supply can in turn normalize the blood supply, venous drainage, and lymphatic supply, which in its turn returns normal digestive function. Correcting the underlying somatic dysfunction will improve the efficacy of other medicinal interventions.

CARDIOPULMONARY PROBLEMS

Congestive heart failure and pulmonary failure are common at end of life and often occur in tandem. The resultant edema, both peripheral and pulmonary, can be treated with lymphatic drainage procedures. "Normally a contraction of the abdominal diaphragm produces changes in the volume between the abdominal and thoracic cavities. When the diaphragm is well domed, the volume changes produce effective pressure gradients between the thoracic and abdominal cavities. In this way a pump action for lymphatic flow is produced. Flattening of the diaphragm seriously decreases volume displacement. This causes decreased lymph flow, which increases congestion of tissues and can decrease cardiac output. Numerous medical and osteopathic research studies have proven that chronic lymphatic congestion with resultant poor oxygenation of cells is associated with increased rates of infection, healing time, fibrosis and scarring, and mortality."[7] Lymphatic pump procedures also add significantly to fluid mobilization and the homeostasis of the patient.

OMT, respiratory therapy, and pulmonary toileting all improve the functional level of a patient. Treatment of somatic dysfunction of the thoracic inlet, thoracic spine, ribs, and thoracoabdominal diaphragm will optimize the mechanics of respiration in the otherwise compromised patient. Treatment of somatic dysfunction of C3, C4, and C5 can optimize phrenic nerve function, further improving diaphragm function.[8]

CONCLUSION

In general, hands-on treatment of the patient has a multitude of benefits. It can correct somatic dysfunctions and provide a positive effect on the emotional state of the patient. It makes a patient feel worthwhile and not just a burden to those around them as they face their final days of earthly being.

Performing OMT helps to decrease pain, improve circulation, and enhance gastrointestinal peristalsis and lymphatic flow. It also says to the patient, "I am here for you, and you are not alone." This hands-on form of medical care makes it so that the inevitable disease process does not have to decrease the quality of any single human second on Earth.

Procedures

OMT may be employed to reduce dysfunction and alleviate discomfort for the terminally ill patient. Because of their compromised condition, these individuals present significant OMT dosage issues. (See Chapter 4.) When the patient is fragile or unstable, it is best to employ limited interventions frequently, often multiple times daily, if tolerated. The amount of OMT will be dictated by the patient's physiologic response during treatment and in the 24-hour period following treatment.

While treating patients, observe them closely for their response, and stop the intervention as soon as one is observed. Relaxation of the soft tissues in the area being treated is a good response. Muscle twitching or spasm during the application of a procedure is an indication that you have exceeded tolerance and should stop the intervention and select a less aggressive procedure. Changes in autonomic nervous activity are also a response. Peripheral vasodilation with redness or increased skin temperature or perspiration indicates it is time to stop. Increased heart or respiratory rate also indicates that you have reached the patient's level of tolerance. If the patient finds the intervention too uncomfortable, stop and choose another approach or wait and try again later.

Avoid causing or aggravating pain during OMT. Immediately after the intervention, the patient will often report symptom reduction. This response is commonly followed briefly by an intensification of the original complaint. Such a rebound reaction should be minimal and should not last more than 24 to 48 hours. If it does, the intensity of the following intervention should be appropriately reduced. As the rebound reaction subsides, a period of resolution typically follows in which the chief complaint is significantly reduced or absent. This period of resolution may last a few hours or longer. Patients should be reevaluated 24 to 48 hours after the treatment and treated again as their response dictates.

The following procedures are examples of OMT that may be employed in the care of the terminally ill patient.

Cervical Soft Tissue/Articulation

For diagnosis, see Chapter 3; for treatment procedure, see Chapter 16.

Cervical, Indirect Balancing

For diagnosis, see Chapter 3; for treatment procedure, see Chapter 16.

These two procedures are employed to decrease cervical tissue tension and enhance the symmetric range of motion of the cervical spine. They can ease tension headaches and reduce cervical dysfunction commonly encountered when patients spend long hours propped up with pillows.

Inhibitory Pressure

This procedure is employed to attenuate an effect upon segmentally related viscera by suppressing the somatic component of a somatovisceral reflex. (For treatment procedure, see Chapter 5.)

Thoracic Inlet Myofascial Release

For treatment procedure, see Chapter 19.

Rib Raising

For treatment procedure, see Chapter 10 and 17.

Thoracoabdominal Diaphragm Release

For treatment procedure, see Chapter 17.

Significant compromise of respiration may occur in the very ill individual as the result of somatic dysfunction.[8] The preceding three procedures are employed to enhance mobility of the entire respiratory mechanism, thereby increasing efficiency of respiration and lymphatic and venous return to the heart.

Transabdominal Stimulation

For treatment procedure, see Chapter 20.

This procedure is employed to treat abdominal somatic dysfunction (ICD 9CM 739.9). It improves bowel function by mechanically stimulating peristalsis, thus increasing gastrointestinal motility while alleviating or preventing constipation (ICD 9CM 564). It is useful when treating hospitalized patients or other bedridden individuals. Because it is most effective when applied several times a day, this procedure may be taught to patients for self-administration if they are sufficiently alert, or it can be taught to a family member.

Thoracic and Lumbar Counterstrain

Counterstrain points are commonly paired as posterior and anterior tender points. This is because they often manifest in this paired relationship. If a thoracic or lumbar tender point is identified, the segmentally related anterior or posterior point should be sought out as well. The two points should then be compared for degree of tissue texture abnormality and tenderness, and the more severe point should be treated first. Following treatment, the treated point should be reassessed, and if it has resolved, the segmentally paired point should be reevaluated. If the paired point is also resolved, the treatment is successful. If the paired point remains tender, it should be treated. Again, following treatment, the second point should be reassessed, and if it has resolved, the paired point first treated should be reevaluated. If the first point treated remains resolved, the treatment is successful. If, however, the first point has returned, a third segmentally related point—an anterior or posterior rib tender point, for example, or an atypical point as described in various counterstrain texts—should be sought out and treated.

ANTERIOR THORACIC TENDER POINTS T1–T6 AND T7–T12 (COUNTERSTRAIN)

These procedures may be employed to reduce pain associated with anterior thoracic tender points. The points (Fig. 13.1) may be found as follows: T1 through T6 are midline points. T1 is located in the suprasternal notch. T2 to T6 descend

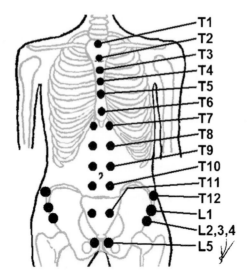

FIGURE 13.1 Counterstrain anterior thoracic and lumbar tender points.

consecutively down the sternum. T7 to L5 are bilaterally paired points. The T7 tender points are inferior to the costal cartilages on either side of the xiphoid process. T9 and T10 surround the umbilicus. The T11 tender points are midway between T10 and the pubis. The T12 tender points are upon the iliac crests at the mid axillary line.[9]

Patient position: supine. Physician position: standing on the side of the tender point (Figs. 13.1 and 13.2).

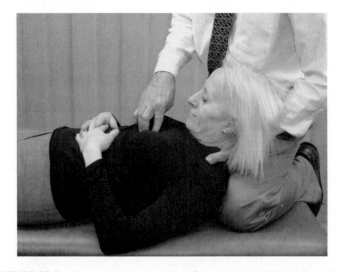

FIGURE 13.2 Counterstrain procedure for an anterior T4 tender point.

Anterior Thoracic Tender Points T1–T6 (Counterstrain)

Because these are midline tender points, you may stand on either side of the patient as dictated by comfort and/or convenience.

Procedure

1. Place the index finger of either hand upon the tender point to be treated. This hand placement must be maintained throughout the procedure.
2. Assess the degree of tissue texture abnormality and tension associated with the tender point. By increasing the amount of digital pressure applied to the tender point, determine the baseline severity of tenderness. Assign this level of tenderness a value of 100% and inform the patient.
3. With your other hand, cradle the patient's occiput and posterior cervical spine. Treatment of anterior tender points involves forward bending of the head upon the chest. The patient's arms and hands should rest comfortably at the sides. To fine-tune the final position, you may have the patient abduct and internally rotate the shoulders. If the patient is lying on a treatment table, this can be accomplished with the arms hanging off the sides of the table. The lower the tender point, the greater the amount of neck and upper torso flexion required. To obtain enough flexion for T5 and T6, you may have to place a pillow or your knee upon the table or bed beneath the patient's neck or upper back.
4. Modify the patient's position by adjusting the amount of flexion and adding side bending and/or rotation to obtain maximum reduction of palpable tissue tension and tenderness. It is generally thought that perceived tenderness should be decreased to not more than 30% of the 100% established in step 2.
5. Hold this position of maximum palpable tissue tension and tenderness reduction for 90 seconds; then slowly return the patient to the original position and reassess. It is important not to remove your monitoring finger during the procedure so that you can be certain that the reduction in tenderness post treatment occurred specifically in the original tender point.
6. Reassess the point for tenderness.

Anterior Thoracic Tender Points T7–T12 (Counterstrain)

As you progress lower down the spine, it becomes necessary to introduce more and more flexion of the torso for the counterstrain procedure to be effective. Treatment of the lower anterior thoracic dysfunctions, which is basically forward bending of the thoracic spine, is done with the patient supine using pillows or a hospital bed to assist in creating flexion. Eventually it is not possible to increase flexion from above, and it becomes necessary to provide the requisite positioning by flexing the patient's hips and pelvis.

Procedure

1. Begin as for anterior thoracic tender points T1 to T6, steps 1 and 2, by establishing contact with the tender point to be treated while identifying the patient's initial subjective level of tenderness (100%) and objective severity of palpable tissue texture abnormality.
2. Introduce flexion of the neck and upper torso as described in the previous instructions. At some point, you will be unable to introduce enough flexion from above to make the procedure effective. At this point additional flexion can be introduced from below by having the patient flex the hips and knees with the feet flat upon the tabletop or mattress.

3. For treating T9 to T12, it becomes necessary to introduce flexion to a greater extent from below. Place your foot upon the table and rest the patient's calves upon your leg. If the patient is in bed, position the pelvis close to the edge of the mattress, while placing your foot upon the box spring or bed frame beneath the mattress. The patient's leg nearest to you is placed upon your thigh first, and the other leg is lifted and placed so that the ankles are crossed and the calves rest upon your thigh.

4. You can now modify the patient's position by adjusting the amount of flexion and adding side bending (typically toward the side of the dysfunction) and/or rotation from below to obtain maximum reduction of palpable tissue tension and tenderness: shift your thigh to increase or decrease flexion of the patient's hips and employ leverage through the patient's legs to side-bend and/or rotate the pelvis. When treating an anterior T12 tender point, more side bending is required than for the other anterior thoracic dysfunctions. It is generally thought that when the patient is properly positioned, perceived tenderness should be decreased to not more than 30% of the 100% established in step 1.

5. Hold this position of maximum palpable tissue tension and tenderness reduction for 90 seconds; then slowly return the patient to the original position and reassess. It is important not to remove your monitoring finger during the procedure so that you can be certain the reduction in tenderness post treatment occurred specifically in the original tender point.

6. Reassess the point for tenderness.

POSTERIOR THORACIC TENDER POINTS T1 TO T4 (COUNTERSTRAIN)

These procedures may be employed to reduce pain associated with posterior thoracic tender points. The points (Fig. 13.3) may be found as follows: the upper thoracic tender points, T1 to T4, are near the midline upon the lateral aspect of the spinous processes. The farther inferior the segment as you descend the tender points may be found more lateral, closer to the tip of the transverse process.[9]

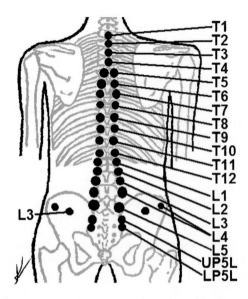

FIGURE 13.3 Counterstrain posterior thoracic and lumbar tender points.

Patient position: lying on the side with the side of the tender point up. Physician position: seated at the side of the table, facing the patient.

Posterior Thoracic Tender Points T1–T4 (Counterstrain) (Figs. 13.3 and 13.4)

Procedure (Example: Right-Sided Tender Point)

1. If the patient is lying on the left side, using the index finger of your left hand, palpate the tender point on the lateral aspect of the upper thoracic spinous process. This hand placement must be maintained throughout the procedure.
2. Assess the degree of tissue texture abnormality and tension associated with the tender point. By increasing the amount of digital pressure on the tender point, determine the baseline severity of tenderness. Assign this level of tenderness a value of 100% and inform the patient.
3. Place your right elbow upon the edge of the table or bed and cradle the left side of the patient's head in the palm of your right hand. Lift the patient's head so that the cervical and thoracic spine is straight.
4. Translate the patient's head and cervical spine posteriorly with your right hand until you sense with the index finger of your left hand that you have obtained maximum reduction of the palpable tissue tension and tenderness. Additional extension may be obtained by having the patient bring both arms above the head. It is generally thought that when the patient is properly positioned, perceived tenderness should be decreased to not more than 30% of the 100% established in step 2.
5. Hold this position of maximum palpable tissue tension and tenderness reduction 90 seconds; then slowly return the patient to the original position. It is important not to remove your monitoring finger during the procedure so that you can be certain the reduction in tenderness post treatment occurred specifically in the original tender point. The standard treatment of posterior T1 to T4 tender points involves direct backward bending of the spine down to the level of dysfunction, with the patient supine and the physician seated at the head of the treatment table. The monitoring finger is placed beneath the patient in contact with the point to be treated, and the patient then slides upward off the end of the table until the tender point is beyond the edge of the table and the patient's head is resting in the physician's lap. Backward bending may be accentuated by lowering the patient's head below the edge of the table: Have the patient bring the

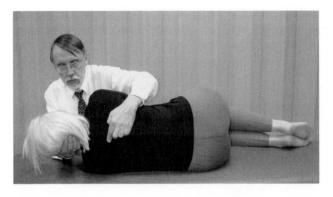

FIGURE 13.4   Counterstrain procedure for a right-side posterior T4 tender point.

hands over the head and put them in your lap; at the same time, have the patient drop the legs off the table on either side. This procedure is not possible if the patient is bedridden.

6. Reassess the point for tenderness.

POSTERIOR THORACIC TENDER POINTS T5–T12 (COUNTERSTRAIN)

The lower tender points are palpable laterally from between the spinous and transverse processes to over the tips of the respective transverse processes (Fig. 13.3).

Patient position: laterally recumbent with the side of the tender point up. Physician position: standing in front of the patient to the side of the table.

Procedure

1. Place your monitoring finger upon the tender point to be treated. Maintain this hand placement throughout the procedure.
2. Assess the degree of tissue texture abnormality and tension associated with the tender point. By increasing the amount of digital pressure applied to the tender point, determine the baseline severity of tenderness. Assign this level of tenderness a value of 100% and inform the patient.
3. Introduce extension from above by sliding the patient's shoulders posteriorly and from below by sliding the patient's hips posteriorly until you have obtained maximum reduction of palpable tissue tension and tenderness. Additional extension may be obtained by having the patient bring both arms above the head. It is generally thought that when the patient is properly positioned, perceived tenderness should be decreased to not more than 30% of the 100% established in step 2.
4. Hold this position of maximum palpable tissue tension and tenderness reduction for 90 seconds; then slowly return the patient to the original position. It is important not to remove your monitoring finger during the procedure so that you can be certain the reduction in tenderness post treatment occurred specifically in the original tender point.
6. Reassess the point for tenderness.

POSTERIOR THORACIC TENDER POINTS, ALTERNATIVE PROCEDURE T9–T12 (COUNTERSTRAIN)

This procedure employs rotation instead of extension.

Patient position: supine. Physician position: standing beside the patient on the side of the tender point.

Procedure

1. Slide one hand palm up beneath the patient, and with your index finger palpate the tender point. Maintain this hand placement throughout the procedure.
2. Assess the degree of tissue texture abnormality and tension associated with the tender point. By increasing the amount of digital pressure applied to the tender point, determine the baseline severity of tenderness. Assign this level of tenderness a value of 100% and inform the patient.
3. With your other hand, grasp the patient's wrist on the side opposite that of the tender point and pull it across the patient's chest until the segment you are monitoring is felt to rotate and you have obtained maximum reduction of palpable tissue tension and tenderness. It is generally thought that when the patient is properly positioned, perceived tenderness should be decreased to not more than 30% of the 100% established in step 2.
4. Hold this position of maximum palpable tissue tension and tenderness reduction for 90 seconds; then slowly return the patient to the original position. It is important

not to remove your monitoring finger during the procedure so that you can be certain that the reduction in tenderness post treatment occurred specifically in the original tender point.

5. Reassess the point for tenderness.

ANTERIOR LUMBAR TENDER POINTS (COUNTERSTRAIN) (FIGS. 13.1 AND 13.5)

These procedures may be employed to reduce pain associated with anterior lumbar tender points. The points (as shown in Fig. 13.1) may be found as follows: The anterior tender point for L1 is either directly over or medial to the anterior superior iliac spine. The L2 tender point is on the inferomedial surface of the anterior inferior iliac spine. The L3 tender point is on the lateral surface of the anterior inferior iliac spine. The L4 tender point is on the inferior surface of the anterior inferior iliac spine. The L5 tender point is on the body of the pubic bone.[9]

Patient position: supine. Physician position: standing on the side of the tender point.

Procedure

1. Place the index finger of either hand upon the tender point to be treated. Maintain this hand placement throughout the procedure.
2. Assess the degree of tissue texture abnormality and tension associated with the tender point. By increasing the amount of digital pressure applied to the tender point, determine the baseline severity of tenderness. Assign this level of tenderness a value of 100% and inform the patient.
3. Place your foot upon the table and rest the patient's calves upon your leg. If the patient is in bed, position the pelvis close to the edge of the mattress, and place your foot upon the box spring or bed frame beneath the mattress. The patient's leg nearer to you is placed upon your thigh first, and the other leg is lifted and placed in such a fashion that the ankles are crossed and the calves rest upon your thigh.

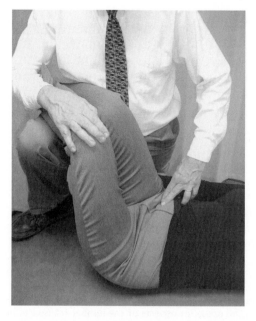

FIGURE 13.5 Counterstrain procedure for a right-side anterior L1 tender point.

4. Modify the patient's position by adjusting the amount of flexion while adding side bending (typically toward the side of the dysfunction) and/or rotation from below to obtain maximum reduction of palpable tissue tension and tenderness: shift your thigh to increase or decrease flexion of the patient's hips and employ leverage through the patient's legs to side-bend and/or rotate the pelvis. It is generally thought that when the patient is properly positioned, perceived tenderness should be decreased to not more than 30% of the 100% established in step 2.

5. Hold this position of maximum palpable tissue tension and tenderness reduction for 90 seconds; then slowly return the patient to the original position. It is important not to remove your monitoring finger during the procedure so that you can be certain that the reduction in tenderness post treatment occurred specifically in the original tender point.

6. Reassess the point for tenderness.

POSTERIOR LUMBAR TENDER POINTS (COUNTERSTRAIN)

These procedures may be employed to reduce pain associated with posterior lumbar tender points. The points (as shown in Figure 13.3) may be found as follows: The posterior lumbar tender points (L1 to L5) are over the posterior aspects of the transverse processes of the respective vertebral segments. Lateral tender points for L3 and L4 may also be found in the gluteal musculature.[9] The lateral tender point for L4 is immediately posterior to the tensor fascia lata and 4 cm below the iliac crest. The tender point for L3 is halfway between the posterior superior iliac spine and the lateral tender point for L4. There are two lateral L5 tender points, an upper pole L5 (UP5L) on the superior medial surface of the posterior superior iliac spine and a lower pole L5 (LP5L) 2 cm below UP5L.[9]

For treatment of the tender points upon the posterior aspects of the transverse processes, the patient lies supine upon the treatment table or bed and the physician stands at the side of the patient on the side of the tender point (Fig. 13.6).

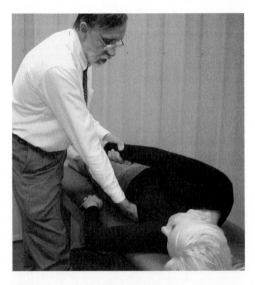

FIGURE 13.6   Counterstrain procedure for the left-side posterior lumbar tender points upon the posterior aspects of the lumbar transverse processes.

Procedure

1. Slide one hand palm up beneath the patient, and with your index finger palpate the tender point. Maintain this hand placement throughout the procedure.
2. Assess the degree of tissue texture abnormality and tension associated with the tender point. By increasing the amount of digital pressure applied to the tender point, determine the baseline severity of tenderness. Assign this level of tenderness a value of 100% and inform the patient.
3. With your other hand, grasp the patient's wrist on the side opposite that of the tender point and pull it across the patient's chest until the segment you are monitoring is felt to rotate and you have obtained maximum reduction of palpable tissue tension and tenderness. It is generally thought that when the patient is properly positioned, perceived tenderness should be decreased to not more than 30% of the 100% established in step 2.
4. Hold this position of maximum palpable tissue tension and tenderness reduction for 90 seconds; then slowly return the patient to the original position. It is important not to remove your monitoring finger during the procedure so that you can be certain the reduction in tenderness post treatment occurred specifically in the original tender point.
5. Reassess the point for tenderness.

LATERAL TENDER POINTS FOR LATERAL L3, LATERAL L4, AND UP5L

Patient position: prone. Physician position: standing on the side of the tender point.

Procedure

1. Place the index finger of either hand upon the tender point to be treated. Maintain this hand placement throughout the procedure.
2. Assess the degree of tissue texture abnormality and tension associated with the tender point. By increasing the amount of digital pressure applied to the tender point, determine the baseline severity of tenderness. Assign this level of tenderness a value of 100% and inform the patient.
3. Reach across the patient with your other hand and grasp the patient's anterior thigh just proximal to the patella. The patient's knee may remain straight, or you can flex the knee to 90 degrees.
4. Lift the patient's knee, drawing it slowly toward you, introducing extension and adduction of the hip until the tender point demonstrates maximum reduction of palpable tissue tension and tenderness. It is generally thought that when the patient is properly positioned, perceived tenderness should be decreased to not more than 30% of the 100% established in step 2.
5. Hold this position of maximum palpable tissue tension and tenderness reduction for 90 seconds; then slowly return the patient to the original position. It is important not to remove your monitoring finger during the procedure so that you can be certain that the reduction in tenderness post treatment occurred specifically in the original tender point.
6. Reassess the point for tenderness.

LATERAL RECUMBENT TREATMENT OF THE LP5L TENDER POINT

Patient position: lying on the side with the tender point up. Physician position: standing at the level of the patient's pelvis.

Procedure

1. Place the index finger of either hand upon the posterior superior iliac spine tender point to be treated. Maintain this hand placement throughout the procedure.
2. Assess the degree of tissue texture abnormality and tension associated with the tender point. By increasing the amount of digital pressure applied to the tender point, determine the baseline severity of tenderness. Assign this level of tenderness a value of 100% and inform the patient.
3. With your other hand grasp the patient's knee ipsilateral to the tender point and draw it toward you, simultaneously introducing flexion to the hip and knee.
4. Flex the hip to 90 degrees and monitor the degree of tissue texture abnormality and tension associated with the tender point. You can further adjust the position by minimally increasing or decreasing hip flexion and adding hip abduction or adduction and internal or external rotation, using the patient's femur as a lever. Finally, you may have to apply a compressive force along the length of the femur toward the pelvis until the tender point demonstrates maximum reduction of palpable tissue tension and tenderness. It is generally thought that when the patient is properly positioned, perceived tenderness should be decreased to not more than 30% of the 100% established in step 2.
5. Hold this position of maximum palpable tissue tension and tenderness reduction for 90 seconds; then slowly return the patient to the original position. It is important not to remove your monitoring finger during the procedure so that you can be certain the reduction in tenderness post treatment occurred specifically in the original tender point.
6. Reassess the point for tenderness.

References

1. Snyder L, Quill TE. Physician's Guide to End-of-Life Care. Philadelphia: American College of Physicians, 2001.
2. Northrup TL, ed. Academy of Applied Osteopathy 1945 Yearbook. Manipulative Therapy Demonstrations. Ann Arbor, MI: Edwards Brothers, 1945. (Now available through the American Academy of Osteopathy, Indianapolis.)
3. Kubler-Ross E. On Death and Dying. New York: Scribner, 1969;7.
4. Northup GW. Osteopathic Medicine: An American Reformation. Chicago: American Osteopathic Association, 1966;64.
5. Deason J. Physiology: General and Osteopathic. Kirksville, MO: Journal Printing, 1913.
6. Bayliss WM, Starling EH. The movements and innervation of the small intestine. J Physiol (Lond) 1901;26:125–138.
7. Kuchera ML, Kuchera WA. Osteopathic Considerations in Systemic Dysfunction. Columbus, OH: Greyden, 1994.
8. Stretanski MF, Kaiser G. Osteopathic philosophy and emergent treatment in acute respiratory failure. J Am Osteopath Assoc 2001;101:447–449.
9. Jones LH. Strain and Counterstrain. Colorado Springs: American Academy of Osteopathy, 1981.

Clinical Conditions

CHAPTER 14

The Patient with Otitis Media

David B. Fuller

INTRODUCTION

Otitis media (infection of the middle ear) is prevalent in children and fairly common in adults. It is amenable to osteopathic diagnosis and treatment, especially if one thinks from a structure and function perspective.

Thinking osteopathically allows one to develop hands-on treatment based on an understanding of each patient's dysfunction and to return that patient to a state of balanced health. Understanding the normal anatomy and physiology and how each patient's pathophysiology presents leads one directly to optimal treatment for each patient. In the case of otitis media, this is well stated in the American Osteopathic Association (AOA) textbook *Foundations for Osteopathic Medicine* in Chapter 22, "General Pediatrics": "Thus, it is important to remember that any infection is a result of a combination of influences: degree of virulence and quantity of an infecting agent, along with host susceptibility. The osteopathic approach favors measures that improve host resistance and recovery concurrent with weakening, or eradicating the infecting agent".[1] Of course, treatment may involve appropriate use of pharmacologic therapy, especially targeted antibiotics when indicated. This section focuses on what can be done from a musculoskeletal perspective to treat patients with otitis media.

A model that helps to organize clinical diagnosis and treatment is one that addresses dysfunction along the lines of structural, neurologic, and fluid aspects of the individual.

ANATOMY AND PHYSIOLOGY

The middle ear is a chamber that sits inside the petrous portion of the temporal bone, with the lateral wall consisting of the tympanic membrane. It contains the auditory ossicles, which transfer sound waves across the middle ear. Pressure is equilibrated with the outside atmosphere via the Eustachian (auditory) tube, which connects anteriorly and inferiorly to the lateral wall of the nasopharynx. The Eustachian tube, like the rest of the upper respiratory tract, is lined with ciliated epithelial cells that move secretions from the middle ear to the nasopharynx.[1,2]

The ear structures are innervated by a sympathetic supply originating from spinal levels at T1 to T4. These sympathetic nerves generally follow the arterial supply to peripheral structures. These same pathways are followed by visceral afferent nerves with information flowing from organs to the spinal cord and central nervous system.[3]

The parasympathetic nerve supply travels via the facial nerve through the pterygopalatine ganglion to the middle ear.[4]

Lymphatic drainage from the ear travels superficially to deep cervical lymphatics via preauricular and postauricular lymph nodes, then inferiorly through the thoracic inlet to the thoracic duct and right lymphatic duct, then to the venous circulation.[5]

Other important structural details are the attachments of the sternocleidomastoid muscles to mastoid processes of temporal bones. The temporomandibular joint sits immediately anterior to the ear.

PATHOPHYSIOLOGY

Acute otitis media is characterized by sudden onset of inflammation of the middle ear. The most common cause of infection is bacteria, although viral infections are common as well. Otitis media usually causes pain, fever, and congestion. Physical examination reveals loss of normal anatomic landmarks (such as the cone of light), inflammation, and bulging of the tympanic membrane.

Sympathetic facilitation is common, with characteristic changes in the mucosal lining of the upper respiratory tract producing increased mucus that becomes thick and tenacious. As sympathetic activity continues, the corresponding spinal segments, T1 to T4, become facilitated.[6] Sympathetic hyperactivity is also believed to be the basis of the Chapman myofascial tender points associated with eye, ear, nose, and throat dysfunction.[7] Posterior Chapman tender points for otitis media are found at the posterior aspect of the tip of the transverse process of the first cervical vertebrae (Fig. 14.1). Associated anterior Chapman tender points are located on the upper edge of the proximal clavicle as it crosses over the first rib.[8] (See Fig. 5.1.)

Dysfunction of the Eustachian tube plays a key role in the development of otitis media. Any structure placing tension on the Eustachian tube will promote dysfunction and obstruction, leading to a pressure gradient in the middle ear chamber as well as fluid accumulation. Hypertonicity of the posterior pharyngeal muscles, the medial pterygoid, and the digastric muscles and dysfunction of the hyoid bone may play an important role in Eustachian dysfunction.[1,9]

Structural factors also include temporal bone dysfunction and sternocleidomastoid hypertonicity. The temporal bones move with the cranial rhythmic impulse in a

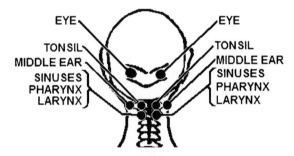

FIGURE 14.1 The posterior Chapman myofascial tender points associated with eye, ear, nose, and throat dysfunction.

continuous cycle of internal and external rotation. This motion assists drainage of the ear. Internal rotation dysfunction of the unilateral temporal has been reported in children with otitis media and is also found in adults.[10] Sternocleidomastoid hypertonicity facilitates this dysfunctional internal rotation of the temporal bone.[1]

Hypertonia in the cervical myofascial tissues can interfere with lymphatic flow.[6]

Lymphatic congestion leads to boggy, edematous tissues that can impair homeostasis and cause discomfort.[11]

The Arnold ear-cough reflex results from stimulation of the auricular branch of the vagus nerve. This is one reason why cough may occur with otitis media, especially when it follows upper respiratory infections. Coughing can aggravate somatic dysfunctions, especially in the upper thoracic, rib and, anterior neck areas.

Chronic otitis media with effusion is inflammation of the ear lasting more than 3 months. Examination often shows a retracted tympanic membrane with decreased hearing. The patient may or may not have pain. Environmental allergies and irritants (especially tobacco smoke) may cause chronic irritation to the middle ear and nasopharynx as well.[1]

Chronic irritation leads to long-term sympathetic facilitation and changes in the upper respiratory epithelium. The number of goblet cells increases and vascular elements decrease, causing the mucosa of the nasopharynx to become thick and sticky.[7] Chronic otitis media can lead to somatic findings similar to those of acute otitis media, but the character of the findings will be consistent with chronic dysfunctions. (See Chapter 3.)

In summary, the pathophysiology of otitis media includes structural dysfunction (Eustachian tube, neck musculature, thoracic and rib), neurologic dysfunction (sympathetic hyperactivity causing mucosal and viscerosomatic changes), and fluid problems (fluid in middle ear, lymphatic congestion of head and neck).

Osteopathic Treatment Paradigm

Osteopathic treatment simply flows from the patient's pathophysiology and specific pattern of somatic dysfunction.

Osteopathic manipulative treatment has been shown to be beneficial in treating patients with otitis media.[9,12]

Osteopathic treatment should address structural, autonomic, and fluid aspects of the dysfunctional process. A course of treatment should address any significant structural somatic dysfunction of the rib, thoracic, and cervical areas along with the cranium. Treatment should address any sympathetic component resulting from facilitated thoracic dysfunction or manifesting as Chapman's points. Treatment should improve fluid mechanics by addressing thoracic inlet, cervical, and head lymphatic components, specifically the Eustachian tube, via ear, mandible, and cranial procedures.

One algorithm that works well is to start with occipitoatlantal release, then address thoracic and rib dysfunction and move cephalad. Of course, every patient has his or her own pattern of dysfunction and needs to be addressed individually. The following is one possible treatment sequence.

With the patient seated, diagnose and treat as follows:

1. Upper thoracic and rib dysfunction to decrease sympathetic facilitation to head and neck as well as improving lymphatic drainage. Procedures can vary with the individual, such as myofascial release; high-velocity, low-amplitude (HVLA) thrust; muscle energy; and counterstrain. (See Chapter 4.)

Move the patient to the supine position, diagnose, and treat as follows:

1. Occipitoatlantal myofascial release (Chapter 16) to address overall tension.
2. Thoracic inlet fascial release (Chapter 19), any clavicular dysfunction (Chapter 16), and specific upper thoracic and rib dysfunction. This procedure will decrease sympathetic facilitation and its effect upon the head and neck and will improve lymphatic drainage from these areas.
3. Posterior Chapman's points and specific dysfunctions at the occipital–C1–C2 complex (discussed later in the chapter).
4. Cervical spine dysfunction with appropriate procedures. (See Chapters 16, 17, and 22.) This procedure addresses mechanical, sympathetic, and fluid components.
5. Anterior neck dysfunction, that is, hyoid, sternocleidomastoid, and anterior vertebral dysfunctions to improve lymphatic drainage and decrease tension on the Eustachian tubes. (See Chapter 16.)
6. Specific procedures for Eustachian tube dysfunction, that is, Galbraith's procedure, traction of the pinna (discussed later in the chapter).
7. Cranial dysfunction, especially cranial torsions and temporal bone dysfunction (discussed later in the chapter).
8. Other head procedure, that is, sphenopalatine ganglion procedure (discussed later in the chapter) and effleurage. (See Chapter 16.) These techniques improve autonomic and fluid functions.

Case Illustration

A 28-year-old patient has ear pain following an upper respiratory infection. After taking a history and performing a physical examination, the physician diagnoses otitis media with accompanying somatic dysfunction that includes T4, rotated and side bent right, extended, with an elevated fourth rib dorsally accompanied by a Jones tender point at the costovertebral angle; fascial restriction at the thoracic inlet; C2 rotated and side bent right; a right cranial torsion; and a fascial restriction at the occipitoatlantal junction.

One appropriate treatment sequence for this patient would be as follows: occipitoatlantal myofascial release, thoracic outlet myofascial release, counterstrain to T4 and fourth rib followed by the HVLA procedure, specific treatment of choice to C2, balance the cranial torsion, and finish with the Galbraith procedure. This sequence takes about 5 minutes, leads to significant improvement in the patient's symptoms, and hastens the resolution of the otitis media.

Procedures

Posterior Chapman's Reflexes from Otitis Media

This procedure is employed to treat posterior Chapman's reflexes associated with otitis media. These are small (2–3 mm) nodular masses that are palpable in soft tissue and that demonstrate sharp pinpoint nonradiating tenderness. The posterior points are located upon the posterior aspect of tips of transverse processes of C1 ipsilateral to the side of the otitis (Fig. 14.1).

Patient position: supine. Physician position: standing or sitting at the head of the table.

Procedure

1. Place your index finger on the palpable nodular mass of Chapman's point on the posterior aspect of the tip of transverse processes of C1, laterally between the angle of the mandible and the tip of the mastoid process.
2. Apply pressure to the point in a circular fashion, massaging it in an attempt to dissipate it. The amount of pressure necessary will be mildly to moderately uncomfortable for the patient.
3. Apply the therapeutic pressure for approximately 10 to 30 seconds. Cease the treatment when the palpable point resolves or is significantly decreased.

Galbraith's Procedure (Fig. 14.2)

This procedure is employed to improve function of Eustachian tube and decongest the middle ear.

Patient position: supine with the head slightly elevated and turned to the right. Physician position: standing at the right side of the table near head level.

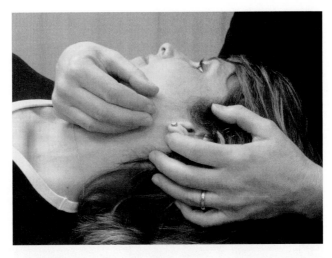

FIGURE 14.2 Galbraith's procedure to improve function of Eustachian tube and decongest the middle ear.

Procedure (Example: Left Eustachian Tube Dysfunction)

1. Stabilize the patient's head by placing the palm of your left hand upon the left side of the patient's head in such a way that your thumb lies superior and anterior to the ear and your index finger lies posterior to the ear on the mastoid process.
2. Place the pads of the middle three fingers of your right hand so that they hook around the angle of the mandible.
3. Pull rhythmically on the angle of the mandible along the line of the mandibular ramus at about 3 cycles per second for 1 minute.
4. You can easily teach patients to perform this procedure upon themselves or their children at home.

Traction on the Pinna (Fig. 14.3)

This procedure is employed to improve function of Eustachian tube and decongest the middle ear. Be careful when performing this procedure in acute conditions because it employs an abrupt application of force that can be very painful. This procedure is more appropriate for adults than for children. (Example: Left Eustachian tube or middle ear dysfunction.)

Patient position: supine with the head turned to the right. Physician position: standing at the head of the table.

Procedure

1. Stabilize the patient's head by placing the palm of your right hand upon the left side of the face so that your thumb lies superior and anterior to the ear.
2. With your left hand grasp the superior aspect of the ear between your thumb and index finger. You may wish to grasp the ear with a small gauze pad to facilitate the firmness of your grasp. The ear must be held firmly, but be careful not to contuse it.
3. Firmly apply intermittent traction to the ear directed superiorly, posteriorly, and laterally. The force should be applied as a tug abrupt enough to move the pinna. An alternative treatment is to apply gentle, steady, continuous traction on the pinna in the same direction without any sudden tug.

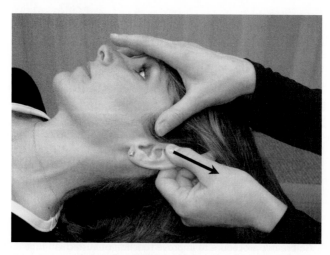

FIGURE 14.3 Traction on the pinna of the ear to improve function of Eustachian tube and decongest the middle ear.

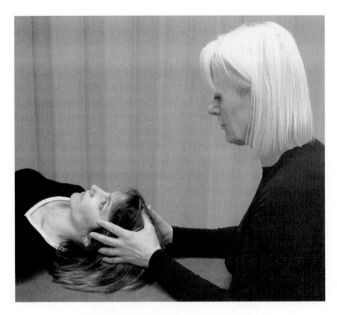

FIGURE 14.4   Cranial vault hold.

The following two cranial procedures are indirect methods that require a sensitive light touch.

Cranial Vault Hold for Spheno-Occipital Synchondrosis Torsion (Figs. 14.4 and 14.5)

The cartilaginous articulation between the sphenoid and occiput, the spheno-occipital or sphenobasilar synchondrosis, remains unfused throughout life in some individuals. In most it does fuse, but not until well into the third decade of life.[13] Various dysfunctional patterns, including torsion, side-bending rotation, extremes of flexion and

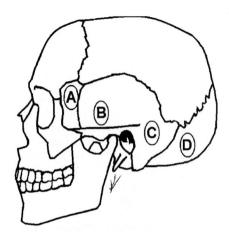

FIGURE 14.5   Placement of fingertips for the vault hold. A, index finger; B, middle finger; C, ring finger; D, little finger.

extension, horizontal strain, vertical strain, and compression, have been described. Their description is beyond the scope of this text. Torsions are discussed here.

Spheno-occipital torsion is, as the name suggests, twisting between the two bones at the synchondrosis. The dysfunction is described in terms of the sphenoid bone relative to the occiput and is named for the side on which the greater wing of the sphenoid is displaced superiorly, toward the vertex of the skull. This area can be palpated with the hand placement referred to as a vault hold. This hand placement allows the physician to palpate the entire cranial base simultaneously. The examiner's hands bilaterally contact the greater wings of the sphenoid, the squamous and petrous portions of the temporal bones, and the occiput.

Patient position: supine. Physician position: seated at the head of the table with the forearms resting on the tabletop.

Procedure

1. Place the distal phalangeal pads of your index fingers bilaterally upon the greater wings of the sphenoid (Fig. 14.5, point A).
2. Place the distal phalangeal pads of your middle fingers bilaterally upon the squamous portion of the temporal bones just anterior to the ears (Fig. 14.5, point B).
3. Place the distal phalangeal pads of your ring fingers bilaterally upon the mastoid portions of the temporal bones just posterior to the ears (Fig. 14.5, point C).
4. Place the distal phalangeal pads of your little fingers bilaterally upon the lateral aspect of the squamous portion of the occipital bone (Fig. 14.5, point D).
5. Your thumbs should rest comfortably over the vault of the skull.
6. Assess for spheno-occipital synchondrosis torsion left by inducing a gentle motion of the sphenoid in a cephalad anterior direction with your left index finger and in a caudal posterior direction with your right index finger. Compliance is consistent with torsion left, resistance with torsion right.
7. Assess for spheno-occipital synchondrosis torsion right by inducing a gentle motion of the sphenoid in a cephalad anterior direction with your right index finger and in a caudal posterior direction with your left index finger. Compliance is consistent with torsion right, resistance with torsion left.
8. Indirect procedure: reproduce the pattern of greatest compliance and hold until the amplitude of cranial rhythmic impulse decreases and stops, a *still point*. When a still point is obtained, release your hold on the mechanism with the next flexion and external rotation phase of the cranial rhythmic impulse.
9. Reassess spheno-occipital motion.

Temporal Bone Dysfunction (Cranial)

This procedure may be employed to treat restriction of motion of the temporal bones as they relate to one another and to the midline bones of the base of the skull, the sphenoid, and the occiput. The dysfunction may be unilateral or bilateral. The motion pattern of the midline bones is flexion and extension. The paired temporal bones externally rotate in association with spheno-occipital flexion and internally rotate with extension. (Readers unacquainted with these mechanics are referred to a basic text on the subject.)[14] This mechanism demonstrates an inherent rhythmicity, the cranial rhythmic impulse, of 6 to 14 cycles per minute and appears to be linked to baroreflex physiology.[15,16] Motion testing is done to identify compliance or resistance between the bones of the cranial base in association with the cranial rhythmic impulse.

Patient position: supine. Physician position: seated at the head of the table with the forearms resting on the tabletop (Figs. 14.6 and 14.7).

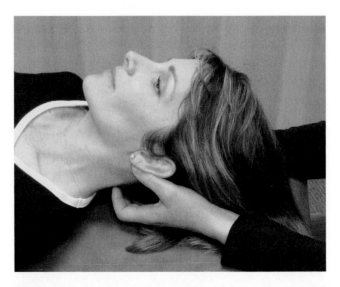

FIGURE 14.6   Treatment of temporal bone dysfunction (cranial).

Readers untrained in cranial manipulation should avoid manipulating the temporal bones because of the sensitivity of the vestibular apparatus.

Procedure

1. Cradle the patient's head in both hands. Your thenar eminences should be in contact with the posterior portion of the temporal bones behind the patient's ears (Fig. 14.7, point A), and your thumbs should be pointing caudally, contacting the tips of the mastoid processes (Fig. 14.7, point B). Be certain that you contact the patient's head laterally to the occipitomastoid suture.
2. With your thumbs, in synchrony with the cranial rhythmic impulse, gently apply medially directed pressure over the mastoid processes (Fig. 14.7, point B). Apply this force as the skull moves into the flexion and external rotation phase of the cranial rhythm.

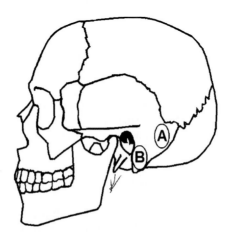

FIGURE 14.7   Points of contact for hand placement during treatment of temporal bone dysfunction. **A** is the contact point for the thenar eminence; **B** is the contact point for the distal thumb.

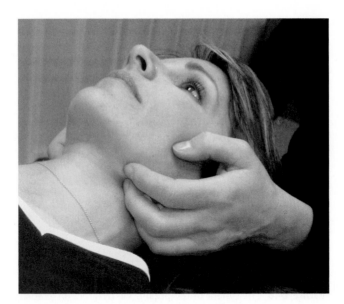

FIGURE 14.8   Hand placement to decongest the pterygoid fossa and improve the nerve function of sphenopalatine ganglion to promote normal Eustachian tube function.

3. As the cranial rhythm moves into extension and internal rotation, decrease the pressure with your thumbs while gently applying medially directed pressure to the temporal bone with your thenar eminences (Fig. 14.7, point A).
4. Follow the cranial rhythmic impulse by synchronously alternating steps 2 and 3.
5. Pay attention to the palpable compliance or resistance of the bones to your applied forces. Compare external rotation, thumb pressure, with internal rotation, thenar pressure. Compare the compliance and/or resistance pattern that you feel for the right temporal bone with that of the left temporal bone.
6. Follow the pattern and gently attempt to amplify it over several cycles of the cranial rhythmic impulse.
7. Reassess temporal bone motion.

Pterygoid Fossa Decongestion, Sphenopalatine Ganglion Procedure (Fig. 14.8)

This procedure is employed to indirectly decongest the pterygoid fossa and improve the nerve function of the sphenopalatine ganglion, thereby allowing normal function of the Eustachian tube. Relaxation of the medial pterygoid muscle also enables the tensor veli palatini muscle to functionally open the Eustachian tube.

Patient position: supine. Physician position: seated at the head of the table.

Procedure

1. Place the pad of the distal phalanx of your middle finger inferior to the angle of the mandible on the side of the otitis.
2. Apply medially and superiorly directed pressure with your finger to contact the edematous tissue along the inner portion of the mandibular ramus.
3. Gently pump the area in a cephalad/caudad direction for 1 minute.
4. Treat the opposite side. This procedure may be taught to the patient for self-treatment twice daily.

References

1. Centers S, Morelli MA, Vallad-Hix C, Seffinger MA. General Pediatrics: Foundations for Osteopathic Medicine. 2nd ed. Philadelphia: Lippincott Williams & Wilkins, 2002;315.
2. Moore KL. Clinically Oriented Anatomy. 2nd ed. Baltimore: Williams & Wilkins, 1985;964.
3. Kuchera M, Kuchera W. Osteopathic Considerations in Systemic Dysfunction. 2nd ed. Columbus, OH: Greyden, 1994;2.
4. Moore KL. Clinically Oriented Anatomy. 2nd ed. Baltimore: Williams & Wilkins, 1985;943.
5. Moore KL. Clinically Oriented Anatomy. 2nd ed. Baltimore: Williams & Wilkins, 1985;43
6. Shaw HH, Shaw MB. Osteopathic management of ear, nose, and throat disease. Foundations for Osteopathic Medicine. 2nd ed. Philadelphia: Lippincott Williams & Wilkins, 2002;372.
7. Kuchera M, Kuchera W. Osteopathic Considerations in Systemic Dysfunction. 2nd ed. Columbus, OH: Greyden, 1994;38.
8. Chapman F. An Endocrine Interpretation of Chapman's Reflexes. 2nd ed. Indianapolis: American Academy of Osteopathy, 1937;27.
9. Shaw HH, Shaw MB. Osteopathic management of ear, nose, and throat disease. Foundations for Osteopathic Medicine. 2nd ed. Philadelphia: Lippincott Williams & Wilkins, 2002:378–379.
10. Steele KM. Clinical management of chronic otitis media/eustachian tube dysfunction. Lecture presented at the Annual Convocation of the American Academy of Osteopathy, 2004; Colorado Springs, CO.
11. Kuchera M, Kuchera W. Osteopathic Considerations in Systemic Dysfunction. 2nd ed. Columbus, OH: Greyden, 1994;6.
12. Mills MV, Henley CE, Barnes LL, et al. The use of osteopathic manipulative treatment as adjuvant therapy in children with recurrent acute otitis media. Arch Pediatr Adolesc Med 2003;157:861–866.
13. Williams PL, ed. Gray's Anatomy. 38th ed. Edinburgh: Churchill Livingstone, 1995;490.
14. King HH, Lay E. Osteopathy in the cranial field. In: Ward RC, ed. Foundations for Osteopathic Medicine. 2nd ed. Philadelphia: Lippincott Williams & Wilkins, 2002;985–1001.
15. Nelson KE, Sergueef N, Lipinski CM, et al. Cranial rhythmic impulse related to the Traube-Hering-Mayer oscillation: Comparing laser-Doppler flowmetry and palpation. J Am Osteopath Assoc 2001;101:163–173.
16. Sergueef N, Nelson KE, Glonek T. The effect of cranial manipulation upon the Traube-Hering-Meyer oscillation as measured by laser-Doppler flowmetry. Altern Ther Health Med 2002;8(6):74–76.

CHAPTER 15

The Patient with Temporomandibular Joint Pain and Dysfunction

John McPartland

INTRODUCTION

Applying an osteopathic perspective to dysfunctions involving the temporo-mandibular joint (TMJ) provides a large toolbox with which we can help our patients. In contrast, the standard medical approach to TMJ dysfunction can be quite limited.[1] The standard medical approach is easily incorporated into the osteopathic perspective, as presented in this review.

TMJ dysfunction is the most frequent source of facial pain after toothache. Current diagnostic criteria divide TMJ dysfunction into three categories: myofascial pain dysfunction (MPD) syndrome, internal derangement (ID) injury, and degenerative joint disease (DJD). MPD syndrome is best characterized as a psychophysiologic disease primarily involving the muscles of mastication, frequently provoked by somatic dysfunctions elsewhere in the body.[2] ID is defined as an abnormal relationship between the articular disc and the mandibular condyle, common examples being acute disc displacement and chronic recurrent dislocations. DJD involves organic degeneration of the articular surfaces within the TMJ. An estimated 10 million people in the United States (1 in 25) have TMJ disorder. The greatest incidence is in adults aged 20 to 40 years. The female-to-male ratio is 4:1.[1]

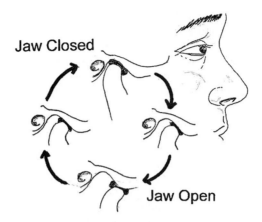

Jaw Closed

Jaw Open

FIGURE 15.1   Time course illustration of TMJ movement: normal position of disc and mandibular condyle during opening and closing of the jaw.

STRUCTURE AND FUNCTION

The TMJ has been described as the most complex joint in the body because it not only acts as a hinge joint but also permits a gliding movement, in which the condyle of the mandible slides along the squamous portion of the temporal bone. The articular surface of the temporal bone is similarly complex, consisting of a convex articular eminence anteriorly and a concave articular fossa posteriorly.

The condyle and the temporal bone are separated by an articular disc that divides the joint cavity into two small spaces. The articular disc, also known as the meniscus, is a biconcave fibrocartilaginous structure. It provides a gliding surface for the condyle, resulting in smooth joint movement. The meniscus has three parts, a thick anterior band, a thin intermediate zone, and a thick posterior band. When the mouth is closed, the condyle is separated from the temporal bone by the thick posterior band. When the mouth is open, the condyle is separated from the temporal bone by the thin intermediate zone (Fig. 15.1). Opening the mouth activates the suprahyoid muscles (mylohyoid, geniohyoid, and digastric muscles), which provide the hingelike movement. Anterior condylar glide is provided by the inferior division of the lateral (external) pterygoid muscles. Elevation of the mandible (closing the mouth) is accomplished by the temporalis, masseter, and medial (internal) pterygoid muscles. Lateral displacement (grinding movement) activates the ipsilateral temporalis and the contralateral medial and lateral pterygoids, with some assistance from the ipsilateral or contralateral masseter muscles. Protraction of the mandible activates the suprahyoid muscles, medial and lateral pterygoids, masseters, and sometimes the temporalis muscles.[3]

ETIOLOGY AND PATHOPHYSIOLOGY OF TMJ SYNDROME

MPD is the most common cause of TMJ pain. Its multifactorial etiology includes somatic asymmetries leading to malocclusion, jaw clenching, bruxism, increased pain sensitivity, and personality disorders, such as stress and anxiety. The bottom-line etiological basis of the symptoms (i.e., pain, tenderness, and spasm of the mastication muscles) is muscular hyperactivity and dysfunction. Whiplash injury and other strains to the neck or upper thoracic spine are frequently overlooked contributors to

MPD-type TMJ syndrome.[2] Although a dental procedure may precipitate MPD, apprehension on the part of the patient may be a more significant factor than the procedure itself.[2] The significance of psychological factors has been recognized during the past few years. Patients with chronic MPD tend to score high on obsessive-compulsive scales and have elevated levels of disease conviction.[1] Although MPD usually starts as a functional disorder, it can lead to organic changes in the joint, in the muscles of mastication, and in the dentition.[3]

ID is caused by a biomechanical problem within the TMJ. Mandibular muscle spasm observed in ID is a response to the dysfunction, not the cause of the problem. Anterior disc displacement is the most common cause of ID (Fig. 15.2). The disc dislocation reduces upon opening of the jaw, which causes an *opening click*. The disc dislocates again upon closing of the jaw, which causes a *closing click*. If the condyle cannot override the displaced disc, jaw locking occurs (described later in the chapter). Disc displacement and interposition of the posterior band between the condyle and the eminence can cause pain and jaw noise.

Degenerative joint disease is often secondary to microtrauma or macrotrauma of the disc, mandibular condyle, or surrounding connective tissues. Dental procedures are a common source of trauma, particularly work on molar teeth. The other causes of DJD are osteoarthritis, rheumatoid arthritis, ankylosis, infections of the bone or joint, and neoplasia.

Clinical History

Patients with TMJ syndrome commonly complain of facial pain, jaw range of motion (ROM) restriction, jaw noise (clicking or popping), and headaches or neck pain. Earache is fairly common. Many patients report a recent history of jaw trauma (e.g., wisdom tooth extraction) and acute or chronic problems with

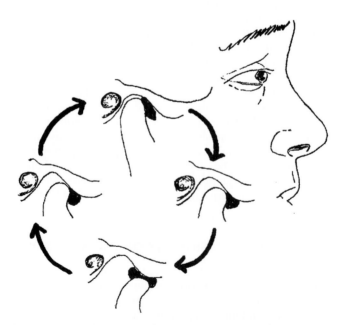

FIGURE 15.2 Time course illustration of TMJ movement: anterior disc dislocation that reduces upon opening the jaw and redislocates upon closing the jaw.

bruxism or the clenching of teeth. Facial pain is usually periauricular, worsened by chewing. Periauricular pain may be unilateral or bilateral. In MPD, the pain may worsen during periods of increased stress. Headaches may be triggered by TMJ syndrome. In patients who have a history of headaches resistant to treatment, the diagnosis and treatment of TMJ syndrome should not be overlooked.

Clicking, popping, and snapping sounds may or may not be associated with pain. (Few nociceptors innervate the disc, so pain may be absent.) An isolated click is very common in the general population and is not a risk factor for development of TMJ syndrome. Reduced jaw ROM and locking episodes are common. The lock can be open or closed. Open lock, or inability to close the mouth, is seen when the condyle dislocates anteriorly in front of the articular eminence; if not reduced immediately, it is very painful. Closed lock, or inability to open the mouth more than 10 mm, is seen when the disc remains anteriorly displaced at all times. Closed lock may be caused by pain or disc displacement.

Physical Examination

The physical examination can be separated into visual and palpatory components. Visually inspect for facial asymmetry (lateral deviation of the mandible), muscle hypertrophy, malocclusion of teeth, and abnormal dental wear. Inspect mandible ROM; normal vertical jaw opening is 50 mm measured between the incisors. Less than 40 mm is hypomobile, and more than 70 mm is hypermobile. Do not be fooled by dentures. (Dentures tend to be short, producing false negatives in hypomobile patients.) Normal ROM for lateral mandibular movement is 10 mm on each side of midline.

Watch for lateral tracking of the mandible away from midline as the mouth is slowly opened. The tip of the chin or the space between the lower incisors serves as a good landmark for observing midline mandible motion. Lateral tracking may present as deflection (lateral deviation en route that corrects when the jaw is fully opened) or as deviation (lateral deviation at end range). Deflection may express a C- or S-shaped pattern. While testing ROM, listen for clicking or popping and feel for crepitus. Less obvious sounds can be auscultated with a stethoscope placed over the TMJ. Visually inspect rotation and side bending of the neck, and check for unusual spinal curves or shoulder elevation.

Palpate the TMJ and surrounding muscles with the patient supine. The TMJ is best palpated directly below the zygomatic arch, 1 to 2 cm anterior to the tragus. The posterior aspect of the TMJ can be palpated through the external auditory canal. Feel for lateral deviation as the mouth is slowly opened, with one condyle moving laterally and the other condyle moving medially. Palpate surrounding muscles for spasm and tender points or trigger points. According to Travell and Simons,[3] trigger points in the lateral pterygoid, medial pterygoid, and masseter muscles frequently refer pain to the TMJ. The temporalis, scalene, sternocleidomastoid, and suprahyoid muscles should also be examined. To exaggerate any dysfunctions, palpate for tenderness while turning the patient's head and neck to one side and then the other. Watch the patient's response to palpation, especially flinching, pain behavior, or lingering pain after palpation.

In a study of 130 TMJ patients, nearly all presented with at least one type of biomechanical cranial dysfunction.[4] Compression of condylar parts of the occiput was most common (27% of patients), followed by compression of the sphenobasilar symphysis (18%), articular strain of the frontosphenoid articulation (12%), and nonphysiologic strain patterns, such as vertical or lateral strain (11%). Extracranial dysfunctions occurred at C3 to C4 (50% of patients), the sacroiliac joints (32%), lumbosacral junction (29%), C4 to C5 (30%), T2 to T3 (14%), T3 to T4 (14%), and occipitoatlantal (9%). About 14% of patients had scoliosis.[4] Interestingly, dysfunctions of the temporal bones were rarely noted in this study, although the temporal bone has been cited as a primary problem in other studies.[2,5,6] Similarly, the study of 130 TMJ patients made no mention of C1 to C2 dysfunction, whereas another study linked unilateral TMJ pain with an anterior rotational of the atlas on the ipsilateral side.[2]

Laboratory Studies

Laboratory studies generally are not indicated. Blood work may be required if systemic illness is suspected to be the cause of TMJ syndrome:

- Complete blood count if infection is suspected
- Calcium, phosphate, and alkaline phosphatase for possible bone disease
- Uric acid if gout is suspected
- Serum creatine and creatine phosphokinase, indicators of muscle disease
- Rheumatoid factor, erythrocyte sedimentation rate, antinuclear antibody panel, and other specific antibodies are checked if rheumatoid arthritis, temporal arteritis, or a connective tissue disorder is suspected.

Imaging Studies

Imaging studies generally are not indicated. If a fracture or bony erosion (DJD) is suspected, conventional radiography is the most widely used imaging study. It is simple, evaluates bony structures, and in most cases is sufficient. Real-time ultrasound allows visualization of the structure and function of the articular discs, mandibular condyles, and surrounding muscles. Computed tomography can explore both bony structures and muscular soft tissues. It can be done with contrast material instilled into the joint cavity. Magnetic resonance imaging (MRI), though costly, is the study of choice if (1) articular or meniscal pathology is suspected and an endoscopic or surgical procedure is contemplated and (2) in a case of traumatic TMJ syndrome.

Other Studies

Dental tapes and dental casts can be used to analyze occlusal strain and stress. Orthodontic strain analysis can diagnose static and kinematic occlusal patterns by detecting bite prematurities and interferences.[6] Arthroscopy is an acute diagnostic approach. It should be reserved for patients with internal TMJ derangements resistant to conservative treatments. A good MRI study should be obtained before contemplating arthroscopy.

Differential Diagnosis of TMJ Syndrome

- Dental infections, mandibular fractures
- Gout, pseudogout, rheumatoid arthritis
- Tension headaches, migraine headaches
- Otitis media, sinusitis
- Temporal arteritis
- Trigeminal neuralgia, postherpetic neuralgia

Treatment

TMJ dysfunction from trauma (e.g., tooth extraction or other dental work) is often self-limiting and responds to simple treatment: osteopathic manipulative treatment

(OMT) and patient education. OMT approaches include soft tissue massage, myofascial release, muscle energy, counterstrain, functional methods, and osteopathy in the cranial field (OCF). Effective OCF methods are described in the procedures section later in the chapter. (See also Chapters 8, 10, and 25.) Patient education includes teaching self-massage, mindfulness while eating, and other forms of self-rehabilitation. Self-massage includes skin pinching, rolling skin between fingers, and stripping massage. The patient should perform self-massage several times per day. Soft tissue massage helps inactivate muscle trigger points and disrupts fibrous adhesions. Moist heat packs are helpful during acute episodes, used not longer than 15 minutes per application. Alternating hot and cold packs may be helpful.

Acute TMJ Pain

Acute TMJ pain from muscle clenching may be relieved by slightly stretching (gapping) the joint capsule, which promotes relaxation of hypertonic muscles. This can be performed by the patient or the practitioner. With the finger pads, apply light caudad traction upon the ramus of the mandible. Alternatively, stretch the joint capsule using a dental appliance. A temporary dental appliance can be fashioned by rolling gauze cotton around the ends of two wood spatulas or tongue blades. Ask the patient to open the mouth about 20 mm, and position the cotton rolls between the molars. Ask the patient to gently close the mouth. The cotton rolls act as fulcra to disengage the TMJs. In the author's opinion, the fulcra also improve temporal bone movement during the inhalation phase (flexion, external rotation) of cranial motion.

Nonsteroidal anti-inflammatory analgesics can be used on a short-term basis (ibuprofen and naproxen are commonly used). Severe muscle spasm may benefit from prescribed muscle relaxants (benzodiazepines, or cyclobenzaprine in patients unable to tolerate benzodiazepines).

Chronic TMJ Syndrome

TMJ syndrome is another kettle of fish. Its treatment can be difficult. Some experts recommend management by a team approach, with the team consisting of an osteopathic physician with good OMT and pharmacologic skills, a dentist, a psychologist, and in a small number of cases, a surgeon. (Surgical indications include internal derangements, adhesions, fibrosis, and DJD.)

Benzodiazepines and codeine have no place in chronic TMJ syndrome. Counsel patients that chronic pain cannot be resolved in the presence of benzodiazepines or opioid pain medications. Relaxation-inducing herbs, such as hops or valerian, may be substituted. Bedtime doses of calcium and magnesium (500 mg each) provide muscle relaxant activity. Tricyclic antidepressants (e.g., amitriptyline and nortriptyline) in low doses have been used effectively for chronic painful conditions. They act by inhibiting pain transmission, by improving axoplasmic flow in nerve fibers, and by reducing nighttime bruxism. Gabapentin (Neurontin) and its new analog pregabalin (Lyrica) have been prescribed for chronic TMJ syndrome. Avoid caffeine, which increases muscle tension, and alcohol, which increases bruxism.

Educate patients about bruxism and the need to avoid clenching and grinding teeth. The key to relaxing jaw muscles is keeping the teeth slightly apart. Prescribe a soft diet for patients with chewing pain, and advise patients to chew more slowly and take smaller bites. Encourage patients to stay away from large, firm food, such as carrots, apples, and stale bagels. Instruct them not to chew gum and to avoid opening the mouth wide while yawning. Teach self-massage (discussed earlier in the chapter), jaw mobilization exercises, and proper posture. The Alexander technique is a good approach for postural reeducation.[7] Other home exercises include passive jaw opening with finger assist, passive jaw stretching with wooden tongue blades, and active ROM exercises. Exercise sheets and other resources can be obtained online from The TMJ Association (www.tmj.org). Exercises should be taught in the office and repeated at home in front of a mirror. Trigger point injections or spray-and-stretch of the lateral pterygoid, medial pterygoid, and masseter muscles may be useful; the reader is directed to Travell and Simons.[3]

Preexisting anxiety, depression, and obsessive-compulsive disorders must be addressed. Any chronic painful condition, such as TMJ syndrome, will worsen any preexisting anxiety or depression. The psychologic component of TMJ can be engaged with cognitive-behavioral treatment.[1] Teach stress reduction strategies and behavior modification. In appropriate settings, psychological counseling may provide benefit. Relaxation training using electromyographic (EMG) biofeedback is helpful if a referral can be found locally.

Occlusal splints (mouth orthotics) are controversial.[8] There are two types of splints. Night guards (also known as bruxism appliances or mouth orthotics) are worn at night. They reduce muscle tension by preventing grinding and clenching of teeth. Repositioning appliances (auto-repositional splints) are worn 24 hours a day. They realign the jaw, usually by anterior repositioning. Splints must be fitted precisely by a dentist; advise against buying ready-made versions sold in drugstores. Significant bite correction may require orthodontic braces or restorative work (e.g., crowns, occlusal adjustments, bridges).

Osteopathic considerations aim at stabilizing the joint and restoring its mobility, strength, endurance, and function. Manipulative treatment should be given before and after fitting for occlusal splints and before and after restorative dentistry. Normalize function of the temporal bone, since the squamous portion of that bone directly affects articular function of the TMJ. Treat sphenobasilar synchondrosis (SBS) compression and nonphysiologic strain patterns. Check the neck, thoracic spine, and the sacroiliac.[9] Do not forget about the causes of scoliosis, such as short leg.[10] (See Chapter 26.)

Procedures

TMJ pain responds best to gentle OMT interventions. Muscle hypertonicity can be treated with counterstrain or indirect myofascial release. Articular dysfunctions in the cervical and thoracic spine respond well to muscle energy procedures. Articular dysfunctions of the cranium should be treated with indirect OCF procedures. Extension of the fourth ventricle (EV-4), perhaps the most indirect procedure available, is described later in the chapter. Indirect OCF may be subtle but may nevertheless produce acute and sometimes unexpected changes, such as ocular alterations.[11] Avoid using intraoral OCF procedures directed at the sphenoid because they frequently cause further problems.[12] In cases of TMJ lock, two direct-action OCF procedures the Strachan procedures, described later in the chapter, are particularly useful.

EV-4 Procedure (Cranial)

Expansion of the fourth ventricle (Fig. 15.3) is the biodynamic counterpart to the CV-4 (compression of the fourth ventricle) procedure developed by Sutherland.[13] (See Chapter 10.) The EV-4 is an indirect procedure that hypothetically works upon the fluid body rather than just ventricular fluids (think globally, not locally). A quick review of indirect OCF procedure may be useful: Pull out some pennies or nickels and place a coin in each palm and on each fingertip. Develop a sense for that amount of pressure. You should never feel more pressure when you apply your hands to

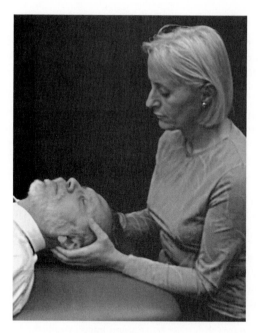

FIGURE 15.3 EV-4.

someone's head using indirect OCF procedures. With the patient supine, sit at the head of the table in a comfortable position, with the seat and the treatment table at correct heights. The patient's head should lie upon the table away from the edge, permitting you to rest your forearms on the table while holding the head. Consider stretching your forearm flexor myofascia to make a light handhold easier to accomplish. Before taking hold of the patient's head, you should be centered—calm, mentally focused upon the moment, breathing from the respiratory diaphragm, seated squarely on the ischial tuberosities, with relaxed hands, arms, shoulders, and neck.

With the patient supine and the practitioner seated at the head of the table, apply the Becker hold. The Becker hold, developed by Rollin Becker is a relaxed alternative to the standard vault hold.[14] Cup your hands, holding the patient's head like a bowl of water. As the weight of the patient's head settles, allow your hands to separate somewhat, so the bottom of the patient's occiput rests upon the padded table. The primary objective is to apply a handhold that is totally unobtrusive to the patient. Imagine that your hands are two water balloons and the head you are holding is another water balloon you are trying to gently balance between your hands. When the Becker hold is properly applied, your thumbs should rest against the patient's sphenoid bones. This facilitates your ability to sense the patient's cranial rhythmic impulse (CRI). The Becker hold also enables the perception of rhythms that are slower and deeper than the CRI, such as the slow wave (the 2- to 3-cycle wave), which moves at 2 to 3 cycles per minute.[13,14] During the patient's inhalation phase (flexion, external rotation) of cranial motion, your intention is to subtly augment a widening of the transverse diameter of the cranium. After several cycles, you may observe a prolonged inhalation phase in your subject or come to a still point, that is, neutral. After time, the rhythm returns and you can disengage during the inhalation phase. When the procedure is complete, reassess the cranial motion pattern and the amplitude of the CRI.

Jaw Lock Corrections

At the other end of the OCF spectrum from the EV-4 procedure are Strachan's procedures for correcting open lock and close lock. The procedures are described and illustrated in Fryette's classic text.[15]

Jaw Lock Open Lock Correction (Example: Right-sided Open Lock)

Strachan called open lock (see Clinical History, earlier in the chapter) an anterior lesion, characterized by an uneven and painful forward glide on the affected side, chin deviation toward the contralateral side, and inability to close the mouth.

Patient position: supine. Physician position: standing or sitting at the end of the table.

Procedure

1. Place your left hand on the left side of the patient's face such that the hypothenar eminence lies against the zygomatic arch and the fingertips extend beyond the chin. The hypothenar eminence stabilizes the patient's head throughout the procedure and prevents it from rolling to the left.
2. Place your right hand on the right side of the patient's face so the fingers wrap around the ramus of the mandible, with two fingers above the angle and two fingers below the angle (Fig. 15.4A).
3. The first phase of the procedure is an indirect (exaggeration) procedure. As the patient relaxes, open the mouth further by applying traction with the fingers of the left hand to depress the chin while the right-hand ring finger and little finger exert forward pressure on the right ramus. This passive movement relaxes the lateral pterygoid muscle.
4. The second phase begins when maximum forward glide has been reached. With the index and middle fingers of the right hand, apply gentle cephalad pressure against the ramus. This presses the condyle into the articular surface of the temporal bone and impinges the disc at its thin central section; maintain the cephalad pressure until the procedure is complete to ensure posterior replacement of the disc.
5. Close the jaw with the fingers of your left hand on the chin. The left hand simultaneously exerts pressure from left to right to cause complete posterior gliding of the right condyle and the impinged disc.
6. When the procedure is complete, reassess the motion of the dysfunctional TMJ.

Jaw Lock Closed Lock Correction (Example: Right-sided Closed Lock)

Strachan called closed lock (see Clinical History, earlier in the chapter) a posterior lesion.[15]

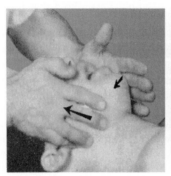
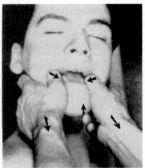

A   B

FIGURE 15.4   TMJ: Strachan's procedures for correcting open lock (**A**) and close lock (**B**). (Reprinted with permission from Fryette HH. Principles of Osteopathic Technic. Indianapolis: American Academy of Osteopathy, 1954, 1980.)

Patient position: supine. Physician position: standing at the side of the table facing the end of the table.

Procedure

1. Instruct the patient to open the mouth enough to permit placement of your thumbs on the occlusal surfaces of the lower molars. Grasp the rami and body of the mandible (Fig. 15.4*B*).
2. With the left thumb, apply sufficient pressure on the right molars to gap the TMJ and stretch the restraining tissues. While maintaining this caudad pressure, use the finger grasping the right ramus to exert a forward pull to overcome the resistance of the lesion. Repeat if necessary.
3. Assess the freedom of forward glide on the right and left sides without changing the position of the hands. With some ingenuity, this procedure can be turned into a muscle energy procedure.[16]
4. When the procedure is complete, reassess the motion of the dysfunctional TMJ.

References

1. Chaudhary A, Appelbaum J. Temporomandibular joint syndrome. Emedicine web page. Last updated June 30, 2004. Available at http://www.emedicine.com/neuro/topic366.htm. Accessed April 10, 2005.
2. Larson NJ. Osteopathic manipulative contribution to treatment of TMJ syndrome. Osteopathic Medicine 1978;10(8):16–26.
3. Travell JG, Simons DG. Myofascial Pain and Dysfunction: The Trigger Point Manual. Vol 1. Baltimore: Williams & Wilkins, 1999.
4. Blood SD. The craniosacral mechanism and the temporomandibular joint. J Am Osteopath Assoc 1986;86:512–519.
5. Magoun HI Sr. The temporal bone: trouble maker in the head. J Am Osteopath Assoc 1974;73:825–835.
6. Royder JO. Structural influences in temporomandibular joint pain and dysfunction. J Am Osteopath Assoc 1981;80:460–467.
7. Brockbank N. Alexander Technique self discovery. Alexander Technique web page. Last updated 2004. Available at http://www.alexandertechnique.com/articles/brockbank. Accessed April 10, 2005.
8. McArdle WD, Goldstein LB, Last FC, et al. Temporomandibular joint repositioning and exercise performance: A double-blind trial. Med Sci Sports Exerc 1984;16:228–233.
9. Hruby RJ. The total body approach to the osteopathic management of temporomandibular joint dysfunction. J Am Osteopath Assoc 1985;85:502–510.
10. Feely RA, Marotz JE. Myofascial pain dysfunction and short-leg syndrome: A retrospective study. J Am Osteopath Assoc 1985;85:663.
11. Weiner LB, Grant LA, Grant AH. Monitoring ocular changes that may accompany use of dental appliances and/or osteopathic craniosacral manipulations in the treatment of TMJ and related problems. Cranio 1985;5:278–285.
12. McPartland JM. Side effects from cranial-sacral treatment: Case reports and commentary. J Bodywork Movement Therap 1996;1(1):2–5.
13. Jealous JS. Emergence of Originality: a Biodynamic view of Osteopathy in the Cranial Field. 2nd ed. Farmington, ME: Biodynamics/Sargent, 2001.
14. McPartland JM, Skinner E. The biodynamic model of osteopathy in the cranial field. In: Liem T, ed. Cranial Osteopathy: Principles and Practice. 2nd ed. Edinburgh: Elsevier Churchill Livingstone, 2004:653–674.
15. Fryette HH. Principles of Osteopathic Technic. Indianapolis: American Academy of Osteopathy, 1954, 1980.
16. Freshwater Z, Gosling CM. The effect of a specific isometric muscle energy technique on range of opening of the temporomandibular joint: a pilot study. J Osteopath Med 2003;6(1): 36 [meeting abstract].

CHAPTER 16

The Patient with an Upper Respiratory Infection

Kenneth E. Nelson

INTRODUCTION

For problems of the upper respiratory tract, osteopathic medicine offers several advantages. Diagnostic palpation reveals tissue texture change, altered structural position, restriction of motion, and tenderness indicative of somatic dysfunction. Somatic dysfunction of the upper thoracic, cervical, and cranial regions can be wholly responsible for functional symptoms and/or pain complaints referable to the upper respiratory tract.

Deep facial pain, which may be interpreted as a symptom of chronic sinusitis, may result from high cervical somatic dysfunction. Anterior occiput dysfunction and anterior atlas dysfunction produce ipsilateral pain in the region of the ear and behind the eye respectively. Upper respiratory symptoms may result from dysfunction involving the base of the skull and face.

Tissue texture change and tenderness without distinct alteration of structural position or restriction of motion are palpated in association with somatic dysfunction of reflex origin, viscerosomatic reflexes. Viscerosomatic reflexes offer useful diagnostic information. A viscerosomatic pattern from the upper respiratory tract corroborates the diagnosis of an upper respiratory tract problem. While viscerosomatic reflexes from the upper gastrointestinal, cardiovascular, or pulmonary system may be associated with musculoskeletal complaints resembling upper respiratory pathology, their presence leads the clinician to inquire about and examine areas in greater depth that might otherwise be given only cursory consideration during evaluation of what appears to be an upper respiratory complaint. The intensity of tissue texture change of a viscerosomatic reflex mirrors the severity of the visceral pathology responsible for it, thereby offering additional diagnostic information.

Primary spinal somatic dysfunction is associated with neurologic hyperirritability, facilitation that can affect the upper respiratory tract. Somatovisceral reflexes have their effect through the autonomic nervous system, resulting in exaggerated reactions mediated by the sympathetic or parasympathetic nervous system.

Osteopathic manipulative treatment (OMT) may be employed to alleviate symptoms of somatic dysfunction that resemble those of upper respiratory complaints. When treating upper respiratory infections, OMT, employed to eliminate somatovisceral activity, modulates the patient's physiology, enhancing recuperation and augmenting the efficacy of any other necessary therapies.[1,2]

The use of OMT to reduce the intensity and duration of illness has been repeatedly documented.[3–6] To understand the osteopathic contribution to the diagnosis and treatment of the upper respiratory tract, it is appropriate to begin with an overview of the anatomy and physiology of the region and the effect of somatic dysfunction upon it.

Structure and Function (and Dysfunction)

The upper respiratory tract is lined with ciliated pseudostratified columnar epithelium, interspersed with goblet cells, columnar cells with microvilli but without cilia, and basal cells. Beneath the epithelium lie groups of serous and mucous glands. Secretions from these glands keep the epithelial surface from desiccating, humidify inspired air, and function as a first line of defense against infections. This protective coat has two layers, an outer mucous layer and an inner serous layer. The sticky mucous layer is intended to entrap particulate matter, including microorganisms. It contains immunoglobulins and the bactericides lysozyme and lactoferrin. The more fluid serous layer allows the cilia of the epithelium to sweep the secretions anteroposteriorly through the nose. This action normally occurs at about 6 mm per minute.[7] As the secretions are swept posteriorly from the nose and sinuses into the nasopharynx, they are imperceptibly swallowed. Typically, 1000 mL of mucus traverses the upper respiratory tract daily.[8]

The nasal mucosa contains cavernous vascular tissue with large venous sinuses that under autonomic control can shrink or swell to affect the size of the nasal passages. As air traverses the nose, the nasal turbinates create turbulence and the air is cleaned, humidified, and warmed.

The efficient function of the upper respiratory tract as a conduit, humidifier, conditioner, and primary defense against infection can be impaired by somatic dysfunction. This impairment predisposes the region to disease and retards recuperation. Somatic dysfunction does this mechanically and through its effect on the nervous system.

The mechanical impact of somatic dysfunction may be direct, from altered functional relationships of the face, calvaria, upper spine, thoracic cage, and associated soft tissues. The mechanical impact may be indirect, through the effect of musculoskeletal dysfunction upon the venous and lymphatic drainage from the head and neck.

Somatic dysfunction results in increased activity within the autonomic nervous system.[9] Efficient function of the upper respiratory tract is predicated upon a dynamic state of balance between sympathetic and parasympathetic control.

Disruption of this balance results in functional symptoms with impaired efficiency of the upper respiratory tract.

This chapter reviews the functional musculoskeletal anatomy, lymphatic drainage, and innervation of the upper respiratory tract and addresses the effect of somatic dysfunction upon upper respiratory physiology.

The Mechanical Impact of Somatic Dysfunction

The upper respiratory tract lies between the anterior bones of the cranium (basiocciput, sphenoid, and frontal) and the bones of the face. The posteroinferior portion of the upper respiratory tract, the pharynx, is suspended from the base of the cranium (basiocciput, sphenoid, and temporal bones) and the anterior aspect of the cervical spine through the precervical fascia. Mechanical dysfunction of the cranial base can result in cranial nerve entrapment. Resultant functional alteration of the facial and vagus nerves affects the upper respiratory tract through altered parasympathetic and pharyngeal motor activity. Dysfunction of the cranial base and facial bones can have a mechanical affect directly upon the upper respiratory tract.[10] Manipulation of these dysfunctions is particularly effective for, although not limited to, the treatment of upper respiratory problems in infants and children. (See Chapter 8.)

The lymphatic vasculature from the nose, sinuses, and pharynx drains predominantly to the submandibular and retropharyngeal nodes and from there through the deep cervical lymphatic vessels to return to the venous circulation. Drainage of lymph from the upper respiratory tract may be encumbered by tension from somatic dysfunction within the precervical muscles and fascia.

Alternating, positive–negative intrathoracic pressure associated with respiration draws lymph centrally into the venous circulation. This mechanism of low-pressure fluid return is an important component of the body's response to the soft tissue congestion often encountered in upper respiratory pathology. Lymphatic drainage of the upper respiratory tract may be impaired when respiratory excursion is reduced by somatic dysfunction effecting the thoracic inlet, thoracic spine, ribs, or thoracoabdominal diaphragm.

The degree of the intrathoracic pressure gradient may also be affected by increased cervical lordosis as the result of upper thoracic flexion or occipitocervical extension. Increased cervical lordosis places traction upon the soft tissues of the anterior neck. This facilitates a shift from nasal to mouth breathing, with untoward affect upon the upper respiratory tract and the patient's total physiology. The resistance to the passage of air through the nose determines to a great extent the gradient of intrathoracic pressure during the respiratory cycle. Because mouth breathing is associated with significantly less resistance than nasal breathing, the intrathoracic respiratory pressure gradient is decreased. Mouth breathing has been shown to result in decreased thoracic cage movement leading to decreased vital capacity, hypoventilation, decreased pulmonary circulation, and a tendency to develop respiratory acidosis.[11]

Nasal congestion resulting from an upper respiratory infection initially increases turbulence of inspired and expired air and the intrathoracic respiratory pressure gradient. This facilitates the cleansing and conditioning of inspired air and lymphatic drainage of the upper respiratory tract, respectively; however, as nasal congestion progresses to relative obstruction, the patient shifts from nasal to mouth breathing. The cleansing and conditioning effect of nasal respiration is lost, and lymphatic drainage of the already congested tissues is reduced. As described previously, somatic dysfunction can add to the pathophysiology of this condition.

Based upon the premise that the functionally unencumbered individual possesses the physiologic basis to reestablish health in the presence of disease, the osteopathic physician works to assist the patient toward optimal functional status. The importance of efficient cardiovascular circulation has been stressed since the beginning of osteopathic medicine. In 1910, Andrew Taylor Still stated, "As you are well versed in anatomy and physiology, I feel a little timid about insisting on the perfect freedom of the arteries that supply and the veins that drain the glandular system of the neck. But the demand for their freedom is absolute and we must be governed accordingly. A sore tongue, sore eyes, sore nose, running ears, the nasal air passages and all the membranes rapidly heal when you have secured perfect drainage."[12]

The importance of the mobilization of passive congestion was reiterated in 1923 by Miller,[13] who described lymphatic pump procedure. He stated that the body develops "auto-anti-toxins" when lymphatic circulation is enhanced. ". . . the body simply absorbed the bacterial toxins which were present and set up a defense against them. This procedure was done regardless of their names or the number of kinds present. The toxins stimulated the defensive mechanism, which in turn produced the auto-anti-toxin. This was the specific cure made directly against the products absorbed. The cure was made, not by any drugs administered, but rather, during the time of the (osteopathic manipulative) treatment." The use of lymphatic pump procedure to stimulate an antibody response has since been documented.[2] The significance of Miller's statement can be fully appreciated when taken in the context of osteopathic outcomes statistics from the influenza epidemic of 1918, in which he actively practiced. The overall fatality rate from influenza in the United States was conservatively between 5 and 7%. Among 110,120 influenza patients reported as receiving osteopathic care, 257 died, a fatality rate of 0.25%, or less than 5% of the national fatality rate.[3]

The Neurologic Impact of Somatic Dysfunction

Somatic dysfunction must be considered in the broader context of dysfunction of the neuromusculoskeletal system and not merely as mechanical kinks. Somatic dysfunction may reflexively result from upper respiratory pathology and as a viscerosomatic reflex provide diagnostic insight. Alternatively, primary somatic dysfunction may exert untoward sympathetic or parasympathetic effects upon the upper respiratory tract as a somatovisceral reflex.

A viscerosomatic reflex results from a peripheral focus of irritation, in this case from the upper respiratory tract, that activates nociceptive general visceral afferent neurons. The ongoing afferent stimulation results in establishment of a state of irritability (facilitation) within the central nervous system. Additional afferent activity from any source results in a response to significantly less stimulus than would normally be required. The response may be parasympathetic, sympathetic, or somatomotor, depending upon the area of the central nervous system affected.[14]

Viscerosomatic reflex tissue texture change and tenderness from upper respiratory pathology is demonstrable in the temporalis muscles. Somatosensory input from the upper respiratory tract is communicated to the central nervous system via the trigeminal nerve. Thus, it is reasonable to find viscerosomatic reflex activity in the muscles that are innervated by the trigeminal nerve.

Tissue texture change and tenderness of the upper cervical paravertebral soft tissues have also been described as a viscerosomatic reflex from the upper respiratory tract. Low-threshold afferent neurons from mechanoreceptors in the facial skin constitute a principal trigeminal input to induce the reflex discharges in the upper cervical nerves that innervate the posterior neck muscles. The amount of reflex cervical muscle spasm depends not only on displacement but also on velocity of mechanical stimulation. Identified neurons were found to be in the magnocellular layer (lamina V) of the trigeminal nucleus caudalis.[15] It can therefore be inferred that neurons in the trigeminal nucleus caudalis, whether from the facial skin or the mucus membranes of the nose and sinuses, project monosynaptically to the upper cervical motor neurons and can be involved in production of the upper cervical viscerosomatic reflex from the upper respiratory tract

The autonomic nervous system is typically thought of as consisting of efferent neurons. Both parasympathetic and sympathetic nerves, however, contain afferent fibers. The cells of origin of these peripheral fibers are unipolar neurons found in their respective cranial and dorsal root ganglia. These sensory neurons travel with their respective parasympathetic and sympathetic nerves.[16]

Parasympathetic innervation of the upper respiratory tract comes from the facial nerve. Preganglionic fibers synapse in the pterygopalatine ganglion. They reach their destination through the palatine, nasal, and pharyngeal nerves in the distribution of the trigeminal nerve. Parasympathetic hyperactivity results in thinning of nasal secretions and rhinorrhea.

The sympathetic innervation of the upper respiratory tract comes from the upper five (predominantly upper three) segments of the thoracic spinal cord. The preganglionic fibers synapse in the superior cervical ganglion. The postganglionic fibers form the carotid plexus. From there, they follow the vascular supply or traverse the pterygopalatine ganglion to reach the upper respiratory tract with branches of the trigeminal nerve. Somatic dysfunction of the upper thoracic spine is associated with spinal segmental facilitation and increased sympathetic tone to the head and neck. A somatovisceral reflex will result in vasospasm and thick, tenacious nasal secretions, impairing the topical cleansing of the nose and paranasal sinuses.

TREATMENT

In contemporary allopathic medicine upper respiratory infections are specifically treated only once the infecting organism has been identified, and then only when the infection is bacterial. Viral infections are treated supportively, with symptom-suppressing pharmaceuticals. Bacterial infections, when recognized, are typically treated empirically. The site of infection, patient's age, and presence or absence of concomitant illness are all taken into account, and the antibiotic with the highest probability of effectively treating the disease is prescribed. The specific infectious agent, its sensitivity, and its resistance come into consideration only when the initial empirical prescription proves to be ineffective. This approach to treatment, specifically designated by the disease process, differs from the approach of classical osteopathic medicine.

As described earlier, the distinctive osteopathic approach considers the disease to be an effect of functional compromise of the patient. It is therefore the osteopathic approach to identify and treat the causes of the functional compromise. The use of OMT to treat somatic dysfunction should enhance the effectiveness of the antibiotic when it is necessary and reduce or eliminate the need for symptom-suppressing pharmaceuticals.

As in all other aspects of medicine, the specific use of OMT is predicated upon the specific diagnosis of somatic dysfunction. The initial examination and manipulative treatment are performed with the patient seated. This can be efficiently integrated into the physical examination of head, eyes, ear, nose, throat (HEENT), heart, and lungs. The thoracic spine, ribs, and clavicles should be examined for somatic dysfunction and appropriately treated. Flexion dysfunction of the upper thoracic spine results in increased cervical lordosis and a propensity for mouth breathing. Upper thoracic, upper rib, and clavicular dysfunctions can compromise lymphatic return through the thoracic inlet.[13,17,18] This adds to upper respiratory passive congestion. General restriction of motion of the thoracic spine and ribs reduces thoracic excursion, further impedes the return of lymph to the general circulation, and possibly impairs the immune response.[2]

Upper thoracic somatic dysfunction with associated spinal facilitation results in a somatovisceral reflex with increased sympathetic tone to the upper respiratory tract. The result is arteriolar constriction and thickening of nasal secretions.

With the patient supine, the cervical region and cranial mechanism may be examined and treated. Additional examination and treatment of the thoracic inlet may also be done, and trigeminal nerve stimulation and lymphatic procedures may be performed.[17–19]

The trigeminal nerve, the sensory innervation of the upper respiratory tract, also carries sympathetic and parasympathetic postganglionic fibers to the upper respiratory tract. Stimulation of the trigeminal nerve (as first described by Bailey in 1922[20]) in association with cervical and thoracic OMT has been demonstrated to reduce nasal congestion and increase secretions for 30 minutes to several hours post treatment.[21]

Anterior cervical soft tissue procedures can be used to facilitate lymphatic drainage of the upper respiratory tract (personal communication from N. J. Larson, Chicago College of Osteopathic Medicine, Chicago, Illinois, 1971). They can be done in association with thoracic lymphatic pump procedures. The efficient return of lymph to the venous system is predicated upon unrestricted mobility of the thoracic inlet, clavicles, thoracic spine, ribs, and thoracoabdominal diaphragm. All thoracic lymphatic pump procedures employ this mobility to augment the intrathoracic pressure gradient between inhalation and exhalation.

A proposed sequence for the diagnosis of somatic dysfunction and the use of OMT when treating a patient with an upper respiratory infection is as follows:

Patient seated, diagnose and treat:

1. Upper thoracic dysfunction
2. Upper rib dysfunction
3. Clavicular dysfunction

Patient supine, diagnose and treat:

1. Cranial dysfunction
2. Cervical dysfunction

Use these procedures:

1. Suboccipital myofascial release
2. Trigeminal nerve procedures
3. Anterior neck soft tissue procedures
4. Thoracic lymphatic pump

This sequence has proved to be effective for me, but it is certainly open to modification, depending upon the needs and tolerances of the patient and the preferences of the individual practitioner.

CONCLUSION

The pharmacologic treatment of common nonbacterial upper respiratory complaints is directed for the most part at supportive symptom suppression, in the belief that if left to their natural course most of these conditions will resolve. That is, the body possesses the inherent ability to heal itself. Osteopathic medicine has long recognized this and offers specific methods to identify and alleviate dysfunction that retards the self-healing process.

Osteopathic medicine has much to offer for diagnosis and treatment of the patient with a complaint referable to the upper respiratory tract. The first question is whether the complaint is truly upper respiratory in origin or is a somatic dysfunction producing symptoms referable to the upper respiratory tract. Pain complaints resembling those of upper respiratory pathology may immediately resolve when somatic dysfunction of the upper thoracic region, upper cervical region, and head is properly treated.

Somatic dysfunction must, however, be considered in the broader context of dysfunction of the neuromusculoskeletal system and not merely as mechanical kinks. Such mechanical impediments do have significant effects upon the patient, but the untoward effect of somatic dysfunction is often altered neurologic activity in the parasympathetic and sympathetic supply to the area affected by illness. Further, general visceral afferent hyperactivity may establish and maintain central dysfunctional areas. Thus, somatic dysfunction resulting from an upper respiratory infection may result in altered physiology that maintains the original problem. This chicken-and-egg dilemma is frequently encountered in osteopathic medicine. Although it may initially appear to be problematic, it allows the clinician to employ seemingly unrelated therapies to address a single clinical problem.

Circulatory dysfunction should also be identified and treated. Manipulation of the thoracic and cervical regions, coupled with the trigeminal procedures of Bailey and the lymphatic pump procedure of Miller can be employed to facilitate the patient's response to the illness. Coupled with all other available methods of therapy, OMT offers a decided therapeutic advantage.

As described previously, the distinctive osteopathic approach considers the disease to be an effect of functional compromise of the patient. It is therefore the osteopathic approach to identify and treat the causes of the functional compromise. The use of OMT to treat somatic dysfunction in the patient with an upper respiratory complaint should reduce or eliminate the need for symptom-suppressing pharmaceuticals and enhance the effectiveness of antibiotics when they are necessary.

Procedures

Upper Thoracic Spine (Muscle Energy) (Fig. 16.1)

This procedure is employed to treat Fryette type II dysfunction, either flexed or extended, in the upper thoracic spine. (For diagnosis, see Chapter 3.)

Patient position: seated upon the side of the treatment table. Physician position: standing behind the patient.

Procedure (Example: T3 Flexed, Side Bent Left, and Rotated Left Upon T4)

1. Place the fingers of your right hand on the patient's right shoulder such that the tip of your thumb lies in contact with the right side of the spinous process of T3.
2. Place your left hand on top of the patient's head.

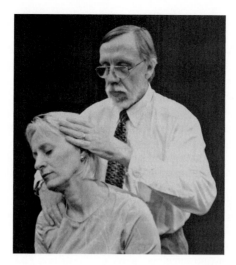

FIGURE 16.1   Muscle energy, upper thoracic spine T3 flexed, side bent left, and rotated left upon T4.

3. With your left hand introduce side bending and rotation of the patient's head, neck, and upper thoracic spine down to your right thumb, contacting T3. This can be accomplished by positioning the head so the patient appears to be looking at the right shoulder.
4. While maintaining the side-bending rotation force against your right thumb, introduce extension down to the level of T3 with your left hand by moving the patient's head so he or she appears to be looking at the ceiling. (If the dysfunction is extended, you can introduce flexion in a similar way by having the patient look at the floor.)
5. With the palm of your left hand against the left posterolateral aspect of the patient's head, instruct the patient to push the head into your hand, and apply a counterforce equal to the patient's force so that you feel pressure of the spinous process of T3 against your right thumb. Experiment by moving the point of contact of your left hand, and you can subtly change the degree of side bending and rotational forces applied to T3. (If the dysfunction is extended, your left hand should contact the left anterolateral aspect of the patient's head.)
6. Have the patient maintain the contraction for 3 to 5 seconds.
7. Instruct the patient to relax while simultaneously ceasing your counterforce and wait 1 to 2 seconds for the patient's muscles to relax.
8. Engage the new barrier by further side bending right, rotating right, and extending as described previously.
9. Repeat steps 5 to 8 until the best possible increase of motion is obtained.
10. Reassess the motion between T3 and T4.

Upper Rib Diagnosis and Treatment

DIAGNOSIS OF ELEVATED FIRST AND SECOND RIBS

The upper ribs, 1 and 2, tend to demonstrate restricted bucket handle motion as their dysfunctional mechanics. That is, their anterior, or sternocostal, articulation and their posterior, or costovertebral, articulations remain relatively fixed, while the lateral portion of the rib body moves up and down like a bucket handle. Upper rib dysfunctions are often positioned as elevated bucket handle mechanics. The posterolateral aspect of the dysfunctional rib is in a slightly cephalad position and resists downward pressure. It may be diagnosed as follows.

Patient position: seated upon the side of the treatment table. Physician position: standing behind the patient.

Procedure

1. Begin by examining the upper thoracic spine for somatic dysfunction. (See Chapter 3.) Segmentally related spinal dysfunction should be treated before any attempt to treat rib dysfunction.
2. Palpate the scalene muscles laterally at the base of the neck in the triangular space superior to the clavicle, posterior to the sternocleidomastoid, and anterior to the trapezius. Spasm of the anterior and middle scalenes will elevate the first rib. The scalenes should be stretched before treatment of an elevated first or second rib.
3. Palpate the lateral aspect of the first rib at the base of the neck. Apply downward force to the rib. An elevated first rib resists this motion.
4. Palpate the angle of the second rib just above the superior border of the scapula.
5. Again, apply downward force over angle of the second rib. An elevated second rib resists this motion.

FIRST RIB (HVLA) (FIG. 16.2)

This procedure is employed to restore normal respiratory excursion of the first rib to establish physiologic range of motion to the T1/rib 1 costovertebral joint.

Patient position: seated. Physician position: standing behind the patient.

Procedure (Example: Elevated First Rib on the Right)

The posterolateral portion of the rib is elevated and resists downward motion from above with surrounding tissue texture change and tenderness.

1. Put your left foot upon the table just to the left of the patient's pelvis.
2. Rest the patient's left arm upon your knee. You may wish to place a pillow between the patient's axilla and your knee.

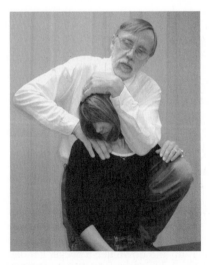

FIGURE 16.2   Elevated first rib on the right, HVLA.

3. Place your right hand at the base of the patient's neck on the right over the elevated first rib such that your index finger is directed anteriorly and your thumb is directed posteriorly.
4. Place your left forearm and hand against the left side of the patient's head and neck to splint the cervical spine.
5. With your left hand, use the patient's head and neck as a lever to rotate and side-bend the cervical spine to the right down to the level of T1 and the first rib.
6. With your right, hand apply downward pressure to rib 1 on the right.
7. Holding the patient's chest between your right hand and left knee, translate the torso to the left to increase right side bending of the cervicothoracic junction.
8. Instruct the patient to inhale deeply and exhale and increase the downward pressure over the first rib with your right hand during the exhalation.
9. The final corrective force is a HVLA thrust directed downward, medially, and anteriorly through your right hand against the dysfunctional first rib.
10. Reassess first rib motion.

SECOND RIB (HVLA) (FIG. 16.3)

This procedure is employed to restore normal respiratory excursion of the second rib to establish physiologic range of motion to the costotransverse joint of rib 2.

Patient position: seated. Physician position: standing behind the patient.

Procedure (Example: Second Rib on the Right)

There is tissue texture change surrounding the angle of rib 2 on the right, which is higher than rib 2 on the left.

1. Put your left foot upon the table just to the left of the patient's pelvis.
2. Rest the patient's left arm upon your knee. You may wish to place a pillow between the patient's axilla and your knee.
3. Place your right hand over the patient's right shoulder, with your thumb contacting the angle of rib 2. You may find it easier to do this if you pull the patient's right arm to the left across the patient's chest. This protracts the shoulder and draws the scapula to the side.

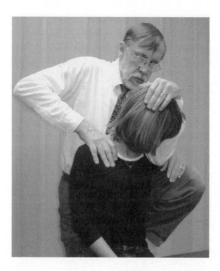

FIGURE 16.3 Elevated second rib on the right, HVLA.

4. Place your left elbow in front of the patient's left shoulder, with your forearm touching the left side of the neck and face. Your left hand should be holding the top of the patient's head. This arm and hand placement allows you to splint the patient's cervical spine with your left forearm.
5. With your left hand, slowly rotate the patient's head and neck to the left, disengaging the rib head from the hemifacet as T1 rotates away from it.
6. With your left hand, and forearm side bend the patient's neck to the right down to the level of rib 2.
7. With your right hand, apply downward pressure to the angle of rib 2.
8. With your left hand, introduce slightly more right rotation of the patient's head and neck while exerting downward pressure on the second rib with your right hand. This further disengages the rib head from the hemifacets. Stop the rotation when you sense that the rib exhibits less resistance to the downward pressure from your right hand.
9. Instruct the patient inhale deeply and exhale and increase the downward pressure over the first rib with your right hand during the exhalation.
10. The final corrective force is an HVLA thrust directed downward, medially, and anteriorly through your right hand against the angle of the dysfunctional second rib.
11. Reassess second rib motion.

Acromioclavicular Dysfunction

ACROMIOCLAVICULAR, ANTERIOR CLAVICLE (HVLA)

This procedure is employed to restore functional motion of the acromioclavicular joint. The patient often complains of shoulder pain. Upon examination, flexion of the glenohumeral joint is limited by discomfort, and the superior surface of the clavicle is rotated anteriorly as opposed to its usual more horizontal position relative to the acromion. The posterior edge of the clavicle is palpably prominent.

Patient position: seated. Physician position: standing behind the patient to the side of the dysfunctional clavicle.

Procedure (Example: Anterior Clavicle on the Right)

1. Grasp the patient's right elbow with your right hand, and using the humerus as a lever, move the elbow anteriorly, flexing the glenohumeral joint. This rotates the acromion process and the superior surface of the clavicle posteriorly (Fig. 16.4).
2. Place your left hand with your fingers directed anteriorly over the patient's clavicle and apply downward force, holding it in the somewhat posteriorly directed position obtained in step 1.
3. Hold the clavicle with your left hand, and with your right hand, draw the patient's elbow posteriorly in an arc that incorporates shoulder abduction and extension, using the arm as a lever to align the acromion and clavicle (Fig. 16.5).
4. Reassess acromioclavicular motion.

ACROMIOCLAVICULAR, POSTERIOR CLAVICLE (HVLA)

This procedure is employed to restore functional motion of the acromioclavicular joint. Many patients complain of shoulder pain. Upon examination, extension of the glenohumeral joint is found to be limited by discomfort, and the superior surface of the clavicle is rotated posteriorly as opposed to its usual more horizontal position relative to the acromion. The anterior edge of the clavicle is palpably prominent.

Patient position: seated. Physician position: standing behind the patient to the side of the dysfunctional clavicle.

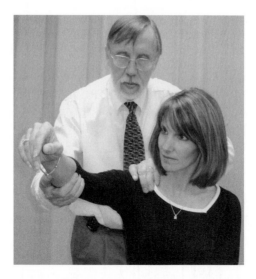

FIGURE 16.4   Starting position for anterior clavicle and final position for posterior clavicle.

Procedure (Example: Posterior Clavicle on the Right)

1. Grasp the patient's right elbow with your right hand, and using the humerus as a lever, move the elbow posteriorly, extending the glenohumeral joint. This rotates the acromion process and the superior surface of the clavicle anteriorly (Fig. 16.5).
2. Place your left hand with your fingers directed anteriorly over the patient's clavicle and apply a downward force, thus holding it in the somewhat anteriorly directed position obtained in step 1.

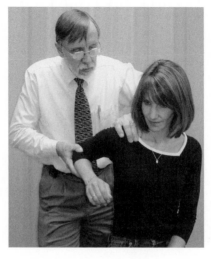

FIGURE 16.5   Starting position for posterior clavicle and final position for anterior clavicle.

3. Hold the clavicle with your left hand, and with your right hand draw the patient's elbow anteriorly in an arc that incorporates shoulder abduction and flexion, using the arm as a lever to align the acromion and clavicle (Fig. 16.4).
4. Reassess acromioclavicular motion.

CERVICAL (SOFT TISSUE/ARTICULATION) (SEE FIG. 10-2)

This procedure is employed to decrease cervical tissue tension and enhance the symmetric range of motion of the cervical spine. (For diagnosis, see Chapter 3.)

Patient position: supine. Physician position: seated at the head of the treatment table.

Procedure

1. With both hands, place the pads of your fingers over the cervical paraspinal tissues at the level of maximal palpable paravertebral tension.
2. Apply bilateral pressure directed in an anterior and cephalad direction until you sense stretch of the cervical paraspinal soft tissues. Applying more pressure will produce articular motion.
3. Hold the position with this degree of applied force until the tissues relax.
4. Slowly release the holding force, exerting care not to unload the muscles too rapidly.
5. Reassess available cervical motion and soft tissue tension. Repeat steps 2 through 4 several times, working up and down the cervical spine until the desired decrease in paraspinal tension is achieved. As you become proficient with this procedure, you will learn to focus specifically upon asymmetric areas of paraspinal tension.

CERVICAL (INDIRECT BALANCING) (FIG. 16.6)

This procedure is employed to decrease cervical tissue tension and enhance the symmetric range of motion of the cervical spine. (For diagnosis, see Chapter 3.)

Patient position: supine. Physician position: seated at the head of the treatment table.

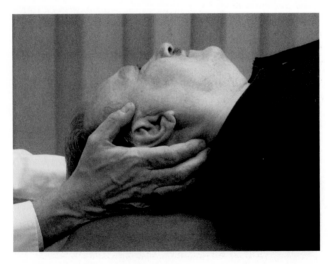

FIGURE 16.6 Cervical indirect balancing to decrease cervical tissue tension and enhance the symmetrical range of motion.

Procedure (Example: C4 Extended, Rotated, and Side Bent Right upon C5)

1. With both hands, place the pads of your fingers over the cervical paraspinal tissues posterior and lateral to the lateral masses of C4.
2. Allow the patient's head to rest upon the table, and with both hands apply anterior force to the posterior aspects of the transverse processes of C4 to introduce extension of C4 relative to C5.
3. Through your right hand, apply lateral force to the left against the right lateral mass of C4 to introduce right side bending of C4 relative to C5.
4. With your left hand, apply anterior force against the posterior aspect of the left transverse process of C4 to introduce right rotation of C4 relative to C5.
5. Sense general tension between C4 and C5 and adjust your holding force until you find the position where the intervertebral tissue tension in all planes is optimally reduced.
6. Hold this position until you perceive a release, a decrease of soft tissue tension between C4 and C5.
7. As the tissues release, you may sense that the C4 seems to move back in the direction of the original barrier. You may follow this sensation, taking C4 through a full range of motion.
8. Reassess motion between C4 and C5.

CERVICAL POSTERIOR (HVLA) (FIG. 16.7)

This procedure is employed to treat articular somatic dysfunction of the typical cervical vertebrae, C2 upon C3 to C7 upon T1. The example, posterior C5 right, consists of C5 upon C6, flexed (forward bent), rotated right, side-bent right (restricted extension, rotation left and side bending left). Tenderness and tissue texture change will be present in the area of the right transverse process of C5. The intent of this manipulation is to reestablish C5 extension, rotation left, and side bending left. (For diagnosis, see Chapter 3.)

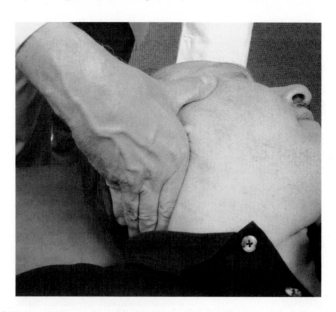

FIGURE 16.7   Cervical: posterior HVLA to treat type II articular somatic dysfunction of the typical cervical vertebrae.

The patient lies supine upon the treatment table, and the physician stands or sits at the head of the table.

Procedure

1. Cradle the patient's head and neck with both of your hands. Contact the posterior component of C5 on the right with the lateral aspect of the proximal phalanx of your right index finger. With the fingertips of your left hand, contact the area of the anterior component laterally over the tip of the left transverse process of C5.
2. Using your right index finger as a fulcrum, introduce extension of the cervical spine between C5 and C6. This extension break must be maintained throughout the remainder of the procedure.
3. With both hands, introduce left side bending of C5 upon C6 translating C5 to the right.
4. Rotate the head and neck to the left down to and including C5 until tension is felt to accumulate between C5 and C6 and the rotational barrier is reached.
5. The final corrective force is a quick, gentle, short rotational movement through your right index finger, directed in an anterosuperior direction toward the patient's right eye along the plane of the articular facets between C5 and C6.
6. Reassess motion between C5 and C6.

ATLAS POSTERIOR (MUSCLE ENERGY) (FIG. 16.8)

This procedure is employed to treat articular somatic dysfunction of C1, the atlas, relative to C2, the axis, to establish symmetric rotation of the atlas upon the axis. (For diagnosis see Chapter 3.)

The patient lies supine upon the treatment table, and the physician stands or sits at the head of the table.

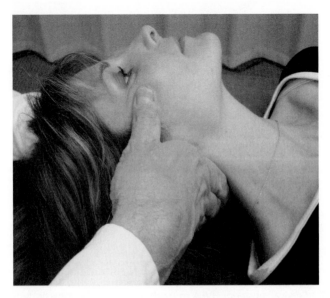

FIGURE 16.8 Muscle energy for posterior atlas on the right.

Procedure (Example: Posterior Atlas Right, Consists of the Atlas Being Rotated to the Right, Restricted Rotation to the Left upon the Axis)

Tenderness and tissue texture change will be present in the suboccipital region on the right. The intent of this manipulation is to reestablish atlas rotation to the left.

1. Begin by cradling the patient's occiput and upper cervical spine in your right hand, with your fingers pointing toward the left and your thumb in contact with the right side of the patient's head pointing toward the patient's cheek.
2. The lateral aspect of your right index finger should contact the posterior right transverse process of the atlas and must remain in this position throughout the remainder of the procedure.
3. Hold the left side of the patient's head in your left hand with your fingers extended downward over the left side of the neck such that your fingertips can palpate the area between the atlas and axis.
4. Lift the head and neck slightly from the table and introduce a small amount of extension between the atlas and axis using the index finger of your right hand as a fulcrum.
5. With both hands, rotate the patient's head and atlas to the left upon the axis to engage the rotational barrier.
6. Maintain tension against the dysfunctional barrier and instruct the patient to gently rotate the head back toward the right against your holding force for 3 to 5 seconds.
7. Pause for 1 to 2 seconds, and then rotate the head further to the left to engage the new barrier.
8. Reassess atlantoaxial motion. Repeat steps 6 and 7 until the best possible increase of motion is obtained.

ATLAS ANTERIOR (HVLA) (FIG. 16.9)

This procedure is employed to treat articular somatic dysfunction of C1, the atlas, relative to C2, the axis, to establish symmetric rotation of the atlas upon the axis. The patient may complain of pain behind the eye on the dysfunctional side. (For diagnosis, see Chapter 3.)

Patient position: supine. Physician position: standing or seated at the head of the table.

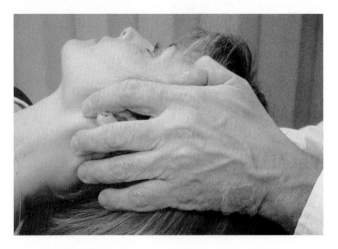

FIGURE 16.9   HVLA for anterior atlas on the left.

Procedure (Example: Anterior Atlas Left)

The atlas is rotated to the right, restricted rotation to the left, upon the axis. Tenderness and tissue texture change will be present in the suboccipital region on the left.

1. Cradle the patient's head with both of your hands such that the tips of your index and middle fingers extend caudally beneath the occiput to contact the transverse processes of the atlas bilaterally. The index finger of each hand should be positioned to contact just anterior and the middle finger just posterior to the tip of the transverse processes of the atlas. The transverse processes of the atlas are palpable bilaterally just posterior and slightly cephalad to the angles of the mandible.
2. With this hand placement, apply traction with your fingertips so that you can hold the atlas up against the occiput, and the two will move as a single unit.
3. With both hands rotate the patient's occiput and atlas to the left to engage the dysfunctional rotational barrier between the atlas and axis.
4. Using your left hand, apply a posterior (rotation left) high-velocity, low-amplitude thrust through the tip of your index finger against the anterior aspect of the left transverse process of the atlas to rotate the atlas to the left upon the axis.
5. When the procedure is complete, reassess the motion between the atlas and axis.

OCCIPUT POSTERIOR (MUSCLE ENERGY) (FIG. 16.10)

This procedure is employed to treat articular somatic dysfunction of the occiput relative to C1, the atlas, to establish symmetric motion between the occiput and the atlas. (For diagnosis, see Chapter 3.)

Patient position: supine. Physician position: standing or seated at the head of the table.

Procedure (Example: Occiput Posterior on the Right)

The occiput is rotated to the right and side-bent to the left upon the atlas, with tissue texture change and tenderness in the suboccipital region on the right.

1. Cradle the patient's head in your right hand with your fingers pointing toward the left and your thumb in contact with the right side of the patient's face pointing toward the cheek.

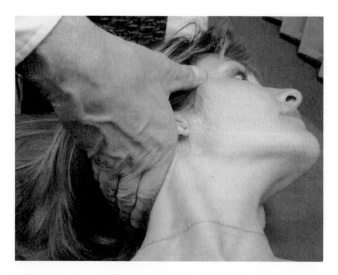

FIGURE 16.10 Muscle energy for posterior occiput on the right.

2. Place the metacarpophalangeal joint of the index finger of your right hand in contact with the posterolateral aspect of the patient's occiput and extend the occiput over your index finger. This establishes an extension break between the occiput and the atlas and helps localize the side-bending and rotational forces introduced to that area during the rest of the procedure. This extension break must be maintained throughout remainder of the procedure.
3. With your left hand, cradle the left side of the patient's face.
4. With both hands, rotate the patient's head to the left until the rotational barrier is engaged between the occiput and the atlas.
5. Introduce side bending to the right between the occiput and the atlas by slightly lifting the patient's head from the table and applying a mild lateral translatory force downward (to the patient's left) through your right index finger.
6. Maintain tension against the dysfunctional barrier and instruct the patient to gently rotate the head back to the right against your holding force for 3 to 5 seconds.
7. Pause for 1 to 2 seconds and then rotate the head further to the left and side-bend to the right (lateral translation to the left) to engage the new barrier.
8. Reassess occipitoatlantal motion. Repeat steps 6 and 7 until the best possible increase of motion is obtained.

OCCIPUT ANTERIOR (MUSCLE ENERGY) (FIG. 16.11)

This procedure is employed to treat articular somatic dysfunction of the occiput relative to C1, the atlas, to establish symmetric motion between the occiput and the atlas. (For diagnosis, see Chapter 3.)

Patient position: supine. Physician position: standing or seated at the head of the table.

Procedure (Example: Occiput Anterior on the Right)

The occiput is rotated to the left and side-bent to the right upon the atlas, with tissue texture change and tenderness in the suboccipital region on the right.

1. Grasp the right side of the patient's face in your right hand in such a way that the cheek rests in your palm and your fingers cup the patient's chin.

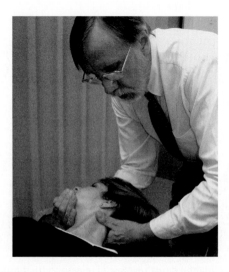

FIGURE 16.11 Muscle energy for anterior occiput on the right.

2. Place your left hand transversely beneath the patient's cervico-occipital junction so that your index finger is over the tip of the transverse process of the atlas on the right and your thumb is over the tip of the transverse process of the atlas on the left. The metacarpophalangeal joint of your left index finger should be touching the atlas on the right side of the midline. This hand placement will allow you to hold the atlas so that you can move the occiput from above with force applied through your right hand.

3. With both hands in position, rotate the patient's head and cervical spine to the right so that the dysfunctional right occipitoatlantal articulation is positioned toward the surface of the treatment table.

4. Introduce a slight amount of occipitoatlantal extension with your right hand by horizontally translating the patient's head posteriorly against the holding force of your left hand. This will increase articular tension and localize the procedure to the occipitoatlantal articulation. The asymmetric placement of your right hand upon the right side of the patient's face and the metacarpophalangeal joint of your left index finger contacting the atlas on the right will also introduce rotation of the occiput to the right upon the atlas.

5. Introduce side bending to the left between the occiput and atlas by applying a lateral translation to the right with your left hand while applying traction in a cephalad direction with your right hand. This step, in combination with step 4, will engage the dysfunctional barrier between the occiput and atlas.

6. Have the patient flex the occiput upon the atlas by pulling the chin toward the chest for 3 to 5 seconds. This is applied as an isometric contraction against the holding force of your left hand upon the atlas.

7. Pause for 1 to 2 seconds, and then rotate the head further to the right and side-bend to the left, as in steps 5 and 6 to engage the new barrier.

8. Reassess occipitoatlantal motion and repeat steps 6 and 7 until the best possible increase of motion is obtained.

Occipitoatlantal (Myofascial Release, Direct) (Fig. 16.12)

This procedure is employed for general treatment of articular and soft tissue myofascial somatic dysfunction of the occiput relative to C1, the atlas, to reduce myofascial tension and establish symmetric motion between the occiput and the atlas. (For diagnosis, see Chapter 3.)

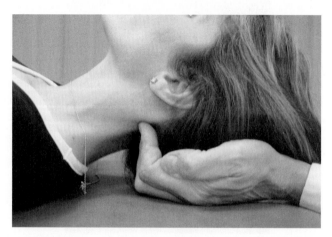

FIGURE 16.12 Occipitoatlantal direct myofascial release to treat articular and soft tissue and myofascial and somatic dysfunction and to establish symmetric motion between the occiput and atlas.

Patient position: supine. Physician position: standing or seated at the head of the table.

Procedure

1. Cradle the patient's head with both of your hands such that the tips of your fingers are at the level of the cervico-occipital junction.
2. Flex your fingers so that your fingertips are directed anteriorly and cephalad between the patient's occiput and atlas. This is the holding position for the remainder of the procedure. In this position your fingers will provide a fulcrum between the patient's occiput and atlas and provide upward traction against the occiput.
3. Allow the weight of the patient's head to rest upon the tips of your flexed fingers.
4. As the suboccipital tissue relaxes, you may alter the direction of the applied pressure against areas of persistent tissue tension.
5. Reassess. The procedure is finished when the suboccipital soft tissues are relaxed and occipitoatlantal articulation has unrestricted motion.

Trigeminal Nerve Procedure of Bailey[20] (Figs. 16.13–16.15)

This procedure employs counterirritation to open the nasal passages and produce drainage of the sinuses. Digital pressure applied over the cutaneous, supraorbital, infraorbital, and mental branches of the trigeminal nerve produces reflex vasoconstriction in the mucous membranes of the upper respiratory tract. This will result in transient decongestion of the nasal mucosa with resultant opening of the orifices of the paranasal sinuses.

Patient position: supine. Physician position: standing or seated at the head of the table.

Procedure

1. Place the pads of your index fingers bilaterally over one of the three paired branches of the trigeminal nerve. Start with the supraorbital nerves and progress to the infraorbital and mental branches.

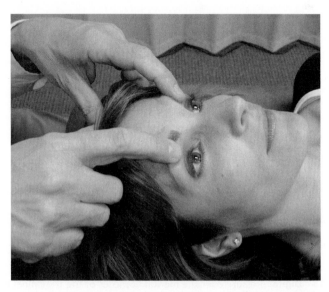

FIGURE 16.13   Digital pressure over the supraorbital branches of the trigeminal nerve to produce a reflex vasoconstriction in the mucous membranes of the upper respiratory tract.

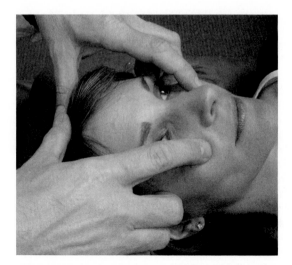

FIGURE 16.14 Digital pressure over the infraorbital branches of the trigeminal nerve to produce reflex vasoconstriction in the mucous membranes of the upper respiratory tract.

2. Apply gradually increasing gentle pressure. When maximum pressure is applied, hold it for 30 seconds and slowly release. Acute tissue texture change is palpable over the supraorbital and maxillary nerves in the presence of frontal and maxillary sinusitis, respectively.
3. Percuss over the frontal and maxillary sinuses. Percussing over the sinuses can produce abrupt drainage of a mucus-filled sinus if the orifice has been opened. It can be likened to hitting the bottom of a catsup bottle. Consequently, the patient should be warned that they might suddenly experience a copious amount of post-nasal mucus.

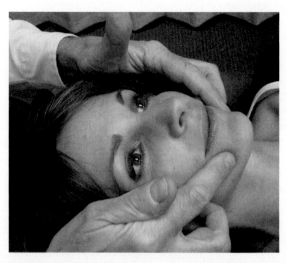

FIGURE 16.15 Digital pressure over the mental branches of the trigeminal nerve to produce reflex vasoconstriction in the mucous membranes of the upper respiratory tract.

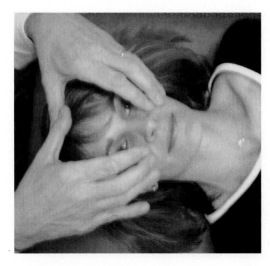

FIGURE 16.16   Facial effleurage to reduce congestion of the superficial soft tissues and enhance lymphatic drainage of the face.

FACIAL EFFLEURAGE (FIG. 16.16)

This procedure is employed to reduce congestion of the superficial soft tissues and enhance lymphatic drainage of the face. The stroking procedure may also be incorporated into the trigeminal sinus procedure of Bailey described previously.

Patient position: supine. Physician position: standing or seated at the head of the table.

Procedure

1. Place the pads of your index fingers bilaterally over the patient's forehead.
2. Apply medial to lateral pressured stroking. This is intended to move interstitial fluid of the soft tissues of the face into the superficial lymphatic drainage.
3. Repeat steps 1 and 2 over the cheeks and chin.

SUBMANDIBULAR PERCUSSION (FIG. 16.17)

This procedure is employed to reduce congestion of the superficial soft tissues and enhance lymphatic drainage of the face.

Patient position: supine. Physician position: standing or seated at the head of the table.

Procedure

1. Hold the patient's chin with your left hand, applying upward pressure being sure the patient's upper and lower teeth are in contact to avoid chipping them.
2. Place the tips of the fingers of your right hand so that they contact the skin over the submental region just medial to the body of the mandible on the right.
3. With your right fingertips, apply a rapidly oscillating percussive force against the submental soft tissues.
4. Repeat steps 1 through 3 on the left side.

ANTERIOR NECK SOFT TISSUE, LYMPHATIC PROCEDURE

This procedure is employed to reduce congestion of the soft tissues and enhance lymphatic drainage of the neck. The fascia of the neck may be considered as an

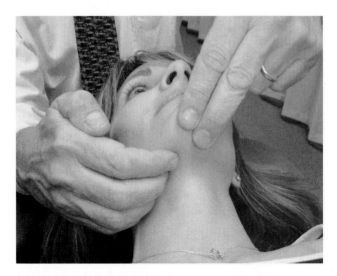

FIGURE 16.17 Submandibular percussion to reduce congestion of the superficial soft tissues and enhance lymphatic drainage of the face.

external cylinder that splits to enclose the sternocleidomastoid and trapezius muscles and surrounds the deep fascia that invests the deeper structures of the neck and fills the space between them. The superficial lymphatic drainage of the head lies outside the external fascial cylinder and must pass through it to drain into the deep cervical lymphatic vessels. The first part of this procedure is directed at moving lymph from the superficial to the deep lymphatic vessels. The second part of this procedure is directed at the deep structures.

Patient position: supine. Physician position: standing or seated at the head of the table.

Procedure

Moving Lymph from the Superficial to the Deep Lymphatic Vessels

1. Grasp the patient such that both of your hands touch the posterior and lateral aspects of their head and neck bilaterally.
2. Apply cephalad traction and rotation of the neck alternately with your hands such that you stretch the most superficial tissues of the neck.

Decongesting the Deep Cervical Structures (Fig. 16.18)

1. Grasp the patient's hyoid bone between the thumb and index finger of your dominant hand.
2. Apply gentle alternating lateral forces to displace the hyoid to the left and right of the midline. Avoid compressing the carotid arteries.
3. Move your hand inferiorly, grasp the thyroid cartilage of the larynx, and repeat the alternating lateral forces in step 2. The patient may be startled by noise produced as the posterior cartilages of the larynx move over structures posterior to them. Do not apply this procedure to the cricoid cartilage or trachea. It will initiate a cough reflex.
4. Reassess anterior cervical soft tissue tension.

Thoracic Lymphatic Pump (Fig. 16.19)

This procedure is employed to facilitate lymphatic and venous return to the heart and reduce pulmonary congestion through the introduction of abrupt negative intrathoracic pressure and improved thoracic cage mobility. It is important to be certain that

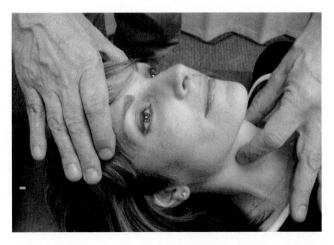

FIGURE 16.18   Anterior neck soft tissue to decongest the deep cervical structures.

the patient does not have anything loose in the mouth (e.g., food, gum, dentures) to prevent aspiration as a result of this procedure. This procedure is inappropriate for patients with chronic obstructive pulmonary disease, such as asthma or emphysema, in which the expiratory phase of respiration is compromised. For a procedure to treat these individuals, see Lymphatic Pump: Oscillatory Modification, Chapter 19.

Patient position: supine. Physician position: standing at the head of the table.

Procedure

1. Place your hands palm down upon the patient's anterior chest wall over the sternum and pectoral muscles. For female patients, the hands should be placed between the breasts.
2. Straighten your arms and lock your elbows.

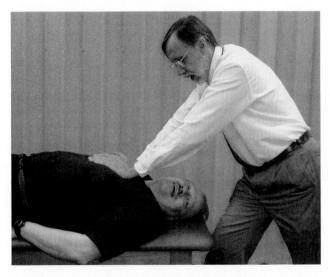

FIGURE 16.19   Thoracic lymphatic pump to facilitate lymphatic and venous return to the heart and reduce pulmonary congestion by introduction of abrupt negative intrathoracic pressure and improved thoracic cage mobility.

3. Instruct the patient to exhale in a relaxed fashion through the open mouth.
4. Lean upon the anterior thoracic cage with your hands and follow the chest into exhalation. Toward the end of exhalation, quickly remove your hands from the chest wall. A resultant inspiratory gasp will occur as a result of the recoil of the thoracic cage.
5. Repeat several times according to patient tolerance.

References

1. Whiting CA. Investigation of the Phagocytic Index. Bulletin 1. A. T. Still Research Institute. Cincinnati, OH: Monford, 1910;61–63.
2. Measel JW Jr. The effect of the lymphatic pump upon the immune response: I. Preliminary studies on the antibody response to pneumococcal polysaccharide assayed by bacterial agglutination and passive hemagglutination. J Am Osteopath Assoc 1982;82(1):28–31.
3. Smith RK. One hundred thousand cases of influenza with a death rate of one-fortieth of that officially reported under conventional medical treatment: 1919. J Am Osteopath Assoc 2000;100:320–323.
4. Pearson WM, Hines NH, Polovich CA, et al. Symposium on respiratory diseases: Etiology, pathology, diagnosis, and treatment. J Am Osteopath Assoc 1938;36:307–331.
5. Purse FM. Clinical evaluation of osteopathic manipulative therapy in measles. J Am Osteopath Assoc 1961;61:274–276.
6. Schmidt IC. Osteopathic manipulative therapy as a primary factor in the management of upper, middle, and pararespiratory infections. J Am Osteopath Assoc 1982;81:382–388.
7. Williams PL, ed. Gray's Anatomy. 38th ed. Edinburgh: Churchill Livingstone, 1995;1634.
8. Proctor DF. Physiology of the upper airway. In: Fenn WO, Rahn H, eds. Handbook of Physiology. Sec. 3, Respiration, vol 1. Washington: American Physiological Society, 1964.
9. Patterson MM, Wurster ED. Neurophysiologic system: Integration and disintegration. In: Ward RC, ed. Foundations for Osteopathic Medicine. Baltimore: Williams & Wilkins, 1997;137–151.
10. Magoun HI. Osteopathy in the Cranial Field. 2nd ed. Kirksville, MO: Journal Printing, 1966;289–291.
11. Ogura JH, Togawa K, Dammkoehler R, et al. Nasal obstruction and the mechanics of breathing: Physiologic relationships and effects of nasal surgery. Arch Otolaryngol 1966;83:135–150.
12. Still AT. Research and Practice. Kirksville, MO: Author. 1910. Reprinted Seattle, WA: Eastland, 1992;47.
13. Miller CE. The mechanics of lymphatic circulation: Lymph hearts. J Am Osteopath Assoc 1923;22:397–398, 415–416.
14. Beal M. Viscerosomatic reflexes: A review. J Am Osteopath Assoc 1985;85:786–801.
15. Sumino R, Nozaki S, Kato M. Central pathway of trigemino-neck reflex. In: Oral-Facial Sensory and Motor Functions. International Symposium, Rappongi, Tokyo. Oral Physiol 1980;28 [abstract].
16. Williams PL, ed. Gray's Anatomy. 38th ed. Edinburgh: Churchill Livingstone, 1995;1293.
17. Rumney IC. Osteopathic manipulative treatment of infectious diseases. Osteopath Ann 1974;2:29–33.
18. Blood HA. Infections of the ear, nose and throat. Osteopath Ann 1978;6:465–469.
19. Harakal JH. Manipulative treatment for acute upper respiratory disease. Osteopath Ann 1981;9:253–257.
20. Bailey JH. Osteopathic treatment of the eye, ear, nose and throat in hay fever, asthma, bronchitis, catarrhal deafness and allied conditions. Lecture 13. Osteopathic treatment of hay fever. Philadelphia: Author, 1922.
21. Kaluza CL, Sherbin M. The physiologic response of the nose to osteopathic manipulative treatment: Preliminary report. J Am Osteopath Assoc 1983;82:654–660.

CHAPTER 17

The Patient with a Lower Respiratory Tract Infection

Zachary J. Comeaux

INTRODUCTION

Clearly the introduction of antibiotics in medical care has become the mainstay of reducing morbidity due to pulmonary infections of many types. Recent guidelines for treatment of community-acquired pneumonia, published by the British Thoracic Society[1] in 2001 with a 2004 update, still hold empiric antibiotic choice and decision about hospitalization to be the key questions in treating the condition. *The Cleveland Clinic Intensive Review of Internal Medicine*[2] lists the same but adds prevention, citing vaccination and averting aspiration as primary prevention strategies. *Foundations for Osteopathic Medicine*[3] mirrors this approach.

Review of the state health department records from the great flu and pneumonia epidemic of 1918, however, reflects a significant reduction in morbidity and mortality in patients attended by an osteopathic physician.[4] The threat of infectious diseases, such as influenza and severe acute respiratory syndrome (SARS), demonstrates that especially in the case of viral illness, supportive care still plays a significant role in recovery from respiratory infection. Add to this the progressive emergence of organisms resistant to antibiotics, which has led to the request for the more judicious use of antibiotics and to implementation of a program of vaccination with newer congregate streptococcal vaccines.[5]

In this context, the use of manual treatment is usually seen as an alternative approach to pharmaceutical treatment. It may, however, be more effective and accurate to see these as complementary therapies, contributing in different ways to enabling the body's self-healing mechanism, or host defenses, to resist and eradicate infection. The loss of elderly patients with multisystem disease to a respiratory tract infection, despite successive courses of paired antibiotics appropriately chosen from culture and sensitivity testing, repeatedly underscores the importance of optimizing the host response component of healing.

What contribution, then, can osteopathic thought and practice make that is relevant to contemporary medical care, especially for the patient with pneumonia?

REVIEW OF PNEUMONIA

Despite the spectrum of potential pathogens, both Centers for Disease Control and Prevention[5] and British Thoracic Society cite *Streptococcus pneumoniae* as the primary pathogen implicated in community-acquired pneumonia. Hospital-acquired pneumonic infection, however, involves a wide spectrum of pathogens, depending on the bacterial climate of the particular institution. In the latter case, attention to supportive organs and systems may be more important. This chapter for the most part addresses uncomplicated streptococcal pneumonia.

The lungs are most often viewed as organs of oxygen exchange, depending primarily on their ability to expand and contract to allow alterations in pressures to drive the system. Certainly this aspect is considered in this discussion. However, the lungs also function as a sensitive low-pressure gaseous and liquid interface, and issues of circulation are as important as oxygenation in function and dysfunction of the respiratory system. The precise analysis of these critical parameters is often the point of placement of a central line in distinguishing pulmonary hypertension from primary heart failure. This logic can be factored into goals of osteopathic treatment.

OSTEOPATHIC CORRELATIONS IN PNEUMONIA

Classical Considerations

Consistent with this idea of the lung's involvement in the circulatory system, Still identified the primary problem in pneumonia as vascular stasis secondary to decreased neural function. His explanation for effectiveness includes the following description: "I usually find the sixth, seventh and eighth ribs pushed above, below or twisted upon the transverse processes, thus closing up the intercostal veins by pressure and disturbing the vasomotors to the lungs. . . . When the ribs are adjusted and the blood and nerve supply freed from pressure, the fever generally goes down and ease will follow."[6] Still wrote in an era when the most advanced science was gross pathology but apparently with positive results from his biomechanical approach to physiology.

Charles Hazzard cites Still's attention to ribs but describes a more general treatment, stressing the harmonious coordination of all affected areas and systems. He describes an approach to a supine patient that is compatible with a hospital bed, beginning with cervical treatment (occipitoatlantal area) for vagal release, scalenes as secondary muscles of respiration, ribs and vertebrae, and also release of abdominal tension.[7] McConnell reiterated the advantage of regional treatment with attention to the thoracoabdominal diaphragm.[8]

Barber, another student of Still's, described a protocol for treating pneumonia beginning with lateral recumbent soft tissue work from cervical to lumbar spine. He followed this with supine cervical articulatory and soft tissue procedure. Next, he performed a variation of rib raising using the arm as a lever in full inspiration.

Following this, he applied 2 minutes of thoracic manual vibration before he finished up with suboccipital inhibitory pressure held for 5 minutes.[9]

Contemporary Considerations

Kuchera and Kuchera[10] recommend a staged application of osteopathic manipulative treatment (OMT) to complement conventional medical care, aimed at increasing the patient's comfort and supporting the patient's self-healing potential. Rib raising coupled with paraspinal muscle stretch is described in detail as a routine initial stage of treatment, treating the thoracic cage as a unit of function. Occipitoatlantal inhibition and compression of the fourth ventricle (CV-4) are recommended to help control fever.

Once the patient is in less distress, the second stage, myofascial release of the fascia associated with the periscapular muscles and the anterior cervical fascia associated with secondary respiratory drive, may be applied. Additionally, attention is paid to any segmental dysfunction from C7 to T4. The third stage, applied during convalescence, consists of continued rib raising, addition of lymphatic pump procedures, and continued treatment of any incidental vertebral dysfunction.

Many of these particulars derive from the respiratory-circulatory model of J. Gordon Zink.[11] For those not familiar with this work, it is well worth the time to review it.

For those interested in refining effectiveness, the approach of J. P. Barral[12] represents an approach to connective tissue release targeting deep tissue. Although presented and taught as a visceral procedure, its application in practice is much broader. Much of it is directed toward diagnosing and treating the cause of a patient's pain. He does not list pneumonia as a treatable condition. But his descriptions of manipulation of the lung and pleura, though not described as treating pneumonia, are of benefit for the pneumonic patient.

Outcome Studies

In the current climate favoring evidence-based choices in medicine, some research supports the use of the osteopathic approach to pneumonia. Smith's[13] report on the osteopathic treatment of influenza patients in 1918, although not rigorous by today's scientific standards, described a 10% mortality rate for patients with pneumonia who received OMT as compared to 33% for those with standard medical care.

Noll and associates performed a series of pilot and clinical trials with elderly patients hospitalized with pneumonia. The largest trial involved 28 in the treatment group and 30 in the control group (control was a light touch protocol). Treatment included a standardized protocol by second-year osteopathic students followed by a visit from an osteopathic manipulative medicine specialist who performed discretionary individualized treatment according to perceived need. Results demonstrated shorter reliance on intravenous antibiotics in the treatment group (implying quicker clinical response) and an overall shorter hospital stay. This was consistent with results from a previous pilot study with 11 and 10 subjects in the treatment and control groups, respectively.[14,15]

Edward Stiles[16] published the results of a retrospective chart review of 25 patients and concluded that in patients hospitalized with chronic obstructive pulmonary disease (COPD), pediatric lower respiratory tract infections, cholecystitis, and hysterectomies, each category had decreased hospital stay with the integration of OMT into their care plan.

Osteopathic Treatment: Mechanism of Action

There is a tendency in medical practice, driven by social accountability, to think in terms of a mechanism of action in selecting any treatment. Used in the field of epidemiology, one general concept that many find useful in dealing with the pneumonia patient is the host disease model. In this application of the model, the individual is stratified according to the risk factors.[17] In the individual case, however, this concept may be inverted to emphasize optimization of function of the different homeostatic or health maintenance systems in the body. As implied in the writings of Still cited previously, the inflammatory or immune response to infection or tissue injury is the primary route of healing; however, this process may be overtaxed or stagnate and benefit from modulation to optimize healing.

In some health circles, the concept of the psychoneuroimmune system has been used to describe this complex interrelated system.[18] (See Chapter 6.) To selectively evaluate the usefulness of a particular osteopathic procedure, especially for visceral disease in the thorax, the following review of interactions may be helpful: potential elements of somatovisceral dysfunction available for osteopathic inputs to normalize the physiologic function of the body—elements of a specially focused physical examination and focused treatment plan based on traditional rationale and theoretical research.[3]

Neuroreflexive

Sympathetic: Stress, including that of acute illness, may cause increased pulse, ineffective tachypnea, and constriction of blood vessels, impeding tissue oxygenation and removal of waste. The proximity of the sympathetic chain ganglia to the rib heads presents an opportunity for external inhibition of sympathetic hypertonicity. The pneumonia patient is often emotionally and physically stressed.

Facilitation: A classical osteopathic concept stating that previously acquired segmental dysfunction may lead to a decreased threshold of reactivity to nociception, resulting in increased myotonia, possibly mediated by sympathetic hyperarousal; facilitation may result in somatovisceral or viscerosomatic reflexes described later in the chapter.

Viscerosomatic and somatovisceral reflexes: Attributed to commonalities in interneuronal communication in the posterior horn of the spinal column, these concepts suggest that dysfunction in the visceral organs can cause segmental somatic dysfunction or that somatic dysfunction may demonstrate itself through visceral pathology. The reciprocal relationships in the pulmonary area involve thoracic segments T2 to T6.[3]

Postural reflexes: The pattern of postural reflexes has led some scientists to postulate postural pattern generators distal to the brainstem and cerebellum.[19] From the osteopathic point of view, these underscore the importance of evaluation and treatment of integrated body regions, not isolated parts or articulations. In this context, the importance of optimizing thoracic expansion is described later in the chapter.

Biomechanical

Articular: For the thorax to function, the complex of costovertebral contacts and intervertebral facet joints and mobility of the spinal column must function normally to accommodate lung expansion.[20] Additionally, the costochondral and chondrosternal joints must be flexible. Articulations of the clavicle and first rib cooperate in mobility of the dome of the lung.

Myofascial: Distensibility of the horizontal diaphragms, tentorium cerebellae, thoracic inlet, thoracoabdominal and pelvic floor, and the fascial elements of the accessory muscles of respiration is required for optimal respiration.

Vascular

Lymphatic: The major route of lymph drainage from the lower body is through the posterior of the thoracic cavity to return to the left subclavian vein. Lymphatic flow is often considered to be passive, totally dependent on the thoracic pressure gradients generated by respiration. This dynamic is important but complements a measurable lymphatic vasomotor oscillation of 0.04 to 0.10 Hz.[21]

Venous: Much venous return relies on the activities of daily living. Acute illness suspends these activities. The vena cava, under activation of the thoracoabdominal diaphragm, acts as a low-pressure pump to expedite return of waste-laden blood to the heart and then the lungs for reoxygenation. The venous stasis of pulmonary disease in conjunction with inactivity from hospitalization may benefit from manipulative assistance. Adjunctive treatments to increase venous return, if not contraindicated in heart failure or pulmonary edema, may assist homeostatic balance.

Interstitial: To clear tissue edema, fluids must find their way to one of the previously mentioned components of the vascular system. External pressure, including myofascial effleurage, may assist in this process.

Pneumatic

Respiratory: An unobstructed respiratory cycle assists bronchial ciliary clearance of debris in the mucous layer, resorption of transudates, gas exchange, and the other processes dependent on the alternating positive and negative intrathoracic pressures.

Impact on Evaluation of the Pneumonia Patient

Sputum and blood cultures with sensitivity describe the nature and invasiveness of the pathogen and help select the antibiotic of choice. Chest radiography describes the amount of pulmonary edema; arterial blood gases describe the compromise to oxygen exchange. Observation of skin tone and state of consciousness of the patient also add information as to the severity.

Similarly, the quality of thoracic compliance (rib mobility and spinal symmetry and flexibility) can help describe physiologic status, chronic host susceptibility, and degree of physiologic stress. Individual rib assessment and segmental spinal diagnosis can help describe predisposing and obstructive factors and organ involvement (viscerosomatic and somatovisceral reflexes).

The role and effectiveness of diaphragmatic excursion may suggest the amount of potential gain from myofascial release. Similarly, but more often to a lesser extent, the thoracic inlet area may offer a point of entry to optimize function.

Posture, tissue quality, psoas muscle tone, and abdominal girth may all suggest aspects of the patient's overall wellness and prognosis. The key to effective treatment is to find changeable features that will promote this patient's health. It is often the temptation to profile the patient as old or diabetic or obese and thereby explain treatment failure. Rather, one should find variables that one can work with. Within the physiology of this patient, what is the rate-limiting step in the return to relative health?

TREATMENT

Following the elements and principles described previously, treat what you find.

Try to be comprehensive and develop a detailed plan with series of discrete intermediate goals and tissues to be affected.

As per Kuchera and Kuchera,[10] staging of treatment is important. All OMT is applied by way of prescription. (See Chapter 4.) Diagnosis gives an initial idea of where to go. And just as antibiotics and oxygen have particular parameters of application and are modified according to certain milestones, so it is with OMT in the pneumonic patient.

The following are possible effective interventions.

Observation and palpation*
Rib raising
Rib articulation
Paraspinal muscle stretch*
Lymphatic pump
Occipitoatlantal release*
Cervical paraspinal muscle release
Cervical articulatory release
Diaphragmatic release*
Oscillatory release

Observation and Palpation

Specific diagnosis is mandatory for effective OMT. Do not start working out of habit. First read the tissues. Start with a broader mental focus than looking for the most restricted articulation. Johnston and Friedman[19] described the sequence of progressive focus in osteopathic diagnosis as "Screen, scan, segmental diagnosis." Begin with a hands-on appreciation of this particular patient. What does the first hand contact tell you about the level of vitality and health of this individual?

To the remark, "It's nice to see you," an elderly gentleman once replied, "It is nice to be seen." Tissue behaves in the same way. Attentive and concerned contact assure patients that they are receiving attention and care and encourages them to cooperate in efforts to rekindle their self-healing capacity. This can contribute to efforts to decrease tone in the sympathetic system.

The first step is to determine the quality of the tissue and make a survey of the area of interest. In the thoracic region, how well does the chest wall move in inspiration? Is the whole shape pliable or rigid? Does the sternum rise or sink with inspiration? Do the ribs cooperatively rise and fall? According to experience with patients and knowledge of anatomy, which tissue is most in need of release and remobilization? Is there a protuberant, crowded abdomen whose contents are restricting descent of the diaphragm? Is a residuum of old trauma affecting the diaphragm? These matters will start to give an indication for prognosis and amount of effort required to approach optimal prognosis.

Analytic assessment of articulations can follow the methods previously learned. It is recommended to be complete and thorough in the thoracic spine and rib cage. Special attention to the thoracic inlet is helpful. Besides its importance in the respiratory-circulatory model, this area can reflect hypertonicity in the scalene muscles that act as accessory muscles of respiration. The first rib has complex

---

*Recommended treatment choices for first contact.

associations and if restricted can impede the pump handle respiratory excursion of all ribs below it. This rib is embedded in the middle cervical fascia that blends with the dome of the lung. Checking tension in the space between the clavicle and the anterior border of the trapezius allows one to affect tension on the dome of the lung.

As noted previously, attention to the thoracoabdominal diaphragm can be crucial. Restriction here can be approached from several vantage points. Within the myofascial model, the diaphragm may be approached as a critical horizontal fascial element. In the Barral model, restriction of the diaphragm can be the result of visceral ptosis, the drag from suspended abdominal viscera. Additionally, a recess in the anterior chest wall just above or below the tenth left rib at its costochondral insertion may in the context of Robert Fulford's approach reflect the residuum of emotional trauma.[22] Use of each of these dimensions of diagnosis and treatment is relevant, especially in severe or treatment-resistant cases. They are helpful in expanding effectiveness and efficiency in routine treatment; however, thorough discussion of them is beyond the scope of this chapter.[12,22]

Other regional influences may be integrated, depending on the degree of compromise of the patient. The pelvic floor interacts reciprocally with the thoracoabdominal diaphragm in developing the reversing pressure gradients that make insufflation of the lungs possible. Therefore, particular pelvic restriction may contribute to respiratory compromise. Also, psoas muscle tension or lumbar restriction of motion may contribute to diaphragmatic excursion through tension on the posterior margin.

In the end, the rule is to treat what you find—but you do not find what you do not look for. Remember, pneumonia is not just an infection of the lungs. You are not just treating the disease; you are treating the patient as a complete, complex functional unit.

Rib Raising

Rib raising can be accomplished with the patient in any of several positions; the supine position is considered first. It is most useful at bedside with the unconscious or otherwise seriously debilitated patient.[3]

Rib Raising, Supine

This procedure is described in Chapter 5 and depicted in Figure 5.6.

Alternative position: Approach the patient from the head of the bed and slide your hands beneath the patient passing beneath each shoulder. Engage rib angles by applying pressure with fingertips below each rib pair. Apply traction by a combination of flexing the fingers and leaning backward.

Rib Raising, Seated

Patient position: seated with arms crossed in front of the chest. Physician position: standing facing the patient. The patient's arms are supported on the physician's chest. The physician's hands reach around the patient to contact the patient's rib angles on both sides.

Activating force: Lean so that gentle extension of the patient's thoracic spine occurs and simultaneously carries the contact with the patient's ribs, anteriorly and superiorly.

Progression: Put the hand on the patient's rib angles above or below the first site and repeat the procedure until all of the patient's ribs have been raised. A focused effort may be placed on any region that exhibits increased restriction.

Alternative positions: The patient's straightened arms, with fingers interlaced, may be placed over either or both of your shoulders.

Either method requires some intimacy with the potential to share air. It is recommended that you work with held inspirations and slowly exhale, then draw breath over your shoulder.

Rotation and Rib Raising (Fig. 17.1)

The following combination method is powerful and convenient. It is used at bedside with the seated patient and with the outpatient examination table or chair. It is a good beginning place and is effective in a busy practice, since it can be done in the time that would otherwise be used for discussion with or instruction of the patient.

Patient position: seated. Physician position: standing behind and at the left side of the patient. The patient's left hand is placed on the patient's right shoulder.

Reach across with your left hand and stabilize the patient's left hand and right shoulder. Place your right palm over the patient's right rib cage at the level needing attention.

Activating force: Apply a right translatory force to the ribs with the right hand while stabilizing or leftward rotating the torso with the left hand. Development of a rhythmic repetition can both be relaxing and soothing and mechanically effective in mobilizing the right hemithorax.

Progression: Reposition and repeat on the other side. With practice, thoracic vertebral articulation can be integrated into this maneuver for optimal effect.

Rib Articulation, Seated

Rib articulation can be achieved by the positioning mentioned just previously. In maximizing articulation, the rhythmic right rotational component in the described underrotation and rib raising example would be modified or enhanced in the following way.

Position: For monitoring purposes the rib or ribs to be articulated are contacted more specifically with the base of the thumb or between the thumb and index finger.

Activating force: Each right translation and left rotation alternates with a returning left translation of the rib and a right rotation and side bending of the torso. Focused attention is on the mobility of the rib or ribs of interest.

Progression: Gentle rhythmic repetition challenges the ligamentous tissue, confining rib motion return to reasonable optimal mobility within this clinical context.

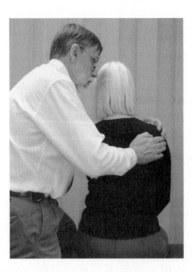

FIGURE 17.1 Rotation and rib raising, patient seated.

Paraspinal Muscle Stretch: Lateral Recumbent (Fig. 17.2)

Recall this basic soft tissue maneuver learned long ago. Just as an aspirin is touted as aborting a myocardial infarction, simple things done at the right time can have helpful results.

Patient position: lateral recumbent. Physician position: standing or seated with finger pads poised to engage the erector spinae musculature.

Activating force: Stabilize the patient if necessary and apply lateral gentle traction effecting lateral cross-stretch to the fascia and muscle tissue.

Progression: Move up and down the spinal column both to test for restriction and to add beneficial stretch to soften and relax tense tissue. Comeaux[23–25] describes further benefits of repetitive application of force.

Lymphatic Pump

Pedal Pump (See Chapter 10, Procedures and Fig. 10.3)

Thoracic Pump (See Chapter 16, Procedures and Fig. 16.19)

Occipitoatlantal Release (See Chapter 16, Procedures and Fig. 16.12)

The intent is to normalize tensions in the vicinity of the jugular foramen and rectus capitis group of muscles affecting the vagus nerve, which provides the parasympathetic supply to the lungs and bronchial tree.

Patient position: supine. Physician position: sitting at the head of the bed or table with forearms gently resting on the bed or table, holding the occiput in the palms of the hands, with fingertips engaged below the inferior occipital border.

Activating force: Straighten your fingers and press the fingertips into the suboccipital muscles.

Progression: Hold this position, allowing the head to be suspended and passively extend into your palms. Allow for maximal relaxation of the muscles, usually 1 to 2 minutes.

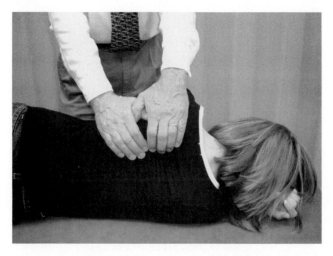

FIGURE 17.2 Paraspinal muscle stretch with the patient in the lateral recumbent position.

Alternative: These principles may be applied at bedside in the uncooperative (unconscious) patient from an anterior approach. Reaching around the neck, place your index fingers at the atlanto-occipital junction and generate forward pressure by gently lifting the neck forward, allowing the head to extend.

Cervical Paraspinal Muscle Release

The intent is to relax some of the accessory muscles of respiration and to treat dysfunction, which may inhibit function of the phrenic nerve.

Patient position: supine. Physician position: standing at the right side of the bed or table facing the head of the bed with the left hand laid across the patient's forehead and the right hand reaching across to grasp the lateral muscle mass of the left side of the neck, with the finger pads engaging the posterior border of the sternocleidomastoid muscle.

Activating force: Use your left hand to stabilize or roll the head to the left while drawing your right hand forward, stretching the engaged muscles.

Progression: Repeat this maneuver rhythmically, gently but effectively until the musculature softens. Repeat the procedure on the opposite side by reversing standing and hand positions.

Variation: A similar relaxation of the superior fibers of the trapezius muscle may be accomplished by placing the right hand over the top of the patient's left shoulder and stretching by pulling your hand and arm down and forward in a way that brings the patient's elbow nearer to the waist.[26]

Cervical Articulatory Release (Fig. 17.3)

The intent is to achieve general articular mobilization and to discover and treat dysfunctional cervical segments whose nerve roots may be involved with the phrenic nerve or other respiratory musculature.

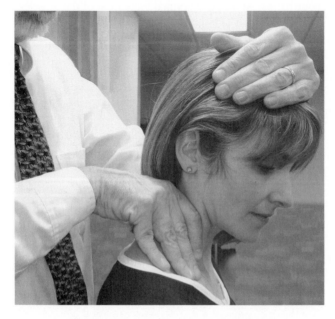

FIGURE 17.3 Cervical articulatory release.

Position: The patient is seated, and diagnosis is made of a segmental or regional side bending (presume C4 flexed, side bend left, rotated left for the description); the physician is standing behind and slightly to the right side of the patient facing the same direction. The physician's left hand is placed across the top of the head, fingers at right angles to midline. The base of the physician's right index finger is placed against the lateral pillars on the right at the level to be treated.

Activating force: Guided by the physician's left hand, the patient drops the head forward, rolls it (side-bending the neck) to the left, extends it, and then rolls it (side-bent right) forward, hoping for articular release in this latter phase.

Progression: Three to four slow, rhythmic repetitions, with the right hand refining the plane of articular mobilization, may be sufficient. Work up and down the spine to determine whether you have the primary segment or there are also others. Usually this procedure is not repeated on the other side.

Variation: This procedure may be performed with the physician at the head of the bed or table if possible. In this position, there is generally more control, with the effect of gravity working with the articulating hand.

Cervical Articulatory Release, Oscillatory Release

As described previously, oscillatory release can be integrated into cervical articular treatment.[22]

Position: The physician stands behind the patient as described for articular treatment. The right hand (metacarpal head) engages the restrictive barrier.

Activating force: Apply gentle pressure to the dysfunctional segment, using the head and superior segments for leverage; side-bend to the right. Once resistance is engaged, the right hand oscillates with a rotary motion at the wrist at about 150 cpm, to enhance release and advance the restrictive barrier.

Progression: Several seconds of oscillation is adequate to begin. Then reassess the barrier; three or four cycles of this are usually enough to assess whether this approach contributes to release.

Variation: The same principles can be applied in the supine patient, with the physician at the head of the bed or table.

Facilitated oscillatory release is a formulation of ideas and maneuvers, many of which are classical, to be used as elements in eclectic or combined procedures with other applications of force. A key idea is the gentle development of a standing wave according to the natural harmonic properties of the tissue involved. Therefore, it should feel natural and relaxing to the patient.

Diaphragmatic Release

Patient position: supine. Physician position: standing facing the side of the patient to be treated. Place one hand across the chondral masses of the lower ribs and the other hand across the posterior lower rib cage.

Activating force (direct treatment): Test the thoracolumbar fascia and diaphragm for ease and bind in flexion and extension, rotation, and side bending. Gently move in three dimensions into the directions of restrictions and apply steady force until tissue give is complete.

Indirect treatment: Test the thoracolumbar fascia and diaphragm for ease and bind in flexion and extension, rotation, and side bending. Gently move in three dimensions into the directions of easy or balanced tension. Follow the shift in balance to maintain this neutral tension until the unwinding process ceases.

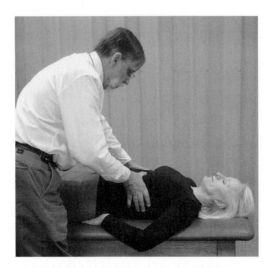

FIGURE 17.4   Diaphragmatic release.

Diaphragmatic Release Alternative (Doming the Diaphragm) (Fig. 17.4)

Patient position: supine. Physician position: standing at side of the bed facing the head. The physician's open palms are placed over the lower margin of the rib cage, with thumbs lateral to the sternum an inch below the tenth rib.

Activating force: Apply slow, progressive pressure to gather the fascia of the anterior abdomen and diaphragm by allowing the thumbs to sink in under the ribs and then press upward.

Progression: Pay attention to taking up any slack with expirations. Maintain pressure through several respiratory cycles until optimal release is obtained.

Case Illustrations

Integrating procedure: In actual practice, one blends procedures based on experience, skill, diagnostic focus, and intent of intervention, as is illustrated in the following case examples.

Additionally, bedside or outpatient protocols can be individualized to patient and practitioner (patient seated, supine, or prone), the physician thinking in terms of principles rather than recipes for imitation.

In the analytic, mechanistic climate of the modern hospital, soothing human contact in the appropriate professional setting can have significant benefit in recruiting the patient's psyche to contribute to healing. Touch communicates concern and builds rapport between physician and patient. Additionally, the delirium and despair of the chronically ill patient is reachable with the hope instilled by caring contact.

Case 1

History

A 67-year-old woman presented to the emergency department with fever and progressive shortness of breath over 2 days. She reported incidental lower thoracic back pain but denied any history of trauma. The patient gave a history of hypertension, moderate intermittent epigastric discomfort, and back pain and had been seen in the primary care setting once every 4 months.

She was a widow of 4 years, living alone. She denied smoking and admitted only occasional social alcohol use. Her usual routine was to be mostly sedentary with occasional housework.

Initial radiographs showed diffuse infiltrate with consolidation in the right lower lobe, and an oxygen saturation of 92%. Vital signs upon admission included a temperature of 103°F rectal, blood pressure of 150/92 mm Hg, respirations at 28 per minute, height 5 feet, six inches, and weight 180 lb.

She was admitted by the emergency physician at 11 P.M. with telephone orders for empiric cefazolin and cultures pending. She was prescribed 4 L oxygen per nasal cannula. Her home medications were continued, and she was reevaluated on the following morning.

Physical Examination the Morning After Emergency Admission

Muscle tone was generally poor. Her heart rate was regular at 84 beats per minute, and respiration was 24 per minute. Her abdomen was protuberant and minimal, and 1+ bilateral pretibial edema was present. Temperature the first morning after admission was 100°F. She had been given ibuprofen upon admission for the back pain. This aggravated her epigastric discomfort, and she refused additional doses.

The musculoskeletal examination, performed with the patient seated and supine in bed, revealed suboptimal thoracic cage compliance without focal rib restriction. The diaphragm and lower ribs revealed restriction secondary to abdominal protuberance. Corresponding to the patient's site of pain, there was tenderness with palpation and increased flexion without rotation of T10. She was also tender in the right suboccipital area without frank rotation of any cervical vertebral segments.

Reevaluation of the admitting radiographs revealed a possible compression fracture at T10 that the radiologist later confirmed as probably an old injury. Moderate degenerative joint changes were also noted throughout.

Assessment

Lobar pneumonia
Back pain
Somatic dysfunction, thoracic and ribs, cervical and abdominal
Gastritis
Old (?) compression fracture

Plan of Treatment

Medical management per standard of care was implemented and is not fully itemized here. Osteopathic manipulation was used in several ways. The initial intent in the thoracic region was to expedite optimal thoracic cage compliance and ease of respiration. In this case, however, there was need to work within the context of her T10 dysfunction and its relationship to her anti-inflammatory use and gastritis. As an old injury, it represented a chronic problem.

With the patient seated at bedside, the T10 vertebral area was approached by applying an articular procedure as described previously. In this application,

(Continued)

however, modification was made to accommodate this patient in several ways. First, the maneuvers were applied using definitive but gentle application of force, emphasizing during the rotational excursion the indirect portion of range of motion, and then only lightly engaging the direct barrier over several repetitions. Special emphasis was placed on solidly supporting the patient so as to give assurance and optimize relaxation.

This process took 30 seconds and was followed by several cycles of seated rib articulation, emphasizing the side bending and lateral glide of the ribs. Then the patient was asked to lie supine. The occipitoatlantal area was loosened with traction, then soft tissue inhibition and articulation (15 seconds): The abdomen was examined for epigastric tenderness. This area was avoided, while traction upon the diaphragm, anterior abdominal muscles, and deeper tissues was applied over the left upper abdomen. The focus of this intervention was to induce diaphragmatic relaxation and also possibly reset the stomach and gastroesophageal junction within the abdominal cavity in the possibility that there might be some aspect of hiatal hernia and associated reflux present (2 to 3 minutes).

That ended the osteopathic manipulative portion of the visit for the first day. Repetition of manipulative procedures by house staff later in the day was requested and propoxyphene was ordered on a short-term basis to replace the ibuprofen.

Progression

On day 2 the patient was resting comfortably on 2 L of oxygen, and oxygen saturation was 96%. Gastric pain and back pain were not present, and the patient had slept comfortably.

Seated examination revealed that the flexion component of the thoracic dysfunction was less prominent. Rib excursion and abdominal protuberance had not changed in appearance. There was less tissue tension in the upper cervical area.

Treatment on day 2 was directed at reinforcing the previous day's treatment. The articular treatment of T10 was slightly more forceful during direct engagement of the barrier.

Days 3 to 5

OMT was continued as the patient gained strength. Generally, abduction of the arms was used to enhance inhalation. During treatment, the use of the arms as long levers optimized flexibility of the upper torso and stretches of accessory muscles of respiration; attention to the serratus anterior and serratus posterior was enhanced by use of connective tissue or myofascial release. The patient was instructed to exercise by raising her arms above her head and taking a deep breath to expand the chest.

Comment

Older patients often accrue a list of musculoskeletal diagnoses attributed to age. If a strategy to optimize function rather than fatalistically accepting arthritic change as age related is adopted, strides can be made to improve functional independence and comfort, requiring less dependence on pharmaceuticals and making their use, when necessary, more effective.

OMT should not be adjunctive. It must be functionally integrated into the treatment of the complex of morbidities that plague the individual patient. The OMT prescription must be tailored to the unique needs of the patient.

This case illustrates that significant improvement can be achieved with limited time on the part of the treatment physician. Adjunctive exercises are a way of expanding the physician's impact while giving independence and motivation to patients. This empowers patients to act on their own behalf and to avoid feeling victimized by the disease and being passive in its treatment. Further, this helps to counter the depression so often associated with chronic or recurrent disease in the elderly.

Case 2

History

A 58-year-old male construction supervisor went to the family clinic complaining of shortness of breath, fever, and chills with progressive onset over the previous 3 hours.

He had a 40 pack-year history of cigarette smoking and had been diagnosed with COPD. Additionally, he had hypertension and stable angina. Cardiac catheterization 1 year previously revealed no total coronary artery occlusion but plaque and 30% occlusion in two vessels. A decision was made in favor of conservative treatment.

The patient's medications included long-acting metoprolol 50 mg daily and salmeterol inhaler 50 µg twice a day.

Physical Examination

Vital signs included the following: height, 5 feet 11 inches; weight, 168 lb; temperature, 103°F; blood pressure, 138/88 mm Hg; and respiration, 28 per minute.

Pulse oximetry showed oxygen saturation of 92%; heart rate was regular; and fine crackles were heard at the end of inspiration, but there was poor expansion of the chest on respiration. Radiography revealed infiltrate in bilateral bases, hyperaeration consistent with COPD, and a nodular density on the right upper lobe unchanged from films taken 2 years ago.

Musculoskeletal examination revealed poor thoracic compliance with heavy involvement of the accessory muscles of respiration. T2 was flexed, side-bent right, rotated right; and T4 was flexed, side-bent left, and rotated left, with marked stiffness and bogginess in this area. Ribs 4 to 8 right were restricted in exhalation. Hypertonia of the sternocleidomastoid and scalene muscles was noted bilaterally.

Assessment

1. Community acquired pneumonia
2. COPD with exacerbation
3. Hypertension
4. History of cardiac disease
5. Nicotine dependence
6. Somatic dysfunction thoracic, ribs, and cervical region

Plan of Treatment

The patient declined hospitalization. Bronchodilator treatment was given in the office and oxygen saturation rose to 94%.

OMT was initiated gently but definitively. In the presence of acute illness and an engaged immune system, there is often an increase in tenderness in

(Continued)

areas of dysfunction. Care should be taken to avoid adding to the stress and discomfort associated with illness by aggressive treatment. Rather, gentle contact can be soothing and comforting. So also in this case osteopathic treatment should progress in stages.

Use of OMT has several purposes in this case. One is if possible to enhance thoracic compliance and tidal volume and decrease sympathetic tone. This patient had a key rib, rib 4 right, that was limiting expansion of the chest cage. Relief of tension in the cervical accessory muscles also offered long-term benefit. Additionally, he had dysfunctions correlated with his hypertension[27] as well as with his coronary disease.[3]

Tolerance being closely monitored, initial OMT included seated paraspinal soft tissue–connective tissue release followed by gentle articular release in the identified dysfunctional segments, with focus on releasing T4 and associated rib dysfunction. Muscle energy is my preferred approach. Supine treatment can be added to do gentle kneading and soft tissue cross-fiber and longitudinal stretch to the cervical musculature. Lateral recumbent periscapular myofascial release follows.

A course of levofloxacin 750 mg daily for 7 days was begun. Arrangements were made to have an office recheck in 2 days. If in the interim things got worse, including onset of chest pain, the patient was instructed to proceed to the emergency department. At follow-up in 2 days, if fever had abated and the patient improved, he would be reassessed at all dysfunctional segments with an eye also to any problem areas missed on the initial cursory examination. Treatment of what is found is the rule. A greater latitude of procedures is available with the increase in patient comfort and tolerance, as long as application is tissue focused and dose appropriate.

Follow-up in a week would be advised to develop a maintenance strategy and treat resistant dysfunctions.

Comment

This case illustrates the fact that osteopathic diagnosis and treatment are integrated into patient management and as such are not just added time. Apparently extra time may add dividends by reducing the number of diagnostic tests by adding additional tracking parameters, as well as directly supporting the body's self-healing capacity. If difficult patients are not given extra care in terms of intensity, they are often instead given extra time over a prolonged treatment course.

Case 3

History

An 89-year-old woman was transferred from a small nursing home because she was not responding to oral cefdinir suspension and had begun demonstrating increased confusion along with an increase in temperature, 101°F rectal; white count, 18,000; and a portable chest radiograph suggesting left lower lobe pneumonia.

The patient was incapable of swallowing medication in pill form and had an advance directive not to resuscitate or apply heroic measures of life support. Discussion with her niece, who had medical power of attorney, however, led to hospitalization for a course of intravenous antibiotics.

Physical Examination

The patient was a cachectic-appearing woman who was responsive only to painful stimuli. Vital signs were temperature, 102°F, rectal; blood pressure, 90/64 mm Hg; respiration, 32, with mouth breathing.

Chest radiographs upon admission revealed left lung infiltrates, blunting of the left costophrenic angle, and overall osteopenia. The leukocyte count was 18,000 with a left shift; culture samples of airway-suctioned fluids and blood were obtained. Arterial blood gas (ABG) on room air demonstrated oxygen saturation 84%; PaO_2, 78 mmHg; HCO_3, 30 mEq/L; pH, 7.48; $PaCO_2$, 32.

The patient's rib cage moved stiffly but with fair expansion. Retractions in intercostal spaces were noted and her abdomen was scaphoid. Cervical spine stiffness overall, with tension in the suboccipital triangle on the right greater than left, was noted.

Assessment

1. Pneumonia
2. Cachexia of chronic disease
3. Somatic dysfunction ribs, cervical and abdomen
4. Dementia

Plan

Medical management of this individual was critical and complex and was modified daily. The details of that management are not germane to this discussion and are not elaborated here.

This patient's ABGs and thoracic structural examination suggest inefficient respiration and uncompensated alkalosis on top of a chronic compensation pattern involving multiple system compromise. OMT can be supportive without the patient's cooperation. During routine rounds, several minutes of doing rib raising from the lateral position and an anterior-approach suboccipital release may contribute to optimizing respiratory effort. These procedures are described previously.

Comment

Dealing with the patient with multisystem failure and possible nearly terminal status is a challenge. Goal setting is sometimes complex and delicate. Knowing one has done the best possible job by being complete and compassionate is gratifying and often productive. It also clearly communicates to the family your dedicated intention to care for this patient.

Life support includes issues of quality of life besides duration. Osteopathic management and attention to the whole person may be directed toward comfort or reassurance measures during a patient's last days or hours. Yes, this costs something in time, but one never knows the full impact of one's limited actions.

SUMMARY

Pneumonia is a diverse clinical arena with common features. In most cases, even with the common streptococcal community-acquired pneumonia, it is helpful to think in terms of optimizing the patient's host resources to self-heal. Pharmacotherapy is a strong player in this situation. Standard-of-care protocols for treating pneumonia emphasize choice of antibiotic and decisions about hospitalization. But the status of the indigenous resources of the patient should not be overlooked.

Osteopathic medicine has traditionally contributed a variety of models aimed at designing a manipulative prescription for the patient with pneumonia. Prescription is the key idea. As with any disease or infirmity, treatment is most effective if specificity of tissue impairment is employed as the rationale for physiologic improvement. Simple things at the right place and time are often important. Not all medicine must be high-tech, high-priced, and heroic.

This chapter is an attempt to be both motivational and practical in suggesting ways to add OMT to the management of the pneumonia patient. CME course review, progression in skills, and use of the chapter references are encouraged.

References

1. British Thoracic Society Guidelines for the Management of Community Acquired Pneumonia in Adults. Thorax [serial online]. Dec 2001;56(suppl 4):iv1–iv64. Update May 2004;59:364–366. Available from Thorax [database online] at http://www.thoraxjnl.com. Accessed February 20, 2005.
2. Stoller JK, Ahmad M, Longworth DL, eds. The Cleveland Clinic Intensive Review of Internal Medicine. 3rd ed. Philadelphia: Lippincott Williams & Wilkins, 2002.
3. Ward RC, ed. Foundations for Osteopathic Medicine. 3rd ed. Philadelphia: Lippincott Williams & Wilkins, 2002.
4. Riley GW. Osteopathic success in the treatment of influenza and pneumonia. Paper before the Chicago session of the American Osteopathic Association, July 1919. J Am Osteopath Assoc 2000;100:315–319.
5. Centers for Disease Control and Prevention. Drug-resistant *Streptococcus pneumoniae* disease. Available at: http://www.cdc.gov/ncidod/dbmd/diseaseinfo/drugresisstreppneum_t.htm. Accessed February 20, 2005.
6. Still AT. Research and Practice. Kirksville, MO: Author, 1910. Reprinted in Seattle: Eastland Press, 1992;83–89.
7. Hazzard C. Pneumonia. In: The Practice of Applied Therapeutics of Osteopathy. 1905. Reprinted at http://meridianinstitute.com. Accessed February 20, 2005.
8. Jordan T, Schuster R, eds. Selected Writings of Carl Philip McConnell, DO. Columbus, OH: Squirrel's Tail, 1994;90.
9. Barber ED. Osteopathy Complete, 1898. Reprinted in: Early American Manual Therapy. Virginia Beach, VA: LifeLine, 1998.
10. Kuchera M, Kuchera W. Osteopathic Considerations in Systemic Dysfunction. 2nd ed. Columbus, OH: Greyden, 1994;45.
11. Zink JG. Respiratory and circulatory care: the conceptual model. Osteopath Ann 1977;5(30):108–112.
12. Barral JP. The Thorax. Seattle, WA: Eastland, 1992;156–159.
13. Smith RK. One hundred thousand cases of influenza with a death rate of one-fortieth of that officially reported under conventional medical treatment. 1919. J Am Osteopath Assoc 2000;100:320–323.
14. Noll DR, Shores JH, Gamber RG, et al. Benefits of osteopathic manipulative treatment for hospitalized elderly patients with pneumonia. J Am Osteopath Assoc 2000;100:776–782.
15. Noll DR, Shores JH, Bryman PN, Masterson EV. Adjunctive osteopathic manipulative treatment in the elderly hospitalized with pneumonia: A pilot study. J Am Osteopath Assoc 1999;99:143–152.
16. Stiles E. Somatic dysfunction in hospital practice. Osteopath Ann 1979;7(1):49–52.
17. Amundson D, Perri J. Community-acquired pneumonia in the managed care environment. J Am Osteopath Assoc 1996;S(4):S16–S19.
18. Adler R, Felten D, Cohen N. Psychoneuroimmunology. 3rd ed. Amsterdam: Elsevier Scientific, 2000.

19. Johnston WL, Friedman HD. Functional Methods: A Manual for Palpatory Skill Development in Osteopathic Examination and Manipulation of Motor Function. Indianapolis: American Academy of Osteopathy, 1994.

20. Stretanski MF, Kaiser G. Osteopathic philosophy and emergency treatment in acute respiratory failure. J Am Osteopath Assoc 2001;101:447–449.

21. Nelson KE. The primary respiratory mechanism. AAO J 2002;12(4):25–34.

22. Comeaux Z. Robert Fulford, DO, and the Philosopher Physician. Seattle: Eastland, 2002.

23. Comeaux Z. Facilitated oscillatory release. AAO J 2002;12(2):24–35.

24. Comeaux Z. Facilitated oscillatory release: A method of dynamic assessment and treatment of somatic dysfunction. AAO J 2003;13(3):30–34.

25. Comeaux Z. The role of vibration and oscillation in the development of osteopathic thought. AAO J 2000;10(3):19–24.

26. Collins FW. Original Osteopathic Moves as Taught by A. T. Still. 9th ed. Pomeroy, WA: Health Research, 1997.

27. Johnston WL, Kelso AF. Changes in presence of a segmental dysfunction pattern associated with hypertension: 2. A long-term longitudinal study. J Am Osteopath Assoc 1995:95:315–318.

CHAPTER 18

The Patient with Hypertension

David M. Driscoll

"Much depends on the heart and great care should be given to its study, because a healthy system depends almost wholly on a normal heart . . ."

A. T. Still[1]

INTRODUCTION

The first person to measure blood pressure was Stephen Hale, a clergyman, who in 1733 inserted a piece of tubing into the carotid artery of a horse.[2] He was astonished to see the blood rise 9 feet in a glass column. This method, however, was not practical for regular use in humans. It was not until 1876 that the sphygmomanometer, invented by Ritter von Basch, was used as a noninvasive device to measure blood pressure. Blood pressure was found to be equal to the pressure in the inflated cuff compressing the arm at the point when the first pulse could be heard as the cuff was deflated—the force of ventricular contraction (systole).[3] In 1905, almost 30 years later, Korotkoff described the region where the pulse sound disappeared as ventricular relaxation (diastole).[4] The measurement of blood pressure as we know it today, therefore, is only 100 years old.

In 1892, A.T. Still eloquently described elevated blood pressure in *The Philosophy and Mechanical Principles of Osteopathy* by viewing disturbances in the heart in terms of increased resistance: "I think any man with anatomical and physiological knowledge will be able to reason and come to the conclusion that if an obstruction in the least toe, and that at the greatest distance from the heart, disturbs its regularity and pulsation, that other causes of irritation and stoppage of either arterial or venous blood will cause demands that the heart use greater energy to force blood through the involved channels, just in proportion to the resistance it has to meet."[1] In today's terms, this is better understood as increased peripheral vascular resistance.

It is estimated that 50 million or more Americans have high blood pressure.[5] Worldwide, that number may be 1 billion; approximately 7.1 million deaths annually may be directly linked to hypertension.[6] Of the 167 countries surveyed, more than 50% of the population aged 60 to 69 have hypertension.[7] The incidence and prevalence continue to increase; it is estimated that 75% of those over age 70 have high blood pressure.[5] A recent analysis from the Framingham Heart Study revealed that a normotensive individual 65 years old had more than an 80% chance of developing high blood pressure within 20 years.[8] Hypertension, therefore, is the most common condition the family physician will encounter in clinical practice.

The Seventh Report of the Joint National Commission on the Prevention, Detection, Evaluation and Treatment of Hypertension (JNC 7) released the latest recommendations in August 2004.[9] Hypertension is defined as systolic blood pressure (SBP) 140 or above, diastolic blood pressure (DBP) 90 or above, or taking antihypertensive medication. The normal range for blood pressure is defined as SBP less than 120 and DBP less than 80 for individuals without certain high-risk cardiovascular conditions.[9] Blood pressure readings between 120/80 and 140/90 are considered prehypertension, and blood pressure readings equal to or greater than 140/90 are classified as hypertension in otherwise healthy individuals without certain high-risk conditions. Home blood pressure readings or self-monitoring readings 135/85 or greater are also classified as hypertension.[10] It is well recognized that early detection and effective treatment of hypertension lead to a significant decrease in cardiovascular mortality and morbidity. According to JNC 7, in individuals 50 years and older, systolic blood pressure above 140 is a more important cardiovascular risk factor than diastolic blood pressure. Starting at 115/75, the cardiovascular risks double for each increment of 20/10. Normotensive individuals at 55 years of age have a 90% lifetime risk of hypertension.[8]

EVALUATION

The evaluation of patients with documented hypertension has four main objectives: (1) Identify a cause of hypertension. (2) Assess the effect of hypertension on target organs. (3) Evaluate the response to therapy. (4) Identify other cardiovascular risk factors or concomitant disorders that may alter prognosis and guide treatment.[9,11] For most individuals with hypertension, the cause is unclear and the disease is classified as essential hypertension. Recent studies have shown several identifying risk factors for the development of hypertension;[12,13] nonetheless, secondary causes of hypertension also should be considered. These include renovascular disease; chronic renal disease; coarctation of the aorta; states of glucocorticoid excess, such as Cushing's syndrome; medications and herbal formulations; primary aldosteronism;[13] mineral corticoid excess; pheochromocytoma; sleep apnea; and thyroid disease.[14]

Certain lifestyles have been shown to contribute to and to enhance the effects of hypertension, while other lifestyles can reverse and prevent some of the devastating affects of hypertension. Smoking, sedentary lifestyle, high sodium intake, and excessive alcohol intake contribute to the development of hypertension.[12] Weight reduction, moderate alcohol use, a high-potassium diet high in fresh fruits and vegetables with low fat, physical activity, and smoking cessation help to prevent and to control high blood pressure.[15,16]

In evaluation of patients for hypertension, the medical history should include the known duration of the hypertension. The direct correlation between duration of hypertension and extent of end-organ damage has been well established. Evidence of longstanding hypertension can be seen in patients with coronary heart disease, congestive heart failure, peripheral vascular disease, renal disease, and sexual dysfunction. A medical history should include weight change, level of physical activity, smoking, and alcohol use. Dietary assessment should take into account intake of sodium, saturated fat, and caffeine. The osteopathic physician should also record musculoskeletal complaints that suggest lumbar, thoracic, cervical, or craniosacral somatic dysfunction.

For diagnosis of hypertension, the physical examination should include the average of at least two blood pressure measurements, separated by 2 minutes, with the patient seated quietly in a chair, feet on the floor, for at least 5 minutes.[17] Caffeine, exercise, and smoking should be avoided for at least 30 minutes prior to the measurements. If home blood pressure monitoring is used, the cuff should be verified for accuracy in the office. If home blood pressure readings are consistently less than 130/80 despite elevated office blood pressure and there is no end-organ damage, treatment is not needed.[18] High readings should be verified in the contralateral arm. If the values are different, the higher reading should be used. Measurements of height, weight, and waist and body mass index (BMI)[19] should be recorded.

$$BMI = weight\ Kg/[height\ M]^2$$

Funduscopic examination should be done to detect retinal hemorrhages, atrioventricular (A-V) nicking, exudates, disc edema, or Hollenhorst plaques. Examination of the neck is done to check for carotid bruits, jugular vein distention, or thyromegaly. Lungs should be auscultated for evidence of rales or bronchospasm. The abdomen should be examined for abdominal bruits and organomegaly; the extremities, for edema and diminished or absent arterial pulsations. The musculoskeletal system should be evaluated for tissue texture changes or other signs of somatic dysfunction, particularly in the cervical and thoracic regions.

Routine laboratory tests are recommended prior to initiating treatment for hypertension. These are done to assess damage to end organs or to identify underlying causes of hypertension. Pertinent tests include urinalysis, complete blood cell count, potassium, sodium, creatinine, fasting glucose, calcium, total cholesterol, high-density lipoprotein (HDL), and an electrocardiogram.[9] Measurement of high-sensitivity C-reactive protein (HS CRP) along with homocysteine levels also may be helpful. Analysis of the Framingham Heart Study revealed that individuals with low HDL levels and elevated HS CRP had a higher risk of developing cardiovascular disease than cohorts with normal or low HS CRP and high HDL.[20]

OSTEOPATHIC APPROACH TO TREATMENT

Once the diagnosis of hypertension has been established, treatment begins with risk stratification. The World Health Organization (WHO) and Joint National Committee on Prevention, Detection, Evaluation and Treatment of High Blood Pressure (JNC) recommend a similar approach to treatment. Major risk factors for the development of cardiovascular disease are smoking, dyslipidemia, diabetes mellitus, age older than 60, sex (higher in males and postmenopausal females), and a family history of cardiovascular disease (women under 65 or men under 55).[21] The risk groups defined for hypertension are given in Table 18.1.

TABLE 18.1

Risk Stratification and Treatment Recommendations[9]

Blood Pressure Stage (mm Hg)	Risk Group A1[a]	Risk Group B2[b]	Risk Group C3[c]
Normal: <120/80			
Prehypertension: 120/80–139/89	Lifestyle modification	Lifestyle modification	Drug therapy
Stage 1: 140/90–159/99	Lifestyle modification (up to 12 months)	Lifestyle modification (up to 6 months)	Drug therapy
Stage 2: >160/100	Drug therapy	Drug therapy	Drug therapy

[a]No organ damage, no cardiovascular disease.
[b]At least 1 risk factor for heart disease not including diabetes mellitus; no organ damage or cardiovascular disease.
[c]Organ damage, cardiovascular disease, and/or diabetes mellitus with or without risk factors.

Lifestyle Modification

Lifestyle modification offers the opportunity to lower blood pressure and cardiac risks without medications. All patients, regardless of what stage or risk group they are in, should be encouraged to participate in aerobic physical activity; the American Council on Aging recommends 30 to 45 minutes a day at least 4 days a week.[22,23] Patients should lose weight if needed. Even a 10-lb loss in total body weight can lead to a significant reduction in cardiac risk.[15,24] Dietary saturated fats and cholesterol should be reduced. Alcohol intake should be limited to 1 oz of ethanol, equivalent to 24 oz beer, 10 oz wine, or 2 oz 100-proof whiskey (vodka) per day for males and half that quantity for females and lighter individuals.[25] Sodium intake should be limited to 2.4 g–6 g sodium chloride—daily.[26,27] Adequate potassium intake (90 mmol daily) is recommended along with adequate intake of calcium and magnesium.[15] A modified DASH (Dietary Approaches to Stop Hypertension) diet, high in fresh fruits and vegetables and low in saturated fats, should be encouraged.[28] Finally, smoking cessation cannot be stressed enough. Smoking cessation aids with nicotine contain a lower amount of nicotine than cigarettes and usually do not significantly raise blood pressure.[26]

Medications

Decreasing blood pressure through the use of medications has been clearly shown to reduce cardiovascular mortality and morbidity in several large long-term population studies.[29–36] It is evident that the most effective medication for treatment of hypertension is the one medication or combination of medications that lowers the blood pressure into a safe range with the least number of side effects. Optimal formulations sustain normal blood pressure for 24 hours with once-a-day dosing. There are several reasons for once-a-day dosing: (1) to provide smoother, persistent blood pressure control instead of fluctuating, intermittent control; (2) to promote better adherence to the (once-a-day) dosing regimen; (3) to protect against the risk of stroke or heart attack secondary to the abrupt increases seen with shorter-acting agents; (4) to reduce the expense for the patient if cost is a factor in compliance.

TABLE 18.2

Conditions to Consider When Selecting or Avoiding Certain Hypertensive Medications[6]

Indication	Medications Reducing Cardiovascular Morbidity and Mortality
Diabetes mellitus	ACE 1, diuretics, beta-blockers, ARB, CCB
Heart failure	ACE I, diuretics, beta-blockers, ARB, aldosterone antagonists
Isolated systolic hypertension (elderly)	Diuretic (preferred), long acting DHP CCB
Post myocardial infarction	Beta-blocker, ACE 1, aldosterone antagonists
Chronic kidney disease	ACE I, ARB
High-risk coronary disease	Diuretics, beta-blockers, ACE I, CCB
Recurrent stroke prevention	Diuretic, ACE I

Indication	Medications That May Have a Favorable Effect on Comorbid Conditions
Angina	Beta-blockers, CCB
Atrial tachycardia and fibrillation	Beta-blockers, CCB (non-DHP)
Cyclosporine-induced hypertension	CCB
Diabetes mellitus type I and II with proteinuria	ACE I, CCB
Diabetes mellitus type II	Low-dose diuretic
Dyslipidemia	Alpha-blockers
Essential tremors	Beta-blockers (non-CS)
Heart failure	Carvedilol, losartan potassium
Hyperthyroidism	Beta-blockers
Migraines	Beta-blockers (non-CS), CCB (non-DHP)
Myocardial infarction	Diltiazem, verapamil
Osteoporosis	Thiazides
Preoperative hypertension	Beta-blockers
Benign prostatic hypertrophy	Alpha-blockers
Renal insufficiency (caution with renal artery stenosis or creatinine ≥3mg/dL [265.2 µmoles/L]	ACE I

Indication	Medications That May Have Untoward Side Effects on Comorbid Conditions
Bronchospasms	Beta-blockers
Depression	Beta-blockers, central alpha-agonists, reserpine
Diabetes mellitus I and II	Beta-blockers, high-dose diuretics
Dyslipidemia	Beta-blockers (non-ISA), high-dose diuretics

(Continued)

TABLE 18.2 (cont.)

Conditions to Consider When Selecting or Avoiding Certain Hypertensive Medications[6]

Gout	Diuretics
2° or 3° heart block	Beta-blockers, CCB (non-DHP)
Heart failure	Beta-blockers (except carvedilol), CCB (except amlodipine, felodipine)
Liver disease	Labetalol, methyldopa
Peripheral vascular disease	Beta-blockers
Pregnancy	ACE 1, ARB
Renal insufficiency	Potassium-sparing diuretics
Renovascular disease	ACE 1, ARB.

According to JNC 7 recommendations, based on the outcome of the Antihypertensive and Lipid Lowering Treatment to Prevent Heart Attack Trial (ALLHAT) study, a thiazide-type diuretic is still considered the initial drug of choice for most cases of stage 1 hypertension.[9,36,37] Patients whose blood pressure is greater than 20 mm Hg above the systolic goal or greater than 10 mm Hg above the diastolic goal should initially take two agents to achieve goal readings. Also, there are compelling reasons to use a different class of antihypertensive medication in patients with diabetes, heart failure, kidney disease, isolated systolic hypertension in the elderly, or ischemic heart disease (Table 18.2).

OSTEOPATHIC APPROACH

The osteopathic approach recognizes the human body as a unit. It is the duty of the osteopathic physician primarily to treat patients, not disease. This is in contrast with practitioners who allow the disease to take center stage, leaving the patient to play a secondary role. When this occurs, the musculoskeletal and psychosocial aspects of the management of the disease entity are lost. Since hypertension has a global effect on the body, all systems must be taken into consideration, including not only the vascular and cardiac systems but the renal, neurologic, endocrine, ocular, and musculoskeletal systems.

Osteopathic manual medicine is traditionally thought of as a method for diagnosing and treating nonsurgical orthopedic problems such as back pain. This simplistic view fails to recognize the role the musculoskeletal system plays in health and disease. The osteopathic approach to hypertension is best used when it draws upon its rich heritage along with implementing the latest in science and technology. By recognizing the role of the musculoskeletal system in cardiac disease, osteopathic physicians can use their keen sense of touch to aid in the diagnosis and treatment of hypertension.[38]

Changes in blood pressure are sensed by the afferent neurons innervating the carotid sinus and aortic baroreceptors. A rise in blood pressure that stimulates the baroreceptor afferent nerve fibers results in both direct and indirect stimulation in the parasympathetic vagal innervation of the heart.[39] The vagus nerve emerges from the medulla of the brain and exits the skull through the jugular foramen. The vagus nerve has four basic components: (1) The brachial motor component (efferent) innervates the striated muscles of the pharynx, tongue, and most of the larynx. (2) The visceral motor component (efferent) innervates smooth muscle and glands of the pharynx, larynx, thoracic, and abdominal viscera. (3) The visceral sensory component (afferent) innervates larynx, trachea, esophagus, and abdominal viscera, the stretch receptors in the aortic arch, and chemoreceptors in the aortic bodies adjacent to the aortic arch. (4) The general sensory (afferent) component innervates the skin at the back of the ear, external acoustic meatus, part of the tympanic membrane, and pharynx.[40]

Dilation of the coronary arteries and heart rate are controlled by the interactions of the sympathetic and parasympathetic nerves. The cardiac sympathetic nerve system arises from the upper five thoracic segments via the cervical ganglia. These sympathetic nerves are responsible for dilation of the coronary arteries and for acceleration of the heart rate. The parasympathetic nerves form from branches of the vagus nerve, which in turn is responsible for deceleration of the heart rate. These autonomic nerves form the superficial and deep cardiac plexuses. Preganglionic sympathetic fibers arise from the nucleus intermediolateralis in the lateral horn at the level of T1 to T5. The higher thoracic segments innervate the ventricles, while the lower innervate the atria.[41] The anatomic location of these nerve fibers and tracts is the basis for looking at the cervical and thoracic vertebrae in the individual with suspected cardiac disease.

RESEARCH BACKGROUND

The effective management of hypertension with medications has changed radically over the past 20 years and continues to evolve. It was not until the 1960s that randomized, controlled double-blind studies started to show the benefits of drug treatment in patients with severe diastolic hypertension (DBP $\geq$ 115). As a result of the Veterans Administration Cooperative Study Group on Antihypertensive Agents (1967), there was a substantial reduction in cardiovascular morbidity.[42] Prior to that, in the early part of the twentieth century, the ability to treat hypertension was limited. Foxglove (digoxin), nitrates, bromides, barbiturates, iodides, reserpine, and other herbal remedies were commonly used.[43] Because of the side effects of many substances and questionable efficacy of several others, many osteopathic physicians resorted to manipulation in the treatment of hypertension. Spinal manipulation was prescribed to decrease sympathetic outflow to the myocardium and arterioles.[44] Visceral manipulation was also used to decrease passive liver congestion.[45] The rational for such treatment was based on studies involving viscerosomatic and somatovisceral reflexes.[46]

In the early 1900s, using human and animal models, Louisa Burns[47] studied viscerosomatic and somatovisceral spinal reflexes. Burns's findings revealed that stimulation of visceral pericardium and the heart resulted in contractions of the second to sixth intercostal muscles and to paraspinal muscles at the level of T2 to T5 in dogs (viscerosomatic). Furthermore, local stimulation at the upper thoracic region resulted in lower systolic blood pressure and lower pulse rate than did local stimulation in the lower thoracic region (somatovisceral). Burns observed that the somatovisceral reflexes were much less circumscribed and direct than were viscerosomatic reflexes. Burns further stated, "Since abnormal conditions of the viscera follow such pressure upon somatosensory nerves as is sufficient to lessen conscious sedation, and since section of somatosensory nerve is followed by abnormal conditions of the viscera, it is inferred that normal visceral activity depends in part upon the stimulation derived from the somatosensory nerves." She further suggested that abnormal viscerosomatic reflexes may be used as an aid to the diagnosis of certain conditions.[47] These studies provided the early foundations for Chapman's reflexes, which would not be published for another 30 years.

Frank Chapman was a practicing osteopathic physician from Tennessee who kept a personal account of his findings. It was not until after his death that his wife, Ada Hickey Chapman, and his brother-in-law, Charles Owens,[48] made them public by publishing *An Endocrine Interpretation of Chapman's Reflexes*. Chapman observed reproducible tender points that were commonly paired anteriorly and posteriorly and that corresponded to specific visceral elements. He discribed these tender points as ganglioform contractions. Not only were these tender points used in the diagnosis of certain conditions, he and others used these reflex points to treat various ailments.[48,49] In 1979, Mannino[50] examined 35 hypertensive and 10 normotensive patients after 7 visits over a 3-week period. Blood pressure and aldosterone levels were measured at each visit after treatment of the posterior adrenal component of Chapman's reflex (T11 and T12). The results showed no significant decrease in blood pressure over the test period. There was a significant decrease in aldosterone levels, however, in patients treated with a "make-break circular motion" at T11 and T12, when compared to patients treated at T8 using the same procedure.[50]

As the profession evolved, a generation of clinical researchers, such as Myron Beal and William Johnston, applied osteopathic principles to clinical medicine. Their efforts provided a framework for osteopathic physicians to record their findings in a reproducible systematic fashion. What is intriguing about these studies by Beal, Johnston, and others are the common findings described in the thoracic and cervical region. In a prospective study of 108 patients conducted in 1983, Beal developed specific palpatory procedures for examining cardiovascular disease.[51] The examination was performed with the patient supine. The cervical and thoracic spine was screened for tissue texture changes and segmental response to deep compression. (See Beal's

x-ref

compression test, Chapter 5.) Areas of somatic dysfunction were recorded in the upper thoracic and at C2 and C6. Changes in tissue texture, vasomotor reactions, temperature changes, skin moisture, muscle hypertonicity, hyperesthesia, and segmental musculoskeletal restriction in the vertebrae and ribs were observed. These changes demonstrated a unique pattern attributable to cardiac disease.[51]

Johnston and his associates[52,53] later reported somatic findings in hypertensive patients over a period of 4 to 8 months in a single (physician) blinded study using a standardized palpatory examination. The 253 patients who participated in the study were classified as normotensive, borderline hypertensive, or hypertensive, according to JNC guidelines. There were 61 normotensive, 25 grade 1 hypertensive, and 167 grade 2 or higher hypertensive patients. Johnston noted a repeated pattern of somatic dysfunction, with asymmetry centered at C6, T2, and T6. During the initial examination, the C6, T2, T6 pattern was observed and recorded in 24 of the 61 normotensive patients (31%), 18 of the 25 grade 1 hypertensive patients (72%), and 134 of the 167 grade 2 or greater patients (80%).[52] A 4- to 8-month follow-up revealed that this pattern was present in 25 of 35 normotensive patients and 133 of 149 hypertensive patients who had continued with the study.[53]

Johnston further observed that the rib or costal component of the corresponding vertebra demonstrated different palpable characteristics depending on whether the examiner was observing a purely somatic component or a viscerosomatic component. If the somatic dysfunction at the vertebral level is a primary dysfunction, the costal segments behave opposite (mirror image) of the corresponding vertebral segment.

TABLE 18.3

Summary of Osteopathic Findings in Patients with Cardiovascular Disease

Reference, Date	T1	T2	T3	T4	T5	T6–T10	C1–C7	Rib
Snyder[55] (1924)	X	X	X	X				
MacBain[56] (1933)		X	X	X	X		C1, C2	
Singleton[57] (1934)		X	X					1, 2, 5
Robuck[58] (1935)			X	X				
Hart[59] (1937)	X	X	X		X		C7	
Pottenger[60] (1938)	X	X	X	X	X	T6		
Becker[61] (1939)	X	X	X	X	X	T6		3, 4, 5, left
Long[62] (1940)	X	X	X	X	X	T6–T10		
Burns[63] (1944)			X	X				
Beasley[64] (1944)								1, 2 left
Korr[65] (1949)	X	X	X	X				
Wilson[66] (1956)	X	X	X	X	X			Left ribs
Patriquin[67] (1957)	X	X	X	X				1–4 left
Koch[68] (1961)		X	X	X	X	T6		
Johnson[69] (1972)				X				2 left
Walton[70] (1972)	X	X	X	X				
Burchett[71] (1976)	X	X	X	X				
Larson[72] (1976)		X	X	X	X		C2 left	
Kelso[73] (1980)	X	X	X	X			C3–C6	
Beal[51] (1983)	X	X	X	X			C2, C6	
Johnston et al.[52,53] (1995)		X				T6	C6	2 left

Modified from Beal MC. Palpatory testing for somatic dysfunction in patients with cardiovascular disease. J Am Osteopath Assoc 1983;82:822–831.

If the primary dysfunction was visceral, such as might be the case in hypertension, the costal segments at C6, T2, and T6 then behave the same as the vertebral segment. These ribs would be linked or demonstrate linkage.[54] Table 18.3 summarizes osteopathic findings in patients with cardiovascular disease.

OSTEOPATHIC MANIPULATION

Osteopathic treatment through manipulation to the thoracic and cervical area should not be controversial if one considers manipulation as adjuvant treatment. To date, no long-term outcomes study has been conducted to determine if indeed manipulation is beneficial in the treatment of hypertension. Morgan and associates[74] carried out an 18-week randomly controlled crossover study with 29 subjects. By the end of 18 weeks, no significant difference in blood pressure was seen in either group.

Other studies have shown a short-term improvement, but these are based on small pilot studies or are anecdotal.[44,45] Larger long-term trials are needed not only to assess reduction of blood pressure but also to look at end-organ damage.[46,75,76] On the other hand, no long-term study has shown manipulation to be harmful with the use of proper procedure. Adverse outcomes have been reported, albeit rarely, with the use of cervical manipulation. The American Academy of Osteopathy has printed a position statement on the subject.[77] When considering cervical spinal manipulation for the adjuvant treatment of hypertension, it is best to avoid high-velocity, low-amplitude and other thrust procedures, especially with older individuals.

Most patients with hypertension have associated paravertebral tissue texture changes.[51,52] These may be a result of viscerosomatic changes involving the kidneys seen in renal artery stenosis, for example. Somatic findings in the thoracolumbar region in hypertensive patients may be associated with altered adrenal or renal function seen in conditions such as pheochromocytoma and renal disease.[46,48] Once hypertension is established, the osteopathic physician should turn his or her attention to the midthoracic, lumbothoracic (kidney, adrenal, splanchnic outflow), and lower cervical regions.

CONCLUSION

Lifestyle modification continues to play an important role in the treatment and management of hypertension. To these ends, physical activity is paramount in maintaining the cardiovascular system. For patients to participate in an exercise program, the musculoskeletal system should be properly aligned. Somatic dysfunction remains a major barrier to the proper development of an exercise program. The osteopathic physician can play a pivotal role with manipulation to improve body dynamics and remove barriers to exercising so that the patient can improve cardiovascular fitness, lose weight, and decrease the dosage and number of hypertensive medications.

Hypertension continues to be the condition most frequently encountered by the osteopathic family physician. The osteopathic diagnosis and treatment of hypertension are unique. The most effective treatment starts with early diagnosis and treatment of the whole person. The use of medications and lifestyle modification guarantees the best outcome for our patients. In addition, the osteopathic physician has a unique role in managing hypertension. The recognition and treatment of the neuromusculoskeletal system by the osteopathic physician provides a unique approach to the management of this common condition.

Procedures

Bill Johnston and his associates[52,53] studied the relationship between spinal somatic dysfunction and hypertension, and although any of the manipulative procedures described in this text can effectively treat somatic dysfunction in the hypertensive patient, it is appropriate to consider the treatment of the somatic component of these patients in the context of his functional approach. He worked extensively to define a mechanical model of spinal somatic dysfunction that differs from the standard description in its appreciation for subtle translatory motions and the recognition of the total body impact of respiratory excursion.[54] Segmental spinal dysfunction (type II) is typically defined in terms of the dysfunctional segment relative to the segment immediately below. (See Chapter 3.) Although the intersegmental spinal mechanics are essentially the same, Johnston[78] considered the dysfunctional segment in relation to the vertebral segment immediately above as well as the segment below. He identified an alternating relationship wherein the segments above and below move in the opposite direction of the mechanics of the dysfunctional segment. Thus, if the dysfunctional segment is rotated right (resists rotation to the left), the segments above and below will be relatively rotated left; that is, they will resist rotation to the right. In the diagnosis of segmental dysfunction, Johnston considered the standard spinal mechanics of flexion and extension, side bending left and right, and rotation left and right. To these he added motion assessment of horizontal translations anterior and posterior and left and right, cephalad traction against caudad compression, and respiratory inspiration against expiration.

The functional assessment begins with a screen for asymmetry of tissue texture, position, and motion. This screen is followed by a local scan of the region to be diagnosed and then by the segmental definition of somatic dysfunction in the context of flexion and extension, side bending left and right, rotation left and right, horizontal translations anterior and posterior and left and right, cephalad and caudad motions, and finally inspiration and expiration. The passive motion testing can be described as an appreciation for articular and soft tissue compliance as much as it is the assessment of actual motion. In the absence of somatic dysfunction, the perception of this motion will be equal and unencumbered for each of the paired motions described previously. Somatic dysfunction, however, results in a sensation of immediate resistance when forces are applied in the direction of the dysfunctional barrier as opposed to unencumbered motion in the opposite paired direction. The forces employed when motion testing are the very lightest that can be applied and still obtain the sensation of resistance or freedom.

Once the intersegmental dysfunctional mechanics have been delineated, treatment is administered using indirect principles. The various motions are combined in the direction of freedom of motion, and at this point the patient is asked to inhale and exhale slowly. One phase of respiration will result in increased tension in the region being examined, while the other phase of respiration will produce more relaxation in the area. It is at this point that the patient is instructed to inhale or to exhale and hold the breath, taking the dysfunctional segment into the position of maximum relaxation and allowing a release to occur. This, when precisely done, requires no more than 3 to 5 seconds.

Because of the association Johnston demonstrated between hypertension and somatic dysfunction at levels C6, T2, and T6, this chapter focuses on the functional treatment of the cervical and thoracic regions. In any patient, the somatic dysfunction that should be treated is dictated by the dysfunctional mechanics of that individual and not by preordained expectations of the examining physician. The following discussion rests on the assumption that the initial screen has been performed and that indications of somatic dysfunction have been identified in the cervical and thoracic regions, respectively.

Local Scan of the Cervical Area (Functional Diagnosis)

Diagnosis

This procedure is employed to screen the cervical spine for segmental somatic dysfunction. It is performed by applying rotational forces to the right and then to the left to each segment of the cervical spine and observing for the alternating left, right, left (or right, left, right) pattern in three adjacent vertebral segments that Johnston identified as the hallmark of segmental somatic dysfunction.

Patient position: seated upon the side of the treatment table. Physician position: standing behind the patient (Fig. 18.1).

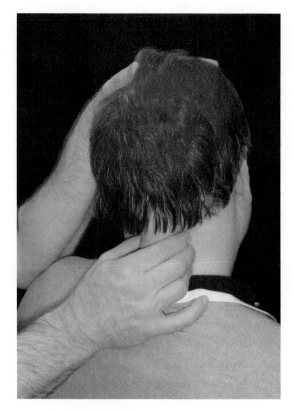

FIGURE 18.1   Functional diagnosis: local scan of the cervical area.

Procedure

1. Place one hand posteriorly upon the patient's neck, in contact with the cervical segment to be evaluated. Palpate one vertebral lateral mass with your thumb and the same point on the other side with your index or middle finger.
2. Place your other hand on the patient's forehead and introduce rotation of the head and cervical spine alternately to the right and left.
3. Observe cervical segmental rotation left and right and determine whether the motion pattern is symmetric or one direction demonstrates greater ease.
4. Move down one spinal segment and repeat steps 1 to 3 until you have screened the entire cervical region.
5. Note any three-segment alternating rotational patterns indicative of somatic dysfunction, and further evaluate these segments.

Segmental Definition of Cervical Somatic Dysfunction (Functional Diagnosis and Treatment)

Diagnosis

This procedure is employed when a primary dysfunctional segment has been identified. It is the method by which motion tests for defining the specific characteristics of the dysfunction are used. Once the diagnosis has been made, the procedure blends seamlessly into an indirect treatment.

Patient position: supine upon the treatment table with the head off the end of the table to facilitate posterior translation during the examination. Physician position: seated at the head of the table (Fig. 18.2).

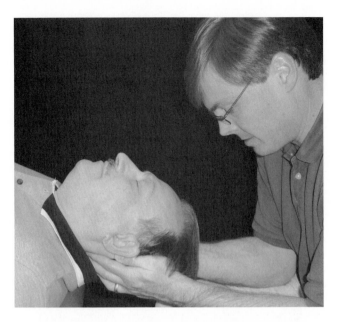

FIGURE 18.2   Functional diagnosis and treatment: segmental definition of cervical somatic dysfunction.

Once a segmental diagnosis has been established, commence indirect treatment in the same position.

Procedure

1. Rest your elbows comfortably upon your thighs and cradle the patient's head in your hands.
2. Place your index fingers bilaterally over the lateral masses of the vertebral segment to be evaluated and your middle fingers in contact with the articular facets.
3. Using minimal force, sequentially introduce flexion and extension, side bending left and right, rotation left and right, horizontal translations anterior and posterior and left and right, and cephalad and caudad traction and compression.
4. At the initiation of each motion test, identify the motion in each of the pairs that results in the perception of resistance. The opposite direction in each pair is the direction of ease.
5. Combine the individual elements to position the dysfunctional segment in the direction of greatest ease, and instruct the patient to inhale slowly and deeply and then slowly exhale. Note the phase of respiration that is accompanied by additional relaxation.
6. The patient, positioned in the direction of greatest ease, should either inhale or exhale deeply (depending upon the phase of respiration that results in the further ease) and hold the breath briefly until a release occurs (3 to 5 seconds). Return the patient to the neutral position and reassess.

Segmental Definition of Thoracic Somatic Dysfunction (Functional Diagnosis and Treatment)

Diagnosis

This procedure is employed when a primary dysfunctional segment has been identified. It is the method by which motion tests to define the specific characteristics of the dysfunction are used. Once the diagnosis has been made, the procedure blends seamlessly into an indirect treatment.

Patient position: seated upon the edge of the treatment table with the arms folded on the chest. Physician position: standing behind the patient.

Procedure

1. Place your index finger and thumb over the thoracic segment to be monitored on either side of the spinous process. This is your monitoring hand.
2. With your other hand, reach in front of the patient and grasp the folded arms. This is your active hand.
3. With your active hand, using minimal force, sequentially introduce flexion and extension, side bending left and right, rotation left and right, horizontal translations anterior and posterior and left and right, and cephalad and caudad traction and compression.
4. At the initiation of each motion test, use your monitoring hand to identify the motion in each of the pairs that results in the perception of resistance and the opposite direction in each pair, that is, the direction of ease.
5. Combine the individual elements to position the dysfunctional segment in the direction of greatest ease, and instruct the patient to inhale slowly and deeply and then slowly exhale. Note the phase of respiration that is accompanied by additional relaxation.
6. The patient, positioned in the direction of greatest ease, either inhales or exhales deeply (depending upon the phase of respiration that results in the further ease) and holds the breath briefly until a release occurs (3 to 5 seconds). Return the patient to the neutral position and reassess.

References

1. Still AT. The Philosophy and Mechanical Principles of Osteopathy. Kansas City, MO: Hudson-Kimberly, 1902;121–128.
2. Hoel D, Howard RB. Hypertension: The silent killer. Postgrad Med 1997;101:116–121.
3. University of California Los Angeles. History of Blood Pressure Measurement. Available at http://www.medphys.ucl.ac.uk/teaching/undergrad/projects/2003/group_03/history.html. Accessed June 21, 2005.
4. Lyons AS, Petrucelli JR. Medicine: An Illustrated History. New York: Harry N. Abrams, 1987;593.
5. Burt VL, Whelton P, Roccella EJ, et al. Prevalence of hypertension in the US adult population: Results from the Third National Health and Nutrition Examination Survey, 1988–1991. Hypertension 1995;25:305–313.
6. World Health report 2002. Available at http://www.who.int/whr/2002. Accessed June 21, 2005.
7. Vasan RS, Larson MG, Leip EP, et al. Assessment of frequency of progression to hypertension in nonhypertensive participants in the Framingham Heart Study: A cohort study. Lancet 2001;358:1682–1686.
8. Vasan RS, Beiser A, Seshadri S, et al. Residual lifetime risk for developing hypertension in middle aged women and men: The Framingham Heart Study. JAMA 2002;287:1003–1010.
9. The Seventh Report of the Joint National Committee on Prevention, Detection, Evaluation and Treatment of High Blood Pressure. Bethesda MD: NIH publication 04–5230, 2004 (JNC 7).
10. White WB, Berson AS, Robbins C, et al. National standard for measurement of resting and ambulatory blood pressures with automated sphygmomanometers. Hypertension 1993;21:504–509.

11. Hajjar I, Kotchen TA. Trends in prevalence, awareness, treatment, and control of hypertension in the United States, 1988–2000. JAMA 2003;290:199–206.

12. Boden-Albala B, Sacco RL. Lifestyle factors and stroke risk: Exercise, alcohol, diet, obesity, smoking, drug use, and stress. Curr Atheroscler Rep 2000;2:160–166.

13. Biglieri EG. Primary aldosteronism. Curr Ther Endocrinol Metab 1997;6:170–172.

14. The Sixth Report of the Joint National Committee on Prevention, Detection, Evaluation and Treatment of High Blood Pressure. Bethesda MD: NIH publication 98–4080, 1997 (JNC 6).

15. He J, Whelton PK, Appel LJ, et al. Long-term effects of weight loss and dietary sodium reduction on the incidence of hypertension. Hypertension 2000;35:544–549.

16. Appel LJ, Champagne CM, Harsha DW, et al. Effects of comprehensive lifestyle modification on blood pressure control: Main results of the PREMIER clinical trial. JAMA 2003;289:2083–2093.

17. Perloff D, Grim C, Flack J, et al. Human blood pressure determination by sphygmomanometry. Circulation 1993;88(5 pt 1):2460–2470.

18. Pickering TG, Coats A, Mallion JM, et al. Blood Pressure Monitoring. Task Force V: White-coat hypertension. Blood Press Monit 1999;4:333–341.

19. Calculate your body mass index. National Heart, Lung, and Blood Institute, National Institutes of Health. http://nhlbisupport.com/bmi/bmicalc.htm. Accessed June 21, 2005.

20. Ridker PM, Rifai N, Rose L, et al. Comparison of C-reactive protein and low-density lipoprotein cholesterol levels in the prediction of first cardiovascular events. N Engl J Med 2002;347:1557–1565.

21. Expert panel on the Detection, Evaluation, and Treatment of High Blood Cholesterol in Adults. Summary of the second report of the national Cholesterol Education Program (NCEP). Expert panel on the detection, evaluation, and treatment of high blood cholesterol in adults (Adult Treatment Panel II). NIH publication 93–3095.

22. Whelton SP, Chin A, Xin X, He J. Effect of aerobic exercise on blood pressure: A meta-analysis of randomized, controlled trials. Ann Intern Med 2002;136:493–503.

23. Kelley GA, Kelley KS. Progressive resistance exercise and resting blood pressure: A meta-analysis of randomized control trials. Hypertension 2000;35:838–843.

24. Trials of Hypertension Prevention Collaborative Research Group. Effects of weight loss and sodium reduction intervention on blood pressure and hypertension incidence in overweight people with high-normal blood pressure: The Trials of Hypertension Prevention, phase II. Arch Intern Med 1997;35:544–549.

25. Xin X, He J, Frontini MG, et al. Effects of alcohol reduction on blood pressure: A meta-analysis of randomized, controlled trials. Hypertension 2001;38:1112–1117.

26. Vollmer WM, Sack FM, Ard J, et al. Effects of diet and sodium intake on blood pressure: Subgroup analysis of the DASH-sodium trial. Ann Intern Med 2001;135:1019–1028.

27. Sacks FM, Svetkey LP, Vollmer WM, et al. Effects on blood pressure of reduced dietary sodium and the Dietary Approach to Stop Hypertension (DASH) diet. DASH-Sodium Collaborative Research Group. N Engl J Med 2001;344:3–10.

28. U.S. Department of Health and Human Services, National Institutes of Heath, National Heart, Lung and Blood Institute. Facts about DASH plan. Available at http://www.nhlbi,nih.gov/health/public/heart/hpl/dash/. Accessed June 21, 2005.

29. Wing LM, Reid CM, Ryan P, et al. A comparison of outcomes with angiotensin-converting-enzyme inhibitors and diuretics for hypertension in the elderly. N Engl J Med 2003;348:583–592.

30. Black HR, Elliott WJ, Grandits G, et al. Principal results of the Controlled Onset Verapamil Investigation of Cardiovascular End Points (CONVINCE) Trial. JAMA 2003;289:2073–2082.

31. Dahlof B, Devereux RB, Kjeldsen SE, et al. Cardiovascular morbidity and mortality in the Losartan Intervention For Endpoint reduction in hypertension study (LIFE): A randomised trial against atenolol. Lancet 2002;359:995–1003.

32. Cutler JA, MacMahon SW, Furberg CD. Controlled clinical trials of drug treatment for hypertension: A review. Hypertension 1989;13(5 Suppl):136–144.

33. Collins R, Peto R, Godwin J, MacMahon S. Blood pressure and coronary heart disease. Lancet 1990;336:370–371.

34. Psaty BM, Smith NL, Siscovick DS, et al. Health outcomes associated with antihypertensive therapies used as first line agents: A systematic review and meta-analysis. JAMA 1997;277:739–745.

35. Psaty BM, Lumley T, Furberg CD, et al. Health outcomes associated with various antihypertensive therapies used as first-line agents: A network meta-analysis. JAMA 2003;289:2534–2544.

36. The ALLHAT Officers and Coordinators for the ALLHAT Collaborative Research Group. Major outcomes in high-risk hypertensive patients randomized to angiotensin-converting enzyme inhibitor or calcium channel blocker vs diuretic: The Antihypertensive and Lipid Lowering Treatment to Prevent Heart Attack Trial (ALLHAT). JAMA 2002;288:2981–2987.

37. Kaplan NM, Gifford RW Jr. Choice of initial therapy for hypertension. JAMA 1996;275:1577–1580.

38. Slick GL. Hypertension. In: Ward RC, ed. Foundations for Osteopathic Medicine. Baltimore: Williams & Wilkins, 1997;319–327.

39. Dodd J, Role LW. The autonomic nervous system. In: Kandel ER, Schwartz JH, Jessell TM, eds. Principles of Neural Science. 3rd ed. Norwalk, CT: Appleton & Lange, 1991;769–771.

40. Wilson-Pauwels L, Akesson EJ, Stewart PA. Cranial Nerves: Anatomical and Clinical Comments. Philadelphia: Decker, 1988;126–132.

41. Willard FH. Autonomic nervous system. In: Ward RC, ed. Foundations for Osteopathic Medicine. 2nd ed. Baltimore: Williams & Wilkins, 2003;90–119.

42. Veterans Administration Cooperative Study Group on Antihypertensive Agents. Effect of treatment on morbidity in hypertension: 1. Results in patients with diastolic blood pressures averaging 115–129 mm Hg. JAMA 1967;202:1028–1034.

43. Beasley HE. Arterial hypertension. Osteopathic Profession 1943;11(1):13–19.

44. Celander E, Koenig AJ, Celander DR. Effects of osteopathic manipulative therapy on autonomic tone as evidenced by blood pressure changes and activity of the fibrolytic system. J Am Osteopath Assoc 1968;67:1037–1038 [abstract].

45. Tilley RM. The somatic component in heart disease. J Am Osteopath Assoc 1970;69:1035–EOA [abstract].

46. Northup TL. Manipulative management of hypertension. J Am Osteopath Assoc 1961;60:973–978.

47. Burns L. Viscero-somatic and somato-visceral spinal reflexes. J Am Osteopath Assoc 1907;7:52–60.

48. Owens C. An Endocrine Interpretation of Chapman's Reflexes. Carmel, CA: American Academy of Osteopathy, 1932.

49. Tettambel MA. Obstetrics. In: Ward RC, ed. Foundations for Osteopathic Medicine. Baltimore: Williams & Wilkins, 1997;349–361.

50. Mannino JR. The application of neurologic reflexes to the treatment of hypertension. J Am Osteopath Assoc 1979;79:225–231.

51. Beal MC. Palpatory testing for somatic dysfunction in patients with cardiovascular disease. J Am Osteopath Assoc 1983;82:822–831.

52. Johnston WL, Kelso AF, Babcock HB. Changes in the presence of a segmental dysfunction pattern associated with hypertension: 1. A short-term longitudinal study. J Am Osteopath Assoc 1995;95:243–255.

53. Johnston WL, Kelso AF. Changes in the presence of a segmental dysfunction pattern associated with hypertension: 2. A long-term longitudinal study. J Am Osteopath Assoc 1995;95:315–318.

54. Johnston WL, Friedman HD, Eland DC. Functional Methods. Indianapolis: American Academy of Osteopathy, 2005;275–292.

55. Snyder CP. Heart conditions commonly found in practice. J Am Osteopath Assoc 1924;24:399–401.

56. MacBain RN. Technic for the treatment of cardiac conditions. J Am Osteopath Assoc 1933;33:68.

57. Singleton RH. Angina pectoris and its manipulative treatment. J Am Osteopath Assoc 1934;34:73–77.

58. Robuck SV. Body mechanics in relation to cardiac conditions. J Am Osteopath Assoc 1935;35:1–4.

59. Hart RC. Angina pectoris: An osteopathic consideration of common and serious heart malady. J Osteop 1937;44:21–25.

60. Pottenger FM. Symptoms of Visceral Disease. 5th ed. St. Louis: Mosby, 1938.

61. Becker AD. Manipulative osteopathy in cardiac therapy. J Am Osteopath Assoc 1939;38:317–319.
62. Long FA. Some observations on spinal motion. J Am Osteopath Assoc 1940;39:405–415.
63. Burns L. Principles governing the treatment of cardiac conditions. J Am Osteopath Assoc 1944;43:231–234.
64. Beasley HE. Osteopathic factors in cause and treatment of heart disease. J Am Osteopath Assoc 1944;44:134–137.
65. Korr IM. Skin resistance patterns associated with visceral disease. Fed Proc 1949;8:87–88.
66. Wilson PT. Osteopathic cardiology. Academy of Applied Osteopathy 1956 Yearbook. Colorado Springs: Academy of Applied Osteopathy, 1956:27–32. (Now available from the American Academy of Osteopathy, Indianapolis.)
67. Patriquin DA. Osteopathic management of coronary disease. Academy of Applied Osteopathy 1957 Yearbook. Carmel, CA: Academy of Applied Osteopathy, 1957:27–32. (Now available from the American Academy of Osteopathy, Indianapolis.)
68. Koch RS. A somatic component in heart disease. J Am Osteopath Assoc 1961;60:735–740.
69. Johnson FE. Some observations on the use of osteopathic therapy in the care of patients with cardiac disease. J Am Osteopath Assoc 1972;71:799–804.
70. Walton WJ. Textbook of Osteopathic Diagnosis and Technique Procedures. 2nd ed. St. Louis: Matthews, 1972.
71. Burchett GD. Somatic manifestations of ischemic heart disease. Osteopath Ann 1976;4:373–375.
72. Larson NJ. Summary of site and occurrence of paraspinal soft tissue changes of patients in the intensive care unit. J Am Osteopath Assoc 1976;75:840–842.
73. Kelso AF, Larson NJ, Kappler RE. A clinical investigation of the osteopathic examination. J Am Osteopath Assoc 1980;79:460–467.
74. Morgan JP, Dickey JL, Hunt HH, Hudgins PM. A controlled trail of spinal manipulation in the management of hypertension. J Am Osteopath Assoc 1985;85:308–313.
75. Bayer JD. An osteopathic approach to the management of hypertension. DO 1971;11:143–151.
76. Anderson RA. An osteopathic method for normalizing blood pressure. J Am Osteopath Assoc 1935;35:128–134.
77. American Academy of Osteopathy. Position paper on osteopathic manipulation of the cervical spine, Indianapolis, Indiana. AAO Newsletter 2003:2–3.
78. Johnston WL. Segmental behavior during motion: I. A palpatory study of somatic relations. J Am Osteopath Assoc 1972;72:352–361.

CHAPTER 19

The Patient with Congestive Heart Failure

Kenneth E. Nelson

INTRODUCTION

Abnormality of cardiac function resulting in the failure to pump blood commensurate with the requirements of the body is congestive heart failure. Diastolic failure occurs when cardiac muscle fiber length (preload) is insufficient for adequate cardiac filling. Systolic failure occurs when the heart's pumping is insufficient to overcome arterial resistance (afterload).

Certain aspects of the pathophysiology of congestive heart failure are found in association with somatic dysfunction. Congestive heart failure is associated with increased beta-adrenergic tone and an altered baroreflex response. Somatic dysfunction of the thoracic spine is known to result in spinal cord–level facilitation, with increased sympathetic efferent stimulation of segmentally related structures.[1,2] The Traube-Hering oscillation, a manifestation of the fluctuating autonomic tone associated with the baroreflex, has been demonstrated to correspond to the palpable observation of the cranial rhythmic impulse (CRI) a fundamental component of cranial osteopathy.[3] Furthermore, cranial manipulation has been shown to increase the Traube-Hering component of blood flow velocity.[4,5]

Restriction of movement of the thoracic cage is known to complicate and even induce congestive heart failure. Somatic dysfunction is associated with articular motion restriction.[6,7] Every adult has some degree of somatic dysfunction of the thoracic spine and ribs with resultant restriction of thoracic cage motion that progresses with age. Somatic dysfunction of the thoracoabdominal diaphragm results in decreased diaphragmatic excursion that further decreases efficiency of thoracic cage movement.

DISCUSSION

Congestive heart failure is the pathophysiologic state in which an abnormality of cardiac function is responsible for the failure of the heart to pump blood at a rate sufficient to meet the requirements of the metabolizing tissues. In some patients with heart failure, however, a similar clinical syndrome is present but without any detectable abnormality of myocardial function. Heart failure should be distinguished from noncardiac and potentially reversible causes of inadequate cardiac output.[8]

Cardiac output is determined by the interplay between the heart and the peripheral circulation. The force of ventricular contraction is a function of the end-diastolic length of cardiac muscle, which is a manifestation of end-diastolic ventricular volume (the Frank Starling relation). Stroke volume correlates directly with cardiac muscle fiber length (preload) and inversely with arterial resistance (afterload). The stroke volume of the ventricle is determined by three influences: (1) length of the muscle at the onset of contraction, that is, preload; (2) the inotropic state of the muscle, that is, the position of its force–velocity–length relation; and (3) the tension that the muscle is called upon to develop during contraction, that is, afterload. Depressed ejection fraction (stroke volume/end diastolic volume = 59 to 75%, normally) and lowered cardiac output may occur in the presence of normal cardiac function if preload is decreased. This is diastolic failure. Decreased inotropic state of the cardiac muscle and/or increased tension required of the cardiac muscle during contraction results in systolic failure.

At any level of inotropic state and afterload, the performance of the myocardium is influenced profoundly by ventricular end-diastolic fiber length and therefore by diastolic ventricular volume. Among the major determinants of preload is distribution of blood volume.[9]

The distribution of blood volume between the intrathoracic and extrathoracic compartments is determined by the following:

1. Body position: Upright posture augments extrathoracic at the expense of intrathoracic blood volume and reduces ventricular work.
2. Intrathoracic pressure: Normally mean intrathoracic pressure is negative, which increases thoracic blood volume and ventricular end-diastolic volume and enhances the return of blood to the heart, particularly during inspiration, when this pressure becomes more negative.
3. Intrapericardial pressure: Constriction of the myocardium from increased intrapericardial pressure (tamponade) decreases cardiac filling and ventricular diastolic volume and, consequently, stroke volume.
4. Venous tone: Venoconstriction occurs, among other times, during muscular exercise and during deep inspiration, and it tends to augment intrathoracic and intraventricular blood volumes and ventricular performance.
5. The pumping action of skeletal muscle: During muscular exercise the muscular pump displaces venous blood centrally, tending (1) to diminish extrathoracic blood volume, (2) to augment intrathoracic blood volume, (3) to augment ventricular end-diastolic volume, and (4) to augment ventricular work.

Factors 1, 2, 4, and 5 are affected by the individual's level of musculoskeletal functional capability. Although factor 1, upright posture, tends to reduce preload and consequently stroke volume, factor 5, the muscular pump, counters this pre-load reduction and augments end-diastolic volume.

Mean Systemic Filling Pressure

The rate of return of blood to the heart is determined by both cardiac and peripheral factors but is proportional to the pressure gradient across the venous bed. The pressure gradient for venous return is the mean systemic filling pressure. Since the capacitance of the veins is 18 to 20 times that of the arteries, this pressure is largely a function of the venous system. If the total peripheral resistance increases by 20% with all of the resistance occurring in the arterioles, venous return is reduced by about 6%. If the 20% resistance change occurs entirely on the venous side, venous return is reduced by about 53% (a ninefold difference).[10]

Pulmonary Circulation

The pulmonary circulation serves a secondary function as a blood volume reservoir for the left heart. It contains approximately 10% of the total blood volume. Its high distensibility allows it to adjust readily to large increases in blood flow.[11] Pressures in the pulmonary circulation are low. The mean pressure in the pulmonary artery is about 15 mm Hg. The mean pressure in the aorta is about 100 mm Hg, more than 6 times that of the pulmonary artery. Pulmonary capillaries receive very little support from the surrounding lung, so they are liable to collapse or distend depending upon the pressures within and around them. The effective pressure outside the capillaries is alveolar pressure; when this rises above the pressure inside the capillaries, they collapse. The pressure around pulmonary arteries and veins tends to be less than alveolar pressure. As the lung expands, these larger vessels are pulled open by the radial traction from the elasticity of the tissue that surrounds them. Pulmonary vascular resistance is a manifestation of the pulmonary pressure gradient divided by pulmonary blood flow. The pressure gradient in the pulmonary system is about 10 mm Hg.

Another determinant of pulmonary vascular resistance is lung volume. Because of the effect of pulmonary parenchyma upon the caliber of extra alveolar vessels, pulmonary resistance is lower during inhalation. Inhalation tends to compress pulmonary capillaries, with resultant increase in vascular resistance.[12]

Noncardiac Congestive Heart Failure

A variety of disorders of the neuromuscular apparatus, diaphragm, and chest wall cause pulmonary hypertension and cor pulmonale secondary to chronic hypoxia and/or compression of the pulmonary vessels.[13]

Chronic Hypoventilation

Chronic hypoventilation can be the result of

- Defective respiratory neuromuscular system, impaired function of the respiratory muscles
- Impaired ventilatory apparatus from restriction of the chest wall, as in kyphoscoliosis and obesity

Obesity Hypoventilation Syndrome

A small proportion of obese persons develop chronic hypercapnia, hypoxemia, and eventually polycythemia, pulmonary hypertension, and right-sided heart failure.[14]

The motivating force that has the greatest effect upon peripheral venous and lymphatic return is the movement of adjacent structures, collectively referred to as the muscular pump (item 5 in the factors affecting distribution of blood volume). To a significant extent but not entirely, this is due to the voluntary action of striated muscle. Movement of the muscles dynamically changes fascial tensions. These movements compress adjacent vessels, moving their contents centrally. The vessels possess valves that prevent retrograde flow of venous blood and lymph.

Circulatory Return to the Heart: The Two-Chambered Pump

The diaphragm is situated between the thoracic and abdominal cavities. This relationship creates a two-chambered pump that draws blood and lymph to the center. During inspiration the thoracic cage actively expands in all of its dimensions. The diaphragm contracts, and its dome descends. This produces the decrease in intrathoracic pressure associated with inspiratory filling of the lungs. At the same time, the descent of the diaphragm compresses the abdominal contents, causing increased intra-abdominal pressure.[15]

During expiration the thoracic cage passively recoils against the air-filled lungs; the diaphragm relaxes and ascends back into the thorax. The result is decreased intra-abdominal pressure and increased intrathoracic pressure. This mechanism, in association with the one-way valves of the veins and lymphatic vessels, squeezes fluid from the abdomen when negative intrathoracic pressure (inspiration) is sucking air and low-pressure fluids into the thorax. Alternately, expiration squeezes air from the lungs and blood and lymph from the veins and thoracic duct as the concomitant drop in intra-abdominal pressure sucks venous blood and lymph from the periphery in preparation for the next cycle.

The driving mechanism of this two-chamber pump is dependent upon the efficient movement of the thoracic cage and diaphragm. Dysfunctional mechanics of either will greatly reduce the pumping effect.

Venous return to the right atrium is affected by dysfunction of the peripheral muscular pump and the mechanics of respiration. This results in increased peripheral venous resistance and decreased cardiac preload.

The low-pressure pulmonary circulation is similarly affected by thoracic cage dysfunction, reducing left-sided preload.

Somatic Dysfunction: Definition

Somatic dysfunction is impaired or altered function of related components of the somatic (body framework) system: skeletal, arthrodial, and myofascial structures and related vascular, lymphatic, and neural elements. Somatic dysfunction is treatable using osteopathic manipulative treatment (OMT). The positional and motion aspects of somatic dysfunction are best described using at least one of three parameters: (1) the position of a body part as determined by palpation and referenced to its adjacent defined structure, (2) the directions in which motion is freer, and (3) the directions in which motion is restricted.[16]

Van Buskirk[17] offers a nociceptively initiated model for spinal somatic dysfunction as follows:

1. A peripheral focus of irritation results in activation of nociceptive neurons. These may be somatosensory or general visceral afferent neurons.
2. These primary afferent neurons synapse in the dorsal horn of the spinal cord with internuncial neurons.

3. Ongoing afferent stimulation of insufficient intensity to reach firing potential establishes a state of irritability (facilitation) of the internuncial neurons.
4. Additional afferent activity from any source results in a segmental response to significantly less stimulus than would normally be required.
5. Such activity from internuncial neurons, which synapse with ventral horn motor neurons, results in segmentally related myospasticity. Stimulation of internuncial neurons, which synapse in the intermediolateral cell column of the thoracic and upper lumbar cord, produce a segmentally related sympathetic response (somatic and/or visceral). The same response to stimulation applies to the parasympathetic efferent system. Moreover, internuncial neurons traverse up and down the spinal cord for several segments and synapse with the spinothalamic tract. Thus, these neurons are capable of initiating a broad response.

Somatovisceral reflexes also occur as the result of facilitation. In this case, the irritability of central nervous system affects a target organ through increased autonomic parasympathetic or sympathetic activity.

Integration of OMT into the Therapeutic Protocol

When treating a patient with congestive heart failure, as when treating a patient with any other problem, the physician can determine how to integrate the treatment of somatic dysfunction into the therapeutic protocol by asking the following questions:

1. How is musculoskeletal dysfunction affecting the patient's ability to respond to the disease process?
2. What sympathetic somatovisceral mechanisms are present? Spinal facilitation with resultant increased sympathetic tone increases vascular tone that decreases tissue perfusion.
3. What parasympathetic somatovisceral mechanisms are present? Spinal facilitation with resultant increased parasympathetic tone slows the heart rate.
4. How is circulatory stasis affecting the patient? The mechanical component of somatic dysfunction restricts motion. Efficient movement of the thoracic inlet, thoracic cage, abdominal diaphragm, mesenteries, and pelvic diaphragm is necessary for optimal low-pressure fluid (lymphatic and venous) dynamics. Inefficiency of this mechanism further adds fluid shift into the venous and lymphatic systems and decreased cardiac preload.

Somatic Dysfunction: Effects on Circulation

Contemporary medicine does not recognize the full extent to which anatomic dysfunction (a reversible condition) contributes to the overall health status and recuperative ability of the patient. The low-pressure venous (and lymphatic) return system is very susceptible to external compromise resulting from pressures placed upon it by dysfunctional musculoskeletal structures. Circulatory efficiency of the venous and lymphatic systems may be enhanced by (1) reducing local myofascial tensions that can compress and obstruct peripheral vessels, (2) ensuring mechanical efficiency of the thoracoabdominal two-chamber pump by treating dysfunction of the thoracic cage, thoracoabdominal diaphragm, thoracic inlet, and pelvis, and (3) treating thoracic somatic dysfunction to reduce the effects of facilitation and increased sympathetic tone upon peripheral vasculature and the heart.

CONCLUSION

OMT is classified as a form of alternative medical therapy.[18] It is applied to overcome a functional restraint to normal anatomic mobility diagnosed through the structural examination. Mechanical force applied to such a restraint results in freeing the anatomic region from that restraint.[6] Somatic dysfunction is associated with increased spinal cord neurologic activity, facilitation.[1] The facilitated spinal segment results in increased segmentally related efferent activity and somatovisceral reflexes. OMT reduces the spinal facilitation and somatovisceral effect.[1,19]

Therefore, a protocol for the application of OMT in the treatment of patients suffering from congestive heart failure was developed. It consists of cervical spine, soft tissue, articulation, and facilitated positional release; scalene release; thoracic inlet release; bilateral scapular release; thoracic lymphatic pump; range of motion upper thoracic region, including rib balancing and rib raising; respiratory diaphragm release and the cranial procedure, compression of the fourth ventricle (CV-4).[20] The sequence of application of the manipulative procedures is not important. Rather, it is appropriate to identify somatic dysfunction as it presents in the individual patient and treat what is found. Certain areas, however, should be specifically looked for. Thoracic cage compliance may be addressed by treating restrictions in the thoracic spine and ribs. Additionally, attention should be paid to the thoracoabdominal diaphragm, the thoracic inlet and the accessory muscles of respiration, particularly the scalene muscles. Diaphragmatic function may be further addressed by treating the cervical spine, C3 to C5, where spinal facilitation can affect the phrenic nerve. The upper cervical spine can be treated to reduce vagal somatovisceral effects, and upper thoracic dysfunction should be treated to reduce sympathetic somatovisceral effects. CV-4 may be performed for its apparent effect upon baroreflex physiology.

Congestive heart failure is a chronic condition with increasing incidence in association with aging. The clinical presentation of congestive heart failure is typically the result of the interplay between cardiac function and peripheral circulation. A significant noncardiac cause of congestive heart failure is restrictive mechanics of the thoracic cage. Aging tends to be accompanied by progressive loss of articular motion, hence progressive functional impairment. Disorders of the respiratory neuromusculoskeletal system can increase the workload of the myocardium through their effects upon pulmonary, venous, and lymphatic systemic circulation. This is encountered in kyphoscoliosis. Similar spinal mechanics, although of lesser degree, are found in most individuals.[7,21,22] Somatic dysfunction of the thoracic spine, ribs, and thoracoabdominal diaphragm results in decreased motion of the thoracic cage with diminished negative intrathoracic pressure during inspiration.[15,23] This in turn results in decreased cardiac preload, which aggravates the cardiac component of congestive heart failure. OMT employed to enhance thoracic cage mechanics should increase preload. Increasing preload and consequently diastolic ventricular volume will increase efficiency of the failing heart, thereby reducing the debilitating symptoms of congestive heart failure.

Upper thoracic somatic dysfunctions with associated spinal facilitation result in an increase of sympathetic tone to the myocardium and lungs.[2] Furthermore, somatic dysfunction of the thoracic spine is associated with increased efferent sympathetic activity that can increase cardiac afterload. Appropriately applied OMT results in peripheral vasodilation.[19] Such vasodilation can contribute to reducing afterload stresses placed upon the failing heart. OMT is not to be considered as primary treatment of congestive heart failure to replace appropriate pharmacotherapy. Appropriately applied OMT should therefore have adjunctive therapeutic value in the treatment of congestive heart failure. It offers benefit without side effects, and in the case of the individual with cardiovascular compromise, a small percentage of functional gain can exert tremendous effects.

Procedures

Cervical (Soft Tissue/Articulation) (See Chapter 10, Fig. 10.2)

This procedure is employed to decrease cervical tissue tension and enhance the symmetric range of motion of the cervical spine. (For diagnosis, see Chapter 3.)

Cervical (Facilitated Positional Release) (See Chapter 19, Fig. 19.1)

This procedure is employed to relax cervical muscle tension and treat articular somatic dysfunction. (For diagnosis, see Chapter 3.)

Patient position: supine. Physician position: seated at the patient's head, one hand employed to actively introduce the corrective positioning while the other hand monitors the area of dysfunction.

Procedure (Example: Paravertebral Muscle Tension on the Right Associated with Fryette II, C5 upon C6, Extended, Side Bent Right, Rotated Right)

1. Place your left hand palm up transversely from left to right at the level of C5.
2. The thumb of your left hand should rest lateral to the patient's neck on the left, and the distal pad of your index finger palpates (monitors) the tight right-sided paravertebral musculature at the level of C5.
3. With your right hand, grasp the top of the patient's head and lift it from the table to straighten the cervical lordosis.
4. In this position use your right hand to apply a compressive force through the patient's head and down the cervical spine to the level of C5. This force should begin to induce paravertebral relaxation at the level of C5 on the right and should be maintained throughout the remainder of the procedure.

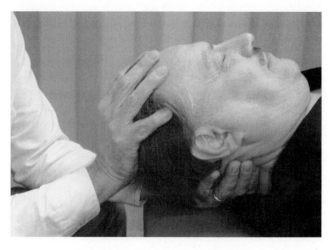

FIGURE 19.1 Cervical facilitated positional release, employed to relax cervical muscle tension and treat articular somatic dysfunction.

5. With your right hand, translate the head and upper cervical spine posteriorly to introduce extension at the level of C5 and monitor the tension in the paravertebral muscles for relaxation.
6. With your left hand, introduce right side-bending by laterally translating C5 to the left and monitor for continued paravertebral relaxation.
7. With your left hand, introduce right rotation by applying anteriorly directed pressure to the patient's left paravertebral musculature with your thenar eminence while continuing to monitor for paravertebral relaxation.
8. Hold C5 in the relaxed position for 3 seconds.
9. Slowly remove the compressive force from your right hand and return the patient's head and neck to the neutral position while monitoring with your left hand to ensure continued paravertebral relaxation.
10. Reassess C5 as it relates to C6.

Ultimately the purpose of this procedure is to induce paravertebral relaxation. The palpable softening of the tissue beneath your monitoring finger is the guide to proper positioning. The specifically localized combination of compression, forward and backward bending, side-bending, and rotation is key. If you introduce forces and the tissues tighten, move in the opposite direction; this will often result in the desired relaxation.

Thoracic Inlet (Myofascial Release) (Fig. 19.2)

This procedure is employed to release restrictions and thereby permit symmetric movement in the transverse fascial tissues of the thoracic inlet. It may be performed either as a direct or indirect procedure.

Patient position: supine. Physician position: seated to the side of the patient at the level of the shoulders.

Procedure (Example: Superficial Fascia of the Anterior Chest Wall Freely Moves to the Left)

1. Place one hand transversely beneath the patient posterior to the thoracic inlet at the level of the first and second ribs.

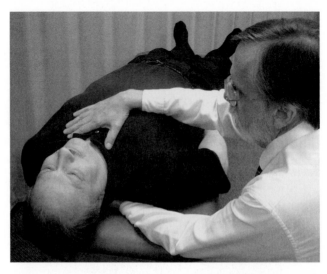

FIGURE 19.2 Thoracic inlet myofascial release, employed to release restrictions and thereby result in symmetric movement in the transverse fascial tissues of the thoracic inlet.

2. Place the other hand at the same level upon the chest wall anteriorly.
3. With the hand on the anterior chest, introduce left and right translation, rotation or twisting, and superior or inferior translation to evaluate available motion for myofascial restrictions.
4. Once asymmetric tension has been identified, the area may be treated indirectly by moving the anterior hand to the position of fascial ease or directly by engaging the soft tissue barrier. Having the patient take a few deep breaths can facilitate a release.
5. With either the direct or indirect method, hold the position and wait for a release, the perception of relaxation of tension, to occur.
6. Reassess the thoracic inlet.

Scapulothoracic (Myofascial Release) (Fig. 19.3)

This procedure is employed to increase the range of motion of the scapula in relation to the thoracic cage.

Patient position: lying upon the side with the dysfunctional side up. Physician position: standing facing the patient at the level of the shoulders.

Procedure (Example: Decreased Range of Motion of the Left Scapulothoracic Relationship)

1. Abduct the patient's left shoulder and place the patient's left forearm upon your left shoulder.
2. Side-bend your neck to the left and hold the patient's forearm between your neck and shoulder.

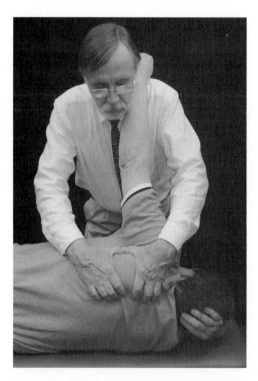

FIGURE 19.3 Scapulothoracic myofascial release, employed to increase the range of motion of the scapula in relation to the thoracic cage.

3. Lean back and apply gentle traction upon the patient's scapula through the arm.
4. Grasp the patient's scapula with both hands and assess its range of motion relative to the posterior chest wall by introducing superior, inferior, medial, and lateral glide and clockwise and counterclockwise motions.
5. Once dysfunctional myofascial tension has been identified, treat the area indirectly by moving the scapula to the position of fascial ease or directly by engaging the soft tissue barrier. Having the patient take a few deep breaths can facilitate a release.
6. With either the direct or indirect method, hold the position and wait for a release, the perception of relaxation of tension, to occur.
7. Reassess the range of motion of the scapula in relation to the thoracic cage.

Lymphatic Pump (Oscillatory Modification) (See Fig. 16.19)

This procedure is employed to facilitate lymphatic and venous return to the heart and to reduce pulmonary congestion through the introduction of alternating positive and negative intrathoracic pressure and improved thoracic cage mobility.

Patient position: supine. Physician position: standing at the head of the table or bed. To prevent aspiration be sure the patient does not have any foreign objects (food, gum, or dentures) in the mouth.

Procedure

1. Place your hands palm down upon the patient's anterior chest wall over the pectoralis major muscles.
2. Straighten your arms and lock your elbows.
3. Instruct the patient to exhale in a relaxed fashion through the open mouth.
4. Lean gently upon the anterior thoracic cage with your hands and follow the exhalation.
5. Toward the end of exhalation, exert a rhythmic pumping action with your hands by an alternating pressure through your hands to produce a slight alternating positive and negative intrathoracic pressure.

Thoracic Soft Tissue Articulation Procedure (Patient on Side) (See Chapter 5 and Fig. 5.3)

This procedure is employed to decrease paravertebral muscle spasm and soft tissue tension of the thoracic spine. (For diagnosis, see Chapter 3.)

Rib Raising (See Chapter 5, Fig. 5.6 and Chapter 17, Fig. 17.1)

This procedure is employed to enhance rib motion and thoracic cage compliance. Consequently it augments venous and lymphatic return to the chest. It is also thought to affect sympathetic tone, initially stimulating regional sympathetic output but eventually resulting in reduction in sympathetic activity from the spinal levels treated.

Thoracoabdominal Diaphragm Release (Fig. 19.4)

This procedure is employed to relax the diaphragm and increase the diaphragmatic component of respiratory excursion.

Patient position: supine. Physician position: standing to the side of the patient at the level of the diaphragm and facing the patient's head.

Procedure

1. Place your hands on either side of the thorax at the level of the diaphragm with your fingers pointing posteriorly toward the thoracolumbar junction and your thumbs pointing anteriorly toward the xiphoid process.

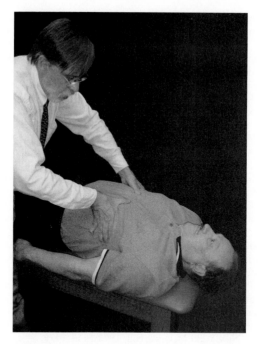

FIGURE 19.4   Thoracoabdominal diaphragm release, employed to relax the diaphragm and increase the diaphragmatic component of respiratory excursion.

2. Instruct the patient to breathe slowly and deeply.
3. Laterally compress the lower ribs between your two hands.
4. Follow respiratory excursion, palpating for asymmetric motion.
5. Once asymmetric tension has been identified, treat the area indirectly by moving your hands in the direction that reduces tension or directly by engaging the soft tissue barrier. Having the patient take a few slow deep breaths or hold the breath to tolerance in exhalation (indirect) or in inhalation (direct) can facilitate a release.
6. With either the direct or indirect method, hold the position and wait for a release, the perception of relaxation of tension.
7. Have the patient breathe deeply and reassess diaphragmatic excursion.

Compression of the Fourth Ventricle (CV-4) (See Chapter 10 And Fig. 10.1)

This procedure is employed to stimulate the body's inherent recuperative ability by promoting fluid interchange. It is thought to especially influence lymphatic and cerebrospinal fluid circulation.

References

1. Korr IM, Wright HM, Chace JA. Cutaneous patterns of sympathetic activity in clinical abnormalities of the musculoskeletal system. Acta Neuroveg (Wien) 1964;25:589–606.
2. Beal MC, ed. Louisa Burns, DO, Memorial. 1994 Yearbook. Indianapolis: American Academy of Osteopathy, 1994.
3. Nelson KE, Sergueef N, Lipinski CM, et al. Cranial rhythmic impulse related to the Traube-Hering-Mayer oscillation: Comparing laser-Doppler flowmetry and palpation. J Am Osteopath Assoc 2001;101:163–173.

4. Sergueef N, Nelson KE, Glonek T. The effect of cranial manipulation on the Traube-Hering-Meyer oscillation as measured by laser-Doppler flowmetry. Altern Ther Health Med 2002;8(6):74–76.

5. Nelson KE, Sergueef N, Glonek T. Cranial manipulation induces sequential changes in blood flow velocity on demand. AAO J 2004;14(3):15–17.

6. Fryette HH. Principles of Osteopathic Technic. Indianapolis: American Academy of Osteopathy, 1954, 1980.

7. Kappler RE. Palpatory skills and exercises for developing the sense of touch. In: Ward RC, ed. Foundations for Osteopathic Medicine. 2nd ed. Philadelphia: Lippincott Williams & Wilkins, 2002;557–565.

8. Braunwald E. Heart failure. In: Fauci AS, ed. Harrison's Principles of Internal Medicine. 14th ed. New York: McGraw Hill, 1998;1287.

9. Braunwald E. Normal and abnormal myocardial function. In: Fauci AS, ed. Harrison's Principles of Internal Medicine. 14th ed. New York: McGraw Hill, 1998;1278–1282.

10. Ross J Jr, Covell JW. Frameworks for analysis of ventricular and circulatory function: Integrated responses. In: West JB, ed. Best and Taylor's Physiological Basis of Medical Practice. 12th ed. Baltimore: Williams & Wilkins, 1990;296–299.

11. Ross J Jr. Introduction to the cardiovascular system. In: West JB, ed. Best and Taylor's Physiological Basis of Medical Practice. 12th ed. Baltimore: Williams & Wilkins, 1990;112.

12. West JB. Pulmonary blood flow and metabolism. In: West JB, ed. Best and Taylor's Physiological Basis of Medical Practice. 12th ed. Baltimore: Williams & Wilkins, 1990;529–531.

13. Braunwald E. Cor pulmonale. In: Fauci AS, ed. Harrison's Principles of Internal Medicine. 14th ed. New York: McGraw Hill, 1998;1327.

14. Phillipson EA. Disorders of ventilation. In: Fauci AS, ed. Harrison's Principles of Internal Medicine. 14th ed. New York: McGraw Hill, 1998;1476–1479.

15. Miller CE. The mechanics of lymphatic circulation: Lymph hearts. J Am Osteopath Assoc 1923;22:397–398, 415–416.

16. Glossary of osteopathic terminology. In: Ward RC, ed. Foundations for Osteopathic Medicine. 2nd ed. Philadelphia: Lippincott Williams & Wilkins, 2002;1249.

17. Van Buskirk RL. Nociceptive reflexes and the somatic dysfunction: A model. J Am Osteopath Assoc 1990;90:797–809 [review].

18. National Institutes of Health. The National Center for Complementary and Alternative Medicine (NCCAM). Strategic Plan (Stephen E. Straus, Director). http://nccam.nih.gov/nccam/strategic. Page expired. For past and present NCCAM strategic plans visit http://nccam.nih.gov/ or contact the NCCAM Clearinghouse, P.O. Box 7923, Gaithersburg, MD 20898-7923.

19. Kappler RE, Kelso AF. Thermographic studies of skin temperature in patients receiving osteopathic manipulative treatment for peripheral nerve problems. J Am Osteopath Assoc 1984;84:76–EOA.

20. Scheunemen GM, Mnabhi AKS, Papp MA, et al. Osteopathic manipulative treatment and congestive heart failure. J Am Osteopath Assoc 2003;103:379–EOA [abstract].

21. Schwab WA. Principles of manipulative treatment: The low back problem. 1965 Yearbook. Vol 2. Indianapolis: American Academy of Osteopathy, 1965;95.

22. Nelson KE. The management of low back pain: Short leg syndrome/postural balance. AAO J 1999;9(1):33–39.

23. Rumney IC. Osteopathic manipulative treatment of infectious diseases. Osteopath Ann 1974;2(7):29–30, 32–33.

CHAPTER 20

The Patient with Gastrointestinal Problems

Kenneth E. Nelson and Ann L. Habenicht

INTRODUCTION

Gastroenterology, as a subspecialty of internal medicine, may not initially appear to lend itself to the application of osteopathic principles. Indeed, if it is approached solely as the diagnosis and treatment of gastrointestinal diseases, it may be exclusive of osteopathic principles.

Osteopathic philosophy in practice is patient oriented rather than disease oriented. The patient is viewed as an integrated manifestation of all the various systems (holism). The nervous and circulatory systems are given particular consideration in this approach because of their contact with all other systems. They link the component parts of the body into a holistic mechanism.

The musculoskeletal system is also of great importance in osteopathic medicine. Dysfunction of the musculoskeletal system, somatic dysfunction, can affect the total health status of the patient. It does this directly through mechanical influences and indirectly through the nervous and circulatory systems. Somatic dysfunction is a reversible condition and is not itself a disease process. It may be the result of mechanical stresses, or it may be a manifestation of neurologic activity, as in the case of viscerosomatic reflexes.

These relationships specifically apply to the gastrointestinal tract. The gastrointestinal tract is obviously linked to the holistic mechanism through the vascular system. The lymphatic and venous drainage of the gastrointestinal tract is a major portal of entry of nutrients and occasionally noxious substances into the body. The gastrointestinal tract is also united with the rest of the body by the nervous system through viscerosomatic, somatovisceral, and viscerovisceral reflexes.

If the patient with a problem of the gastrointestinal system is approached from this perspective, this subspecialty subject is easily linked into the holistic practice of osteopathic medicine.

Nutrition is an important component of a holistic approach to health care. There is a particularly obvious relationship between diet, gastrointestinal function, and nutritional status. It is easy to see how gastrointestinal dysfunction can untowardly affect nutritional status and how dietary intolerance can result in gastrointestinal dysfunction. It is also easy to see how nutritional deficiencies and excesses affect health status.

If the term *functional* precedes a disease process (e.g., functional gastritis), it implies a condition without demonstrable organic pathology. Symptoms such as dyspepsia, nausea, vomiting, belching, flatus, and diarrhea may be functional or the result of some organic pathology.[1]

The patient with cholecystitis has an organic cause for the symptoms. The patient with postcholecystectomy syndrome has persistent symptoms after the organic pathology has been effectively removed.[2] This functional condition appears to be the result of a persistent somatovisceral reflex. Anecdotal evidence indicates that when osteopathic manipulative treatment (OMT) is employed to treat somatic dysfunction of the low thoracic region, the symptoms of postcholecystectomy syndrome quickly resolve.[3]

Similarly, constipation is typically the result of inadequate consumption of dietary fiber and water, possibly exacerbated by diminished peristalsis. Increased sympathetic tone can decrease peristalsis. Thoracolumbar somatic dysfunction can have this effect upon the intestines through somatovisceral reflex activity.[4]

Physical activity mechanically stimulates peristalsis. Discomfort associated with somatic dysfunction interferes with ease of movement. In elderly individuals who are predisposed to constipation, diminished activity because of treatable somatic dysfunction can contribute significantly to intestinal stasis. Prolonged gastrointestinal transit time is associated with the development of pathology, including diverticulosis of the colon.[5]

This chapter addresses the osteopathically distinctive component of the diagnosis and treatment of gastrointestinal disorders.

VISCEROSOMATIC AND SOMATOVISCERAL REFLEXES

Viscerosomatic reflexes are distinctively osteopathic diagnostic tools. Tissue texture change and tenderness to palpation are found in soft tissue as a reflex manifestation of segmentally (spinal cord) related visceral pathology. Viscerosomatic reflexes occur as follows:[6]

1. A peripheral focus of irritation (e.g., visceral pathology) results in increased general visceral afferent (GVA) neural activity. These are the afferent nerves of the autonomic nervous system. They travel with the sympathetic and parasympathetic nerves.
2. GVA neurons synapse in the dorsal horn of the spinal cord with internuncial neurons. The increase in GVA activity produces a condition of irritability (facilitation) of the internuncial neurons and consequently of that spinal segment. In severe conditions, the facilitation will spread up and down the cord through the internuncial neurons to involve adjacent segments.

3. The segmental facilitation manifests itself as increased efferent activity to all areas innervated by that spinal segment, with resultant paravertebral changes in muscular and—in the thoracolumbar region—vasomotor tone (tissue texture change). This same physiology produces somatovisceral and viscerovisceral reactions through sympathetic and parasympathetic efferent neurons.
4. Spinal facilitation also makes segmentally related tissues more sensitive to exogenous stimulation (tenderness).
5. These manifestations are directly proportional to the intensity of input from the visceral focus of irritation and therefore are quantifiable.

Because viscerosomatic reflex patterns are relatively segmentally specific and demonstrate proportionate reactivity, they provide diagnostic information as to the site and severity of the underlying condition. The quantitative aspect of the reflexes also offers the osteopathic practitioner a simple method to monitor the progress of the disease process. Viscerosomatic reflexes augment diagnosis and are not intended to replace other aspects of physical diagnosis or laboratory and radiological studies.

As an example, an awareness of viscerosomatic patterns may assist in differentiating between upper gastrointestinal symptoms resulting from myocardial disease (T1–T5 left-sided) and gastric disease (T5–T10 left-sided).[6]

Somatovisceral reflexes also occur as the result of facilitation. In this case, the irritability of the central nervous system affects a target organ through increased parasympathetic or sympathetic autonomic activity.

Viscerosomatic reflexes are classified as parasympathetic or sympathetic according to the somatovisceral reflexes segmentally associated with them.

Viscerosomatic reflex findings with parasympathetic association are palpable in the paravertebral soft tissues of the high cervical and sacral regions.

The high cervical parasympathetic viscerosomatic reflex is the vagal reflex. After exiting the skull, the vagus nerve interdigitates with C1 and C2 within the cervical plexus.[7] Vagal reflexes are found at the level of the occiput, C1, and C2, with greater tendency for a right-sided reaction from pancreas, liver, gallbladder, small intestine, ascending colon, and the right half of the transverse colon. The left-sided upper cervical reaction occurs classically with upper gastrointestinal problems (esophagus, stomach, and duodenum).

The sacral parasympathetic reflex (S2, S3, S4) is associated with conditions affecting the left half of the transverse colon, descending colon, sigmoid, and rectum.

Viscerosomatic reflex findings with sympathetic association are palpable as tissue texture change and tenderness in the thoracolumbar paravertebral soft tissues as follows:

T3 to T6, right-sided reaction	Esophagus
T5 to T10, left-sided reaction	Stomach
T6 to T8, right-sided reaction	Duodenum
T5 to T9, bilateral block reaction	Pancreas; in chronic pancreatitis area tends to be fixed in extension
T5 to T10, right-sided reaction	Liver
T9 to T10, right-sided reaction	Gallbladder
T8 to T10, bilateral reaction (R > L)	Small intestine
T9 to T12, right-sided reaction	Appendix; associated with tenderness over the tip of the 12th rib on the right (anterior Chapman's tender point)
T11 to L1, right-sided reaction	Cecum and ascending colon
L1 to L3, left-sided reaction	Descending colon

The combination of C2 left, T3 to T6 right, T5 to T10 left, and T6 to T8 right is referred to as the *upper gastrointestinal* pattern.

The locations of the somatic manifestations of visceral dysfunction or pathology are generally predictable. The intensity of the tissue texture change mirrors the severity of the visceral problem. Viscerosomatic reflexes add greatly to physical diagnosis and may also be used to follow the clinical progression of a disease. Neoplastic diseases do not produce typical viscerosomatic reflex responses. The cord level response for the involved viscus will occur, but because neoplasm typically develops without innervation, there is no direct source of afferent input. Reflex activity occurs as a result of visceral displacement and inflammation from the presence of the neoplasm, not from the neoplasm itself. As such, the reflex, when encountered, is often less intense than would be anticipated considering the severity of the disease.

Chapman's reflexes, another viscerosomatic-somatovisceral system, are a group of palpable nodular areas of tissue texture change that have diagnostic and therapeutic significance. They are considered to be a neurolymphatic reaction. Treatment of these points using inhibitory pressure is reported to be an effective treatment of visceral complaints.[8] The posterior reflex points in Chapman's system in many instances approximate the locations of the viscerosomatic reflexes listed previously.

The integration of the treatment of somatic dysfunction into the therapeutic protocol with OMT is indicated for the specific treatment of somatic dysfunction. As stated previously, somatic dysfunction is functional impairment of the neuro-musculoskeletal system. Although it may exist in the presence of pathology, it is not in itself pathology. OMT for treatment of somatic dysfunction is used to increase available motion, modify activity of the nervous system, or increase tissue perfusion.

The integration of the diagnosis and treatment of somatic dysfunction into the practice of gastroenterology may initially seem superfluous. The severity of illnesses encountered and the fact that the gastrointestinal system is considered to be separate from the musculoskeletal system make the diagnosis of somatic dysfunction seem inconsequential. Furthermore, OMT is not directly used for the treatment of gastrointestinal disease processes. Why then should one diagnose and treat somatic dysfunction in the patient with gastrointestinal complaints and/or pathology?

It is beneficial, if a patient complains of a pain that resembles a gastrointestinal problem, to determine whether it is actually a primary musculoskeletal problem amenable to OMT.

If the problem is gastrointestinal, is it functional or organic? Functional complaints that result from somatovisceral reflexes respond to the treatment of underlying somatic dysfunction.

When treating a patient with an organic gastrointestinal disease process, the physician can determine how to integrate the treatment of somatic dysfunction into the therapeutic protocol by answering the following questions:[4]

1. How is musculoskeletal dysfunction affecting the patient's ability to respond to the disease process?
2. What sympathetic somatovisceral mechanisms are present? Spinal facilitation with resultant increased sympathetic tone increases vascular tone, hence decreases tissue perfusion and nutrient and oxygen supply to tissues and thereby increases any need for anaerobic glycolysis. It relaxes the gallbladder and biliary ducts and decreases the glandular secretions and peristalsis, producing constipation or ileus.

3. What parasympathetic somatovisceral mechanisms are present? Spinal facilitation with resultant increased parasympathetic tone increases the secretion of the digestive enzymes amylase and lipase. It causes contraction of the gallbladder and biliary ducts and increased glandular secretions and peristalsis, producing diarrhea.
4. How is circulatory stasis affecting the patient? The mechanical component of somatic dysfunction results in restriction of motion. Efficient movement of the thoracic inlet, thoracic cage, abdominal diaphragm, mesenteries, and pelvic diaphragm is necessary for optimal low-pressure fluid (lymphatic and venous) dynamics and tissue perfusion. Inefficiency of this mechanism further adds to the tendency toward tissue congestion.

Viscerosomatic reflexes cause muscle spasm, tenderness, and pain. Part of the diagnostic dilemma is the differentiation between a viscerosomatic reflex and primary somatic dysfunction. The pelvic diaphragm is innervated by the pudendal nerve (S2–S4) of the pelvic splanchnic nerves. Pain in this area may be viscerosomatic, pelvic parasympathetic, or simply the result of sacropelvic somatic dysfunction. Proper application of OMT resolves primary somatic dysfunction. Although viscerosomatic reflexes can be affected by OMT, the associated somatic findings will not resolve until the underlying visceral condition is treated. Failure of somatic dysfunction to respond to OMT should lead to the consideration of a viscerosomatic etiology. Indeed, part of the evaluation of any somatic dysfunction should include inquiry about segmentally related viscera. Appendicular complaints may result from viscerosomatic-somatic reflexes, as in the example of left arm pain resulting from myocardial ischemia.

CHOOSING AND USING THE PROCEDURE

Having decided what to treat and how the treatment is intended to affect the patient, the physician must decide upon the manipulative procedure to employ. Patient tolerance dictates the level of aggressiveness of the procedure chosen. A somewhat artificial continuum of procedure can be created based upon the relative aggressiveness of the procedure.

• High-velocity, low-amplitude (HVLA)—most aggressive
• Articulation
• Soft tissue
• Direct fascial release
• Muscle energy
• Counterstrain
• Facilitated positional release
• Indirect fascial release
• Inhibitory pressure
• Indirect cranial—least aggressive

As stated, this list is quite arbitrary and open to debate, but the idea is valid. Also, besides the aggressiveness of the procedure type, the time required for application affects patient tolerance. The longer a procedure takes, the less the patient may be able to tolerate it. As a rule, the more aggressive the procedure, the less time required for its application.

How much OMT is enough? Treat the patient until a response occurs. What kind of response? Relaxation of the soft tissue in the area being treated is a good response. Altered autonomic tone is also an indication of a response. Peripheral vasodilation resulting in increased skin temperature or redness and increased sudomotor (sweating) activity indicate it is time to stop. Increased heart or respiratory rate also indicates that the patient's level of tolerance has been reached. If the patient feels that intervention is too uncomfortable, the physician should stop and choose another approach or return later and try again.

Clinical Example: Pancreatitis

The Disease

Pancreatitis is classified as acute or chronic. Acute pancreatitis is most frequently encountered as the result of gallstone obstruction of the common duct (choledocholithiasis). The condition resolves clinically and histologically once the obstruction is eliminated. Chronic relapsing pancreatitis, which typically results from alcohol abuse, persists histologically after cessation of the etiologic circumstance. Both acute and chronic relapsing (histologic) pancreatitis are most often encountered clinically as acute pancreatitis. There are many other causes of pancreatitis. Choledocholithiasis and alcoholism, however, account for most cases.[9]

The patient has severe constant upper abdominal pain and referred pain that radiates through to the mid to low thoracic region of the back. There may be cephalgia. There is nausea, vomiting, diaphoresis, tachycardia, and shallow tachypnea. The patient's temperature may be normal or slightly elevated. The abdominal wall may be rigid, with rebound tenderness. Bowel sounds are hypoactive. In severe cases, the liberation of pancreatic enzymes results in pancreatic autolysis and shock.

The Pain Pattern

Initially, the acutely inflamed pancreas is perceived as a deep dull pain. As the inflammatory process involves the pancreatic visceral peritoneum, which contains unmyelinated nociceptive nerve endings, the pain becomes severe. At this point, peritoneal signs develop. Further spread of the inflammatory process involves the parietal peritoneum of the anterior abdominal wall. This results in the rigid abdominal wall splinting seen in pancreatitis. The patient perceives referred pain in the interscapular region. Occipital headache may also be present.

The generalized upper abdominal pain associated with acute pancreatitis seems easy to understand. The pancreas is an upper abdominal midline organ. The viscerosomatic reflex from pancreas makes this pain distribution even more logical. The pancreas reflex is bilateral from T5 to T9. The T5 through T9 dermatomes supply the upper abdominal wall. Spinal facilitation produces segmental hyperalgesia. The bilateral involvement of the pancreas reflex results in sensitization of the entire upper abdominal wall. Pancreatic referred pain in the mid to low thoracic region is a direct manifestation of the location of the pancreas in association with the bilateral T5 through T9 paravertebral tenderness of the viscerosomatic reflex. The occipital headache is a result of the vagal viscerosomatic reflex through the greater and lesser occipital nerves that originate from C2 and C3.

The Musculoskeletal Palpatory Findings

The sympathetic viscerosomatic reflex from the pancreas is found bilaterally from T5 to T9. Paravertebral tissue texture change is palpable at these levels. The more severe the condition, the greater the area of tissue texture change. In longstanding cases of chronic pancreatitis, this area becomes extended, demonstrating flattening or reversal of the thoracic kyphosis. The parasympathetic (vagal) viscerosomatic reflex is found in the upper cervical region (occiput to C2). It is unilateral, with a greater incidence on the right. This reflex is particularly useful for monitoring progression of the illness because its suboccipital location makes it easily accessible in the bedridden patient. If pancreatitis develops as the result of cholecystitis and choledocholithiasis, a gallbladder reflex will be present at T10 right. If it develops in association with alcoholic hepatitis, a slightly broader reaction, T9 to T10 right, can be expected. With the development of ileus, a small intestinale reflex will be present, T8 to T10 bilateral, right greater than left. The upper gastrointestinal irritation associated with the nausea and vomiting that accompany pancreatitis produces an upper gastrointestinal reflex pattern of occiput to C2 left (vagus), T3 to T6 right (esophagus), T5 to T10 left (stomach), and T6 to T8 right (duodenum). The accompanying peritonitis involves the parietal and visceral peritoneum. The parietal peritoneum is innervated by somatic nerves; therefore, parietal peritonitis produces a somatosomatic paravertebral reflex with palpable findings in the low thoracic and mid cervical (phrenic) regions.

The somatic findings paravertebrally in the upper cervical region and from T5 to T9 bilaterally in association with the signs and symptoms of pancreatitis are very useful information. As can readily be seen, the more complex the presentation and the more intense the pathology, the greater the area of viscerosomatic reflex paravertebral tissue texture change. In severe pancreatitis, the entire cervical, thoracic, and upper lumbar regions may become reactive.

Viscerosomatic reflex findings are a part of the complete physical examination. They are not intended to replace examination of the rest of the patient. On the contrary, the palpatory skill level necessary to perform the osteopathic musculoskeletal examination has great value for palpating the acute abdomen and elsewhere. A complete history and physical examination give the information necessary to formulate differential diagnoses. The more information available, the more precise the diagnosis. Diagnoses are confirmed or ruled out using technological methods (e.g., laboratory, ultrasound, radiography, computed tomography, magnetic resonance imaging). The more precise the diagnoses are, the more cost effective the use of techno-diagnostic procedures.

Treatment

Acute pancreatitis may vary in intensity from mild to life threatening. The basic treatment is supportive, with specific treatment directed at underlying conditions. OMT used at this time is intended to reduce the intensity of the acute condition. The patient's tolerance is reduced, and care must be taken not to use a procedure that is unnecessarily stimulating.

The sympathetic viscerosomatic reflexes associated with pancreatitis and consequently the areas that are treated for somatovisceral effect are found in the mid to low thoracic region. The parasympathetic reflexes are found in the upper cervical and suboccipital region. The intensity of the visceral pathology determines the amount of spinal facilitation present. Paravertebral tissue texture change is directly proportional to the severity of visceral pathology. The use of OMT to produce a somatovisceral response is not simply "pushing the button" at the anticipated reflex level. Osteopathic physicians must use their palpatory skills to determine the areas of maximum tissue texture change, then, with an appreciation for the degree of tolerance of the patient, decide upon the type of procedure to use.

For treating an acute viscerosomatic reflex for somatovisceral effect, inhibitory pressure is useful. Inhibitory pressure is a direct procedure that may be described as extremely low velocity and low amplitude. Pressure is applied over the area of maximum tissue texture change using the distal phalangeal pad of the finger or thumb. The pressure is increased very slowly as the target tissues relax. The development of reactive muscle spasm indicates that the procedure is too aggressive and should be stopped. When tolerated, the pressure is applied and held until pressure anesthesia develops in the treating physician's thumb or finger. (If pressure anesthesia is sensed by the treating physician, it is probable that pressure anesthesia also has been produced in the tissues being treated.) At this time, the pressure is very slowly released. This procedure may be repeated in 1 or 2 hours depending upon the patient's tolerance. It may be employed in the thoracic region for sympathetic effect and in the upper cervical region for parasympathetic effect.

The peritonitis associated with acute pancreatitis limits diaphragmatic excursion. This predisposes the patient to lower pulmonary atelectasis and pneumonia. Gentle thoracic and costal mobilization and rib raising to tolerance are appropriate here. As the peritonitis begins to subside, myofascial procedures for the abdominal wall, diaphragmatic release, and thoracic pump procedures should be employed.

The limitation of thoracic cage and abdominal wall mobility and decreased diaphragmatic excursion severely limits the return of lymph to the general circulation. This has enormous consequences when pancreatic inflammation has shifted fluid into the interstitial space. The presence of cellular debris and macromolecules in the fluid exert significant osmotic force, making lymphatic drainage the only route of egress. The procedures identified previously are also appropriate therapy here. As soon as patient tolerance permits, lymphatic (pedal pump and thoracic pump) procedures should be initiated.

Clinical Example: Cholecystitis

The Disease

Cholecystitis is very common in the United States. Approximately 90% of patients with cholecystitis have gallstones with the potential for obstruction.[10] In 1996, 30 million people were diagnosed with cholecystitis with lithiasis and nearly 900,000 cholecystectomies were performed. The remaining 10% of these patients are described as having acalculous cholecystitis, or cholecystitis without gallstone formation.[11] It is this 10% of cases of cholecystitis that the osteopathic physician may often diagnose through the use of viscerosomatic reflexes.

The diagnosis of cholecystitis is often difficult, as its common symptoms of belching, bloating, heartburn, fatty food intolerance, chronic right upper quadrant pain, right shoulder pain, and mid epigastric pain may also be symptoms of peptic ulcer disease, appendicitis, ileitis, and hepatitis. Also, cholecystitis may cause right lower quadrant pain, left upper quadrant pain, and even chest pain as atypical presentations.[11,12] Gallbladder disease is often considered only after the patient with symptoms of peptic ulcer disease is unresponsive to the use of H_2 blockers or proton pump inhibitors.

Cholecystitis does not have any specific laboratory markers to help with diagnosis. If a biliary duct obstruction has been persistent, mildly elevated transaminases with leukocytosis may result, but alcoholic hepatitis will also produce these changes.[11] Procedures such as hepatic and gallbladder ultrasounds may help with the diagnosis when gallbladder wall thickening and stones are present. The presence of gallstones does not necessarily mean the patient has clinically significant disease. Many patients have gallstones without acute disease.[11]

Nuclear imaging may also be useful in the diagnosis. Biliary tract imaging, hipoto-iminodiacetic acid (HIDA), para-isopropyl acetanilido-iminodiacetic acid (PIPIDA), or diisopropyl iminodiacetic acid (DECIDA, pronounced des-ī-da) scans are useful in determining obstruction of the biliary tract. If cholecystitis is present, the gallbladder will not fill with radioactive contrast by retrograde flow through the cystic duct. The assumption is that the cystic duct wall is too edematous and inflamed to permit flow of the radionucleotide from the common duct through the cystic duct and into the gallbladder. When used in conjunction with ultrasound findings of thickened duct and gallbladder walls, this information carries a high probability that the diagnosis of acute cholecystitis is correct, but it is not always conclusive.[13]

The Musculoskeletal Palpatory Findings

The viscerosomatic reflex from liver and gallbladder has been identified as right-sided paravertebral tissue texture change from T5 to T10 posteriorly.[6,14–17]

Recently, Miller and associates[18] studied the relationship of the visceral gallbladder afferent projections in the mouse to determine the neuroanatomical relationship of visceral gallbladder neurons to somatic intercostal neurons via the dorsal root ganglion. Fast blue dye was placed in the gallbladder of the experimental mice. A second dye, nuclear yellow, was placed on severed ends of thoracic intercostal nerves. The dyes traveled retrograde along the axons via axonal transport. After 48 to 72 hours, the mice were killed. Of the experimental mice, 80% revealed the presence of dyes from both the gallbladder and the intercostal nerves in the dorsal root ganglia at the T9 to T12 levels on the right. The findings of this experiment confirm the presence of bifurcating viscerosomatic dorsal root ganglion cells (bifurcating peripheral processes from individual dorsal root ganglion cells to the gallbladder and intercostal nerves) in the mouse. Thus, Miller's findings demonstrate that at least for mice the viscerosomatic reflex from gallbladder is between the levels of T9 to T12 on the right.

The palpatory examination during an acute episode of cholecystitis will reveal tissue texture changes in the areas of the costotransverse articulation and the rib angles on the right, most intensely at T9 and T10. These changes include moisture, puffiness, tenderness, warmth, and redness. The patient may also have findings consistent with the viscerosomatic pattern from upper gastrointestinal irritation (C1–C2 left, T3–T6 right, T5–T10 left). They may also demonstrate a restriction of motion of the right hemidiaphragm.

Spinal cord segment facilitation thus allows the trained osteopathic physician to differentiate between different disease processes. This is particularly useful when standard physical and laboratory findings are inconclusive.

Treatment

Initial treatment of the patient with cholecystitis depends on the severity of the patient's symptoms. Symptomatic patients who are ambulatory and afebrile, without dehydration or signs of an acute abdomen, may be given dietary restrictions as the first line of treatment. Reduction of fatty foods may prevent further gallbladder attacks, especially in patients without stone formation. Treatment of areas of somatic dysfunction will also improve neural function to the areas.

Some patients with disease accompanied by stone formation can be maintained with the fatty food restrictions, but often the chronic irritation of the gallbladder from the stones and the chance of expulsion of stones and possible obstruction of the cystic or common ducts remains quite high. As a result, small amounts of fatty foods may trigger an attack precipitating a surgical emergency with increased morbidity as opposed to an elective surgical intervention. Surgical removal of the gallbladder, therefore, is often recommended to patients with gallbladder disease and stone formation.

The diagnosis of somatic dysfunction is not only important in the effective treatment of musculoskeletal complaints but also useful in diagnosing visceral pathology. Viscerosomatic reflexes result in somatic dysfunction that is resistant to OMT.

OMT works only after the visceral component is treated. Reoccurring areas of somatic dysfunction, especially when the areas are consistent with a viscerosomatic reflex pattern, should alert the physician that underlying visceral pathology may be present. This is true especially with the recurrent gastrointestinal pattern. A complaint of persistent right shoulder pain in the absence of trauma should be a red flag to the osteopathic physician and raise a high suspicion of underlying gallbladder disease.

Surgical removal of the diseased gallbladder may remove the cause of the patient's discomfort, but often some of the patient's symptoms remain or return. Careful evaluation of the thoracic area will reveal the persistent reflex pattern. Treatment of the residual viscerosomatic reflex using OMT will help resolve the patient's symptoms. Treatment of the reflex areas will help to reset the neural input and normalize the facilitated areas.

CONCLUSION

Little has been said here about the importance of nutrition in the care of the gastrointestinal patient. While this is an extremely important subject, its inclusion here would have greatly expanded the size of this chapter. This discussion stresses musculoskeletal diagnosis and treatment, the focus of this chapter.

Musculoskeletal diagnosis and treatment must be integrated into the total diagnostic and therapeutic protocol for the patient with gastrointestinal pathology. OMT is not intended as a replacement therapy. It is intended to enhance therapy by facilitating the body's inherent capacity to heal itself. The use of osteopathic diagnosis and treatment procedures should reduce the morbidity and mortality associated with gastrointestinal pathology. Although this makes sense, the statistical support for it does not yet exist. Much of what has been presented here is anecdotal, based upon more than 100 years of osteopathic clinical empiricism. The challenge to substantiate this distinctive approach to patient care rests upon the osteopathic profession. It is hoped that by describing the integration of the diagnosis and treatment of somatic dysfunction for patients with gastrointestinal pathology the profession can identify protocols upon which to base future outcomes studies.

Procedures

Please note: The procedures that follow are examples of manipulative treatment that you may wish to employ. The actual choice of procedures used should be determined by the unique circumstances of each individual patient.

The following procedures are useful when treating the somatic dysfunction as it relates to the gastrointestinal patient.

Thoracic Soft Tissue, Deep Articulation

PATIENT ON SIDE

See the procedure description in Chapter 5 and Figure 5.3.

This procedure is employed to decrease paravertebral muscle spasm and soft tissue tension of the thoracic spine.

Thoracic Soft Tissue Deep Articulation

PATIENT PRONE

See the description of the procedure in Chapter 5 and Figure 5.5.

This procedure is employed to decrease paravertebral muscle spasm and soft tissue tension of the thoracic spine.

Patient position: prone on the treatment table. Physician position: standing beside the patient opposite the side to be treated.

Rib Raising for Thoracic Cage Dysfunction

This procedure is employed to enhance rib motion and thoracic cage compliance. Consequently it augments venous and lymphatic return to the chest. It is also thought to affect sympathetic tone, initially stimulating regional sympathetic output but eventually resulting in reduced sympathetic activity from the spinal levels treated. (See the description of the procedure in Chapter 5 and Fig. 5.6.)

Patient Supine for Flexed or Extended Thoracic Somatic Dysfunction, HVLA (Fig. 20.1)

This procedure is employed to treat articular somatic dysfunction, type II mechanics, in the mid to low thoracic spine. It may be employed for flexed or extended dysfunctions. In either case, the physician's hand placement is the same. The patient positioned with the hands behind the neck works well for a patient with long arms and a thin torso; this is the position described next. Folding the arms across the chest works better, however, if the patient is stocky with short arms.

Patient position: supine. Physician position: standing beside the patient, on the side toward which the dysfunction is side bent and rotated, facing the patient's head at approximately the level of the abdomen.

Procedure (Example: Nonneutral Type II Articular Dysfunction of T5 upon T6, Flexed, Side Bent Left, and Rotated Left)

1. Tell the patient to clasp the hands together behind the neck and to approximate the elbows.
2. Stand on the patient's left side and grasp the elbows with your right forearm and hand. This will allow you to use the patient's pectoral girdle to introduce side bending and extension or flexion.

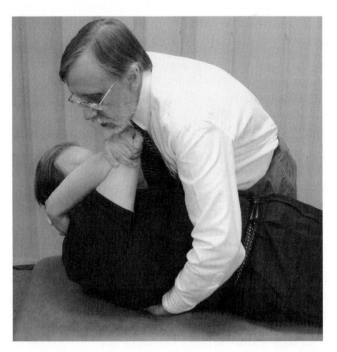

FIGURE 20.1   Patient supine thoracic HVLA for flexed or extended thoracic somatic dysfunction.

3. Roll the patient's upper body to the left so that only the left shoulder is in contact with the table.
4. Reach across with your left arm and place your left hand, palm up, upon the table at the level of T6. In this position, with your left hand open, your fingers should be pointing toward the patient's left shoulder.
5. Roll the patient's shoulders and upper torso back onto the table and position the thenar eminence of your left hand so that it is in contact with the right transverse process of T6. This asymmetric placement of your left hand beneath the patient will introduce extension and right rotation of T5 upon T6.
6. Additional side bending may be introduced with your right arm and hand through the patient's arms and pectoral girdle.
7. Place your chest firmly against the patient's elbows and pin them to the table. You may wish to place a pillow between the patient's elbows and your chest to protect your chest.
8. The final corrective force is applied as a quick thrust down the shaft of the patient's humerus, introducing extension and rotation to the right and side bending to the right over the asymmetrically placed fulcrum of your left thenar eminence.
9. Reassess the dysfunctional area.

To treat an extended dysfunction (T5 upon T6 extended, side bent left and rotated left) with this procedure, the positioning of both the patient and the physician remains exactly the same. The final corrective force, however, is delivered by using the patient's arms as levers to introduce flexion by bringing the elbows closer to the chest.

Transabdominal Stimulation

This procedure is employed to treat abdominal somatic dysfunction (ICD-9CM 739.9). The procedure improves bowel function by mechanically stimulating peristalsis, thus increasing gastrointestinal motility and alleviating or preventing constipation (ICD-9CM 564). It is useful for hospitalized patients or other bedridden individuals. Because it is most effective when applied several times a day, this procedure may be taught to patients for self-administration if they are sufficiently alert, or it can be taught to a family member.

Patient position: supine. Physician position: standing beside the bed.

Procedure

1. Place the pads of the fingertips of one hand upon the left lower quadrant of the patient's abdominal wall over the sigmoid colon.
2. Place the fingers of the other hand over the first for reinforcement.
3. Apply rhythmic pressure with the pads of the fingers, slowly and deeply through the abdominal wall to stimulate the colon.
4. Next apply a deep stroking pressure cephalad to caudad along the accessible portion of the sigmoid colon.
5. Repeat steps 3 and 4, progressing proximally along the length of the descending, transverse, and ascending colon.

For individuals who are debilitated or who have abdominal tenderness, the procedure may be modified as an indirect manipulation:

1. Beginning in the left lower quadrant, place one hand over the other upon the abdominal wall, as in steps 1 and 2.
2. Palpate with as much pressure as will be tolerated by the patient.
3. Sequentially apply alternating cephalad–caudad, left–right, and clockwise–counterclockwise pressures.

4. Move the abdominal wall and underlying abdominal contents in the direction of least resistance.
5. Hold until you perceive a sense of further loosening or relaxation in the tissues beneath your hands.
6. Repeat this procedure sequentially throughout the abdomen, right upper quadrant, left upper quadrant, and left lower quadrant, in that order.

Pedal Dalrymple Pump

See the description of the procedure in Chapter 10 and Figure 10.3.

This procedure is employed to enhance venous and lymphatic low-pressure return to the heart and thereby reduce passive congestion of the lower extremities, abdominal contents, and lungs.

References

1. Rothstein RL. Functional gastrointestinal disease. In: Noble J, Greene HL, Levinson W, et al, eds. Textbook of Primary Care Medicine. 3rd ed. St. Louis: Mosby, 2001;999–1009.
2. Abu Farsakh NA, Stietieh M, Abu Farsakh FA. The postcholecystectomy syndrome: A role for duodenogastric reflux. J Clin Gastroenterol 1996;22:197–201.
3. Wilson PT, Miller ES. Internal medicine: An osteopathic approach. Osteopath Ann 1979;7:259–273.
4. Kuchera ML, Kuchera WA. Osteopathic Considerations in Systemic Dysfunctions. 2nd ed. Columbus, OH: Greyden, 1994.
5. Camilleri M, Lee JS, Viramontes B, et al. Insights into the pathophysiology and mechanisms of constipation, irritable bowel syndrome, and diverticulosis in older people. J Am Geriatr Soc 2000;48:1142–1150 [review].
6. Beal MC. Viscerosomatic reflexes: A review. J Am Osteopath Assoc 1985;85:786–801.
7. Williams PL, ed. Gray's Anatomy. 38th ed. Edinburgh: Churchill Livingstone, 1995;1251–1252.
8. Patriquin DA. Chapman's reflexes. In: Ward RC, ed. Foundations for Osteopathic Medicine. 2nd ed. Philadelphia: Lippincott Williams & Wilkins, 2002;1051–1055.
9. DiMagno EP, Suresh C. Acute pancreatitis. In: Feldman M, Friedman LS, Sleisenger MH, Schorschmidt BF, eds. Sleisenger and Fordtran's Gastrointestinal and Liver Disease. 7th ed. Philadelphia: Saunders, 2002;913–942.
10. Tierney LM Jr, ed. Current Medical Diagnosis and Treatment. 39th ed. New York: Lange, 2000;685.
11. Noble J, Greene HL, Levinson W, et al., eds. Textbook of Primary Care Medicine. 3rd ed. St. Louis: Mosby, 2001;920–927.
12. Tintinalli J, Ruiz E, Krome RL. Emergency Medicine: A Comprehensive Study Guide. 5th ed. New York: McGraw Hill, 2000;577.
13. Adcock D. Nuclear medicine. University of South Carolina School of Medicine home page. Accessible at http://radiology.med.sc.edu/4nucmedabc.htm. Last updated July 11, 2002. Accessed April 10, 2005.
14. Conley GJ. The role of the spinal joint lesion in gallbladder disease. J Am Osteopath Assoc. 1944;44:121–123.
15. Malone EP. Manipulative therapeutics for gallbladder disease. In: Northup TL, Osteopathic Manipulative Therapeutic and Clinical Research Association. Morristown, NJ: American Osteopathic Association, 1941;4:44–45.
16. Wilson PT. Gall bladder disease. In: American Academy of Applied Osteopathy 1949 Yearbook. Ann Arbor, MI: Edwards Bros, 1949:182–184. (Now available through the American Academy of Osteopathy, Indianapolis.)
17. Becker AR. Conservative treatment of gallbladder disease. J Am Osteopath Assoc 1951;51:104–107.
18. Miller WJ, Collins G, Kosinski RJ, et al. The dorsal root ganglion cell as a potential model for viscerosomatic reflexes. J Am Osteopath Assoc 1997;97:480–EOA.

CHAPTER 21

The Patient with Thyroid Disease

Douglas J. Jorgensen

INTRODUCTION

A key relationship in osteopathic medicine since its inception has been systemic pathology and somatic dysfunction, meaning subluxation or mechanical interruption of the spinal nerve supply as described in the early osteopathic texts and literature—the osteopathic model. Still sought to achieve a health care model focused on health and the body's inherent self-regulatory and self-healing physiologic capacities, not simply identification and/or treatment of disease, the allopathic model. To understand health, however, intimate knowledge of the pathologic mechanisms and their sequelae are paramount. Normal physiology includes a dynamic system of health responsive to protection and/or immune defense coupled with rudimentary housekeeping functions. This system is orchestrated via neurophysiologic mechanisms, with the endocrine system being a primary driving force because of its ubiquitous systemic effects. Early osteopathic literature focused on the thyroid gland as a somatovisceral responder and as a viscerosomatic source of diffuse somatic dysfunctions.[1,2] Modern medicine has affirmed this early observation, as the thyroid gland influences virtually every organ system in the body.

This chapter is a review of thyroid development, physiology, pathology, systemic interactions, and pathophysiologic responses as they relate to somatic dysfunction and other tissue changes from viscerosomatic and somatovisceral relationships and to treatment approaches. An exhaustive compilation of neuroendocrine thyroid pathophysiology is beyond the scope of this chapter, but basic structure and function are reviewed as a foundation on which the understanding of systemic structural changes must be grounded.

Thyroid Development and Histology[3-5]

Developing from the root of the tongue by the middle of the first trimester of fetal development, the distal end of the rudimentary thyroid remains as the mid and proximal portions dissipate, leaving the thyroid gland located anteriorly, paramidline to the trachea. In the 10-week-old fetus, thyrotrophic cells in the anterior pituitary begin secreting thyroid-stimulating hormone (TSH), which regulates thyroid size, biosynthesis, and storage and release of thyroid hormones. By adulthood, the thyroid can be H shaped to U shaped and can extend anteriorly from the level of C1 to the level of T1 or somewhere in between. It typically weighs 20 to 30 g (slightly heavier in females), with two lateral lobes and a broad midline isthmus. Each lobe is further divided into lobules via septa derived from the inner thyroid capsule.

The fibrous isthmus is typically 12 to 15 mm in height and occasionally is associated with a pyramidal or conical lobe superiorly. The levator of the thyroid, a myofascial element more common on the left, may attach to the hyoid bone and create a direct anatomic relationship and be a factor in somatic dysfunction from both a viscerosomatic and somatovisceral perspective. Should vestigial tubular tissue remain, there is the potential for development of thyroglossal duct cysts. Additionally, multiple variants from incomplete embryological descent or deviation beyond normal anatomical positioning can result in the gland being abnormally displaced, prompting workup for a suspicious mass.

Histologically, the lobules are divided into follicles, the functional units of the gland. The follicles are composed of spherical cells and lined with epithelium consisting of regular cuboid cells enclosing a colloid-filled cavity. There are two types of epithelial cells: principal (i.e., follicular) and parafollicular. The principal epithelial cells develop colloid, which contains iodothyroglobulin, the precursor to thyroid hormones. The parafollicular epithelial cells develop C cells, described later. The typical organelles are present, and fine microvilli extend into the follicular colloid. Dense sympathetic fibers, lymphatic vessels, and fenestrated capillaries create a sophisticated, ubiquitous, and highly regulated neurovascular plexus for trophic and feedback function in this follicular mix. Thyroglobulin stores the thyroid hormone, and the microvilli assist in its mobilization. The follicles are separated by stroma or fibrous septa. C cells, derived from the neuroectoderm, are calcitonin-secreting cells They predominate in the upper and middle third of the lateral lobes. They are located in the basal lamina adjacent to the follicles. Their presence is significant in the pathology of hypercalcemia and hypergastrinemia, and they are prominent in neonatal development. The parafollicular cells are central players in systemic calcium homeostasis by virtue of their calcitonin production.

The active thyroid hormones are triiodothyronine (T_3) and thyroxine (T_4). They are merely a combination of the amino acid tyrosine with either three or four iodine atoms, respectively. Their synthesis is controlled by a negative feedback inhibitory process moderated by TSH (pituitary) and thyrotropin-releasing hormone (TRH), secreted from the hypothalamus. Briefly, the biochemistry is as follows. Iodide is trapped within the follicular thyroid cells and then oxidized (iodide peroxidase) to become capable of iodinating tyrosine residues in the thyroglobulin. After iodinating at the level of the microvilli, monoiodotyrosine (MIT) and diiodotyrosine (DIT) form.

Coupling results in T_3 or T_4, depending on whether two DITs make a T_4 or an MIT and a DIT make a T_3. Then, by endocytosis, T_3 and T_4 are released from the thyroglobulin. Roughly 80% of thyroid hormone is T_4, and the balance is T_3. Because of its availability, however, the predominantly active thyroid hormone is T_3. Once in the blood, T_4 is heavily protein bound (mostly to alpha-globulin), leaving little available for hormonal activity.

SYSTEMIC EFFECTS FROM AN OSTEOPATHIC PERSPECTIVE

In general, the osteopathic model of spinal segmental facilitation and subsequent hypersympathetic output and tone were the basis for etiologic explanations even in the early 1900s.[1] Visceral abnormalities (somatovisceral reflex), in terms of hormonal response, are primarily seen as an autonomic dysfunction or in some cases a reflexive secondary etiology.[7] In the thyroid gland, histopathology shows a predominance of sympathetic autonomic fibers, and the tenth cranial nerve, the vagus nerve, provides the parasympathetic portion. In response to stress, the thyroid enlarges; the cuboid cells elongate to columnar cells, and the gland increases in size. If the stressor (e.g., menses, peripheral nociception of pain, trauma, illness) abates, the hyperplasia is transient; the cells resorb and normal histology is restored.[3]

Without proper osteopathic treatment of somatic dysfunction, distortion of normal innervation occurs secondary to the facilitated segment. This stressor alters physiologic function of the thyroid, hence its response and ability to respond to endogenous or exogenous stimuli (e.g., chemotherapeutics, T_3, T_4, TSH). Because of the heavily sympathetically mediated modification of normal innervation secondary to somatic dysfunction, this can result in facilitated spinal segments, which cause persisting abnormal thyroid autonomic innervation. This autonomic dysfunction is primarily hypersympathetic, which would follow based on the predominance of sympathetic fibers found histologically.[3,8]

In the allostatic model, long-term facilitation impedes hypothalamic-pituitary-adrenal (HPA) axis function via amygdala stimulation with catecholamine increases. This establishes a feed-forward loop in which the facilitated segment remains indefinitely. The pathologic relationship, with its visceral structure, propagates further abnormal viscerosomatic stimulation. Thus, the thyroid pathology worsens the somatic dysfunction and, in turn, the somatic dysfunction continues to worsen the thyroid function, further worsening the neuroendocrine crisis and potentially making it a chronic, irreversible pathologic relationship.[9]

Webster[1] described a series of experiments on humans and animals demonstrating the premise for somatovisceral reflexes. Subsequently, Larson[10] detailed the physiologic mechanisms involved, specifically looking at the thyroid. Research to prove these reflexive relationships is nearly as old as osteopathic medicine itself. Two notable figures, McConnell and Burns, who were Still's students and subsequently his colleagues, provided some of this research grossly linking the viscerosomatic and somatovisceral relationships.

As early as 1906, C. P. McConnell experimented with an animal model creating segmental lesions (spinal somatic dysfunction) at the site of origin for visceral innervation. Vertebral and rib dysfunctions induced in healthy dogs resulted in segmentally related visceral pathology. Among the specifically noted induced pathologies were goiters. Subsequent treatment of the induced dysfunctions was followed by goiter resolution, while goiter in control animals did not resolve.[1,11]

At the same time, Louisa Burns[12] used both animal and human models to study viscerosomatic relationships. Using anesthetized cats, dogs, guinea pigs, and white rats, she induced vertebral lesions with digital pressure and recorded the effects of the experimental somatic dysfunction upon segmentally related viscera. The results of the animal studies were compared to the effect of pressure applied to the vertebral spinous processes in human subjects and to retrospectively reviewed clinical records. Of particular interest was the observed relationship between somatic dysfunction involving C4 to C7 and response observed in the thyroid.[13] She observed increased susceptibility to infection in the affected organs. She also noted restoration of tissue and function following treatment of the somatic dysfunction, with symptom resolution at the target sites.[1]

While some of these studies did not report how long the somatic (segmental) dysfunction was maintained, one could postulate that these were not longstanding dysfunctions, for tissue restoration did occur except where frank destruction was noted. Lacking the histopathologic techniques available today, this was exceptional and really timeless work, for these results have pragmatic application nearly a century later.

Thyroid Function and Dysfunction

Hypothalamic (medial division of paraventricular nuclei of the median eminence) TRH stimulates release of pituitary (anterior) TSH in the face of low serum T_3 and T_4. This results in stimulation of the follicular colloid with resulting increases in T_3 and T_4, as described previously. In normal thyroid physiology, this is a dynamic relationship, and the inhibitory and stimulatory functions are autoregulated. Normal subjects typically have a TSH of 0.5 to 5.0 μU/mL, with higher levels noted nocturnally. TRH, in addition to TSH stimulation, causes the release of prolactin.[14]

In the hypothyroid state, TRH will stimulate TSH to increase biosynthesis and release of thyroid hormone. Simultaneously, prolactin levels will increase secondary to the hypothalamic response to low thyroid hormone and its effect on pituitary lactotroph. Hypothyroidism can be primary or secondary, depending on the etiology.

Primary Hypothyroidism (Thyroprivic or Goitrous)

Primary hypothyroidism is thyroid gland failure and is the most common form of hypothyroidism, accounting for 95% of cases. The most common cause is ablative therapy (radioactive or surgical) for Graves' disease, but thyroprivic hypothyroidism can be congenital or idiopathic. Biosynthetic defects, iodide deficiency, fetal-maternal antithyroid transmission, and drug-induced, iatrogenic, and immune-mediated causes fall into the goitrous category. Inadequate gland synthesis occurs despite maximal stimulation and can lead to secondary or compensatory thyrotrophic hypertrophy in the pituitary. This can lead to pituitary-mediated crowding in the sella turcica with possible visual field deficits. Hyperprolactinemia may occur here too, secondary to the process noted earlier. If medical thyroid replacement therapy resolves the hyperprolactinemia, the diagnosis is essentially confirmed. Other pituitary-mediated disease (pituitary myxedema) can occur in severe primary hyperthyroidism, but again it is reversible with thyroid replacement therapy. Children left untreated can develop cretinism. In iatrogenic causes, the implicated medications are amiodarone, lithium, aminosalicylic acid, and iodine.[14,15]

Secondary Hypothyroidism (Trophoprivic)

Secondary (central) hypothyroidism is due to hypothalamic or pituitary dysfunction; it is suprathyroid in local etiology. In the primary disease, TSH is elevated before T_3 or T_4 declines. Moreover, simple thyroid replacement medication will not correct the scenario. TSH may be mildly elevated. Exogenous TRH stimulation will result in TSH increases. Furthermore, the mild TSH elevation is typically associated with a marked decrease in T_4 concentration. This is the reverse effect that elevation of TSH should have, and this scenario strongly suggests central hypothyroid disease. Because of the unreliability of TSH here, T_4 must be used to monitor this state. The euthyroid-hypothyroid patient typically falls into this category, but euthyroid sick syndrome can have many manifestations.[14,15]

Hyperthyroidism[3,5,15–17]

Graves' disease, the most common form of hyperthyroidism, is relatively common, with a 0.4% prevalence in the United States. It is thought to be multifactorial in its etiology, but the exact cause is not known save that it is an autoimmune disorder. The result is a hyperfunctioning thyroid gland that becomes diffusely hypertrophic, an associated infiltrative ophthalmopathy, and sometimes infiltrative dermopathy. It affects women more than men (5:1 to 8:1, female to male), with a peak incidence in the fourth and fifth decades; it rarely occurs after 50 years of age. There is a strong familial predisposition with specific human leukocyte antigen (HLA) markers noted by race. It can be preceded by Hashimoto's thyroiditis and has been associated with other autoimmune disorders, such as pernicious anemia, systemic lupus erythematous, rheumatoid arthritis, Sjögren's syndrome, and chronic hepatitis. It is a gamma-globulin–mediated autoimmune reaction on the plasma membrane resulting in hypertrophic thyroid tissue with increased colloidal T_3 and T_4 production. As with Hashimoto's thyroiditis, there is a defect in the antigen-specific suppressor T cells. Since hyperthyroidism worsens T cell function, this process may be self-perpetuating.

Diagnosis of thyrotoxicosis is not difficult, as problems affect multiple systems. Weakness, weight loss despite good appetite, palpitations, hyperdefecation, tremors, nervousness, sweating, and heat intolerance are all symptomatically related. These coupled with a goiter with an undetectable TSH and elevated thyroid hormones make it difficult to miss. If detected early or in relatively mild cases, particularly those lacking palpable goiter or ophthalmic manifestations, suspicion must be high for associated symptoms. Goiter too, which is not always uniform or symmetric in Graves' presentation, must be distinguished from other causes of thyroid masses. Symptoms can be relapsing and remitting, so index of suspicion should remain high to diagnose and commence treatment.

Treatment for Graves' disease is to address the thyroid hypertrophy, with medical or surgical management focused on limiting thyroid hormone production. Antiadrenergics have been used to assist in symptom control as well. Antithyroid medications (i.e., propylthiouracil) inhibit thyroid synthesis but work only when the medication is given. Leukopenia is the primary adverse effect of the antithyroid medications, so serologic monitoring must be performed. Radioactive iodine is ablative but is seen as simpler and more economic. It too carries risks, especially if used in children, as carcinogenesis must be vigilantly monitored. Even in adults, if radioactive treatment is used, the longer the life expectancy post treatment, the greater the risk of carcinoma. Surgery is a more permanent solution than nonradioactive pharmaceutical management, but it poses risks perioperatively. Postoperatively, indefinite thyroid replacement will be necessary, and there is the potential for inadvertent parathyroidectomy because of the parathyroid's intimate anatomic relationship to the thyroid gland. Thyrotoxic crisis or storm used to be precipitated by surgery (emergency) or a complicating illness (i.e., sepsis). Proper preoperative and intraoperative medical management and appropriate timely diagnosis can control this life-threatening associated syndrome, making death a rare outcome today.[17]

Pituitary (TSH-induced) hyperthyroidism is not the typical etiology for a hyperthyroid state. There are two types: pituitary tumors and pituitary resistance to thyroid hormone. The tumors (macroadenomas) autonomously secrete TSH outside of the normal feedback inhibition process of the anterior pituitary, resulting in excess thyroid hormone. The resistance to T_3 and T_4 results in a failure to inhibit TSH production once satisfactory levels of hormone are present. Thus, the pituitary fails to shut off TSH production (again not following the negative feedback loop) and a hyperthyroid state results.

Thyroiditis[3,14,16,17]

Thyroiditis, or inflammation of the thyroid, has many etiologies. Subacute, chronic, and Hashimoto's thyroiditis are the most common forms.

Subacute thyroiditis (de Quervain's, giant cell, or granulomatous thyroiditis) is viral. Typically, this follows an upper respiratory infection, and the patient has marked weakness and malaise with pain over the thyroid gland. Usually, these symptoms are present for weeks, but acute cases, though rare, do occur. In these rare instances, fever and thyroid pain are the primary complaints, and the potential for thyrotoxicosis exists. Although thyroid pain is the most common presentation, some patients have no thyroid pain despite the other symptoms.

Chronic thyroiditis is a disorder in which self-limited thyrotoxicosis occurs without previous thyroid issues, and histology subsequently shows chronic lymphocytic thyroiditis distinct from Hashimoto's thyroiditis. Laboratory values for the erythrocyte sedimentation rate usually stay below 50 mm/hour, and antithyroid antibodies have a low titer. The thyrotoxicosis typically abates in 2 to 5 months, but some patients have recurrent episodes. The etiology is unclear, favors women, and can occur at any age. Postpartum, this is the most common form of thyroiditis.

Hashimoto's thyroiditis is lymphadenoid goiter, with autoimmune events being the primary etiology. As the most common form of goitrous hypothyroidism in regions with sufficient iodine, it was first described by Hashimoto in 1912. It is most common in middle-aged women and in children; it is the most common cause of sporadic goiter. Goiter is the most prominent feature, affecting the entire gland, though it is not necessarily uniform or symmetric. The autoimmune evidence exists serologically, with lymphocytic proliferation and immunoglobulins raised against several components of thyroid tissue. Early laboratory findings may indicate euthyroid, but the gland eventually burns out and TSH increases. A correlation with concurrence of Graves' disease and Hashimoto's thyroiditis exists. Here ablative therapy is used less often, as the autoimmune response in Hashimoto's thyroiditis typically slows the progression of the hyperthyroid state associated with Graves' disease.

Pyogenic thyroiditis usually has antecedent pyogenic infection somewhere other than the thyroid. The patient has tenderness and warm erythema over a swollen thyroid gland and the typical constitutional signs of systemic infection. It is fortunately rare but must be considered in immunocompromised patients. Treatment consists of antibiotics and drainage if a flocculent area exists.

The following discussion is a breakdown of the body systems and their relationships to and with the thyroid physiology and/or pathology. Some are observations from Still and his students and colleagues; others are pathophysiologic explanations interwoven with longstanding osteopathic concepts. Many of the early observations, although well documented and repeatedly observed, had no quantifiable or measurable proof. Where possible, pathophysiologic data have been supplied to explain or elucidate the likely physiologic dynamics that were observed but lacked objective explanations in early osteopathic research and teachings.

Constitutional

A case study of goiter status post tonsillectomy resulted in sleep disturbance and a general sense of emotional lability.[2] Postsurgical treatment of the somatic dysfunctions resulted in improved mood and normalization of sleep. Notable in this case was the inability of high-velocity, low-amplitude (HVLA) procedures to result in a favorable outcome. "Relaxation, movement (and) flexibility"[2] were the key to somatic dysfunction resolution in what would be best described today as myofascial release. This patient presented for care because of the cosmetic appearance of the goiter and the thyroid, and subsequent somatic dysfunctions were found via history and physical examination.

Hypothyroidism can result in weakness, lethargy, sleepiness, fatigue, weight gain, cold intolerance, and/or general malaise. With appropriate treatment, these symptoms are potentially reversible.[15]

Eyes

Still regarded exophthalmic goiter (exophthalmos, proptosis) as being secondary to venous congestion. However, in doing so he specifically referenced the lack of knowledge at that time regarding the hypothalamic and pituitary interaction in thyroid disease and function, which has since been elucidated. Nevertheless, he reported cases of successful treatment of exophthalmos, presumably thyroid mediated, via decongesting venous return to the heart which proved effective.[6] Proptosis, or protuberant eyes, occurs secondary to immunoinflammatory changes that are part of the inflammation or congestion to which Still referred but did not histologically note in his diagnosis or treatment.[6]

To address this, he began with the inquiry of the etiology behind the "congestion." Beginning at the clavicles, he moved medially to the sternoclavicular junction and then laterally to the coracoid processes, treating myofascial structures as he found impaired tissue motion. He then moved his attention to the ribs, with the first two being his primary focus. Focus next moved to the upper thoracic and cervical spine and then the occipitoatlantal joint, hyoid, and maxillae, investing tissue, and related vascular structures.[6]

Eye involvement in thyroid disease is typically thought of in the hyperthyroid state, specifically Graves' disease, and is again autoimmunologic, with histologic confirmation possible. Proptosis, noted by Still, is the most associated feature, but early in the course of the disease there may be no apparent ophthalmic effects. As the disease progresses, however, periorbital soft tissue, periorbital muscle, eventually the cornea, and finally the optic nerve can all be adversely affected if the diagnosis is missed or treatment not initiated.[17]

In hypothyroidism, there are myxedematous periorbital changes and slow muscular response. The face has been described as cretinoid because of the associated cretinism if hypothyroidism is left untreated indefinitely. Despite an edematous look, there are likely fine wrinkles, particularly in pituitary-based hypothyroidism.[18]

Ear, Nose, and Throat

Vascular congestion of the thyroid has been implicated in tonsillar hypertrophy and pain as well as dysphagia secondary to mass obstruction of the esophagus.[2,6] Goiter demands serologic and/or radiographic work up, with the potential for surgical intervention should the histopathology and/or radiographic findings warrant it. Caution is essential in addressing an abnormal thyroid mass with osteopathic manipulation, as enhancing vascular and lymphatic drainage has the potential to metastasize cells. Fine-needle biopsy and/or surgical referral is paramount if tumor is suspected.[4,6]

The deep cervical fascia forms a sheath around the thyroid gland, firmly attaching it to the laryngoskeleton. Ligamentous attachments stick each lobe to the cricoid and thyroid cartilage, and the posteromedial portion attaches to the side of the cricoid cartilage and the first and second tracheal ring. During swallowing, these attachments create adherent thyroid movement. The recurrent laryngeal nerve typically passes inferior to the posterolateral ligamentous attachments. Lateral to the nerve is a posteromedial portion of the thyroid lobe that can be forgotten during thyroid surgery.[5]

Goiter is the most common ear, nose, and throat (ENT) issue associated with the thyroid gland other than the anatomy described previously. Goiter is simply enlarged thyroid gland, and the etiologic event is indeed variable. History, examination, and laboratory or imaging (when warranted) workup are important in determining the etiology so that appropriate treatment can be rendered. Treatment is based on understanding the pathology and anatomy well enough to allow for application of osteopathic procedures uniquely suited for a particular patient's malady.

Cardiovascular

The earliest osteopathic writings speak of Still's saying that the "rule of the artery remains supreme." Regarding thyroid vascular supply, impeded arteriovenous flow is fundamental to the osteopathic approach to the thyroid. Before the neuroendocrinology was understood, the anatomic abnormalities spoke volumes to the base pathologic mechanisms affecting the thyroid; that is, congestion of venous drainage or impeded arterial supply resulted in abnormal thyroid tissue with systemic effects. This was confirmed in vivo and postmortem by Still and his students. Thus, keeping cervicothoracic vascular (and presumably lymphatic) anatomy patent, particularly in the anterior neck and thoracic outlets, was paramount. This approach, combined with normalization of the surrounding structure and function, resulted in documented success in the treatment of goiter, exophthalmos, myxedema, and thyroiditis.

Although only general arteriovenous normalization was recommended for goiter, thyroiditis was specifically noted to need unimpeded flow of "blood and lymph from the thyroid gland into the internal jugular and innominate veins"[19] on to the superior vena cava and the right auricle of the heart.[6] In myxedema, relief from obstruction of the thyroid and/or carotid arteries has been associated with symptomatic improvement.[3] The likely reason for success in these patients was that despite not knowing the exact histopathology or neuroendocrine cause behind the symptoms, the treatment allowed for the immune-mediated inflammation to drain. In some of these maladies, the disease was self-limited. In others, the thyroid tissue would eventually burn out, allowing the lymphatic and vascular structures to flow unimpeded, permitting remarkable symptomatic improvement. For the physician to do this effectively, an understanding of the anatomy is again paramount.

The specific vascular anatomy of the thyroid includes three pairs of veins. Adjacent to the superior thyroid artery is the superior thyroid vein, which drains into the internal jugular vein. The left inferior thyroid vein goes to the brachiocephalic vein, and the right takes one of two paths. On the right, the inferior thyroid vein could drain either to the left or right brachiocephalic veins, depending on its course. Another variant for both the inferior veins, however, is to join and form the thyroid ima vein, draining into the left brachiocephalic vein.[5]

The arterial supply to the thyroid gland comes from the superior and inferior thyroid arteries and occasionally the thyroid ima. Bilateral collateral circulation is abundant here. The superior thyroid artery runs adjacent to the omohyoid and sternohyoid muscles, and typically the external branch of the recurrent laryngeal nerve runs with this artery. This artery is cut during thyroidectomy, which puts this nerve branch at risk during this procedure. Additionally, this is the arterial vessel that can be cut during an emergency cricothyroidotomy. The inferior thyroid artery is intimately related to the recurrent laryngeal nerve, but its anatomic relationship is highly variable. Furthermore, what is found on one side in terms of this relationship between nerve and artery is not necessarily the same relationship contralaterally. Again, surgical impairment of this nerve is possible because of its variable course. This is likely to manifest as phonation problems.[5,16]

In hypothyroid disease, pulse rate, stroke volume, and cardiac output are diminished. If the disease is left untreated, pericardial effusion and hypertrophic myocardium can result. In hyperthyroid states, dysrhythmias, cardiomegaly, hypertension, and thyrotoxic cardiomyopathy are all possible secondary to the hypersympathetic state that results from increased catecholamine in circulation. Electrocardiogram, echocardiogram, and hemodynamic changes also consistent with sustained catecholamine states can be found. Some studies have suggested a marked increase in mitral valve prolapse in thyrotoxic patients. The usual cause of death from thyroid storm is cardiac arrest.[16–18]

Pulmonary

The lungs provide a site for metastatic lesions of papillary thyroid adenocarcinoma. Pulmonary symptoms in the face of a new thyroid mass or a thyroid nodule of long standing warrants a chest radiograph or other pulmonary imaging to rule out related pathology. Pulmonary metastasis of thyroid carcinoma worsens the overall prognosis.[6]

Pulmonary arterial hypertension (PAH) has been found to be strongly associated with autoimmune thyroid disease. If a patient is diagnosed with PAH, part of the systemic workup should include thyroid function studies to examine for occult disease.[19]

In the thyroid storm, respiratory distress is an important and life-threatening complication.

Gastrointestinal

Thyroid effects on the gastrointestinal system in general terms are hypermobility in the hyperthyroid and hypomobility in the hypothyroid state. Hypothyroid patients have anorexia, flatus, and constipation. Gastric emptying is slow, with long intestinal transit time, decreased absorption, and occasionally ileus. Ascites may be present, as may elevated liver function test findings; the gallbladder may have insufficient tone. Finally, autoimmune hypergastrinemia is associated with autoimmune thyroid disease as much as previously mentioned autoimmune pathologies that tend to group together. In a patient with achlorhydria, thyroid workup again is indicated.[20]

Genitourinary

While current literature does not emphasize the relationship between thyroid and the genitourinary system, early osteopathic literature noted an ovarian connection. One may speculate that our osteopathic predecessors had a better understanding of the HPA axis and endocrine-related issues than we have evidence to prove or disprove. It has been confirmed, however, that thyroid size fluctuates with pregnancy and menses. Furthermore, early literature noted improvement of menstrual regularity once goiter was resolved with osteopathic treatment.[2–6] Struma ovarii, an ovarian teratoma, is made up of mature thyroid tissue. Moreover, this monodermal teratoma can result in hyperthyroidism. There is no evidence to suggest the case studies in the early osteopathic literature had such tumors or related carcinoid syndromes; this could have been part of the differential diagnosis in addition to the affected and dysfunctional endocrine system.[3]

Musculoskeletal

The musculoskeletal system has been noted to be very rigid in the hyperthyroid state, with poor mobility and range of motion. At the very least, this represents autonomic dysfunction, but most of the literature suggests that the pathologic results are sympathetically mediated. Increased musculoskeletal tone is likely secondary to the hypersympathetic stimuli associated with cyclic enhancement of somatic segmental irritation by the viscera and subsequent increased sympathetic response upon the viscera. These two cycles, if not interrupted, continuously enhance one other in a feed-forward mechanism that is a truly pathologic relationship locally and systemically. Specific findings in terms of the musculoskeletal system are found, with the sternum often twisted and with posterior displacement potentially impeding vascular flow.[3] Another specific finding is the rotation of C2 to the left. Unlike the sympathetically mediated effects, this finding is thought to be parasympathetically mediated via cranial nerve 10 (vagus) at the second spinal segment.[6]

Hypothyroidism can present as myalgia and arthralgias, and thyroid work up for nonspecific myofascial and/or joint pain is warranted in addition to the usual rheumatologic tests.[3,14]

Neurologic

Of anatomic importance are the relationships of the recurrent laryngeal nerve. Thyroid surgery can harm this nerve, especially when a parathyroidectomy, intentional or not, occurs with a complete or partial thyroidectomy. Phonation problems postoperatively are often the first sign of recurrent laryngeal nerve damage. The anatomic basis for this is outlined in the section on the ENT.

While the recurrent laryngeal nerve is of anatomic interest and importance, the primary innervation for the thyroid gland is autonomic. Cranial nerve 10 provides parasympathetic innervation, while the superior, middle, and inferior ganglia of the cervical sympathetic trunk distribute the sympathetics.[10] The latter are, again, the most highly concentrated histologically and are intimately related to the vascular and lymphatic supply.[3] The sympathetic nerves can be further broken down into afferent and efferent supplies. The afferent supply to the thyroid is derived from cerebral and meningeal blood vessels, and the nerve fibers follow branches of the internal carotid and vertebral arteries traversing the upper cervical spinal nerves. The visceral afferents are carried along the vagus nerve or get to the sympathetic trunk via the pharyngeal plexus and then pass through the rami communicantes to C5 to C6 spinal nerves and/or the upper thoracic spinal nerves.

The sympathetic efferents have three ganglia, the superior cervical, middle cervical, and stellate. The superior cervical ganglion is the largest in the cervical sympathetic system, with the first two spinal nerves more active than are the third and fourth. The middle cervical ganglion (fifth and sixth spinal nerves, or the thyroid nerves) create a plexus inferior to the inferior thyroid artery. The stellate ganglion is a combination of the inferior cervical and the first thoracic sympathetic ganglia. It connects via the gray rami of the sixth, seventh, and eighth cervical spinal nerves and the first two thoracic spinal nerves.[10,21]

A denervated thyroid gland retains its capacity to respond to central nervous system triggers. In this state, however, it is not adaptive, and the response is excessive, both temporally and in hormone output.[10] Further, without central regulation, protein synthesis is interrupted. Once innervation is restored, normal protein synthesis returns, suggesting a trophic response to the autonomic nervous system.[10]

Hypothyroidism may present as hyporeflexia, deafness, and/or memory impairment.[16] Hyperthyroidism can be associated with hyperreflexia.

Psychiatric

A distinction should be made between anxiety as its own disorder and hyperthyroidism. Similarly, hypothyroidism should be considered as a possible etiology of depression. Thyroid testing should be included in the workup for either psychiatric condition. In the hypothyroid state, fatigue may appear anhedonic; thus, hypothyroidism may manifest as psychiatric disease too. Delirium in thyrotoxicosis is also a possibility and part of an acute mental status change; thyroid laboratory tests are clearly indicated.[14]

Endocrine and Immunologic[3,7,10,14]

A key feature of the endocrine system is thyroid function and its systemic manifestations. The thyroid gland itself, if subject to multiple forms of immune-mediated inflammatory diseases and thyroiditis, is the most common pathologic site associated with immune function and dysfunction. In the immunocompromised state, *Staphylococcus aureus,* streptococci, *Salmonella,* Enterobacter, tuberculosis, and fungi are the most frequent causes of infectious thyroiditis. These are rare. Treatment is incisional drainage and organism-specific antibiotics. Viral thyroiditis also can occur and is discussed briefly later. The most common and clinically important yet less well defined thyroiditis problems are the autoimmune forms. Of these, Hashimoto's thyroiditis is the best known. Other types include subacute granulomatous, subacute lymphocytic, and Riedel's thyroiditis.

The exact etiology of Hashimoto's thyroiditis is unknown, but it is thought to be genetic and mediated via antigen-specific suppressor T cells. Subsequently, there is an unimpeded attack on follicular cells, with resulting lymphoid cellular proliferation. The colloid becomes atrophic and sparse, decreasing facilitation of T_3, T_4, or thyroglobulin production. Thus, typically it is associated with a hypothyroid state. Yet although most long-term sufferers develop a hypothyroid state, some become thyrotoxic (hashi-toxicosis) in mid course. Again, the etiology here is unclear.

Hashimoto's thyroiditis is the most common etiology of goitrous hypothyroidism in regions with iodine deficiency and a major cause of nonendemic goiter in children. Female to male predilection is 10:1, and it typically occurs between 30 and 50 years of age. The genetic relationship is associated with human leukocyte antigen DR5, and there is a strong correlation among these patients in that they are likely to have other autoimmune disorders as well.

Of the other thyroiditis subtypes, subacute granulomatous thyroiditis is thought to be secondary to specific viral infections with resulting painful goiter. Female to male predilection is 3:1, with prevalence in the second to fifth decades. Subacute lymphocytic thyroiditis is different in histology, and it is painless compared to the granulomatous form. These may be present for months, but eventually normalization of the thyroid returns. Aspirin alone suffices for mild cases; however, in severe forms, oral steroids may be necessary. A beta-blocker also may be indicated to prevent thyroid storm. T_4 and radioactive iodine treatment should be monitored, and once normalized, therapy can be stopped.

Riedel's thyroiditis is rare but important in that it must be in the differential with thyroid carcinoma when a hard thyroid mass or gland is found. It is a fibrosing reaction that essentially destroys the thyroid gland and some of the surrounding soft tissue. It exhibits the same 3:1 female-to-male predilection but occurs in the fourth to seventh decades of life. As with the other autoimmune thyroiditis problems, its etiology is unknown.

Osteopathic treatment can help to expedite healing and normalize thyroid endocrine function. In one study, unilateral electrical stimulation of cervical sympathetic ganglia resulted in TSH-induced thyroid hormone production. This was secondary to ipsilateral vasoconstriction, with subsequent parasympathetically controlled enhanced follicular sensitivity to the TSH itself.[10] Thus, sympatheticotonia from somatic dysfunction could result in a similar physiologic response. Furthermore, it would suggest that osteopathic manipulative treatment (OMT) can shorten courses of thyroid disease. This was found by Still, as noted earlier, in addition to others. Hashimoto's thyroiditis specifically responded with a shortened course of illness. A high index of suspicion for thyroid disease must be present when other autoimmune disease is present.

Hematological and Lymphatic

Still based most of his treatment in this area on the palpatory finding of congestion in the thyroid and surrounding tissues. Proximity to parathyroid makes this area particularly vulnerable to metastatic or inflammatory dissemination.[3] Thyroid lymphatic drainage is extensive and multidirectional. The immediate drainage follows along the recurrent laryngeal nerve via the periglandular, pretracheal, prelaryngeal, and paratracheal nodes onto the mediastinal nodes. Metastatic spread typically moves cephalad along the internal jugular vein due to paraglandular obstruction blocking inferior drainage.

Dermatologic[3,7,14,17]

Insufficient thyroid hormone can result in hypothyroidism or myxedema. Treatment is focused on thyroid replacement. Myxedema is a local thickening over the lateral distal lower extremity superior to the ankle. It is typically bilateral, with the surface usually shiny, but it may be scaly or even puckered, like the skin of an orange. The legs appear edematous but do not have pitting edema. Myxedema can also occur on the dorsum of the feet or phalanges and rarely the stomach. Pretibial dermopathy with Graves' disease occurs in approximately 10 to 15% of cases. It is insidious in presentation, but once it is evident, damage is irreversible. Along with skin findings, there is evidence for cognitive delay. In children, cretinism manifests as physical and mental slowing, both of which can be avoided with vigilant screening and treatment. Iodine-deficient communities are most at risk. There can be sporadic cases without iodine deficiency; however, these cases typically are the result of a genetic disease affecting thyroid hormone synthesis. Since thyroid disease can accompany other pathology, particularly autoimmune, patients with sarcoid may have thyroid involvement as well.

Manipulative Treatment of Thyroid Disease States[2,7,8,10]

The use of OMT is intended to address somatic dysfunction that is found in association with thyroid disease. It is intended to augment and not to replace standard medical therapies.

Treatment as described by Still was focused on opening arteriovenous, nervous, and lymphatic flow. It is well described in his encounters with exophthalmos. This was described by him as treatment under eye-related thyroid disease, as eye manifestations were likely the first presenting symptoms other than a goiter. Without the current serologic, histopathologic, and imaging advancements, the historical treatment was nevertheless remarkably accurate. Today the main treatment, however, should be to resolve the underlying pathologic mechanism. This will allow structure and function to return to their normal interplay. Osteopathic manipulation does have a potentially significant role in this arena. However, caution must be exercised to match the dosage of the manipulative intervention to the disease process, so that no harm is done. (See Chapter 4.)

In the hyperthyroid state, manipulative procedures must not be aggressive or stimulatory. Furthermore, the more acute the illness, the more limited the procedure should be, and appropriate medical prophylaxis (e.g., beta-blockers) should be prescribed. In the case of hyperthyroidism, literature directs us to C4 to C6, with the likelihood of a single-segment dysfunction being found. A myofascial release, facilitated positional release, and/or Still technique may be effective; articulatory or high-velocity procedures are contraindicated. Treatment intervals can be as frequent as two to three times a day as needed.

In the chronic thyroid state, treatment is again aimed at resolving the underlying hormonal, immune, or infectious etiology. Simultaneous initiation of osteopathic procedures as deemed appropriate should be implemented. The upper thorax is predominantly involved here, with a flexion dysfunction of T2 being most commonly noted.[6] Frequency and intensity of treatment are individualized until resolution of the chronic symptoms and/or disease state. While local treatment is appropriate, the thyroid is a major endocrine organ. As such, cranial dysfunction and treatment must be addressed because of the pituitary's proximity to the sphenobasilar synchondrosis and the consequent effect of the cranial mechanism on the HPA axis. Again, osteopathic treatment should include a comprehensive treatment of the underlying pathology and the associated symptoms.

Thyroid malignancy (primary or metastatic) should not be addressed with osteopathic treatment because of the risk of metastases. Pyogenic infection should be addressed on a case-by-case basis, but similar caution should be noted, as most cases of pyogenic thyroid disease are in immunocompromised individuals, and systemic dissemination can result in sepsis and/or multiorgan involvement.[7]

Common sites of thyroid-related somatic dysfunction are listed in Table 21.1.

TABLE 21.1

Common Sites of Thyroid-Related Somatic Dysfunction

Maxillae[6]

Occipitoatlantal joint[2,6]

Atlantoaxial joint[2]

Hyoid[6]

Cervical spine (C2 rotated left)[6]

Cervicothoracic (CT) junction[2]

Clavicles[2,6]

Ribs 1 and 2[6]

T1–T4 (myxedema)[6]

T1–T8 (goiter)[6]

Sacroiliac joint[2]

Procedures

Please note: The procedures that follow are examples of manipulative treatment that you may wish to employ. The actual choice of procedures used should be determined by the unique circumstances of each individual patient.

The use of OMT to treat the somatic component for patients with thyroid disease should, therefore, logically include the following:

- Upper thoracic HVLA
- Thoracic inlet release
- Ribs 1 and 2
- Deep cervical fascia, muscular, and ligamentous attachments to the hyoid and cricoid, and thyroid cartilages
- C4 to C6 myofascial release
- Occipitoatlantal myofascial release

Upper Thoracic on Side, Extended: HVLA and Articulatory Treatment (Fig. 21.1)

This procedure is employed to treat type II articular somatic dysfunction of the upper thoracic spine. In learning to do this procedure, it is often easier to employ it generally to introduce articular range of motion. (For diagnosis, see Chapter 3.)

Patient position: lying on the side. Physician position: standing at the level of the patient's shoulders, facing the patient.

Procedure (Example: T2 on T3 Extended, Side Bent Left, and Rotated Left)

1. The patient lies on the left side so that the relatively posterior transverse process of T2 is down.
2. Cradle the left side of the patient's head in the palm of your right hand.
3. With your left hand, firmly grasp the spinous process of T3 between your thumb and index finger. Your left hand must remain tightly in contact with T3 throughout the remainder of the procedure to ensure that forces introduced with your right hand are localized between T2 and T3.

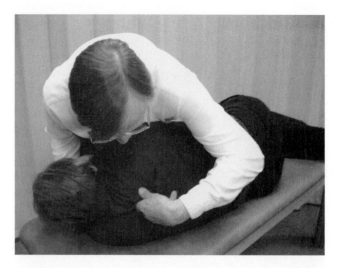

FIGURE 21.1   Patient on side, upper thoracic type II, extended, high-velocity, low-amplitude.

4. Roll the patient slightly toward you and lean forward, pinning the patient's upper torso to the table by placing your chest against the patient's right shoulder. You may wish to place a small pillow between your chest and the shoulder.
5. While cradling the patient's head with your left hand (step 2) introduce right side bending by lifting the head away from the table until you feel right side bending occurring between T2 and T3.
6. Translate the patient's head and cervical spine anteriorly with your right hand until with your left hand you feel flexion between T2 and T3.
7. Rotate the patient's head and cervical spine to the right with your right hand until with your left hand you feel right rotation between T2 and T3. It is important that you consciously maintain the right side bending described in step 5 above during this part of the procedure.
8. Apply the final corrective force through your right hand as an HVLA increase of flexion, right side bending, and right rotation of T2 against the holding force of your left hand upon T3.
9. Reassess the motion between T2 and T3.

Upper Thoracic on Side, Flexed: HVLA and Articulatory Treatment (Fig. 21.2)

This procedure is employed to treat type II articular somatic dysfunction of the upper thoracic spine. In learning to do this procedure, it is often easier to employ it generally to introduce articular range of motion. (For diagnosis, see Chapter 3.)

Patient position: lying on the side. Physician position: standing at the level of the patient's shoulders, facing the patient.

Procedure (Example: T2 on T3 Flexed, Side Bent Right, and Rotated Right)

1. The patient lies on the left side so that the relatively posterior transverse process of T2 is up.
2. Cradle the left side of the patient's head in the palm of your right hand.

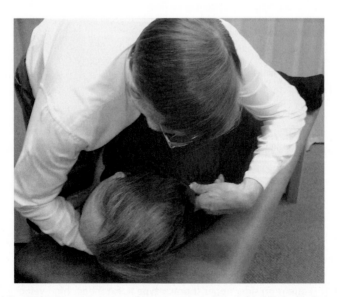

FIGURE 21.2   Patient on side, upper thoracic type II, flexed, high-velocity, low-amplitude.

3. With your left hand, firmly grasp the spinous process of T3 between your thumb and index finger. Your left hand must remain tightly in contact with T3 throughout the remainder of the procedure to ensure that forces introduced with your right hand are localized between T2 and T3.

4. Roll the patient slightly toward you and lean forward, pinning the patient's upper torso to the table by placing your chest against the right shoulder. You may wish to place a small pillow between your chest and the shoulder.

5. While cradling the patient's head (step 2), allow the dorsum of your right hand to rest on the treatment table. This introduces side bending to the left. It is important to keep your right hand as close to the table as possible throughout the remainder of the procedure to ensure that the side bending is correctly applied.

6. Translate the patient's head and cervical spine posteriorly with your right hand until with your left hand you feel extension between T2 and T3. It is important that this movement be applied as a straight posterior translation to prevent hyperextension of the low cervical spine.

7. Rotate the patient's head and cervical spine to the left with your right hand until with your left hand you feel left rotation between T2 and T3. It is important that you consciously maintain the left side bending described in step 5 during this part of the procedure. Also, for practitioners with relatively short forearms, it is important not to compress the patient's face between your forearm and upper arm.

8. Apply the final corrective force through your right hand as an HVLA increase of extension and left rotation of T2 against the holding force of your left hand upon T3.

9. Reassess the motion between T2 and T3.

Thoracic Inlet Myofascial Release

See the procedure description in Chapter 19 and Figure 19.2.

This procedure is employed to release restrictions of the thoracic inlet and thereby produce symmetric movement of the transverse fascial tissues. It may be performed either as a direct or indirect procedure.

Upper Rib Diagnosis and Treatment

DIAGNOSIS OF ELEVATED FIRST AND SECOND RIBS

The upper ribs, 1 and 2, tend to demonstrate restricted bucket handle motion as their dysfunctional mechanics. That is, their anterior sternocostal articulation and their posterior costovertebral articulations remain relatively fixed, while the lateral portion of the rib body moves up and down like a bucket handle. Upper rib dysfunctions are often positioned as elevated bucket handle mechanics. The posterolateral aspect of the dysfunctional rib is in a slightly cephalad position and resists downward pressure. It may be diagnosed as follows:

Patient position: seated. Physician position: standing behind the patient.

Procedure

1. Begin by examining the upper thoracic spine for somatic dysfunction. (See Chapter 3.) Segmentally related spinal dysfunction should be treated before rib dysfunction.

2. Palpate the scalene muscles laterally at the base of the neck in the triangular space superior to the clavicle, posterior to the sternocleidomastoid, and anterior to the trapezius. Spasm of the anterior and middle scalenes will elevate the first rib. The scalenes should be stretched before you treat an elevated first or second rib.

3. Palpate the lateral aspect of the first rib at the base of the neck. Apply downward force to the rib. An elevated first rib resists this motion.

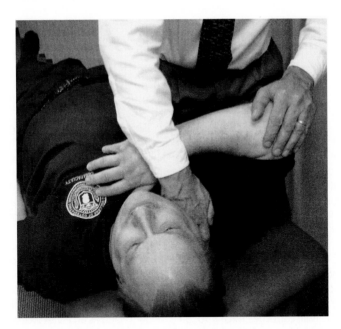

FIGURE 21.3   First rib facilitated positional release to reduce muscle tension associated with a dysfunctional first rib.

4. Palpate the angle of the second rib just above the superior border of the scapula. Again, apply downward force over the angle of the second rib. An elevated second rib resists this motion.

FIRST RIB, FACILITATED POSITIONAL RELEASE (FIG. 21.3)

This procedure is employed to reduce muscle tension associated with a dysfunctional first rib.

Patient position: supine. Physician position: standing beside the treatment table on the side of the dysfunctional rib and facing the patient's head.

Procedure (Example: Elevated First Rib on the Right)

1. Standing on the patient's right side, position the patient in such a way that the right shoulder is slightly flexed and adducted and the right elbow is flexed so that the right hand lies upon the anterior chest near the left shoulder.
2. Place your right hand upon the patient's right shoulder with your index finger touching the area of tissue texture change over the angle of the first rib on the right. Maintain your hand in this position throughout the remainder of the procedure to monitor the first rib.
3. With your left hand, grasp the flexed right elbow.
4. Flex the patient's right shoulder until the right forearm is brought into contact with your right forearm.
5. With your left hand, apply a compressive force to the patient's right elbow through the humerus until with your right index finger you feel decreased tension in the soft tissue over the first rib. This compressive force should be maintained throughout steps 6 and 7.
6. Slowly further extend the patient's right shoulder, bringing the right forearm firmly into contact with your right forearm, thereby introducing internal rotation of the right shoulder.

7. Extend the patient's shoulder as much as possible and then abduct it, moving the right elbow in an arc of circumduction, first cephalad, then laterally, and finally returning to the position of step 1.
8. Reassess available first rib motion.

FIRST RIB, HVLA

See Figure 16.2.

This procedure is employed to restore normal respiratory excursion of the first rib to establish physiologic range of motion to the costovertebral joint between T1 and rib 1.

Patient position: seated. Physician position: standing behind the patient.

Procedure (Example: Elevated First Rib on the Right)

The posterolateral portion of the rib is elevated and resists downward motion, with surrounding tissue texture change and tenderness.

1. Put your left foot upon the table just to the left of the patient's pelvis.
2. Rest the patient's left arm upon your knee. You may wish to place a pillow between the patient's axilla and your knee.
3. Place your right hand at the base of the patient's neck on the right over the elevated first rib so that your index finger is directed anteriorly and your thumb is directed posteriorly.
4. Place your left forearm and hand against the left side of the patient's head and neck to splint the cervical spine.
5. With your left hand, use the patient's head and neck as a lever to rotate and side-bend the cervical spine to the right down to the level of T1 and the first rib.
6. With your right hand, apply downward pressure to rib 1 on the right.
7. Holding the patient's chest between your right hand and left knee, translate the torso to the left to increase right side bending of the cervicothoracic junction.
8. Instruct the patient to inhale deeply and exhale, and increase the downward pressure over the first rib with your right hand during the exhalation.
9. Apply an HVLA thrust downward, medially, and anteriorly through your right hand against the dysfunctional first rib.
10. Reassess available first rib motion.

SECOND RIB, HVLA

See Figure 16.3.

Second rib HVLA is employed to restore normal respiratory excursion of the second rib to establish physiologic range of motion to the costotransverse joint.

Patient position: seated upon the treatment table. Physician position: standing behind the patient.

Procedure (Example: Second Rib on the Right)

There is tissue texture change surrounding the angle of rib 2 on the right, which is higher than rib 2 on the left.

1. Put your left foot upon the table just to the left of the patient's pelvis.
2. Rest the patient's left arm upon your knee. You may wish to place a pillow between the patient's axilla and your knee.
3. Place your right hand over the patient's right shoulder, with your thumb contacting the angle of rib 2. You may find it easier to do this if you pull the patient's right arm to the left across the chest. This protracts the shoulder and draws the scapula laterally.
4. Place your left elbow in front of the patient's left shoulder, with your forearm touching the left side of the neck and face. Your left hand should be holding the top of

the head. This arm and hand placement allows you to splint the patient's cervical spine with your left forearm.

5. With your left hand, slowly rotate the patient's head and neck to the left, disengaging the rib head from the hemifacet as T1 rotates away from it.

6. With your left hand and forearm, side-bend the patient's neck to the right down to the level of rib 2.

7. With your right hand, apply a downward directed pressure to the angle of rib 2.

8. With your left hand, introduce slightly more left rotation of the patient's head and neck while exerting simultaneous downward pressure on the 2nd rib with your right hand. This further disengages the rib head from the hemifacets. Stop the rotation when you sense that the rib exhibits less resistance to the downward pressure from your right hand.

9. Instruct the patient to inhale deeply and exhale, and increase the downward pressure over the first rib with your right hand during the exhalation.

10. The final corrective force is an HVLA thrust directed downward, medially and anteriorly through your right hand against the angle of the dysfunctional second rib.

11. Reassess available second rib motion.

Anterior Neck Soft Tissue (Lymphatic) Procedure

See the description of the procedure in Chapter 16 and Figure 16.18.

This procedure is employed to reduce congestion of the soft tissues and enhance lymphatic drainage of the neck. The fascia of the neck may be considered as an external cylinder that splits to enclose the sternocleidomastoid and trapezius muscles and surrounds the deep fascia that invests the deeper structures of the neck and fills the space between them. The superficial lymphatic drainage of the head lies outside the external fascial cylinder and must pass through it to drain into the deep cervical lymphatic vessels. The first part of this procedure is directed at moving lymph from the superficial to the deep lymphatic vessels. The second part of this procedure is directed at the deep structures and may also be employed to decrease tension in the suprahyoid and infrahyoid muscles.

Cervical, Indirect Balancing

See the description of the procedure in Chapter 16 and Figure 16.6.

This procedure is employed to decrease cervical tissue tension and enhance the symmetrical range of motion of the cervical spine.

Occipitoatlantal Direct Myofascial Release

See the description of the procedure in Chapter 16 and Figure 16.12.

This procedure is employed to treat general articular and soft tissue, myofascial, somatic dysfunction of the occiput relative to C1, the atlas, to reduce myofascial tension, and to establish symmetric motion between the occiput and the atlas.

References

1. Webster GW. Concerning Osteopathy. Revised ed. Norwood, MA: Plimpton, 1917;102–104, 136–142.
2. Unverferth EC. Goiter: A case report. Applied Academy of Osteopathy 1940 Yearbook. 1940. Vol 3;102–108. (Now available through the American Academy of Osteopathy, Indianapolis.)
3. Robbins SL, Kumar V, Cotran RS. Robbins Pathologic Basis of Disease. 4th ed. Philadelphia: Saunders, 1989;1214–1242.

4. Norman Endocrine Surgery Clinic. How Your Thyroid Works. Available at http://www. endocrineweb.com/thyfunction.html. Accessed May 28, 2005.

5. Lamaire D, Dorion D. Thyroid anatomy. http://www.emedicine.com/ent/topic532.htm; last updated May 3, 2005. Accessed May 28, 2005.

6. Still AT. Research and Practice. Kirksville, MO: Author, 1910;82–83, 106–115.

7. Kuchera M, Kuchera W. Osteopathic Considerations in Systemic Dysfunction. 2nd ed. Columbus, OH: Greyden, 1994;4–6, 11, 17, 187, 192.

8. Willard FH, Mokler DJ, Morgane PJ. Neuroendocrine-immune system and homeostasis. In: Ward RC, ed. Foundations for Osteopathic Medicine. Baltimore: Williams & Wilkins, 1997;107–135.

9. Willard FH, Mokler DJ, Morgane PJ. Neuroendocrine-immune system and homeostasis. In: Ward RC, ed. Foundations for Osteopathic Medicine. Baltimore: Williams & Wilkins, 1997;126–131.

10. Larson NJ. Osteopathic approach to thyroid disease. In: Physiology, Disease and Management of the Thyroid. Evanston, IL: A. Retlaw, 1976;10–19.

11. Further proof of the osteopathic theory: Dr. McConnell's experiments. J Osteopathy 1906;13:160–161.

12. Burns L. Viscero-somatic and somato-visceral spinal reflexes. J Am Osteopath Assoc 1907;7:51–60.

13. Burns L. The immediate effect of boney lesions. A. T. Still Bulletin 1. Cincinnati, OH: ER Booth Press, Montfort, 1910;30–44.

14. Isselbacher KJ, Kasper DL, Martin JB. Harrison's Principles of Internal Medicine. Vol 2. New York: McGraw Hill, 1994;1883–2058.

15. Jelovsek FR. Women's diagnostic cyber disease profile: Primary hypothyroidism. Available at http://www.wdxcyber.com/dxbld001.htm. Last modified November 2001. Accessed May 28, 2005.

16. Norman Endocrine Surgery Clinic. Hyperthyroidism: Overactivity of the thyroid gland: 2. Causes of Hyperthyroidism. Available at http://www.endocrineweb.com/hyper2.html. Accessed May 28, 2005.

17. Hennemnan G. Graves' disease: Complications. Revised November 25, 2003. In: The Thyroid and Its Diseases. Available from Endocrine Education at http://www.thyroidman-ager.org/chapter12/12–text.htm. Accessed May 28, 2005.

18. Wiersinga WM. Adult hypothyroidism. Revised March 4, 2004. In: The Thyroid and Its Diseases. Available from Endocrine Education at http://www.thyroidmanager.org/Chapter9/9–frame.htm. Accessed May 28, 2005.

19. Chu JW, Kao PN, Faul JL, Doyle RL. High prevalence of autoimmune thyroid disease in pulmonary arterial hypertension. Chest 2002;122:1668–1673.

20. Radebold K. Achlorhydria. Available at http://www.emedicine.com/med/topic18.htm. Last updated July 11, 2002. Accessed May 28, 2005.

21. Clemente CD. Anatomy: A Regional Atlas of the Human Body. 4th ed. Baltimore: Lippincott Williams & Wilkins, 1997;237–340.

CHAPTER 22

The Patient with Parkinson's Disease

Charles J. Smutny, III

INTRODUCTION

The Parkinson's disease (PD) patient represents a unique opportunity for osteopathic medicine to demonstrate its ability to affect the central nervous system via the musculoskeletal system. The fundamentals of a strong osteopathic treatment plan will individualize the treatment of a patient's somatic dysfunctions, with selected procedures working toward balancing the tone in the somatic system. This movement toward balance in the soma is associated with simultaneous changes toward balance in the autonomic nervous system. These changes can be measured in the patient with PD by physiologic markers including decreased hypertension, decreased muscle tone, decreased ligamentous tension (measured as passive joint range of motion), and when present, decreased cogwheeling. The target of the treatment plan is to demonstrate a decrease in the severity of the physical expression of the disease that can be measured as an increase in activities of daily living (ADL) and an increase in quality of life measures.[1]

Lessons learned from treating PD can be extrapolated to the treatment of other neurodegenerative disorders, given that the principles are similar, though the physical expressions of the varied diseases differ.[2] This chapter discusses recent osteopathic research that has demonstrated statistically significant improvement in patients' quality of life, increased independence in ADL, and reduction of a number of risk factors for injury.[3,4] Gait was improved, stiffness and rigidity were reduced, and patient psychologic states were shown to be improved. Of 35 patients, 25 (71%) had measurable positive changes in all areas of assessment.[3] The total number of falls during the study was lower than both fall frequency prior to the study's start and to age-matched and severity-ranked PD patient controls. No patient required an increase in medication dosage during the 3-month initial phase, while 9 of 35 controls (26%) had at least one increase and/or additional medicines added to their treatment protocol. Also, 5 patients in the treatment group successfully decreased their dosage of combined carbidopa and levodopa during the same phase (author's unpublished research). Findings associated with cranial dysfunctions improved dramatically.

The purpose of another study was to compare the recorded observations of cranial strain patterns of patients with PD for the detection of common cranial findings. Records of cranial strain patterns from physician-recorded observations of 30 patients with idiopathic PD and 20 age-matched normal controls were compiled. This information was used to determine whether different physicians observed particular strain patterns in greater frequency between PD patients and controls. Patients with PD had a significantly higher frequency of bilateral occipitoatlantal compression (87% versus 50%; $P < .02$) and bilateral occipitomastoid compression (40% versus 10%; $P < .05$) compared with normal controls. Over subsequent visits and treatments, the frequency of both strain patterns were reduced significantly (occipitoatlantal compression, $P < .01$; occipitomastoid compression, $P < .05$) to levels found in the control group.[5]

Osteopathic assessment and treatment of the neuromusculoskeletal system as a unit of function has more clearly defined the total physical expression of PD in terms that provide treatment options not considered in the past. Osteopathic physicians are uniquely qualified to deliver these treatments by virtue of their specialized training in manipulative skills applied according to highly disciplined medical training in neuromusculoskeletal relationships and pharmacologic interventions. Combined osteopathic manipulative treatment (OMT) with closely supervised physical therapy, strength training, flexibility training, proprioceptive awareness training, neuromuscular reeducation, and the restructuring of basic nutrition provided the strongest treatment outcomes in all patients.

PARKINSON'S DISEASE

PD is a chronic progressive neurodegenerative disease in which dopaminergic cells in the substantia nigra begin to die prematurely (apoptosis), affecting the motor system's ability to control fine motion and to maintain balanced muscular tone (posture), eventually leading to gross motor dysfunction and cognitive dysfunction. PD has an estimated prevalence of 31 to 328 per 100,000 people worldwide. It is estimated that more than 1% of the population over age 65 are afflicted with PD; incidence and prevalence increase with age.[6] Disease onset is most often unilateral, progressing to bilateral within a widely variable time span. It affects people of all ages and is often misdiagnosed in its early stages.

The diagnosis of PD is nearly always based on clinical signs and symptoms. A typical presentation would be a patient with unilateral resting tremor, reduced arm swing, and slowed hand movement who has noticed a change in gait, dexterity, and energy level. The clinical diagnosis may be less certain for a patient with bradykinesia without a resting tremor. In this case, other parkinsonian disorders, such as progressive supranuclear palsy, multiple system atrophy, or vascular parkinsonism must be considered. Ultimately, the best indicator of PD is a robust response to levodopa or one of the dopamine agonists.[7]

The three cardinal signs of PD are resting tremor (3–6 Hz), cogwheel rigidity, and bradykinesia. Postural instability, typically not recognized until late in the progression of the disease, is the fourth cardinal sign. This fourth sign is a central parameter of the osteopathic structural examination. Physicians trained as doctors of osteopathy are in a unique position to assess postural dysfunction because they have extensive education in applied anatomy and the structure and function relationship. Therefore, PD may be uncovered earlier in its onset by doctors of osteopathy than by medical physicians. Additional common findings are asymmetric onset of symptoms and symptomatic response to levodopa (levodopa). Diagnosis of PD is problematic because of the lack of a reference standard test. The diagnosis is generally made clinically, although up to 25% of patients with clinical diagnoses of PD have received different pathologic diagnoses at autopsy.[6]

By the time the disease symptoms are clearly delineated, most patients have substantial cell loss in the substantia nigra that is visible on positron emission tomography and single proton emission computed tomography.[8] "Pathologic studies suggest that patients may be symptom free until 60 to 80% of substantia nigral neurons have degenerated."[9] Interestingly, early detection of the disease is unlikely, even with a variety of radiologic procedures, as reported in a review of randomly controlled trials evaluating PD diagnostics in an Agency for Healthcare Research and Quality review article.[6]

- 3 studies of magnetic resonance imaging: insufficient evidence to determine role in diagnosing PD
- 8 studies of positron emission tomography: insufficient evidence to determine role in diagnosing PD
- 13 studies of single photon emission computed tomography: insufficient evidence to support role in diagnosing PD
- 2 studies of other scans (nuclear magnetic resonance, ultrasound): insufficient evidence to support role in diagnosing PD[6]

There continues to be great speculation as to the causes of PD, and as yet there are no clear answers. Therapy targeted at dealing with the muscular tone and tremors has consisted primarily of various pharmacologic agents. "Levodopa was the first agent shown to significantly impact the disease and has remained the gold standard."[8] Most physical modalities have been used with some short-term gain. A review of randomized controlled studies by the Cochrane Collaboration could not find sufficient evidence for or against physical therapy, occupational therapy, or a best-practice guideline.[10] Dopamine agonists (DAs) are also used, either alone or in combination with levodopa. DAs act directly on dopamine receptors, mimicking endogenous dopamine. Monoamine oxidase B inhibitors act by inhibiting dopamine catabolism thereby increasing dopamine levels in the basal ganglia. Catechol O-methyl transferase inhibitors act by inhibiting catabolism of dopamine, thereby extending levodopa's peripheral half-life. Despite the large selection of medications available to treat PD, all PD patients ultimately require levodopa.

In patients with early PD, the goal of treatment is to alleviate symptoms and maintain independent function. In advanced PD, the focus is on maximizing "on time" (time when medication is effective), minimizing "off time" (time when medication is not effective), and treating medication-related complications, such as dyskinesias, motor fluctuations, and psychiatric problems.[6] None have been shown to affect long-term function or progression of the disease, though most do improve quality of life and ADL in the interim. Surgical treatment for PD is generally considered for patients who respond to medications but have intolerable side effects. Surgical options include ablative procedures (pallidotomy or thalamotomy), deep brain stimulation, and tissue transplantation (e.g., pluripotent stem cells).

"The total annual cost for PD in the United States is estimated to be approximately $26 billion, including direct and indirect costs and lost productivity."[11]

"Clearly, PD places a major burden on both individual and societal healthcare resources."[12]

It is clear that Parkinson's patients are not going to be cured by pharmacologic or osteopathic manipulative treatments at today's level of understanding of the disease. Why, therefore, give these treatments at all? It is simply because the quality of life for patients and their caregivers must be considered. What reasons do insurance payers consider justification for continued repetitive treatment? The reduction of costs of treating falls and other accidents should be sufficient. What benefits do the patients receive? The improved quality of life for the early and intermediate stages of the disease is undeniable. Caregivers may be given back, for a time, the individual taken from them, and one cannot place a price on decreasing a loved one's suffering. Improvement of these treatments is the largest portion of current investigations. Osteopathy has contributed some interesting pilot research showing trends in improving overall outcomes, and these findings bear further investigation.

Research on more than 300 physician–patient interactions covering a 1-year period and using the Rand 36 Short Form ADL survey, the GHAA satisfaction survey, the UPDRS Parkinson's assessment protocol, in combination with 3D gait analysis,[13] have provided some initial evidence that osteopathic manipulative treatment (in combination with standard drug therapy intervention) had better quality-of-life measures than did standard medicines alone (author's unpublished research).

Common Osteopathic Problems

With a quick look at the classic posture of a parkinsonian gait, several somatic dysfunctions are clearly identified as major problems. Psoas, hamstring, quadratus lumborum, sternocleidomastoid, and the occipitoatlantal muscles are commonly hit hard by the neurogenic dystonia of the disease. Reciprocal muscles attempting to counter this increase in tone expend large amounts of energy. This feed-forward failure of imbalanced reflex arcs contributes to the pathophysiologic process. Joint breakdown from asymmetric tone and chronic joint destabilization ensues. As a result, the early-onset osteoarthritis and scoliosis that are common early degenerative changes associated with this pathophysiology are more easily understood.[14] The frequency of other musculoskeletal findings, though lower in number, still exhibit significant correlations with the visceral systems' dysfunctions and comorbid disease states that are usually presented as sequelae of PD. Somatovisceral responses may play a much larger role in the development of sequelae, and trends in initial observational studies indicate several associations that should be investigated further (author's unpublished research).

Changes in chest wall restriction, diaphragmatic excursion, and thoracolumbar postural relationships frequently preceded episodes of a variety of pneumonias, exacerbation of chronic obstructive pulmonary disease and asthma, and complaints about gastroesophageal reflux disease. Destabilization of hypertension, congestive heart failure, and the incidence of syncope were preceded by changes in the kyphoscoliosis of the upper thorax and cervical regions. Major falls associated with severe sprains (above grade 3) and/or moderate to severe fractures were associated

TABLE 22.1

Hoehn and Yahr Scale

1	Unilateral disease
2	Bilateral disease
3	Postural instability, mild
4	Postural instability, marked
5	No independent walking

with acceleration of the degenerative process by one order of magnitude without recovery to baselines before injury in patients over 65 years of age with initial Hoehn and Yahr scales of 3 or higher (Table 22.1). Any process requiring 6 or more weeks of immobilization or severe restrictions in activity ended with similar results (author's unpublished research).

Quality of Life

Quality of life was a significant and reliable measure of the severity of the disease, but rigorous reviews of the gait analysis maps, charts, and 3D video overlays provided far more objective measures and were extremely powerful tools for demonstrating to the patients during treatment that they were improving. This made it possible to overcome many psychological barriers to improving or maintaining quality of life and ADL in the face of the depression associated with the disease. This also led to trends of lower dosing of antidepressants, a higher likelihood of coming out of reclusive behaviors, and a higher degree of participation in social activities both inside and outside the immediate family and friends. There was also a higher degree of participation in self-help groups and support group activities. Patient satisfaction levels increased significantly over the initial 12-week period and maintained high scores even a year later (author's unpublished research).

Treatment Methods and Reasoning

Neurologic disease, PD in particular, lends itself very well to applications of the tenets of osteopathic medicine. The most effective treatments rely on carefully integrated medical and musculoskeletal knowledge. Treatments follow thorough diagnosis and the application of all appropriate treatment modalities as soon as possible, with the goal of achieving longer retention of quality of life and ADL. Standard osteopathic structural examinations have been combined with basic neurologic examinations, regular general physical examinations, periodic gait analyses, and regular interviews with patients and caregivers to create the foundation of decision making for the use of OMT (author's unpublished research).

Each treatment begins with a reassessment of the entire patient at every visit, monitoring changes in medicines, falls, progress with ADL, exercise programs, nutritional status, blood pressure, and a review of any other active health care issues. The osteopathic practitioner examines gait, and the degree of dysfunction is estimated. A 3D gait analysis is completed in the biomechanics laboratory on the initial visit, twelfth visit, and then every 3 months. This provides a single standard that has a higher degree of precision and interexaminer correlations than goniometry. Cybex strength testing for power output and endurance is obtained on the same schedule. This objective assessment is compared to the physician's impression before the results of the tests are discussed during periodic quality assurance chart reviews. Then these measurements and calculations extracted from them are used to document comparisons to the baseline function of the patient before OMT begins.

The OMT used was predominantly (alphabetically listed) balanced ligamentous tension, facilitated positional release, muscle energy, myofascial release, and osteopathy in the cranial field. First rib restrictions were most often treated with facilitated positional release, while other rib restrictions were initially treated with balanced ligamentous tension followed by respiratory-assisted muscle energy and myofascial release. Osteopathy in the cranial field was applied when cranial, facial, or upper cervical musculature demonstrated asymmetric tone either anteroposteriorly or laterally or when craniofacial articulations had palpable asymmetric movement patterns. In advanced cranial applications in which speech was affected, intraoral procedures were usually added to the treatment when the provider was appropriately trained. Choices were based on the patient's initial response to the application of a procedure. If the initial execution became difficult to apply or if there seemed to be resistance to the application in the initial tissue response phase as William Johnston describes in his textbook on functional technique.[15] The procedure was halted and another tried. This process was used at each body site and at each visit. Procedures that provided good initial tissue responses (nearly immediately decreased TART [tissue texture abnormality, asymmetry of position, restriction of motion, tenderness] findings) tended to be reused, increasing the ease of treatment while decreasing the time needed to complete treatment.

Statistical analyses of these measures were used to quantify what had been observed anecdotally. All patients treated during that 1-year period had at least 1 of 75 measurements improve significantly. Most patients maintained improvement in more than half of the measures. In a comparison of patterns of movement to age-standardized and gender-standardized controls, all patients treated shifted their movement patterns back toward normal movement patterns, though the amplitude of movements remained somewhat reduced. None of the solely pharmacologically treated patients improved their patterns of motion.

Posture is assessed in the structural examination, with additional attention to the long axis twist often present in PD patients. Scoliosis is common, as is some of the traditional parkinsonian posturing similar to psoas contracture posture. This posture was nearly always associated with severe psoas and sternocleidomastoid hypertonicity restrictions. This also improved on 3D gait analysis in the population treated with OMT.

Physical Therapy

Strength training, proprioceptive training, stretching, and cardiovascular endurance training were helpful adjuncts to the program. Patients who were missing even one of these modalities had poorer outcomes than those who received the full spectrum of training.

Integration of Osteopathic Diagnosis and Treatment and Pharmacologic Considerations

Tactile communication is a standard part of the interaction between the osteopathic physician and the patient. It is a method of communication that often exceeds patients' ability to express the severity of their complaints, the sites of the greatest problems, and their daily difficulty in just sitting or standing. In addition, pharmacotherapy affects tissue texture and postural tone. These drugs that change postural tone, may induce dyskinesia, shift water content from various compartments, and profoundly alter range of motion, gait, and balance. All of these changes can be perceived early in their development by trained hands far in advance of the changes that must take place to register on the various scales and measures customarily used to follow the progress of the disease. The medical necessity for repetitive evaluation and management in the hands of an osteopathic physician is eminently clear in this light.

Considerations for Students, Interns, Residents, and Attending Physicians

The MSIII (third-year osteopathic medical student) level of training is sufficient to have significant influence on this disease state. At that level of training, the basic skills required for executing simple yet sufficient osteopathic manipulative treatment interventions are exactly what is required. Experience with the disease itself and its subtle nuances of change require a good deal more experience in interpretation. Outcomes in more skilled hands showed trends toward longer on-periods between treatments and higher-quality movement patterns. Earlier diagnosis and intervention provide longer quality-of-life periods in most diseases, and the osteopathic practitioner has skills that can detect symptoms of the disease earlier via the traditional osteopathic structural examination and osteopathic gait analysis. Radiologic testing and blood work have been shown to be inconclusive in the early stages. Allopathically trained physicians are not ordinarily as skilled with structural diagnostic methods as are osteopathic physicians. They are therefore less likely, because they miss this undergraduate training, to diagnose PD as early as an osteopathic physician does. Treatments require little time once the initial treatment series is completed, though the requisite follow-up evaluations before each treatment can become more time consuming as the severity of the disease increases.

Trends identified in these studies warrant further investigation, but because the treatment modalities can do no harm, they should be continued until further studies indicate more precisely which are statistically stronger and under what circumstances they are the preferred treatment modality. The effects on duration of pharmacologic therapy and on dosage of medication trends are perhaps the most important subjects of further investigation. The chance that OMT may assist the internal environment in prolonging a patient's ability to take a drug and to use it effectively at lower doses has profound economic and social ramifications. The cost of patient care could go down in the short term, while the sales of a specific agent might go up or at least be prolonged before intolerances require changes. Because "the goal of treatment should be to obtain an optimal reduction of parkinsonism with a minimal risk of long-term side effects,"[16] osteopathic interventions should clearly continue to be a part of the treatment process.

DISCUSSION

Trends indicated strongly that patients who received OMT averaged faster improvement, longer retention of quality movement, decreased drug use, longer tolerance of their medications, a reduction in side effects, lesser degrees and severity of side effects, and they had less frequency and severity of additional visceral disease than those who did not. Patterns of movement based on length–velocity relationships assessed in gait analysis returned to near normal, though the amplitude of gait factors remained smaller than those of standardized age- and gender-matched "normals." Osteopathic treatment initially appears to have an impressive effect in the treatment of parkinsonian disorders and warrants further investigation. Practitioners at all levels of training should be including OMT in their treatment paradigm as details of mechanism of action and efficacy studies continue.

Procedures

Please note: The procedures that follow are examples of manipulative treatment that you may wish to employ. The actual choice of procedures used should be determined by the unique circumstances of each individual patient.

The following procedures are useful when treating somatic dysfunction as related to the patient with PD. All treatment must include continuous tactile feedback to modulate the minimum degree of force required to achieve a neuromuscular release response (a change in TART qualities). Execution of this process with attention to matching the forces within the tissues lets the patient's system gradually return to more normal movement patterns. Excessive force consistently yields the opposite effect. Increased precision yields increased symmetry of motion.

Occipitoatlantal Release

This procedure is employed to decrease cervical tissue tension and enhance the symmetric range of motion between the base of the skull and the cervical spine. (See the procedure description in Chapter 8 and Fig. 8.7. Also see the procedure description in Chapter 16 and Fig. 16.12.)

Occipitomastoid Decompression

This procedure is employed to enhance motion of the cranial mechanism at the occipitomastoid suture. (See the procedure description in Chapter 8 and Figure 8.8.)

Cervical (Soft Tissue)

See Figure 10.2.

This procedure is employed to decrease cervical tissue tension and enhance the symmetric range of motion of the cervical spine. (For diagnosis, see Chapter 3.)

Patient position: supine. Physician position: seated at the head of the treatment table.

Procedure

1. With both hands, place the pads of your fingers bilaterally over the cervical paraspinal tissues at the level of maximal palpable paravertebral tension.
2. Symmetrically apply anterior and cephalad pressure until you sense the stretch of the cervical paraspinal soft tissues. Applying more pressure will produce articular motion.
3. Hold with this degree of applied force position until the tissues relax.
4. Slowly release the holding force, exerting care not to unload the muscles too rapidly.
5. This sequence should be repeated several times, working up and down the cervical spine, until the desired decrease in paraspinal tension is achieved. As you become proficient with this procedure, you will learn to focus specifically upon asymmetric areas of paraspinal tension.
6. When the procedure is complete, reassess cervical paravertebral soft tissue tension and range of motion.

Cervical (Muscle Energy) (Fig. 22.1)

This procedure is employed to treat articular somatic dysfunction of the cervical vertebrae, C2 upon C3 to C7 upon T1, caused by asymmetrical muscle tension. (For diagnosis, see Chapter 3.)

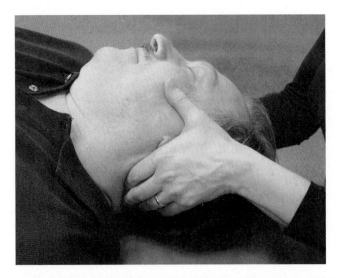

FIGURE 22.1. Cervical muscle energy is employed to treat articular somatic dysfunction of the cervical vertebrae, C2 upon C3 to C7 upon T1, caused by asymmetric muscle tension.

Patient position: supine. Physician position: standing or seated at the head of the table.

Procedure (Example: C4 Flexed, Rotated Left, Side Bent Left upon C5)

1. Hold the patient's head and neck with both hands. Contact the transverse process of C4 on the left with the lateral aspect of the proximal phalanx of your left index finger. With the fingertips of your right hand, contact the area laterally over the tip of the right transverse process of C4.
2. Using your left index finger as a fulcrum, introduce extension of the cervical spine between C4 and C5. This extension, which localizes forces to the vertebral level being treated, must be maintained throughout the remainder of the procedure.
3. With both hands, introduce right side bending of C4 upon C5 by horizontally translating C4 to the left until you feel tension accumulating between C4 and C5 and the side-bending barrier is reached.
4. Rotate the head and neck to the right, down to and including C4, until you feel tension accumulating between C4 and C5 and the rotational barrier is reached.
5. Maintain tension against the dysfunctional barrier and instruct the patient to gently rotate the head and neck back to the left against your holding force for 3 to 5 seconds.
6. Pause for 1 to 2 seconds, and then side-bend and rotate further to the right to engage the new barrier.
7. Repeat steps 5 and 6 until the best possible increase of motion is obtained.
8. When the procedure is complete, reassess C4 upon C5.

Thoracic and Lumbar Soft Tissue, Articulation; Patient Prone

This procedure is employed to decrease paravertebral muscle spasm and soft tissue tension of the thoracic and lumbar spine. (See the procedure description in Chapter 5 and Figure 5.5.)

Thoracic Inlet Myofascial Release

This procedure is employed to release restrictions and thereby result in symmetric movement of the in the transverse fascial tissues of the thoracic inlet. It may be performed either as a direct or an indirect procedure. (See the procedure description in Chapter 19 and Figure 19.2.)

Rib Inhalation and Exhalation Muscle Energy

This procedure is employed to optimize the respiratory motion of individual ribs. You can assess the motion of a specific rib with the patient seated or supine, by placing one of your hands posteriorly upon the angle of the rib to be evaluated, placing the other hand anteriorly upon the costochondral junction of the same rib, and palpating motion as the patient inhales and exhales. An inhalation rib moves freely during inhalation but stops moving before adjacent ribs stop at the end of exhalation. As such, an inhalation rib may appear to be displaced, up in front, at the costochondral junction, and down in back at the rib angle. Conversely, an exhalation rib moves freely during exhalation but stops moving before adjacent ribs stop at the end of inhalation, and it may appear to be displaced, down in front and up in back. If several adjacent ribs are perceived to be similarly restricted, a single rib may be responsible. If the group is in inhalation, the most inferior rib in the group may be preventing the rest of the group from moving freely into exhalation. If the group is in exhalation, the most superior rib in the group may be responsible. Consequently, when treating a group of dysfunctional ribs, the procedure should first be directed at mobilizing the rib most likely to be responsible for maintaining the group pattern. In any attempt to treat rib dysfunction, any and all concomitant somatic dysfunction of the thoracic spine should be diagnosed and treated first. Frequently, mobilization of thoracic somatic dysfunction will eliminate any associated rib dysfunctions.

The following procedures employ isometric muscular contraction to mobilize the ribs. Because different muscle groups are employed to affect different ribs, the thoracic cage is divided into upper, middle, and lower regions, each region requiring a slightly different procedure to achieve the desired effect.

INHALATION, ELEVATED, FIRST RIB

The inhalation dysfunction of the uppermost ribs, particularly the first rib, occurs as lateral elevation of the rib, an elevated rib. A facilitated positional release procedure for an elevated first rib is described in Chapter 21 and shown in Figure 21.3.

INHALATION SECOND TO SIXTH RIBS (MUSCLE ENERGY) (FIG. 22.2)

Patient position: supine. Physician position: standing at the head of the patient and toward the side of the dysfunctional rib.

Procedure (Example: Inhalation Third Rib on the Left)

1. Standing at the head of the table, place the thenar eminence of your left hand upon the patient's anterior chest wall contacting the dysfunctional third rib.
2. With your right hand, lift the patient's head and neck from the table, thereby introducing flexion down to and including T2 upon T3.
3. Have the patient inhale and exhale deeply.
4. As the patient exhales, apply an inferoposterior force to the anterior aspect of the third rib with your left hand to move the rib into exhalation against the restrictive barrier.
5. At the end of exhalation, hold the rib against the restrictive barrier, wait 2 to 3 seconds, and instruct the patient to inhale deeply again. The inspiratory effort against the holding force from your left hand provides the isometric contraction for the procedure.

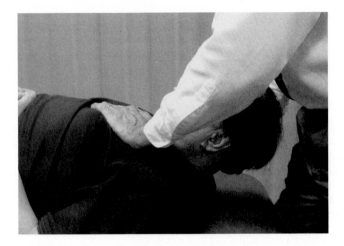

FIGURE 22.2   Muscle energy for an inhaled third rib on the left.

6. Repeat steps 4 and 5 until the best possible increase of motion is obtained.
7. When the procedure is complete, reassess the respiratory motion of rib 3.

INHALATION SEVENTH TO TENTH RIBS (MUSCLE ENERGY) (FIG. 22.3)

Patient position: supine. Physician position: standing at the side of the patient on the side of the dysfunctional rib.

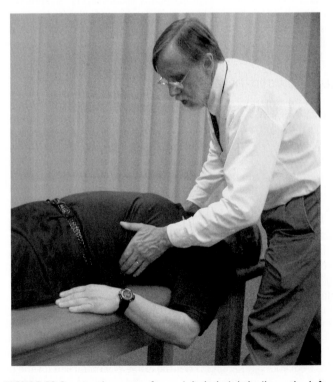

FIGURE 22.3   Muscle energy for an inhaled eighth rib on the left.

Procedure (Example: Inhalation Eighth Rib on the Left)

1. Standing on the left side of the patient, using your left hand, palpate the lateral chest wall at the level of the dysfunctional eighth rib. Grasp the patient's right shoulder with your right hand and slide it toward you, introducing side bending of the patient's upper torso to the left, until you palpate decreased tension at the level of the dysfunctional rib. Maintain this position throughout the remainder of the procedure.
2. Place the thenar eminence of your left hand on the lateral aspect of the dysfunctional eighth rib.
3. Have the patient inhale and exhale deeply.
4. As the patient exhales, apply an inferomedial force with your left hand to move the dysfunctional rib into exhalation against the restrictive barrier.
5. At the end of exhalation, hold the rib against the restrictive barrier, wait 2 to 3 seconds, and instruct the patient to inhale deeply again. The inspiratory effort against the holding force from your left hand provides the isometric contraction for the procedure.
6. Repeat steps 4 and 5 until the best possible increase of motion is obtained.
7. When the procedure is completed, reassess the respiratory motion of the eighth rib.

EXHALATION FIRST AND SECOND RIBS (MUSCLE ENERGY) (FIG. 22.4)

Patient position: supine. Physician position: standing at the side of the patient on the side opposite the dysfunctional rib.

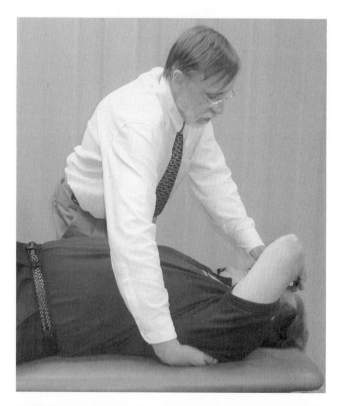

FIGURE 22.4 Muscle energy for an exhaled second rib on the left.

Procedure (Example: Exhalation Second Rib on the Left)

1. Have the patient rotate the head slightly to the right, fully flex the left elbow, and abduct and externally rotate the left shoulder, placing the back of the left hand upon the forehead.
2. With your left hand, grasp the patient's left wrist and hold it against the patient's forehead while maintaining the rotational position of the head.
3. Reach across the patient's chest and slide your right hand, palm up, beneath the patient's upper torso so that your fingers contact the posterior angle of the dysfunctional second rib.
4. Have the patient inhale deeply and attempt to lift the head from the table while you resist the effort with your left hand and simultaneously apply caudolateral traction to the posterior aspect of the second rib with your right hand for 3 to 5 seconds. Rotating the rib angle downward elongates the levator costarum, directly moving the rib further into an inhalation position.
5. Have the patient exhale and relax as you relax your counterforce.
6. Wait 2 to 3 seconds and repeat steps 4 and 5 until the best possible increase of motion is obtained.
7. When the procedure is complete, reassess the respiratory motion of the second rib.

EXHALATION THIRD TO FIFTH RIBS (MUSCLE ENERGY) (FIG. 22.5)

Patient position: supine. Physician position: standing at the side of the patient on the side opposite the dysfunctional rib.

Procedure (Example: Exhalation Fourth Rib on the Left)

1. The patient flexes the left elbow and abducts and externally rotates the left shoulder, placing the left hand palm up behind the head, cradling the occiput.

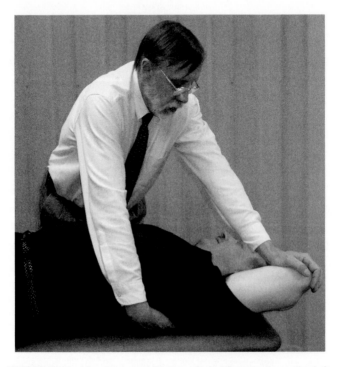

FIGURE 22.5   Muscle energy for an exhaled fourth rib on the left.

2. With your left hand, grasp the patient's left elbow, holding the patient's left shoulder in the externally rotated abducted position obtained in step 1.
3. Reach across the patient's chest and slide your right hand, palm up, beneath the patient's upper torso so that your fingers contact the posterior angle of the dysfunctional fourth rib.
4. Have the patient inhale deeply and attempt to lift the left elbow while you resist the effort with your left hand and simultaneously apply caudolateral traction to the posterior aspect of the fourth rib with your right hand for 3 to 5 seconds.
5. Have the patient exhale and relax as you relax your counterforces.
6. Wait 2 to 3 seconds and repeat steps 4 and 5 until the best possible increase of motion is obtained.
7. When the procedure is completed, reassess the respiratory motion of the fourth rib.

EXHALATION SIXTH TO TENTH RIBS (MUSCLE ENERGY) (FIG. 22.6)

Patient position: supine. Physician position: standing at the side of the patient on the side of the dysfunctional rib.

Procedure (Example: Exhalation Seventh Rib on the Left)

1. Grasp the patient's left arm with your right hand and abduct the shoulder 90 degrees. Maintain the arm in this position by holding it against the anterolateral aspect of your right thigh with your right hand.
2. Slide your left hand, palm up, beneath the patient's torso so that your fingers contact the posterior angle of the dysfunctional seventh rib.
3. Have the patient inhale deeply and attempt to adduct the left arm while you resist the effort with your right thigh and simultaneously apply caudolateral traction to the posterior aspect of the seventh rib with your left hand for 3 to 5 seconds.
4. Have the patient exhale and relax as you relax your counterforces.
5. Wait 2 to 3 seconds and repeat steps 3 and 4 until the best possible increase of motion is obtained.
6. When the procedure is complete, reassess the respiratory motion of the seventh rib.

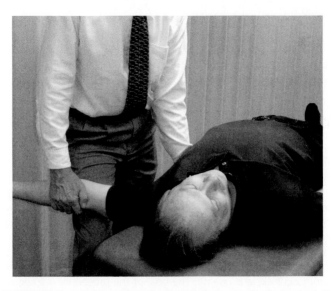

FIGURE 22.6 Muscle energy for an exhaled seventh rib on the left.

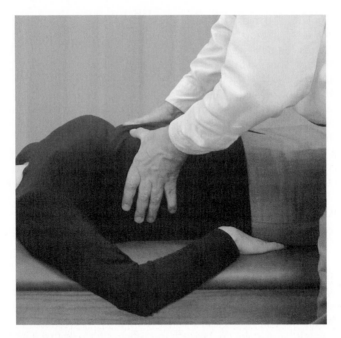

FIGURE 22.7   Indirect balancing of the thoracic cage to optimize range of motion of the chest.

Thoracic Cage Balancing (Indirect) (Fig. 22.7)

This procedure is employed to optimize range of motion of the chest cage. It is extremely effective in patients whose ability to contract muscle is severely limited because of neurologic hypertonicity. In this procedure, the right and left halves of the thoracic cage are balanced against each other.

Patient position: supine or prone. Physician position: standing on either side of the table facing the patient's head.

Procedure

1. Firmly grasp the patient's thoracic cage with both hands, your fingers comfortably spread, so that your thumbs are directed cephalad and your fingers curl around their chest on either side.
2. Slightly rotate the thoracic cage to the left and to the right about the vertical axis and identify the direction of least resistance.
3. With similar force, introduce lateral translation of the thoracic cage to the left and right, and again identify the direction of least resistance.
4. Introduce anteroposterior translation of the thoracic cage and again identify the direction of least resistance.
5. Position the thoracic cage away from the identified rotational, left, right, anterior, and posterior barriers in such a way that you that feel the least amount of tension between your two hands. This sensation is the point of balance (balanced ligamentous tension and/or myofascial neutral).
6. Hold the chest in this position of balance and patiently wait. After seconds to 1 to 2 minutes, you will feel a further relaxation of the patient's thoracic cage, a palpable neuromusculoskeletal release. The goal of the procedure is a decrease in TART.

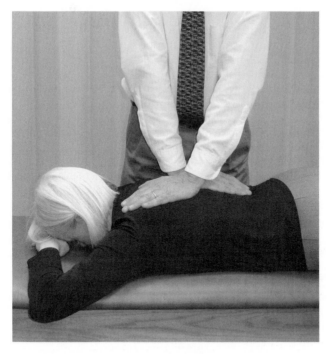

FIGURE 22.8   Cross pisiform (Texas twist) HVLA to treat T5 flexed, side bent left, rotated left.

7. As the release occurs, maintain the patient's thoracic cage in the position of balance and repeat steps 2 to 6 until the most symmetric thoracic cage motion is obtained.
8. When the procedure is complete, reassess the motion of the thoracic cage.

Cross Pisiform or "Texas Twist" (HVLA) (Fig. 22.8)

This procedure may be employed to treat type II thoracic dysfunction from the level of T3 to the thoracolumbar junction.

Because there is a high incidence of osteoporosis and vertebral compression fracture in the PD patient population, bone density screening may be considered a reasonable precaution. There appears to be a higher correlation between calcium loss and duration of the disease than the traditional age–severity relationship. Cross pisiform HVLA is a simple procedure that is easy to accomplish but presents with notable limitations. If significant kyphosis is present, the patient will be unable to lie prone as required without placing undesirable stress upon the cervicothoracic junction. Because the procedure compresses the patient's thoracic cage against the treatment table, there is the possibility of rib fracture if excessive force is used. This procedure is effective only for flexed dysfunctions and consequently can painfully aggravate an extended type II dysfunction.

Patient position: prone. Physician position: standing on either side of the table.

Procedure (Example: T5 Flexed, Side Bent Left, Rotated Left)

1. Standing on the patient's right side, place the hypothenar eminence (pisiform bone) of your left hand over the left transverse process of T5 in such a way that your fingers are pointed cephalad.

2. Place the hypothenar eminence (pisiform bone) of your right hand in contact with the right transverse process of T6 in such a way that your fingers are pointed caudally.
3. Introduce side bending to the right by translating T5 laterally to the left. This is accomplished by applying a cephalad and left lateral force over the left transverse process of T5 with your left hand.
4. Obtain rotation and extension by applying a ventral force toward the table with both of your hands.
5. When the extension, side bending, and rotation barriers have been specifically engaged, apply the final corrective force as a minimal quick high-velocity, low-amplitude cephalad thrust with your left hand upon the left transverse process of T5, accompanied by a caudad holding force with your right hand upon the right transverse process of T6.
6. When the procedure is complete, reassess the motion between T5 and T6.

Psoas Muscle Energy, Patient Prone

This procedure is employed to stretch prevertebral hip flexors, particularly psoas major. It increases hip extension and reduces compressive forces at the lumbosacral junction. (See the procedure description in Chapter 26 and Figure 26.22.)

Psoas Release (Balanced Ligamentous Tension) (Fig. 22.9)

Because some disease is so severe that patients cannot lie down, a seated treatment protocol is included.

Patient position: seated, arms draped over the physician's shoulders. Physician position: standing.

Procedure

1. Place your thumbs above the iliac crests in the posterolateral compartment adjacent to the quadratus lumborum's most lateral edge.

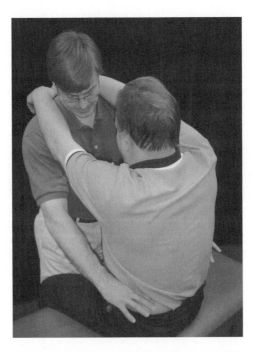

FIGURE 22.9   This procedure may be employed to reduce psoas tension for patients whose disease process is so severe that they cannot lie down.

2. With the thumb pads facing medially and posteriorly with the *internal* edge of the quadratus lumborum along the pad surface, allow the patient to lean forward, flexing the trunk, relaxing the abdominal muscles, and allowing the thumbs to move more medially and somewhat caudally.
3. Respiratory excursion facilitates the process, with relaxation on exhalation.
4. Repeat the process until the tip of the thumb comes into contact with the psoas.
5. Indirect fine-tuning of the position takes place, and psoas tone is decreased with 2 to 5 ensuing exhalations.
6. Passive side bending and rotation can be added as the patient's arms are suspended across the physician's shoulders with digits interlocked or interlaced behind the physician's neck. Both sides are treated to restore symmetry and tone.
7. When the procedure is complete, reassess psoas tension (hip extension).

References

1. Wells MR, Giantinoto S, D'Agate D, et al. Standard osteopathic manipulative treatment acutely improves gait performance in patients with Parkinson's disease. J Am Osteopath Assoc 1999;99:92–98.
2. Kandel ER, Schwartz JH, Jessell TM. Principles of Neuroscience. 4th ed. New York: McGraw Hill, 2000.
3. Smutny CJ, Wells WR, Bosak A. Osteopathic considerations in Parkinson's disease. J Am Osteopath Assoc 1998;98:389–EOA.
4. Wells MR, McCarty CL, Smutny CJ, et al. Osteopathic manipulation in the management of Parkinson's disease: preliminary findings. J Am Osteopath Assoc 2000;100:521–EOA [meeting abstracts].
5. Rivera-Martinez S, Wells MR, Capobianco JD. A retrospective study of cranial strain patterns in patients with idiopathic Parkinson's disease. J Am Osteopath Assoc 2002;102: 417–422.
6. Levine CB, Fahrbach KR, Siderowf AD, et al. Diagnosis and Treatment of Parkinson's Disease: A Systematic Review of the Literature. Agency for Healthcare Research and Quality publication 03-E040. Rockville, MD: US Department of Health and Human Services, June 2003.
7. Tetrud JW. Highlights of the 8th International Congress of Parkinson's Disease and Movement Disorders (Sunnyvale, California; The Parkinson's Institute; Portola Valley, California; Director, Movement Disorders Treatment Center). Rome, Italy, June 13–17, 2004.
8. Hauser RA. Conference report. Highlights of the 8th International Congress of Parkinson's Disease and Movement Disorders (Sunnyvale, California; The Parkinson's Institute; Portola Valley, California; Director, Movement Disorders Treatment Center). Rome, Italy, June 13–17, 2004. Posted on Medscape July 8, 2004.
9. Agid Y, Ruberg M, Javoy-Agid F, et al. Are dopaminergic neurons selectively vulnerable to Parkinson's disease? Adv Neurol 1993;60:148–164.
10. Deane KHO, EllisHill C, Playford ED, et al. Occupational therapy for Parkinson's disease. The Cochrane Collaboration, Cochrane Rev Abstract 2004. Posted on Medscape July 1, 2004; date of most recent substantive amendment, February 27, 2001.
11. Berchou RC. Maximizing the benefits of pharmacotherapy in Parkinson's disease. Pharmacotherapy 2000;20(1 Pt 2):33S–42S [review].
12. Dodel RC, Singer M, Kohne-Volland R, et al. The economic impact of Parkinson's disease. Pharmacoeconomics 1998;14:299–312.
13. Scandalis TA, Bosak A, Berliner JC, et al. Resistance training and gait function in patients with Parkinson's disease. Am J Phys Med Rehabil 2001;80:38–43; quiz 44–46.
14. Duvoisin RC, Marsden CD. Note on the scoliosis of Parkinsonism. J Neurol Neurosurg Psychiatry 1975;38:787–793.
15. Johnston WL, Friedman HD. Functional Methods: A Manual for Palpatory Skill Development in Osteopathic Examination and Manipulation of Motor Function. Indianapolis, IN: American Academy of Osteopathy, 1994.
16. Miyasaki JM, Martin W, Suchowersky O, et al. Practice parameter: Initiation of treatment for Parkinson's disease: An evidence-based review. Report of the Quality Standards Subcommittee of the American Academy of Neurology. Neurology 2002;58:11–17.

CHAPTER 23

The Patient with Larson's Syndrome: Functional Vasomotor Hemiparesthesia Syndrome

Frank C. Walton, Sr.

INTRODUCTION

Norman J. Larson described a clinical presentation of patients with a unilateral complex of symptoms and physical changes associated with discrete paravertebral somatic dysfunction of the ipsilateral upper thoracic area. He went on to describe the response of these patients to osteopathic manipulative treatment (OMT) directed to the upper thoracic somatic dysfunction.[1] Patients with similar clinical findings, somatic correlation, and response to osteopathic manipulative treatment have been observed by other osteopathic clinicians.[2–7]

CLINICAL PRESENTATION

The presenting clinical history typically includes subjective complaints involving one-half of the patient's body, with description of sensory disturbance, dysesthesia, pain, and physical changes in peripheral somatic tissues. Some patients have the same clinical complaints and findings, but with variations of pattern distribution of symptoms and findings, as discussed elsewhere in this chapter.

The sensory disturbance may include numbness, tingling, tissue or limb heaviness, inaccurate sensation of local heat, or inaccurate sensation of local cold. Some patients complain of diminished limb position awareness (proprioception) and disturbed perception of body part position and motion tracking.

The dysesthesia may include the skin or deeper tissues, a sensation of crawling, tightness, hypersensitivity to light touch, hypersensitivity to minimal compression or palpation pressure, and abnormal sensitivity to harmless levels of exposure to radiant heat or sunlight. The patient may describe an unpleasant awareness of non-specific stiffness of the soft tissues of the affected area or of remarkable resistance to compliance with active or passive motion of joints in the affected areas.

The pain complaint commonly includes a burning pain and may be described as noxious dys-ease, ache, sharp pain, or dull pain. The pain may be described as steady, variable, or shooting along typical neurotome patterns or portions of nerve distributions. However, especially if the condition becomes well established, the pain may be described in other patterns, such as affecting the upper extremity from the mid forearm distally, including all of the hand and fingers (sometimes clinically described as glovelike) or all of the lower extremity from just below the knee or just above the ankle distally to include all of the foot and toes. The structures described as painful may include some or all of the skin, subcutaneous fascia, muscle, joint, or bone components.

Patients' freehand images of symptom patterns and distribution (numbness, tingling, cold sensation, hot sensation, and various qualities of pain) drawn on body parts paper have been found to be remarkably useful for defining and following subjective descriptions.[8] It is remarkable how well subjective symptom pattern changes (drawings) can be correlated with objective findings of perceived changes in the associated upper thoracic somatic dysfunction.

Objective physical changes in tissues involving the affected peripheral and extremity areas include several especially consistent elements. Skin of the area of greatest subjective complaint will show early erythema. The skin will begin to manifest increased turgor or intracellular swelling, slight initially and greater with time. Typically, no actual extracellular edema is present unless later associated with toxic changes, necrotic changes, or infection in compromised tissue. This tissue turgor can be appreciated by palpation of the affected skin and associated subcutaneous tissue. Longstanding peripheral manifestations begin to show chronic tissue changes. Fibrotic changes thicken the skin and underlying tissues, making them harder and still less compliant to active movement and passive movement testing.

Compromise of microcirculation in the tissues of the affected area is visible in the skin. Rapid capillary blanching and delayed refilling are evident. As the condition becomes established, especially if it becomes chronic, discoloration of the skin (greater in the more distal areas) that may suggest slight to increased cyanosis develops. In a rare and atypically dramatic presentation, some patients exhibit a remarkable skin tissue structural disruption, deterioration, and even superficial rawness and sloughing that may appear early or after the condition progresses. Clinical experience suggests that the same changes are occurring in other tissues not visible under the skin. Thermographic studies have been used to document and evaluate changes in skin and local tissue temperature and circulation in the paravertebral area, trunk, and extremities.[9]

Swelling of deeper connective tissues, fascia, and muscles develops as the untreated or ineffectively treated clinical condition matures. As a consequence of the cellular swelling, compliance of the involved tissues decreases. The patient recognizes the decreased compliance as subjective complaints and the clinician can appreciate it with physical examination. When the muscles are involved, their girth initially increases, the tissue yield to pressure decreases, voluntary active movement is compromised, and passive quality of motion and range of motion are diminished. If it is not treated effectively, prolonged pathology will begin to manifest as muscle atrophy and fibrotic scarring changes. Swelling of the connective tissues of joints, ligaments, and tendons begins to cause diminished compliance to motion and stretch, resulting in further reduced active and passive movement.

If the condition remains chronically present, additional trophic changes become evident in the affected tissues. These appear to be associated with inadequate circulation, oxygenation, nutrition, and toxin and waste product removal. The physical changes in the tissues also suggest additional changes explainable by compromised cell health, resulting from deprivation of neurotrophic protein substances (discussed later in the chapter).

There is a correlation of objective findings in the tissues and structures where subjective clinical complaints manifest. Physical examination, assessing for tenderness to light and firm palpation, pain manifestations on tissue manipulation and joint motion testing, and tissue swelling and/or edema offer valuable information. Traditional testing for confirmation of light touch, pinprick, and two-point discrimination sensation status are useful. Soft tissue assessment of swelling, compliance to compression, and subtle compliance to myofascial guiding procedures allows interpretation of the status of the vitality of the tissues.

Distribution Patterns Other Than Full Half of the Body

Variations of the clinical presentation may include other distributions of symptoms and objective findings that may not include one entire side of the body. In any of these variations, however, there typically is paravertebral somatic dysfunction in the ipsilateral upper thoracic region.

One fairly common variation includes only one upper quadrant of the body, including half of the head, face, neck, and upper torso and including the ipsilateral upper extremity. Obvious clinical complaints and findings may be limited to some or all of the upper extremity, with much-reduced symptoms and findings in the remainder of the upper extremity or upper quadrant. Less frequently, only the more distal portions of both extremities on half of the body may be affected.

The clinical presentation may include only a lower quadrant of the body, including half of the lower torso and the ipsilateral lower extremity. There may be clinical complaints and findings limited to some or all of the lower extremity, with reduced symptoms and findings in the remainder of the lower quadrant, hip, or lower extremity.

Occasionally, manifestations on both sides of the body are observed. The presentation may involve essentially all of the body distal to the cervicothoracic junction of the torso. When this is present, it is likely that the predominance of the clinical findings will be limited to the extremities, with the torso less affected. A pattern affecting only bilateral upper extremities does occur. A pattern affecting only bilateral lower extremities is less common.

Not a common presentation but more frequent with increased severity and duration of the condition is that a patient may also complain of head and cranial nerve unilateral sensory changes (vision, pupil, hearing, tinnitus, taste, smell, and/or face skin sensation), secretory functional changes (disturbed lacrimation, disturbed nasal secretion), and/or motor functional changes (diminished paraorbital and eyelid muscle tone and strength, diminished paraoral muscle tone and strength, diminished tongue extension strength). When these variations are present, there typically is a distinct finding of paravertebral somatic dysfunction in the ipsilateral higher upper thoracic level. These head and cranial manifestations may mimic facial palsy and must be differentiated from shingles and herpes.

Somatic Dysfunction of the Upper Thoracic Spine and Upper Ribs

Somatic dysfunction findings in the upper thoracic area are specific to this clinical condition. Somatic dysfunction and paravertebral soft tissue reactivity findings are typically present at T2, T3, or T4 on the side of the peripheral manifestations. There are essentially always additional costotransverse soft tissue findings and rib somatic dysfunctions associated with the paravertebral thoracic findings. Less common are paravertebral findings at the level of T1, although these are more likely if the peripheral manifestations include the head or neck. Somatic dysfunction the level of T5, although also less commonly encountered, is most likely if the peripheral manifestations include only the lower extremity.

The paravertebral soft tissue changes of thoracic somatic dysfunction and the rib and costotransverse findings are easily identified, but the soft tissue findings commonly are not as intense as might seem consistent with the pronounced degree of the peripheral presentation. Focal pressure during palpation of the dysfunctional paravertebral and costotransverse tissues commonly reproduces the patient's pain and other subjective dysesthesias in the area of the peripheral complaint.

A dramatic confirmation of these upper thoracic somatic dysfunctions and associated rib somatic dysfunctions' relationships to the peripheral disturbances is the consistency, degree, and rapidity of response of the peripheral disturbances when OMT is administered effectively to alleviate the somatic dysfunction. Even conditions that have manifested for extended periods respond impressively to OMT, often showing distinct improvement as quickly as immediately after a single treatment. Continued improvement of peripheral findings and symptoms can be identified to correlate with the degree of improvement of the somatic dysfunction after initial and subsequent OMT.

The findings of upper thoracic and upper rib somatic dysfunction may be defined using physical examination, allowing interpretation of their role in the clinical presentation and for the appropriate treatment approach needed. Using the mnemonic TART (tenderness, asymmetry, range or quality of motion, and tissue texture changes) when describing the paravertebral and costotransverse findings allows for an organized method of description for somatic dysfunctions.[10] Palpatory tissue assessment and defined motion testing findings of posterior vertebral, costotransverse, and rib tissues and structures provide the descriptions needed to define and name somatic dysfunction. The findings associated with the clinical condition described in this chapter commonly include characteristics that are different from more typical paravertebral somatic dysfunction.[11]

Tenderness (t) as an element of somatic dysfunction as delineated by palpation and pressure applied to tissue is typically present within the skin and soft tissues overlying the posterior thoracic skeletal elements lateral to the spinous process and superficial to the transverse process. In the presentation of Larson's syndrome, significant tenderness may manifest deeper in the paravertebral soft tissues than is the case with more typical somatic dysfunction. Palpation of the tissues in this presentation may delineate the area of deep dull ache (as described by the patient) in deep tissues in the areas of the costotransverse junction and the posterior rib tubercle. Tenderness commonly is remarkable and may be found as deep as the ligaments of the costotransverse joint capsule.

Asymmetry (**a**) refers to the description of the tissues and structures on either side of the midline of the involved vertebral segments. These findings may be visible or palpable as the following changes:

- Skin: color, texture, temperature, capillary circulation, congestion, edema, turgor, and trophic character
- Underlying soft tissue (including subcutaneous, fascial, muscular, ligamentous, tendinous, lymphatic, and vascular): fullness, swelling, congestion, edema, tension, spasm, turgor, and trophic character
- Paravertebral bony elements: change of position in relation to original neutral normal position or to other bony elements (see discussion of rotation and side bending later in the chapter)
- Neck, torso, spine, or other structures: lateral curvature, scoliosis, or focal angulation

Description of vertebral and paravertebral bony asymmetry includes definition of vertebral positional changes described separately from the description of motion freedom and restriction of motion. (See the description of range of motion and quality of motion.) If there is a significant sustained rotated or side-bent position of the involved vertebral segments, there will be an observable difference on each side of the midline consistent with mechanical positional changes of the vertebral elements. These position changes may include the following:

- Posterior positioning of the transverse process on the side of sustained rotation, thus a more posterior prominence of this transverse process than of the contralateral transverse process (rotated posterior dysfunction)
- Anterior positioning of the transverse process on the side opposite to the sustained rotation, thus a more anterior (deeper) position of the transverse process on the side opposite the rotation (rotated anterior dysfunction)
- Caudad positioning of the transverse process and approximation to the transverse process of the next lower vertebra on the side of sustained side bending, thus a crowding approximation of the transverse processes on the side of side bending (side-bent toward dysfunction)
- Cephalad positioning of the transverse process and movement away from the transverse process of the next lower vertebra on the side opposite the sustained side bending, thus a separation or widening of the space between the transverse processes on the side opposite the side bending (side bent away from dysfunction).
- Combination positioning of the transverse process or processes as determined by sustained rotated and side-bent positional changed elements that may be produced by or during the development of the somatic dysfunction, the presence or absence of flexed or extended position or forces affecting the pattern of combinations of motion and positioning

When somatic dysfunction is present at a thoracic vertebral level, there typically is manifest definable altered position and motion within the normal range of motion of the affected vertebra.[12] The dysfunctional sustained position is poorly yielding to passive motion testing and may result in loss of motion or significant compromise of quality of motion. The dysfunctional position is typically significantly distant from the normal neutral point. The dysfunctional position may be anywhere within the normal range of motion, however, from an extreme to essentially the normal neutral position.

There may be *no* skeletal or vertebral asymmetry. Other disturbances of physical findings and functional changes may be evident without distinct rotated and/or side-bent changes, that is, no clearly posterior transverse process on the side of the somatic dysfunction. This is possible even with a distinct alteration of the pattern, range, or quality of rotation and/or obvious abnormality of the soft tissue findings. Careful attention should be directed to evaluating the possible role of a viscerosomatic mechanism in the production of the original somatic dysfunction, its recurrence, or its perpetuation. (See Chapter 5.)

Range and Quality of Motion in Vertebral Somatic Dysfunction

Range (r) and quality of motion of the vertebral segments and spinal regions are assessed and described in terms of somatic dysfunctions as a part of the physical examination of the paravertebral area. Regional motion and individual vertebral segmental motion should exhibit normal and full range of motion in each of the three primary motions. The three primary motions of the vertebrae include flexion and extension (forward and backward bending), rotation, and side bending. Various motions and motion patterns of the vertebrae commonly include combinations of these primary motions. They must be considered as both single and combined motions in descriptions of normal and abnormal motions of the vertebrae. Other lesser motions that may be significant in determining the character and clinical import of somatic dysfunction are also sometimes described. These lesser motions are not discussed in this chapter but may be reviewed in other writings.

Normal range of motion is expected for each of the specific movements of the vertebral segments, including symmetric rotation and side bending. When the range is reduced (or less frequently, increased) toward one or both sides, notation is taken. An assessment is made to determine whether the change in motion range is related to anatomic bony or ligamentous changes or to soft tissue physical and functional changes. Muscular contraction and tension changes and effects of nerve input to motor function are assessed. Muscular effects and the effects of other soft tissues may produce alteration of both range of motion and quality of motion or only of quality of motion.

In the somatic dysfunctions related to Larson's syndrome, the motion change may be a less common type. The motion may be compromised in such a way that the bony element (transverse process, spinous process, facets, rib) position remains near the normal, neutral, resting position, with a definable resistance to movement of the element during active motion effort and passive motion testing. This distinct loss of range of motion and position held near the neutral position, alone or combined with other quality of motion changes, may be a reason that OMT directed to the somatic dysfunctions typically found in Larson's syndrome are likely to be most effective if they specifically include emphasis on vertebral–rib element mobilization procedures, in particular including high-velocity, low-amplitude (HVLA) procedures.

Range and Quality of Motion in Rib Somatic Dysfunction

Range of motion, quality of motion, and asymmetry of the ribs as they relate to the vertebral column, to the sternum and costosternal elements, to the other ribs, and to the diaphragm and abdominal wall are assessed and defined as a part of the physical examination of structural aspects of somatic dysfunctions. The upper five ribs are important in this discussion. Ribs in general terms move with inspiration, expiration, and mechanical movements of the vertebral units and thorax. Ribs exhibit motion patterns including the following:

- Upward and downward movement of their most lateral aspect (sometimes named *bucket-handle motion*)
- Upward and downward movement of the most anterior aspect (sometimes named *pump-handle motion*)

- Twisting motion of the head of the rib at its attachment to the vertebral body about an anteromedial to posterolateral axis
- Upward and downward movement of the posterior tubercle or angle of the rib about an approximately side-to-side horizontal axis modulated by the ligamentous attachments to the associated vertebrae and accentuated or diminished by an effect of the movement or restriction of movement of the transverse process of the associated vertebrae
- Small gliding anterior or posterior movement in a horizontal plane, as the rib moves with the vertebral transverse process during spine, trunk, and vertebral rotation

Normal motion of the ribs is directly influenced by the other structural elements adjoining and attached to the rib elements. Rib motion may likewise directly influence the motions of the other structural elements.

When somatic dysfunction involves a rib, there typically is a definable altered position (held in an inhaled, inspired, elevated position or an exhaled, expired, depressed position) and altered motion within the normal range of motion of the affected rib.[13,14] The dysfunctional sustained position yields poorly to passive motion testing, with loss of motion and/or significant compromise of quality of motion. The dysfunctional position is typically significantly distant from the normal neutral point; however, the dysfunctional position may be anywhere within the normal range of motion from the extreme to essentially the normal neutral position.

Alteration of rib motion may reflect a situation similar to that sometimes seen in vertebral motion, in which the rib element is held at or near the normal neutral position with definable resistance to movement of the rib during active motion effort and/or passive motion testing. The range of motion may be minimal in one or more directions. A more detailed discussion of rib motion, in particular a discussion of the uniqueness of motion patterns of particular rib pairs at various levels of the rib cage, can be found in other writings.

Quality-of-motion assessment of the vertebra and rib may demonstrate normal, smooth active and passive movement throughout the range of motion, normal to the structures being assessed. Normal quality of motion is expected for each of the specific movements of the vertebral segments, including symmetry of rotation and side bending. When the quality is altered on one side or both sides, notation is taken. If quality of motion is altered, this may offer information useful in describing abnormal findings.

The altered quality of motion of the somatic dysfunction can be identified from the following characteristics: (1) It can yield resistance to motion throughout all or most of the range of motion. (2) It can demonstrate resistance to motion that becomes remarkably greater as the extreme of normal range is approached. (3) It can demonstrate resistance that becomes greater as movement approaches a point well before the anticipated normal end of the range of motion. Each of these characteristics offers different information that is useful for clinical interpretation. In the somatic dysfunction that is a part of Larson's syndrome, it is common that a distinct resistance is noted very early as passive motion is attempted in any direction away form the static point.

Tissue Texture Changes

Changes in soft tissue texture (t) in the paravertebral and rib areas can be assessed by palpation and other physical examinations that allow gathering of information and a means of interpreting the findings. Soft tissue status, including skin, fascia, and subcutaneous, vascular, lymphatic, ligamentous, tendinous, muscular, periarticular, and periosteal tissues, can be appreciated for acute and chronic changes. Changes may reflect soft tissue physical, physiologic, and functional status. Acute tissue congestion, swelling, edema, metabolic, and toxic changes may be recognizable: Tension changes of muscular contraction, effects of motor nerve input, effects of sensory nerve feedback and response, and metabolic status may be identified by palpation. Chronic tissue changes, fibrotic changes, and trophic changes may affect tissue circulation, compliance, and vitality. Soft tissue changes affect movement of the soft tissues and associated joints, including quality and range of motion. Consideration should be directed at an effort to determine whether the paravertebral soft tissue findings (reactivity) have characteristics that strongly suggest an underlying viscerosomatic reflex etiology. (See Chapter 5.)

Role of the Sympathetic Nervous System

Somatic dysfunction in the upper thoracic segmental levels is observed to have an integral role in the clinical condition described here as Larson's syndrome.[1] One plausible explanation of this relationship correlates with the observation that the sympathetic autonomic nervous system demonstrates a remarkable concentration of interactive neurons (intermediolateral cell columns) in the cord levels of T1 to T5.[15] This suggests a relationship between normal function of the upper thoracic cord segments and normal sympathetic effects on the related peripheral tissues and structures. A reasonable extension of this observation would be that a significant disturbance of function of the upper thoracic cord segments can be expected to contribute to an abnormal functional state of the associated sympathetic nerves, possibly producing an abnormal sympathetic effect on the related peripheral tissues and structures.

The manifestations of upper thoracic somatic dysfunctions and their relationships to other neurointeractive musculoskeletal and autonomic mechanisms play a role in the vulnerability to, development of, and perpetuation of sympathetically mediated peripheral disturbances. The relationship of primary somatic dysfunction to the development and accentuation of secondary somatovisceral and reflex peripheral vasomotor disturbances plays a significant role in development of peripheral sympathetic disturbances.[16]

Original external insult or primary and secondary internal neurologic dysfunction have been demonstrated to contribute to development of sustained somatic dysfunction in the thoracic spinal cord segments that thereafter contribute to the development of acute and of sustained peripheral vasomotor (sympathetic) disturbances. Other peripheral disturbances are associated with altered nerve stimulation and compromised delivery of neurotrophic proteins and other nerve-transmitted nutritional elements.

Osteopathic clinicians and researchers have observed a relationship between upper thoracic spinal cord function or somatic dysfunction and sympathetic function or dysfunction that offers a mechanism to describe a role of the sympathetic nervous system in Larson's syndrome.[17] This description includes the following:

- Spinal cord–level (upper thoracic) somatic dysfunction contributing to distorted functional status of associated sympathetic nervous elements
- Distorted input of sympathetic innervation to vascular tissues and to other nerve tissues
- Altered arterial circulation to larger peripheral nerves precipitated by distorted sympathetic motor input
- Altered tissue health of the nerves resulting in distorted nerve impulse transmission
- Altered target tissue (arteries and other peripheral cells and tissues) response to nerve impulse input
- Altered trophic status of target tissues (arteries and peripheral cells and tissues) due to lack of neurotrophic substances production, centrifugal movement, and release to tissues

- Functional distortion of nerve function related to compromised efficacy in response to sensory neurotransmission
- Altered tissue health of the nerves resulting from compromised uptake and retrograde transfer of nutrient and tissue trophic substances
- Altered tissue health of the nerves resulting in distorted production of neuropeptides and their centripetal movement

This cascade of effects and events seem capable of producing the clinical conditions discussed. It remains to be seen whether adequate data to result in general acceptance of such an explanation can be obtained.

Other Clinical Entities

Some of the clinical presentation discussed by Larson in his description of functional vasomotor hemiparesthesia syndrome shares characteristics with other described conditions. Specifically, peripheral causalgia, reflex sympathetic dystrophy, and Horner's syndrome can be considered.[18] Each of these conditions is attributed to a disturbance of function or anatomic disruption of sympathetic nervous elements. None of these entities, as discussed in traditional medical literature, address the potential of spinal cord functional disturbance as the likely etiology. Correlation has been drawn by osteopathic physicians for a proposed causal relationship between somatic dysfunction, associated disturbance of the sympathetic nervous supply, and the symptoms and signs in the peripheral somatic structures.

Osteopathic Manipulative Treatment

Effective application of OMT to somatic dysfunction depends upon accurate diagnostic interpretation of the paravertebral and rib findings. Treatment must appropriately address mechanical, functional, and reflex neurologic elements. Distinct response to initial osteopathic manipulation, as expected, is a confirmation of accurate diagnosis, correct selection of treatment approach, and effective application of the treatment.

Of particular note in selection of osteopathic manipulation procedures for treatment of somatic dysfunctions as typically found in Larson's syndrome is the character of range or quality of motion disturbances. Distinct loss of range of motion and position held near the neutral position alone or with other quality of motion changes may be a reason that OMT directed at the somatic dysfunctions typically found in Larson's syndrome is likely to be most effective if it specifically includes emphasis on vertebral and rib element mobilization. OMT, particularly HVLA and other direct procedures using low-velocity, high-amplitude insistent range-of-motion forces, also may be needed to facilitate the motion of the dysfunctional musculoskeletal elements.

The patient typically reports rapid reduction of symptoms, sometimes immediately after the first effective OMT. Subjective symptoms may remain abated or may return over a few to several days. Reported improvement after one or two treatments may be as great as complete resolution of subjective symptoms and may be permanent. It is common that subjective symptoms are dramatically improved after four to six treatments. Tissue physical changes and trophic changes in the affected peripheral areas may take substantially longer to improve and resolve. This process may be recognizable within the first few treatments but may take as long as several months, depending on the duration and severity of tissue compromise.

Reassessment at 2 to 3 days after the initial OMT allows evaluation of the effect of treatment. Some patients have an accentuation of symptoms after treatment, either after an initial improvement or without any initial positive response. Such accentuation of symptoms tends to be transient, resolving in 24 to 48 hours, and is not typical after subsequent treatments. At 2 to 3 days after the initial treatment or after regression of any significant exacerbated symptoms, further OMT can be done. Symptom improvement rather than accentuation, is the expected result.

A failure of significant sustained improvement after initial OMT should lead the clinician to look for another principal etiology or other unaddressed primary or secondary etiologies, including medical, psychological, somatic, viscerosomatic, structural, and mechanical conditions. Other medical treatment, including prescription analgesic, anti-inflammatory, antibiotic, antifungal, cardiac, gastrointestinal, and muscle spasm medications, may be necessary. Patients respond better if they are successful in reduction or elimination of tobacco usage and use of caffeine.

Procedures

Using OMT is a matter of dosage, as discussed in Chapter 4. The following procedures are direct HVLA procedures that Larson commonly used to treat upper to mid thoracic somatic dysfunction. Once mastered, they can be quickly performed, lending themselves well to busy clinical practice. However, sometimes the patient cannot tolerate the more aggressive forms of manipulation, and procedures based upon indirect principles, such as facilitated positional release or functional procedures, are more appropriate.

Counterstrain, based upon indirect principles, is useful when treating the patient with Larson's syndrome because it is one of the few forms of manipulation that specifically addresses the pain component of somatic dysfunction. Consequently, it may be employed alone or in combination with direct procedures. Counterstrain procedures are useful to address residual discomfort that occasionally remains after the articular component of the somatic dysfunction has been successfully treated. The counterstrain procedures for posterior (elevated) and anterior (depressed) rib tender points, described later in this chapter, are particularly useful.

Please note: The procedures that follow are examples of manipulative treatment that you may wish to employ. The actual choice of procedures used should be determined by the unique circumstances of each individual patient.

Spinous Process Thrust (HVLA) (Fig. 23.1)

This procedure is employed to treat upper thoracic, T1 upon T2 to T4 upon T5, type II vertebral somatic dysfunction. (For diagnosis, see Chapter 3.)

Patient position: seated. Physician position: standing behind the patient.

Procedure (Example: T2 upon T3, Flexed, Side Bent Right, Rotated Right)

1. Place your right foot upon the table just to the right of the patient's pelvis.
2. Rest the patient's right arm upon your right knee. You may wish to place a pillow between the patient's axilla and your knee.
3. Place your left hand upon the patient's left shoulder with your fingers directed anteriorly and your thumb directed medially, contacting the left lateral aspect of the spinous process of T2.
4. Hold the patient's torso firmly between your left hand and right knee. This will help to localize forces between T2 and T3 and must be maintained throughout the remainder of the procedure.
5. Introduce left side bending between T2 and T3 from below by laterally translating the patient's torso to the right with your left hand and right knee.
6. Place the palm of your right hand, with your fingers extended upward, in contact with the right side of the patient's neck. Alternatively, you may wish to place your right elbow upon the patient's right shoulder and your right hand on top of the

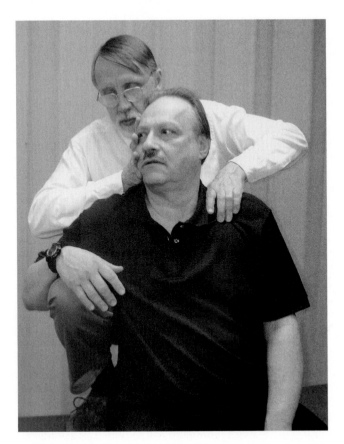

FIGURE 23.1   Spinous process thrust (HVLA) for T2 upon T3, flexed, side bent right, and rotated right.

     patient's head, allowing your right forearm to contact the right lateral aspect of their neck. Both of these hand positions allow you to introduce forces down to T2 upon T3 while splinting the cervical spine.

7. Using your right hand, introduce extension down to T2 upon T3 by translating the patient's head and neck posteriorly. (For extended dysfunctions, follow the same sequence, but translate the head and neck anteriorly to introduce flexion down to the dysfunctional segment.)
8. With your right hand, introduce side bending of the head and neck to the left down to T2 upon T3.
9. Again, using your right hand, introduce left rotation of the head and neck down to T2 upon T3.
10. The final corrective force is a HVLA thrust toward the right with your left thumb against the left side of the spinous process of T2, which increases left side bending, left rotation, and extension (or flexion, step 7) of T2 upon T3.
11. Reassess the relationship between T2 and T3.

Fixed Point, Rotation (HVLA) (Fig. 23.2)

This procedure is employed to treat thoracic (T3 or lower) type II somatic dysfunction. (For diagnosis, see page 3.)

     Patient position: seated. Physician position: standing behind the patient toward the side of the dysfunction.

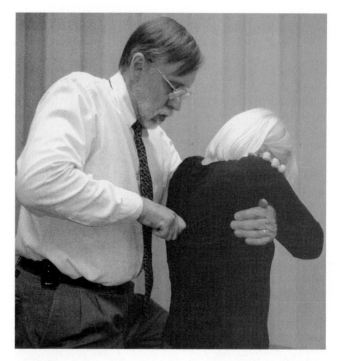

FIGURE 23.2 Fixed point, rotation (HVLA) for T5 on T6, flexed, rotated left, side bent left.

Procedure (Example: T5 on T6, Flexed, Rotated Left, Side Bent Left)

1. Flex your left hip and knee and place your left leg upon the table so that the full length of your shin is in contact with the tabletop just to the left of the patient's pelvis.
2. Have the patient loosely fold the arms across the chest, and with your left arm reach under the patient's left axilla, across the chest, and under the right axilla so that the fingers of your left hand contact the patient's right lateral thorax. For female patients, some practitioners elect to place a small pillow between their left forearm and the patient's chest.
3. While holding the patient firmly between your left arm and your chest, introduce extension down to and including T5 on T6 by applying upward traction with your left arm. (When treating an extended dysfunction, flexion is introduced by forward-bending the patient's torso down to and including T5 on T6.)
4. With your right hand, firmly grasp the spinous process of T6 between your thumb and index finger. This is the fixed point.
5. Use your left arm to introduce side bending to the right and rotation to the right from above down to T5 on T6.
6. Apply the final corrective force as a HVLA increase of right rotation of the patient's upper torso with your left arm and hand against the holding force of your right hand.
7. Reassess the relationship between T5 and T6.

Reverse Rib (HVLA) (Fig. 23.3)

This procedure is employed to treat costovertebral somatic dysfunction that can affect the second, third, or fourth ribs. The dysfunctional relationship occurs between a thoracic vertebra and the rib of the segment below. Rotation of the

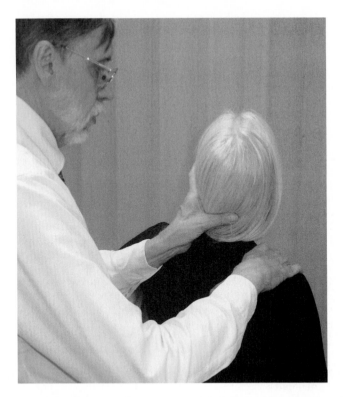

FIGURE 23.3   Reverse rib (HVLA) for treatment of dysfunction between T1 and the second rib on the right.

vertebra causes the inferior vertebral hemifacet to impinge upon the head of the rib. This in turn drives the rib posterior, impinging upon the costotransverse articulation and causing palpable prominence, tissue texture change, and tenderness over the angle of the dysfunctional rib. This is a secondary dysfunction, the result of a primary thoracic type II vertebral dysfunction. As such, the primary thoracic dysfunction should be treated before this procedure is employed.

Patient position: seated. Physician position: standing behind the patient.

Procedure (Example: Dysfunction Between T1 and the Second Rib on the Right)

The rib angle is prominent, with tissue texture change and resistance to an anteroinferior force.

1. Begin by placing your left foot upon the table just to the left of the patient's pelvis.
2. Place the patient's left arm over your left knee. You may wish to place a pillow between your knee and the patient's axilla.
3. With your left hand, reach in front of the patient, grasp the right wrist, and pull the right arm across the lap to protract the right scapula, exposing the angle of the second rib.
4. Place your right hand upon the patient's right shoulder so that your fingers are directed anteriorly and your thumb points inferiorly, contacting the angle of the dysfunctional second rib.
5. With your right hand apply an inferomedial force, holding the patient's torso firmly between your right hand and left knee. This holding force must be maintained throughout the remainder of the procedure.

6. With your left hand, grasp the left side of the patient's head so that your widespread fingers are directed anteriorly, contacting the patient's left cheek, and your thumb contacts the posterior skull at or just inferior to the external occipital protuberance.
7. Using your left hand, posteriorly translate the patient's head to straighten the upper thoracic and cervical spine. This spinal positioning must be maintained throughout the remainder of the procedure.
8. With your left hand introduce rotation of the head and cervical spine to the left until forces accumulate at the level of T1.
9. The final corrective force is a HVLA increase in left rotation of the patient's head and cervical spine against the holding force of your right thumb upon the second rib angle.
10. Reassess the relationship between T1 and the second rib.

Counterstrain Procedures for Posterior (Elevated) and Anterior (Depressed) Rib Tender Points

Counterstrain points are commonly paired as posterior and anterior points. This is because they often present clinically in this paired relationship. If a posterior tender point is identified, as might be anticipated over the rib angle in a patient with Larson's syndrome, the segmentally related anterior point should be sought out too. The two points should then be compared for degree of tissue texture abnormality and tenderness, and the more severe point should be treated first. Following treatment, the treated point should be reassessed, and if it has resolved, the segmentally paired point should be reevaluated. If the paired point is also resolved, the treatment procedure is successful. If the paired point remains tender, it should be treated. Again, following treatment, the second point should be reassessed, and if it has resolved, the segmentally paired point (the first point treated) should be reevaluated. If the first point treated remains resolved, the treatment procedure is successful. If, however, the first point has returned, a third segmentally related point, an anterior or posterior thoracic point, or an atypical point (as described in various counterstrain texts) should be sought out and treated.

The counterstrain points associated with the upper six ribs that may be encountered in the patient with Larson's syndrome (Fig. 23.4) are described here. The posterior (elevated) counterstrain tender points are found bilaterally over the posterior rib angles of their respective ribs. The anterior (depressed) rib tender points are located bilaterally over the anterior aspect of the chest. The tender point for the first rib is at its costosternal junction, just inferior to the sternoclavicular joint. The tender point for the second rib is over the anterior aspect of the second rib at the mid clavicular line. The tender points for the third and lower ribs are located upon the respective ribs at the anterior axillary line.

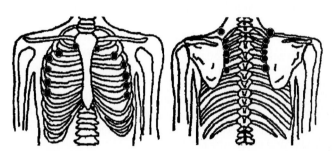

FIGURE 23.4 *Left:* Anterior (depressed) rib tender points for ribs 1 to 6 bilaterally over the anterior aspect of the chest. *Right:* Corresponding posterior (elevated) counterstrain tender points for ribs 1 to 6, found bilaterally just medial to the scapula, over the posterior rib angles of their respective ribs.

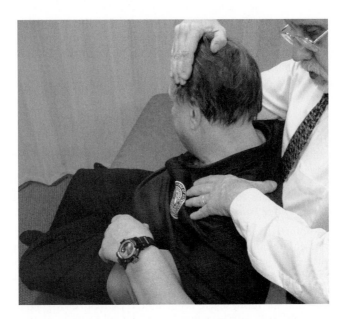

FIGURE 23.5 Counterstrain for posterior third rib tender point on the left.

Ribs Posterior (Elevated) Tender Points, Patient Seated (Counterstrain) (Fig. 23.5)

This procedure is employed to reduce tenderness and pain associated with a counterstrain tender point. The locations of the respective tender points are described previously. The patient may be diagnosed while seated or prone by palpation for the tissue texture abnormality and associated tenderness in the tender points.

Patient position: seated on the side of the treatment table. Physician position: standing behind the patient.

The physician monitors the tender point continuously throughout the procedure, using light touch and intermittent increased palpatory pressure to determine the degree of tissue texture abnormality and tenderness. As the patient is positioned for the procedure, the tissue texture abnormality and tenderness associated with the tender point should be reduced to no more than 30% of that encountered at the outset of treatment. This is determined by palpating the tissue texture and asking the patient for their perception of tenderness to increased palpatory pressure. The duration of the procedure is classically 90 seconds, although if you are capable of palpating a release, this may be employed as an indicator that the treatment is finished.

Procedure (Example: Posterior Third Rib Tender Point on the Left)

1. Palpate the posterior tender point upon the angle of the third rib on the left with the index finger or thumb of your left hand. This hand placement must be maintained throughout the procedure.
2. Assess the degree of tissue texture abnormality and tension associated with the tender point. By increasing the amount of digital pressure applied to the tender point, determine the baseline severity of tenderness. Assign this level of tenderness a value of 100% and inform the patient.
3. Tell the patient to place the left foot upon the table beneath the right thigh. The left hip should be fully flexed and externally rotated with the left knee flexed. The lateral aspect of the left thigh and leg should be in contact with the tabletop.

4. Place your left foot upon the table lateral to the patient's left hip.
5. Place the patient's left arm over your left thigh. Placing a pillow between your thigh and the patient's axilla while flexing the patient's left elbow and placing the forearm upon your left knee will reduce pressure upon the brachial plexus and reduce the tendency to develop paresthesias during the remainder of the procedure.
6. Translate the patient's upper torso to the left by side-shifting your pelvis and left knee to the left.
7. Have the patient allow the right arm to hang over the side of the table behind them.
8. With your right hand, grasp the patient's head and introduce rotation and side bending of the cervical and upper thoracic spine to the right. Introduce flexion of the cervical and upper thoracic spine by dropping the chin toward the chest. The cumulative effect of steps 3 to 8 should be a progressive reduction of tissue tension and tenderness associated with the tender point.
9. Further modify the patient's position, particularly by adjusting the positions introduced in steps 6 and 8, to obtain maximum palpable tissue tension and tenderness reduction. It is generally felt that patient-perceived tenderness should be decreased to no more than 30% of the 100% established in step 2.
10. Hold this position of maximum palpable tissue tension and tenderness reduction 90 seconds, then slowly return the patient to the original position. It is important not to remove your monitoring finger during the procedure so that you can be certain the reduction in tenderness post treatment occurred specifically in the original tender point.
11. Reassess the point for tenderness.

Ribs Anterior (Depressed) Tender Points, Patient Seated (Counterstrain) (Fig. 23.6)

This procedure is employed to reduce tenderness and pain associated with a counterstrain tender point. The locations of the respective tender points are described previously. The patient may be diagnosed seated or supine by palpating for the tissue texture abnormality and associated tenderness in the location of the tender points.

Patient position: seated on the side of the treatment table. Physician position: standing behind the patient.

The physician monitors the tender point throughout the procedure, using light touch and intermittent increased palpatory pressure to determine degree of tissue texture abnormality and tenderness. As the patient is positioned for the procedure, the tissue texture abnormality and tenderness associated with the tender point should be reduced to no more than 30% of that encountered at the outset of treatment. This is determined by palpating the tissue texture and asking the patient for his or her perception of tenderness to increased palpatory pressure. The duration of the procedure is classically 90 seconds, although if you are capable of palpating a release, this may be employed as an indicator that the treatment is finished.

Patient position: seated on the side of the treatment table. Physician position: standing behind the patient.

Procedure (Example: Anterior Third Rib Tender Point on the Right)

1. Palpate the tender point upon the third rib at the anterior axillary line on the right with the index finger of your right hand. This hand placement must be maintained throughout the procedure.
2. Assess the degree of tissue texture abnormality and tension associated with the tender point. By increasing the amount of digital pressure applied to the tender point,

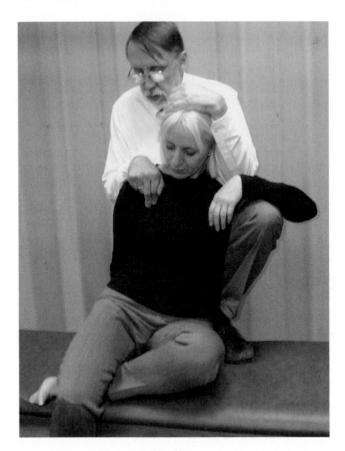

FIGURE 23.6 Counterstrain for anterior third rib tender point on the right.

determine the baseline severity of tenderness present. Assign this level of tenderness a value of 100% and inform the patient.

3. Tell the patient to place the left foot upon the table beneath the right thigh. The left hip should be fully flexed and externally rotated with the left knee flexed. The lateral aspect of the left thigh and leg should be in contact with the tabletop.

4. Place your left foot upon the table lateral to the patient's left hip.

5. Place the patient's left arm over your left thigh. Placing a pillow between your thigh and the patient's axilla while flexing the patient's left elbow and placing the forearm upon your left knee will reduce pressure upon the brachial plexus and reduce the tendency to develop paresthesias during the remainder of the procedure.

6. Laterally translate the patient's upper torso to the left by side-shifting your pelvis and left knee to the left.

7. Have the patient allow the right arm to hang over the side of the table behind him or her.

8. With your left hand, grasp the patient's head and introduce rotation and side bending of the cervical and upper thoracic spine to the right. Additionally, introduce flexion of the cervical and upper thoracic spine by dropping the chin toward the chest. The cumulative effect of steps 3 to 8 should be a progressive reduction of tissue tension and tenderness associated with the tender point.

9. Further modify the patient's position, particularly by adjusting the positions introduced in steps 6 and 8, to obtain maximum palpable tissue tension and tenderness

reduction. It is generally thought that patient-perceived tenderness should be decreased to no more than 30% of the original 100% established in step 2.

10. Hold this position of maximum palpable tissue tension and tenderness reduction 90 seconds, then slowly return the patient to the original position. It is important not to remove your monitoring finger during the procedure so that you can be certain that the reduction in tenderness post treatment occurred specifically in the original tender point.

11. Reassess the point for tenderness.

For additional manipulative procedures for rib somatic dysfunction, see Chapters 21 and 22.

References

1. Larson NJ. Functional vasomotor hemiparesthesia syndrome. Academy of Applied Osteopathy 1970 Yearbook. Carmel, CA: Academy of Applied Osteopathy, 1970:39–44. (Available through the American Academy of Osteopathy, Indianapolis.)

2. Larson NJ. A study of the response of uncomplicated peripheral sensory disturbances to specific osteopathic manipulative treatment. J Am Osteopath Assoc 1972;72:62–EOA.

3. Kappler RE. Addendum July 1970; Larson NJ. Functional vasomotor hemiparesthesia syndrome. Academy of Applied Osteopathy 1970 Yearbook. Carmel, CA: Academy of Applied Osteopathy, 1970:44. (Available through the American Academy of Osteopathy, Indianapolis.)

4. Larson NJ, Walton MW, Kelso AF. Effectiveness of manipulative treatment for paresthesias with peripheral nerve involvement. J Am Osteopath Assoc 1980;80:216–EOA.

5. Larson NJ, Walton MW, Hunt HH, Kelso AF. A double-blind clinical study of the effects of manipulative treatment of patients with peripheral nerve complaints. J Am Osteopath Assoc 1976;76:209–EOA.

6. Sprafka SA. Clinical problem solving: Case six. In: Ward RC, ed. Foundations for Osteopathic Medicine. 2nd ed. Philadelphia: Lippincott Williams & Wilkins, 2002;269.

7. Larson NJ. Osteopathic manipulation for syndromes of the brachial plexus. J Am Osteopath Assoc 1972;72:378–384.

8. Larson NJ. A study of the response of uncomplicated peripheral sensory disturbances to specific osteopathic manipulative treatment. J Am Osteopath Assoc. Sep 1972;72(1):62–EOA.

9. Kappler RE, Kelso AF. Thermographic studies of skin temperature in patients receiving osteopathic manipulative treatment for peripheral nerve problems. J Am Osteopathic Assoc 1984;84:76–EOA.

10. Glossary of osteopathic terminology. In: Ward RC, ed. Foundations for Osteopathic Medicine. 2nd ed. Philadelphia: Lippincott Williams & Wilkins 2002;1229–1253.

11. Walton FC. Palpation and motion testing in acute and chronic disease. Osteopath Med 1977;2:80–83, 86.

12. Walton WJ. Textbook of Osteopathic Diagnosis and Technique Procedures. 2nd ed. Chicago: Chicago College of Osteopathic Medicine, 1970;114–119.

13. Hruby RJ. The rib cage. In: Ward RC, ed. Foundations for Osteopathic Medicine. 2nd ed. Philadelphia: Lippincott Williams & Wilkins 2002;718–726.

14. Walton WJ. Textbook of Osteopathic Diagnosis and Technique Procedures. 2nd ed. Chicago: Chicago College of Osteopathic Medicine, 1970;338.

15. Willard FH. Autonomic nervous system. In: Ward RC, ed. Foundations for Osteopathic Medicine. 2nd ed. Philadelphia: Lippincott Williams & Wilkins, 2002;90–119.

16. Korr IM. The spinal cord as organizer of disease processes: IV. Axonal transport and neurotrophic function in relation to somatic dysfunction. J Am Osteopath Assoc 1981;80:451–459.

17. Patterson MM, Wurster RD. Neurophysiologic mechanisms of integration and disintegration. In: Ward RC, ed. Foundations for Osteopathic Medicine. 2nd ed. Philadelphia: Lippincott Williams & Wilkins, 2002;120–136.

18. Nelson KE. Osteopathic medical considerations of reflex sympathetic dystrophy. J Am Osteopathic Assoc 1997;97:286–289.

CHAPTER 24

The Patient with Fibromyalgia/Chronic Fatigue Syndrome

Anette K. Schilling Mnabhi

INTRODUCTION

Everyone gets tired, and everyone has occasional aches and pains. The difference for people with chronic fatigue syndrome and/or fibromyalgia is that the fatigue and the aches and pains do not just go away after a few nights of sleep or a break from the usual activities or even with time. The challenges for individuals with one of these syndromes are compounded for several reasons: First, the causes of these syndromes are still not clear; there is much debate as to their etiology and pathophysiology. Second, many physicians and health professionals still do not recognize these syndromes. Third, because of the complexity of symptoms and unknown causes, research into effective treatment is challenging. Without diagnosis, little effective treatment can follow. Individuals with chronic fatigue syndrome or fibromyalgia have many needs and often require a variety of therapeutic approaches. It is increasingly apparent that both syndromes involve an interaction of dysfunction across systems, including immune, endocrine, cardiovascular, digestive, and autonomic nervous systems. Osteopathic medicine is ideally suited to provide an integrated approach to the somatic and visceral dysfunction experienced by these individuals.

Chronic fatigue syndrome is a serious problem affecting many individuals. It is estimated that 400,000 to 800,000 Americans of all ages, races, socioeconomic groups, and genders may be affected by this disorder. Chronic fatigue syndrome is most common in women in their 40s and 50s. Some studies have shown the highest rates are in Latinos and African-Americans, followed by whites and Asians. Similar illnesses have been seen in adolescents and children, but prevalence data are limited for this population. Internationally, some societies are just beginning to recognize the disorder. The etiology and pathophysiology of chronic fatigue syndrome are not known, but evidence is growing that a neuroendocrine dysfunction cascading into multiple-system dysfunction is a key factor.[1,2]

Fibromyalgia is estimated to have a prevalence of 3.4% for women and 0.5% for men. While the causes of fibromyalgia are still unclear, it appears that alterations in sleep patterns and changes in neuroendocrine transmitters play significant roles.[3]

THE DIAGNOSTIC PROCESS

As a starting point to effective diagnosis and treatment of chronic fatigue syndrome or fibromyalgia, it is essential to know what symptoms are present and how the conditions are defined. Both are primarily clinical diagnoses and must be diagnoses of exclusion; both are treated empirically, although some small clinical studies have looked at the use of low-dose antidepressants, exercise, and cognitive therapy. Research into causes and treatments is ongoing, and this is a constantly evolving field. Chronic fatigue syndrome and fibromyalgia are separate conditions, yet often individuals in either group will share similar characteristics or exhibit both conditions simultaneously. Treatment interventions overlap, so the two conditions are usually treated together. Although known by many names (chronic fatigue and immune dysfunction syndrome, myalgic encephalopathy or encephalomyelitis, postviral fatigue, chronic Epstein-Barr syndrome, neurasthenia, fibrositis), these syndromes are characterized by the following:[4–6]

- Headache
- Frequent infections, such as sinus or respiratory infections
- Lymphadenopathy
- Urinary bladder infections or candidiasis
- Myalgia and arthralgia
- Inability to concentrate, or brain fog
- Exhaustion
- Disordered sleep
- Bowel disorders
- Increased thirst
- Low libido
- Low temperatures
- Anxiety and depression
- Weight gain

This constellation of symptoms reflects significant visceral and somatic dysfunction that the osteopathic physician is well equipped to handle.

Chronic Fatigue Syndrome

Chronic fatigue syndrome is characterized by severe and debilitating fatigue that has been present for more than 6 months and has associated muscle aches, tender and swollen lymph nodes, chills, arthralgias, sore throat, headaches, postexertional malaise, and unrefreshing sleep. The Centers for Disease Control (CDC) has established that a case of chronic fatigue syndrome is defined by the presence of the following:

- Clinically evaluated, unexplained, persistent, or relapsing chronic fatigue that is of new or definite onset (has not been lifelong); is not the result of ongoing exertion; is not substantially alleviated by rest; and results in substantial reduction in previous levels of occupational, educational, social, or personal activities
- Concurrence of four or more of the following symptoms, all of which must have persisted or recurred during 6 or more consecutive months of illness and must not have predated the fatigue:
  - Self-reported impairment in short-term memory or concentration severe enough to cause substantial reduction in previous levels of occupational, educational, social, or personal activities
  - Sore throat
  - Tender cervical or axillary lymph nodes
  - Muscle pain
  - Multijoint pain without joint swelling or redness
  - Headaches of a new type, pattern, or severity
  - Unrefreshing sleep
  - Postexertional malaise lasting more than 24 hours

This research definition excludes many individuals because of its restrictive nature.[7] Fatigue is common in many illnesses. For this reason, the differential diagnosis includes an extensive list of diseases that must be excluded.

Fibromyalgia

Fibromyalgia is characterized by sleep disturbance; spontaneous, widespread soft tissue pain; fatigue; and widespread tender points. The American College of Rheumatology has set the following criteria for a definition of fibromyalgia:

- A history of widespread pain. The patient must have pain or achiness, steady or intermittent, for at least 3 months. At times, the pain must have been present
  - On both the right and left sides of the body
  - Both above and below the waist
  - Mid body, for example, in the neck, mid chest, or mid back, or in the head
- Pain on pressing at least 11 of the 18 spots on the body that are known as tender points (Fig. 24.1).[8]
- The presence of another clinical disorder, such as arthritis, does not rule out a diagnosis of fibromyalgia.[9]

For a tender point to be considered positive, the subject must state that the palpation was painful; *tender* is not to be considered painful. The tender points are paired and are located as follows: 1 and 2, occiput, bilateral, at the suboccipital muscle insertions; 3 and 4, low cervical, bilateral, at the anterior aspects of the intertransverse spaces at C5 to C7; 5 and 6, trapezius, bilateral, at the midpoint of the upper border; 7 and 8, supraspinatus, bilateral, at origins, above the scapula spine near the medial border; 9 and 10, second rib, bilateral, at the second costochondral junctions, just lateral to the junctions on upper surfaces; 11 and 12, lateral epicondyle, bilateral, 2 cm distal to the epicondyles; 13 and 14, gluteal, bilateral, in upper outer quadrants of buttocks in anterior fold of muscle; 15 and 16, greater trochanter, bilateral, posterior to the trochanteric

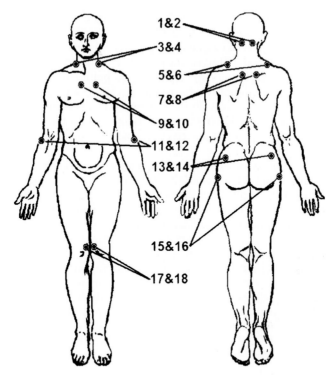

FIGURE 24.1 Fibromyalgia is suspected if pain can be elicited in 11 of 18 tender point sites with digital palpation using an approximate force of 4 kg.

prominence; 17 and 18, knee, bilateral, at the medial fat pad proximal to the joint line.[8]

Disturbance in the neuroendocrine axis is implicated in the etiology of fibromyalgia as well. In sleep studies, patients with fibromyalgia have a disturbance of the non-REM sleep phase by intrusions of alpha waves, with infrequent progression to stage 3 and stage 4 sleep.[10] Several conditions besides chronic fatigue syndrome are associated with fibromyalgia, including migraine headache, irritable bowel syndrome, and depression.[11]

Diagnosis of either chronic fatigue syndrome or fibromyalgia involves eliciting a detailed history from the patient, a thorough physical examination, and ruling out any underlying conditions that may mimic the symptoms of either chronic fatigue syndrome or fibromyalgia (discussed later in the chapter).

Theories, Causes, and Contributing Factors

Although for some time individuals who complained of chronic fatigue syndrome or fibromyalgia were considered to have an emotional disturbance (and by some practitioners many still are), it is becoming clear that chronic fatigue syndrome and fibromyalgia cannot be understood on the basis of a single dysfunction; rather, the function of all essential systems must be considered in an integrated manner. Evidence exists for immune, endocrine, cardiovascular, and autonomic nervous system dysfunction in patients with chronic fatigue syndrome.

In fibromyalgia, in addition, there is evidence of sleep disturbance and neuroendocrine dysfunction. Leaders in the field advocate for multidisciplinary research.[4] This situation is analogous to having a car with four flat tires and a dead battery. If you change one tire, you will have one good tire but still three flats and a dead battery. If you change the battery, the car will start, but it will still be a rough ride with flat tires, and you will not be able to go very fast. All four tires and the battery must be changed for success. In the same way, it is beginning to appear that multiple systems are involved in both chronic fatigue syndrome and fibromyalgia, and successful intervention means treating and supporting multiple systems simultaneously.

Regarding the etiology of these disorders, a strong neuroendocrine connection is emerging. In one study, it was found that patients with chronic fatigue syndrome had reduced gray matter volume in the bilateral prefrontal cortex. The volume of reduction in the right prefrontal cortex paralleled the severity of the subject's fatigue.[12] In another study, chronic fatigue syndrome patients were found to have a decreased density of serotonin transporters, indicating an alteration of the serotonergic system in chronic fatigue syndrome.[13]

The hypothalamus controls sleep, hormonal patterns, autonomic function, and temperature. Hypothalamic dysfunction is often a common denominator in chronic fatigue syndrome and fibromyalgia.[14] Hypothalamic dysfunction may come from mitochondrial dysfunction. How do the mitochondria become dysfunctional? Autonomic dysfunction, various infections, stresses, and hormonal deficiencies can exhaust the mitochondria, leading to mitochondrial dysfunction. That in turn leads to hypothalamic dysfunction, leading further to chronic fatigue, sleep disturbance, and fibromyalgia.

In a survey of the literature regarding the biology of chronic fatigue syndrome, Komaroff[15] and Komaroff and Buchwald[16] summarized the following findings in patients with chronic fatigue syndrome:

- Magnetic resonance imaging has revealed punctate areas of high signal in the white matter.
- Single photon emission computed tomography signal abnormalities are often found in patients with chronic fatigue syndrome; abnormalities of the sympathetic and parasympathetic systems that are not explained by depression or deconditioning have been revealed through autonomic nervous system testing.
- Hypothalamic and pituitary studies have revealed abnormalities not seen in healthy control subjects; a central down-regulation of the hypothalamic-pituitary-adrenal axis is often present, resulting in a mild hypercortisolism.
- Disruption of the serotonergic and noradrenergic pathways has been identified.
- Many chronic fatigue syndrome patients have been found to be in a state of chronic immune activation, with increased numbers of CD8+ cytotoxic T cells with antigenic markers of activation and depressed function of natural killer cells, leading to a hypothesis of reactivation of latent viruses or of chronic low-grade viral infection.
- A novel 37-KDa protein has been found in about 70% of patients with chronic fatigue syndrome.
- Aberrations in the 2-5A synthetase pathway (that has antiviral roles) have also been seen.

While these findings have not yet been synthesized into a single theory that explains the etiology or pathophysiology of chronic fatigue syndrome, there is clearly an abundance of evidence pointing to an underlying biological process.

Neurologic and endocrinologic findings in patients with fibromyalgia include the following:

- Elevation of cerebrospinal fluid substance P levels to three times normal levels[17]
- Low overall production of cortisol and alteration of the hypopituitary-adrenal axis[18]
- A significant prevalence of neuronally mediated hypotension evidenced by provocation of symptoms during tilt-table testing[19]

The musculoskeletal system, the neuroendocrine system, and the central nervous system, particularly the limbic system, appear to play major roles in the pathogenesis of fibromyalgia as well.[20] (See Chapter 6.)

If we consider what is known about nervous system function from a neuroendocrine perspective and from the body's drive to maintain homeostasis, this seemingly random cascade of symptoms and findings fits together as parts of an integrated whole. Moreover, these findings are consistent with the consequences of excessive allostatic load or a chronic state of allostasis.

Structure and function are interrelated. If function is impaired, structure will ultimately be impaired; if structure is impaired, function ultimately will be affected. Somatic dysfunction is a part of this process. In addition to activating related spinal cord circuits, somatic dysfunction releases humoral factors. Summation of these two events occurs at the level of the brainstem to initiate general arousal and protective endocrine and neural reflexes. In acute situations, these responses, which result in a state of allostasis or compensation, are protective; however, chronic exposure to allostasis is pathologic. Allostasis is the response by the neuroendocrine and immune network to stimuli, with a consequent rapid release of chemicals that alter the normal homeostatic patterns: norepinephrine, adrenal cortical steroids, and cytokines. Allostasis is distinct from homeostasis, and when prolonged, allostasis produces harmful effects. Chronic somatic or visceral dysfunction can have pathologic consequences arising from continuous stimulation of the arousal system.[21] Allostasis is a defensive state. Long-term activation of the allostatic mechanism or increasing allostatic load leads to extensive wear and tear on the organ systems of the body. Some consequences of prolonged activation of the allostatic system include memory loss, depression, immunosuppression, and enhanced Th2 cytokine activity, allowing yet more antibody-mediated autoimmune and allergic types of diseases to be expressed. In the gastrointestinal system and skin, elevated cortisol and catecholamines increase the responsiveness of delayed-type hypersensitivity reactions, insulin resistance, atherosclerosis, and hypertension.[21]

The sympathetic nervous system and the hypothalamic-pituitary-adrenal axis are coupled to the arousal system. With increased input to the arousal system, there is a release of catecholamines from the sympathetic nervous system and adrenal corticosteroids from the hypothalamic-pituitary-adrenal axis. Cortisol and norepinephrine work to modify the production of the cytokines from the immune system. The neural, endocrine, and immune systems all work together in response to threat to alter homeostasis to the compensatory state of allostasis. If the body is unable to return to homeostasis, whether because of chronic exposure to threat or failure of the neural or humoral pathways, the body exists in a chronic compensatory state. As we know in the case of congestive heart failure, the compensatory mechanisms ultimately create further pathology if homeostasis is not restored.

How does this relate to chronic fatigue syndrome and fibromyalgia? The consequence of existing in a chronic compensatory state or allostasis reflects many of the problems encountered by the individual with chronic fatigue syndrome or fibromyalgia. If one examines the wide array of symptoms and the biologic findings previously noted, they are clearly indicative of a state of chronic allostasis.

Differential Diagnosis

A multitude of conditions can lead to symptoms of long standing chronic fatigue and must be considered in the differential diagnosis and ruled out. In the future, some may even be found to be causative factors. Disorders in all systems can be a factor. The following must be considered (Table 24.1).

The differential diagnosis must include careful consideration of infectious, neuroendocrine, psychiatric, neuropsychiatric, hematologic, rheumatologic, cardiovascular, pulmonary, and gastrointestinal disorders.

Psychological causes of fatigue also act as triggers of allostasis. Fear, sorrow, guilt, depression, anxiety, anger, resentment, bitterness, frustration, worry, jealousy, hatred, and grief all depress bodily functions and can lead to somatic dysfunction. Negative factors include the following:

- Boredom drains energy and is stressful.
- Compulsions can lead to continuous fatigue.
- Depression can be the cause of or the result of fatigue.
- Noise pollution, including background noise in large cities and constant TV, radio, or music in the workplace or home, can be wearying.
- Stress—lack of balance in the lifestyle—leads to fatigue as the body is no longer able to react to the stress when the stress-reaction mechanisms become exhausted (excessive allostatic load).

Positive emotions, such as joy, on the other hand, induce dilation of the capillaries and arteries, increasing blood supply throughout the body. The eyes brighten, thinking becomes clearer, respirations deepen, heartbeats strengthen, and digestion becomes more efficient.

Allergy and Fatigue

Allergens act as stressors, triggering allostasis; energy is depleted with every allergic reaction. Allergy symptoms can mimic chronic fatigue syndrome and fibromyalgia. Muscle and bone pain, paleness, dark circles under the eyes, irritability and tension, headaches, stomachaches, and respiratory tract symptoms (repeated colds, asthma, or allergic rhinitis), fatigue, irritability, mental confusion, unhappiness, nervousness, emotional instability, and inability to concentrate are characteristic of allergies. Identifying allergens and treating and eliminating the causes can be helpful. Sources of allergens include foods, the environment, workplace exposure, and household toxins. Common food allergens include milk, kola (includes cola drinks and chocolate, which both contain much caffeine), corn, eggs, and legumes. (The pea family includes peanuts, soybeans, and licorice.) Mature dry peas and beans are more likely to induce reactions than are green or string beans or green peas. People sensitive to legumes are often sensitive to honey. (In the United States, honey is collected mostly from plants in the legume family.) Other allergen-inducing agents include citrus, apple, tomato,

TABLE 24.1

Causes of Longstanding Chronic Fatigue

System Dysfunction	Causative Factors		
Immune	Collagen-vascular disease	Food allergies	Infectious mononucleosis
		Malignancy, cancer	Multiple chemical sensitivities
	Occult infection	Rheumatic fever	Sarcoidosis
	Streptococcal infections	Systemic lupus erythematosus	Tuberculosis
	Viral diseases		
Endocrine, hematologic	Anemias	Diabetes	Endocrine abnormalities
	Hyperthyroidism	Hypoglycemia	Hypothyroidism
	Menstrual disorders	Obesity	Pregnancy
	Sickle cell disease		
Pulmonary	Asthma	COPD	Emphysema
	Hyperventilation, hypoventilation	Sleep apnea	
Cardiovascular	Congestive heart failure	Hypertension	Low cardiac output
	Mitral valve dysfunction		
Digestive tract, hepatic	Chronic constipation	Gluten intolerance, celiac disease	Hepatitis
	Inflammatory bowel disease	Irritable bowel syndrome	Ulcer disease
Neurologic	Amyotrophic lateral sclerosis	Dementia	Insomnia
	Multiple sclerosis	Myasthenia gravis	Narcolepsy
	Parkinson's disease	Post concussion syndrome	
Genitourinary	Glomerulonephritis	Lower urinary tract infection	Menorrhagia
Metabolic, nutritional	Alcoholism	Caffeine use	Chemical dependency, drug abuse
	Chronic dehydration	Fasting	Hypokalemia
	Medications	Severe dietary deficiencies	Severe dietary restrictions
Musculoskeletal	Hypermobility	Osteoarthritis	Rheumatoid arthritis
Environmental, social	Environmental stress	Inadequate rest	Lack of exercise
	Poor ventilation	Recent illness	Recent surgery
	Sick building syndrome	Sleep disturbance	

COPD, chronic obstructive pulmonary disease.

grains (wheat is the most allergenic; rye, the least), food additives and spices, and meats. (Pork is a common meat allergen; all other meats and seafood can be also.) Environmental allergies, such as plants, molds, gases, animals and their hair and dander, chemicals, drugs, cosmetics, and synthetic fabrics also must be considered.

Prognosis

Little is known about long-term outcomes of chronic fatigue syndrome or fibromyalgia. Most patients seem to improve within 5 years, but most continue to struggle with some symptoms and some degree of impairment on an ongoing basis. In light of understanding the consequences of a chronic compensatory state, unless the body achieves homeostasis, the negative effects of chronic exposure to allostasis will progress.

Initial Workup

The initial workup for patients who complain of fatigue and/or widespread musculoskeletal pain should include the following:

- A detailed history elucidating onset of symptoms and a thorough evaluation for evidence of underlying conditions or contributing factors
- A detailed physical examination, including neurologic and psychologic evaluations and musculoskeletal and structural examinations
- Urinalysis
- Complete blood count with leukocyte differential
- Sedimentation rate or C-reactive protein
- Alanine amino transferase and aspartate transaminase
- Globulin
- Alkaline phosphatase
- Glucose
- Calcium
- Phosphorus
- Thyroid function test (thyroid-stimulating hormone, free T_4, total T_3)
- Rheumatoid factor and antinuclear antibodies

If there are indications of nutritional concerns, serum B_{12} is useful, and if allergic symptoms are predominant, an immunoglobulin-E may be helpful. Often the history and examination will indicate further tests that may explain the fatigue state, for example a sleep study for suspected sleep apnea. An early morning cortisol level, hepatitis serology, rapid plasma reagin, Lyme serology, and a tuberculin purified protein derivative with an anergy panel may be indicated if other laboratory and clinical findings are negative.[22]

Key symptoms to evaluate on the initial visit include sore throat, painful cervical or axillary lymph nodes, unexplained generalized muscle weakness, prolonged (more than 24 hours) generalized fatigue, generalized headaches, migratory painful joints without swelling or redness, areas of lost or depressed vision, photophobia, forgetfulness, excessive irritability, confusion, difficulty thinking, inability to concentrate, depression, and unrefreshing sleep. It is helpful to have the patients grade the symptoms as mild, moderate, severe, or absent.

The chronic fatigue syndrome Diagnostic Decision-Making Model provides a basic guide to working through the diagnostic process[7] (Fig. 24.2).

For more information or to obtain continuing education credits, please visit www.cfids.org/treatcfs or phone 1-704-364-0016.

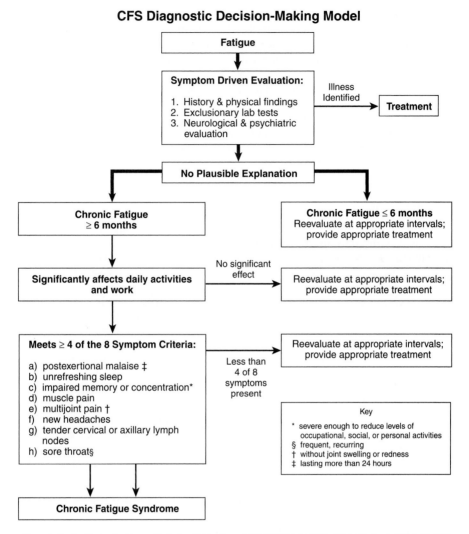

CFS Diagnostic Decision-Making Model

Fatigue

Symptom Driven Evaluation:

1. History & physical findings
2. Exclusionary lab tests
3. Neurological & psychiatric evaluation

Illness Identified → **Treatment**

No Plausible Explanation

Chronic Fatigue ≥ 6 months

Chronic Fatigue ≤ 6 months
Reevaluate at appropriate intervals; provide appropriate treatment

Significantly affects daily activities and work

No significant effect → Reevaluate at appropriate intervals; provide appropriate treatment

Meets ≥ 4 of the 8 Symptom Criteria:

a) postexertional malaise ‡
b) unrefreshing sleep
c) impaired memory or concentration*
d) muscle pain
e) multijoint pain †
f) new headaches
g) tender cervical or axillary lymph nodes
h) sore throat§

Less than 4 of 8 symptoms present → Reevaluate at appropriate intervals; provide appropriate treatment

Key

* severe enough to reduce levels of occupational, social, or personal activities
§ frequent, recurring
† without joint swelling or redness
‡ lasting more than 24 hours

Chronic Fatigue Syndrome

Supported by the Centers for Disease Control and Prevention and the CFIDS Association of America * www.cfids.org/treatcfs

FIGURE 24.2 The chronic fatigue syndrome diagnostic algorithm was designed for the chronic fatigue syndrome Provider Education Project, which is supported by the Centers for Disease Control and Prevention and the Chronic Fatigue and Immune Dysfunction Syndrome Association of America.

THE INTERRELATIONSHIP OF STRUCTURE AND FUNCTION IN CHRONIC FATIGUE SYNDROME AND FIBROMYALGIA

In osteopathic practice, the objective is to find the underlying causes of illness and remove barriers to healing. While there is no clearly defined cause of chronic fatigue syndrome or fibromyalgia, the constellation of symptoms is consistent with a state of chronic allostasis. There is evidence of abnormal neuroendocrine function in chronic fatigue syndrome and fibromyalgia. The physician can use knowledge of structure and function interrelationships to facilitate homeostasis and eliminate sources of input activating allostasis. The finding of viscerosomatic reflexes on structural examination can offer useful information and direct clinical investigation. Specific organ systems identified can help the physician evaluate for underlying organic pathology. (See Chapter 5.) Two drives affect the arousal–allostatic mechanism: physical, through somatic dysfunction and visceral dysfunction, and psychological, through emotional and cognitive influences.[21] Individuals with chronic fatigue syndrome or fibromyalgia are clearly in a chronic compensatory state, a state of allostasis rather than homeostasis. By addressing somatic, visceral, emotional, and cognitive dysfunction, the physician can help facilitate the patient's return to a state of homeostasis.

Management

Individuals with chronic fatigue syndrome and fibromyalgia often have been struggling with symptoms for years and require much support from the physician. A willingness to try novel therapies in difficult cases is useful. The goals of treatment are to alleviate allostatic load, support return to homeostasis, decrease fatigue and pain, and increase daily functional abilities by supporting dysfunctional systems while eliminating identifiable contributing factors. Effective and supportive therapy must be directed toward key areas providing symptomatic treatment and relief. Teitelbaum,[5] based on a double-blind study, has published an extensive list of interventions ranging from nutritional supports and herbal interventions to pharmaceutical interventions for each of the systems that may be in dysfunction in chronic fatigue syndrome or fibromyalgia. Emphasized for the beginning of treatment are five key areas: sleep treatments, pain treatments, hormonal treatments (adrenal, thyroid and sex hormones), nutrition, and infections.

Some key interventions for these four areas are summarized in Table 24.2, which provides an excellent resource when seeking options for symptomatic treatment.[5]

Osteopathic manipulative treatment (OMT) is useful for enhancing immune function and has proved helpful in reducing the intensity and duration of illness.[23–25] Goals of treatment include the following:[26]

- Normalizing nerve function, including all cranial and spinal nerves as well as the autonomic nervous system
- Balancing sympathetic and parasympathetic tone
- Normalizing function of the cerebrum, thalamus, hypothalamus, and pituitary body
- Normalizing cerebrospinal fluid fluctuation
- Releasing membranous tension
- Modifying gross structural patterns
- Counteracting stress-producing factors
- Alleviating pain
- Improving lymphatic function and improving circulation

In this author's experience, patients respond best to gentle indirect OMT procedures, and while they may derive some temporary relief from direct procedures and high-velocity, low-amplitude (HVLA), these approaches often result in a flare of symptoms later in the day that may persist for several days. Myofascial release, gentle muscle energy, facilitated positional release, balanced membranous tension, balanced ligamentous tension, the Fulford percussor, gentle soft tissue, and articulation are all helpful approaches.

TABLE 24.2

Selected Treatment Interventions for Chronic Fatigue Syndrome or Fibromyalgia

Sleep Treatments

Zolpidem (Ambien) 10 mg 1/2–11/2 at HS; may take an extra 1/2 during the night

Trazodone (Desyrel) 50 mg 1/2–6 at HS

Revitalizing Sleep Formula (herbal blend by Enzymatic Therapies and PhytoPharmica) 1–4 at HS; can be used during the day for anxiety

Tizanidine (Zanaflex) 2–8 mg at HS

Clonazepam (Klonopin) 0.5–3 mg at HS; very effective for sleep, restless leg syndrome, pain

Doxylamine (Unisom), over-the-counter antihistamine, 25 mg 1/2–1 tablet

Carisoprodol (Soma) 1/2–1 at HS; can be useful if pain is severe

Cyclobenzaprine (Flexeril) 10 mg 1/2–2 at HS

Zaleplon (Sonata) 10 mg 1 at HS—may repeat during the night if awake before 3 a.m.

Melatonin 0.5–1 mg at HS

5-HTP (5-hydroxytryptophan) 200–400 mg at HS; natural stimulator of serotonin

Mirtazapine (Remeron) 15 mg 1–3 tablets at HS

Amitriptyline (Elavil) 10 mg 1/2–5 tablets at HS; good for nerve pain and vulvodynia

Doxepin (Sinequan) 5–10 mg 1–3 capsules at HS

Alprazolam (Xanax) 0.5 mg 1/2–4 tablets at HS

Pain Treatment

Glucosamine sulfate 500 mg t.i.d. for patients with arthritis

Lidocaine 15% in PLO gel; rub on painful areas

Lidocaine patch; can be cut to size and left on for 12 hours

Methocarbamol (Robaxin) 750 mg 1 or 2 capsules t.i.d.–q.i.d. as needed

Tramadol (Ultram) 50 mg 1 or 2 tablets up to q.i.d.

Metaxalone (Skelaxin) 400 mg 1 or 2 tablets q.i.d. as needed

Gabapentin (Neurontin) start with 100–300 mg at HS; may increase dose as needed to maximum of 3600 mg/day

Hormonal treatments (All dosages adjusted to patient's response)

Adrenal

Hydrocortisone (Cortef) 5-mg tablets 1/2–21/2 tablets at breakfast, 1/2–11/2 tablets at lunch, 0–1/2 tablet at 4 P.M.; lowest dose that feels best for patient

Panax ginseng 100–200 mg twice a day

Increase salt, water, potassium for low blood pressure (12 oz V8 juice, 1 banana/day)

Thyroid

Levothyroxine (Levoxyl or Synthroid) 50 µg—titrate dose as needed

Thyroid desiccated (Armour Thyroid) 30 mg (1/2 grain = 30 mg); if taking Cortef, begin Cortef 1–7 days prior to start of thyroid support

Liothyronine (Cytomel pure active T$_3$) 5-µg tablets

(Continued)

TABLE 24.2 (CONT.)

Selected Treatment Interventions for Chronic Fatigue Syndrome or Fibromyalgia

Nutrition

Magnesium glycinate 75 mg/malic acid 300 mg 2 tablets t.i.d. for 8 months then 2 tablets daily (decrease dose if diarrhea occurs)

Magnesium malate 100 mg 3 t.i.d.

Zinc picolinate or zinc sulphate 25 mg b.i.d. for 6 weeks then stop

Vitamin C 500–1000 mg b.i.d.

Vitamin B_{12} 1000–15,000 mcg/ml IM 3–5 times a week for up to 10 weeks

N-Acetyl-L-cysteine 500–650 mg per day

Chromagen FA (R_x) one tablet daily (for low iron levels)

Omega 3 fish oils 1/2–1 tablespoon per day

Vitamin E 400 IU per day

Calcium 500–1000 mg daily with 400 IU vitamin D

B-complex one tablet or capsule daily

Complete amino acids, nutrients, vitamins and minerals (Daily Energy Enfusion Powder formulated by Enzymatic Therapies) 1/2–1 scoop daily in morning; take with B-complex

Digestive enzymes (Complete Gest Enzymes by Enzymatic Therapies or Similase by PhytoPharmica) 2 capsules with each meal to help digestion

Antiviral and Antibacterial Treatments

Famciclovir (Famvir) 750 mg t.i.d.

Amantadine (Symmetrel) 100 mg b.i.d.

Ciprofloxacin (Cipro) 750 mg b.i.d.

Doxycycline 100 mg b.i.d.

Sinusitis nasal sprays, ordered from a compounding pharmacist: itraconazole (Sporanox), xylitol, mupirocin (Bactroban), beclomethasone (Beconase), nystatin

HS, hour of sleep; IM, intramuscular; PLO, pluronic lecithin organogel; t.i.d., three times a day; q.i.d., four times a day; b.i.d., twice a day.

Data from Teitelbaum J. From Fatigued to Fantastic. New York: Penguin Putnam, 2001.

Many patients with chronic fatigue syndrome or fibromyalgia are extremely sensitive; therefore, when beginning osteopathic treatment, care should be taken not to overdose. (See Chapter 4.) Too much treatment will result in an exacerbation of pain symptoms that may last for days. When in doubt, be conservative and evaluate the patient's response before proceeding with more extensive treatment. Osteopathic treatment of somatic dysfunction can provide the patient with relief of often relentless and intense pain. While the effects may not always be long lasting, OMT is a nonpharmacologic intervention with limited side effects and is often soothing to the patient. Moreover, it has demonstrated immunologic benefits.[25]

A sequence to consider for the use of OMT when treating a patient with chronic fatigue syndrome or fibromyalgia is presented next. (Again, this sequence would be modified by the patient's condition, individual needs, and structural findings.)

It is a nine-step treatment regimen for a gentle basic treatment emphasizing the neuroendocrine, myofascial, and lymphatic systems. Patient is supine.

- Release of myofascial restrictions of the feet, knees, and lower extremities
- Pelvic diaphragm release
- Sacrum
- Relax or dome the abdominal diaphragm
- Respiratory diaphragm release
- Rib balancing, rib raising, and/or paraspinal inhibition (T1–L2)
- Release of thoracic inlet
- Lymphatic pump (thoracic or pedal, depending on patient's tolerance and level of pain)
- CV-4

See other procedures described at the end of this chapter.

Individual structural findings can be addressed on an ongoing basis. Focus treatment on key somatic dysfunctions that will improve and balance sympathetic and parasympathetic tone, improve lymphatic flow, improve circulation, and improve neuroendocrine function.

An important adjunct to hands-on treatment is a realistic plan of physical activity for the patients. Often patients are too fatigued or in too much pain to do anything, yet decreased activity contributes to the cycle of pain and fatigue. Beginning with gentle stretches that can be done in bed and breathing exercises, patients must be taught to titrate their activity and include frequent rest periods; they must learn to stop before they begin to feel tired. As symptoms improve, they will be tempted to overdo exercise and will consequently often regress. It is important to teach patients to stop early and rest often but then to get moving again.

Sleep

The goal is for the patient to get 7 to 9 hours of refreshing sleep each night without feeling hung over. Sleep is an essential part of healing. Many of the restorative processes take place at night. Without adequate sleep, it is difficult to achieve homeostasis. It is essential to work on establishing normal sleep architecture. Have the patient eliminate caffeine and alcohol, both of which interfere with sleep. Instruct the patient to get out of bed at the same time each morning to promote a healthy circadian rhythm. Referral to a sleep specialist may be helpful if there is an underlying sleep disorder. Most sleeping pills in common use worsen the quality of sleep by increasing the amount of light-stage sleep and decreasing the deep stages of sleep. It is important to avoid the use of such agents. Some helpful options include zolpidem, zaleplon, trazodone, clonazepam, doxylamine, carisoprodol (for patients in severe pain), cyclobenzaprine, mirtazapine, amitriptyline, and alprazolam.[27] Start with low doses. Often a low dose of two agents is more effective than a high dose of just one. Since research into the pharmacology of these agents at the applied clinical level is limited, the physician will have to work on an approach that fits the patient best and achieves the goal of 7 to 9 hours of refreshing sleep.

Pain

Osteopathic treatment, warm baths, and acetaminophen are helpful. Use of opioids has not been found helpful, but in extreme cases of pain, they may be necessary. More benefit has been found from the use of a muscle relaxant such as cyclobenzaprine. The causative mechanism of pain is not fully understood, so interventions are geared to support. Biofeedback, transcutaneous neural stimulation, massage, and ultrasound are some of the techniques that individuals have found to be helpful. Pain relief at bedtime is important to facilitate adequate rest and sleep.

Neuroendocrine Imbalances

Dysautonomias are sometimes helped with increased fluid and salt intake. Hypoadrenal function has been shown to benefit from low-dose hydrocortisone (5–25 mg daily up to 24 months, then taper dosage as necessary). Fatigue was improved and disability was reduced without significant short-term adverse effects or suppression of the hypothalamic-pituitary-adrenal axis.[28-31] Thyroid and ovarian function often improve once adrenal function is supported, but at times, the patient will still be borderline or low in thyroid or ovarian function and require treatment as indicated by the individual condition. Sleep, pain, brain fog, and energy levels have all been found to improve with adrenal support.

Infections

Any underlying infections should be treated. Chronic sinus infections, fungal skin infections, vaginal yeast infections, and chronic viral and bacterial infections all act as stressors on the system. While there is no consensus as to the best approach to treat these chronic infections, we do know that the ongoing presence of untreated infections acts as a stressor and pushes the system toward allostasis and away from homeostasis. A review of past treatment attempts, current available options, and a willingness to try new interventions will be most helpful to the patient.

Nutrition

Adequate water intake and good nutrition are essential. Adequate intake of protein, fruits, and vegetables is important to provide the essential vitamins, minerals, and amino acids needed to repair and restore body functions. Consultation with a nutritionist will be helpful if the physician desires assistance regarding nutritional issues.

Psychological Support

Several interventions can be helpful. Stress management, relaxation techniques, and emotional support are all important parts of treatment. Some clinical studies have found cognitive therapy to be helpful; it should, however, be carried out by a trained clinician.[22] Most important is the psychological support provided by the treating physician. Living with chronic fatigue syndrome or fibromyalgia is difficult, and many patients have been told they are crazy or that nothing is wrong with them. They need and deserve the support of a compassionate physician who is willing to work with them to find solutions for their symptoms, even as researchers attempt to explain why and find solutions.

It is important to evaluate new symptoms or any changes or deterioration for possible onset of other illnesses. When treating the patient, focus on all of the symptoms, not just the fatigue. Provide support for the patient, family, and significant others. Symptomatic treatment can improve the quality of life for people with chronic fatigue syndrome or fibromyalgia.[7] Working with these patients will require an ongoing supportive physician–patient relationship.

While there is still much to understand about chronic fatigue syndrome and fibromyalgia, the osteopathic physician has the opportunity to support the patient's return to homeostasis through osteopathic treatment, mitigating and eliminating somatic dysfunction as a stressor, and providing ongoing clinical support for the myriad of symptoms and comorbid conditions affecting these individuals.

Procedures

Please note: The procedures that follow are examples of manipulative treatment that you may wish to employ. The actual choice of procedures used should be determined by the unique circumstances of each individual patient.

The following is a gentle basic treatment emphasizing the neuroendocrine and lymphatic systems.

- Release of the thoracic inlet (See the description of the procedure in Chapter 19 and Fig. 19.2.)
- Rib raising (See the description of the procedure in Chapter 5 and Fig. 5.6.)
- Paraspinal (T1–L2) inhibition in the same positions as rib raising (See Chapter 5.)
- Relax or dome the thoracoabdominal diaphragm (See the description of the procedure in Chapter 19 and Fig. 19.4.)
- Lymphatic pump, thoracic (See the description of the procedure in Chapter 16 and Fig. 16.19.)
- Pedal pump (See the description of the procedure in Chapter 10 and Fig. 10.3.)
- Treat the pelvic diaphragm (See the description of the procedure in Chapter 9 and Figs. 9.11 and 9.12.)
- CV-4 (See the description of the procedure in Chapter 10 and Fig. 10.1.)

For a more extensive treatment, add the following:

- Release of myofascial restriction of the feet, knees and lower extremities (discussed later in the chapter)
- Sacrum (See the description of the procedure in Chapter 12 and Fig. 12.5.)
- Piriformis (discussed later)
- Psoas (if indicated) (See the description of the procedure in Chapter 9 and Fig. 9.3.)
- Facilitated positional release or counterstrain for thoracic and lumbar regions dysfunction (See Figs. 13.2 and 13.4–13.6.)
- Rib balancing (See Fig. 22.8.)
- Cervical spine procedures (See Figs. 12.1, 16.6, and 25.6.)
- Occipitoatlantal joint (See Figs. 16.12 and 25.7.) Cranium (See Figs. 8.5–8.9, 14.4–14.7, and 25.8–25.10.)

Piriformis Muscle Tender Point (Counterstrain) (Fig. 24.3).

This procedure is employed to alleviate tenderness of the piriformis muscle.

Patient position: prone. Physician position: seated beside the table at the level of the patient's pelvis on the side of the dysfunctional piriform muscle.

Procedure

1. With the index finger of one hand, locate the tender point commonly found centrally within the body of the piriformis muscle approximately midway between the inferolateral angle of the sacrum and the greater trochanter of the femur. This hand placement must be maintained throughout the procedure.
2. Assess the degree of tissue texture abnormality and tension associated with the tender point. By increasing the amount of digital pressure applied to the tender point, determine the baseline severity of tenderness present. Assign this level of tenderness a value of 100% and inform the patient.
3. Have the patient slide the pelvis toward you so that the hip on the side of the dysfunctional piriformis muscle is at the edge of the treatment table.
4. With your other hand, grasp the patient's ankle closer to you, flex the knee, and lower it off the side of the side of the treatment table, flexing the hip. At this point,

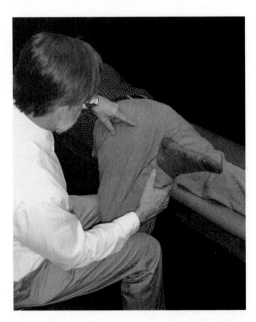

FIGURE 24.3   Piriformis tender point, counterstrain, employed to alleviate tenderness of the piriform muscle.

you may find it easiest to support the patient's thigh by holding their knee between your knees.

5. Further adjust hip flexion and extension, abduction and adduction, and internal and external rotation by moving the patient's knee with your knees to obtain maximum reduction of palpable tissue tension and tenderness. It is generally thought that when the patient is properly positioned, perceived tenderness should be decreased to no more than 30% of the 100% established in step 2.

6. Hold this position of maximum palpable tissue tension and tenderness reduction 90 seconds, then slowly return the patient to the original position. It is important not to remove your monitoring finger during the course of the procedure so that you can be certain the reduction in tenderness post treatment occurred specifically in the original tender point.

7. Reassess the tender point for residual tenderness.

Hamstring Release (Myofascial Release) (Fig. 24.4)

This procedure is employed to decrease hamstring hypertonicity. It employs the principles of counterstrain to treat dysfunction between agonist and antagonist muscle groups. A specific tender point is not necessarily present. The physician loads the antagonist and unloads the agonist. This may be considered a direct myofascial release to the antagonist or an indirect technique to the agonist.

Patient position: prone. Physician position: standing at the side of the treatment table on the side of the dysfunctional hamstring muscle or muscles.

Procedure

1. Using both hands, palpate the dysfunctional hamstring muscle to identify increased muscular tension. Keep one hand in contact with this area throughout the remainder of the procedure.

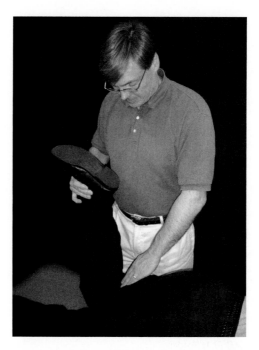

FIGURE 24.4   Hamstring release, employed to decease hamstring hypertonicity.

2. With your other hand, grasp the ankle of the dysfunctional lower extremity and slowly flex the patient's knee until you palpate decreased tension in the dysfunctional hamstring muscle. In this position, the patient should feel tension in their anterior thigh musculature. Thus, you have unloaded the hamstring (agonist) muscles and loaded the quadriceps (antagonist).
3. It may be necessary to introduce small amounts of internal or external rotation of the tibia, or translation of the hamstring group medially or laterally with your monitoring hand until you feel the least amount of tension in the hamstring. The purpose of the procedure is to identify the position of greatest reduction of tissue tension.
4. Hold the position and wait for a release, the perception of relaxation of tension, to occur. Slowly return the leg down to the table.
5. Reassess hamstring muscular tension and tenderness.

Knee (Myofascial Release) (Fig. 24.5)

This procedure is employed to alleviate fascial restriction and improve knee function. It is particularly beneficial for treating tibial torsion, a dysfunction in which the tibia is internally or externally rotated relative to the femur. This procedure may be performed with either direct or indirect treatment principles.

Patient position: supine. Physician position: standing at the side of the treatment table on the side of the dysfunctional knee.

Procedure

1. Standing with your weight upon one leg, flex your other hip and knee and place that knee upon the treatment table with your thigh beneath the patient's dysfunctional knee, thus introducing slight flexion of the patient's knee. You may also accomplish this by placing a pillow beneath the patient's knee.

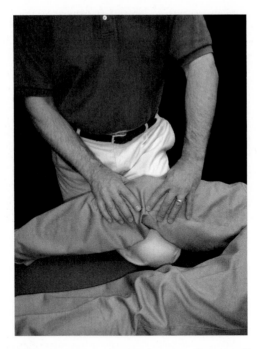

FIGURE 24.5   The position for this procedure may be employed to alleviate fascial restriction and improve knee function and to treat dysfunction between the tibia and femur.

2. Place one of your hands upon the patient's anterior thigh just proximal to the patella and your other hand upon the anterior tibia at the level of the tibial tuberosity.
3. Use this hand placement to assess myofascial tension of the knee by gently applying alternating left and right lateral translation, internal and external rotation, and compression and distraction between the tibia and femur. For each of these motion pairs, identify the directions of ease and of restriction.
4. To perform direct myofascial release, engage the restrictive barrier or barriers, moving the tibia in relation to the femur in the direction of the restrictions of lateral translation, rotation, and compression and distraction. Hold this position and wait for an inherent release or softening of tissue tension.
5. To perform indirect myofascial release, move away from the restrictive barrier or barriers, moving the tibia in relation to the femur in the direction of ease of lateral translation, rotation, and compression and distraction. Hold this position and wait for an inherent release or softening of tissue tension.
6. Reassess the dysfunctional knee.

Tibiofibular Balancing (Indirect) (Fig. 24.6)

Patient position: supine. Physician position: standing at the side of the treatment table on the side of the dysfunctional knee.

Procedure

1. Standing with your weight upon one leg, flex your other hip and knee and place that knee upon the treatment table with your thigh beneath the patient's dysfunctional

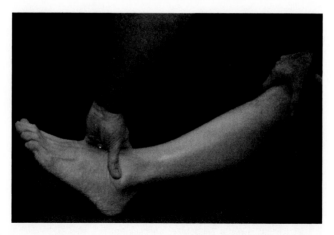

FIGURE 24.6 This procedure is employed to treat dysfunction between the tibia and fibula.

knee, thus introducing slight flexion of the patient's knee. You may also accomplish this by placing a pillow beneath the patient's knee.

2. Place one of your hands upon the patient's anterior tibia at the level of the tibial tuberosity with your thumb positioned laterally to monitor motion of the proximal fibula. This is your passive, monitoring hand.

3. Place your other hand on the anterior aspect of the patient's ankle in such a manner that you can grasp the ankle between your thumb and index finger. This is your active hand.

4. Use your active hand to introduce internal and external rotation between the tibia and the fibula around the longitudinal axis of the leg and identify the direction of ease and of restriction. The relationship between the tibia and fibula is such that as you introduce internal rotation of the leg at the distal tibiofibular articulation, the lateral malleolus will be drawn anteriorly, and simultaneously, at the proximal tibiofibular articulation, the fibula should move posteriorly.

5. Conversely, as you introduce external rotation of the leg at the distal tibiofibular articulation, the lateral malleolus will be pushed posteriorly, and simultaneously, at the proximal tibiofibular articulation, the fibula should move anteriorly.

6. To perform indirect myofascial release move away from the restrictive barrier or barriers, moving the fibula in relation to the tibia in the direction of ease. Hold this position and wait for an inherent release or softening of tissue tension.

7. Reassess the motion between the tibia and fibula.

Plantar Fascial Tender Point (Counterstrain) (Fig. 24.7)

This procedure is employed to alleviate tenderness of the plantar fascia at its insertion on the calcaneus.

Patient position: supine. Physician position: seated at the foot of the treatment table.

Procedure

1. With the index finger of one hand, locate the tender point on the inferior surface of the calcaneus, where the plantar fascia inserts. This hand placement must be maintained throughout the procedure.

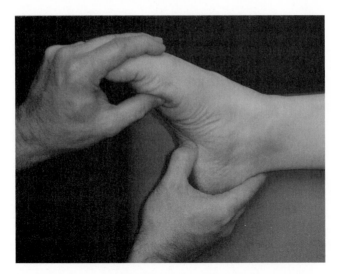

FIGURE 24.7   Plantar fascial tender point, counterstrain, employed to alleviate tenderness of the plantar fascia at its insertion on the calcaneus.

2. Assess the degree of tissue texture abnormality and tension associated with the tender point. By increasing the amount of digital pressure applied to the tender point, determine the baseline severity of tenderness. Assign this level of tenderness a value of 100% and inform the patient.
3. Grasp the distal portion of the painful foot with your other hand, plantar flex the ankle, and flex the toes to obtain maximum reduction of palpable tissue tension and tenderness. Supination or pronation of the foot may also be required to obtain the optimal positioning. It is generally thought that when the patient is properly positioned, perceived tenderness should be decreased to no more than 30% of the 100% established in step 2.
4. Hold this position of maximum palpable tissue tension and tenderness reduction 90 seconds, then slowly return the patient to the original position. It is important not to remove your monitoring finger during the course of the procedure so you can be certain the reduction in tenderness post treatment occurred specifically in the original tender point.
5. Reassess plantar fascial tenderness and tissue texture.

References

1. Chronic fatigue syndrome: Diagnosis and Management. Training Manual. Rev ed. A collaborative effort of the Centers for Disease Control and Prevention and the CFIDS Association of America. Atlanta: CFIDS Association of America; Centers for Disease Control and Prevention, 2003;8.
2. Craig T, Kakumanu S. Chronic fatigue syndrome: Evaluation and treatment. Am Fam Physician 2002;65:1083–1090, 1095.
3. Millea PJ, Holloway RL. Treating fibromyalgia. Am Fam Physician 2000;62:1575–1582, 1587.
4. Gerrity TR, Papanicolaou DA, Amsternam JD, et al. Immunologic aspects of chronic fatigue syndrome. Report on a Research Symposium convened by the CFIDS Association of America and cosponsored by the US Centers for Disease Control and Prevention and the National Institutes of Health. Neuroimmunomodulation 2004;11:351–357.

5. Teitelbaum J. From Fatigued to Fantastic. New York: Penguin Putnam, 2001;1.
6. Chronic fatigue syndrome Fact Sheet. National Institute of Allergy and Infectious Diseases Website. Last updated May 2004. Available at http/www.niaidh.nih.gov/factsheets/cfs.htm. Accessed May 4, 2005.
7. Chronic fatigue syndrome: Diagnosis and Management. Training Manual. Rev ed. A collaborative effort of the Centers for Disease Control and Prevention and the CFIDS Association of America, Inc. Atlanta, GA: CFIDS Association of America; Centers for Disease Control and Prevention, 2003:1.
8. Wolfe F, Smyte HA, Yunus MB, et al. The American College of Rheumatology 1990 Criteria for the Classification of Fibromyalgia. Report of the Multicenter Criteria Committee. Arthritis Rheum 1990;33:171.
9. Wolfe F, Smythe HA, Yunus MB, et al. The American College of Rheumatology 1990 Criteria for the Classification of Fibromyalgia. Report of the Multicenter Criteria Committee. Arthritis Rheum 1990;33:160–172.
10. Lentz MJ, Landis CA, Rothermel J, Shaver JL. Effects of selective slow wave sleep disruption on musculoskeletal pain and fatigue in middle aged women. J Rheumatol 1999;26:1586–1592.
11. Hudson JI, Goldenberg DL, Pope HG Jr, et al. Comorbidity of fibromyalgia with medical and psychiatric disorders. Am J Med 1992;92:363–367.
12. Okada T, Tanaka M, Kuratsune H, et al. Mechanisms underlying fatigue: A voxel-based morphometric study of chronic fatigue syndrome. BMC Neurol 2004;4(1):14.
13. Yamamoto S, Ouchi Y, Onoe H, et al. Reduction of serotonin transporters of patients with chronic fatigue syndrome. Neuroreport 2004;15:2571–2574.
14. Nampiaparampil DE, Shmerling RH. A review of fibromyalgia. Am J Manag Care 2004;10(11 Pt 1):794–800.
15. Komaroff AL. The biology of chronic fatigue syndrome. Am J Med 2000;108:169–171.
16. Komaroff AL, Buchwald DS. Chronic fatigue syndrome: An update. In: Coggins CH, Hancock EW, Levitt JJ, eds. Annual Review of Medicine. Palo Alto, CA: Annual Reviews, 1998;49:1–13.
17. Russell IJ, Orr MD, Littman G, et al. Elevated cerebrospinal fluid levels of substance P in patients with the fibromyalgia syndrome. Arthritis Rheum 1994;37:1593–1601.
18. Demitrack MA, Crofford LJ. Evidence for and pathophysiologic implications of hypothalamic-pituitary-adrenal axis dysregulation in fibromyalgia and chronic fatigue syndrome. Ann NY Acad Sci 1998;840:684–697.
19. Bou-Holaigah I, Calkins H, Flynn JA, et al. Provocation of hypotension and pain during upright tilt table testing in adults with fibromyalgia. Clin Exp Rheumatol 1997;15:239–246.
20. Demitrack MA, Dale JK, Straus SE, et al. Evidence for impaired activation of the hypothalamic-pituitary-adrenal axis in patients with chronic fatigue syndrome. J Clin Endocrinol Metab 1991;73:1224–1234.
21. Willard FH. Nociception, the neuroendocrine immune system, and osteopathic medicine. In: Ward RC, ed. Foundations for Osteopathic Medicine. 2nd ed. Philadelphia: Lippincott Williams & Wilkins, 2002;137–156.
22. John JF, ed. A Consensus Manual for the Primary Care and Management of chronic fatigue syndrome. Academy of Medicine of New Jersey, University of Medicine and Dentistry of New Jersey, and New Jersey Department of Health and Senior Services. March 2002;11.
23. Whiting CA. Investigation of the phagocytic index. Bulletin 1. AT Still Research Institute. Cincinnati, OH: Monford, 1910;61–63.
24. Smith RK. One hundred thousand cases of influenza with a death rate of one-fortieth of that officially reported under conventional medical treatment. J Am Osteopath Assoc 1920;19:172–175.
25. Measel JW Jr. The effect of the lymphatic pump upon the immune response:. I. Preliminary studies on the antibody response to pneumococcal polysaccharide assayed by bacterial agglutination and passive hemagglutination. J Am Osteopath Assoc 1982;82:28–31.
26. King HH, Lay EM. Osteopathy in the cranial field. In: Ward RC, ed. Foundations for Osteopathic Medicine. 2nd ed. Philadelphia: Lippincott Williams & Wilkins, 2002; 985–1001.
27. Teitelbaum J, Bird B. Effective treatment of chronic fatigue syndrome and FMS: A randomized, double-blind placebo controlled study. J Chronic Fatigue Syndrome 2001;8(2).

28. Cleare AJ, Heap E, Malhi GS, et al. Low-dose hydrocortisone in chronic fatigue syndrome: A randomised crossover trial. Lancet 1999;353:455–458.

29. Teitelbaum J, Bird B. Effective treatment of severe chronic fatigue: A report of a series of 64 patients. J Musculoskeletal Pain 1995;3(4):91–110.

30. Jefferies WM. Safe Uses of Cortisol. 2nd ed. Springfield, IL: Charles C. Thomas, 1996 [monograph].

31. Jefferies WM. Low-dosage glucocorticoid therapy: An appraisal of its safety and mode of action in clinical disorders, including rheumatoid arthritis. Arch Intern Med 1967; 119:265–278.

CHAPTER 25

The Patient with Chronic Pain, Headache

Thomas M. Richards

INTRODUCTION

More than 50 million workdays are lost each year to pain, the second leading cause of medically related work absenteeism.[1] In addition to absenteeism, most pain-related lost productive time has been shown to occur in the form of reduced performance while at work.[2]

In the United States, the use of complementary and alternative medicines (CAM) are on the rise.[3] Most people use CAM to prevent and/or treat musculoskeletal or other conditions associated with chronic or recurring pain. These conditions afflict one-quarter to one-third of the adult U.S. population.[4–9]

Many forms of chronic pain resist conventional medical treatment, so it is not surprising that so many seek alternative treatments.[10,11] In 1997 (the most recent year for which data are available), it was estimated that between $36 billion and $47 billion was spent by the U.S. public on CAM therapies.[5] Between $12.2 billion and $19.6 billion was paid out of pocket for the services of professional CAM health care providers (e.g., chiropractors, acupuncturists, and massage therapists). This is more than the U.S. public paid out of pocket for all hospitalizations and about half that paid out of pocket for all physician services that same year.[12] Health plan providers report that the cost effect of chronic pain is greater than that for all other typically diagnosed chronic conditions.[13] Thus, the costs of acute and chronic pain to society, through consumption of health care services and lost productivity, are enormous. Emotional costs and suffering are inestimable.

The ideal way to treat any malady is to identify and treat the cause. Somatic dysfunction is a frequent primary, secondary, and/or sustaining cause of both acute and chronic pain. Optimum pain management requires the identification and appropriate treatment of somatic dysfunction.[14–19]

Somatic dysfunction is defined as impaired or altered function of related components of the somatic (body framework) system: skeletal, arthrodial, and myofascial structures and related vascular, lymphatic, and neural elements.[15,17] It is characterized by palpation of tissue texture abnormality, asymmetry, restriction of motion, and tenderness (the standard osteopathic TART [tissue texture abnormality, asymmetry of position, restriction of motion, tenderness] criteria of somatic dysfunction).[20]

TABLE 25.1

Somatic Dysfunction Codes from the *International Classification of Diseases, 9th Clinical Modification, 2005*

739 Nonallopathic lesions not elsewhere classified
Includes segmental and somatic dysfunctions

739.0 Head region
Occipitocervical region

739.1 Cervical region
Cervicothoracic region

739.2 Thoracic region
Thoracolumbar region

739.3 Lumbar region
Lumbosacral region

739.4 Sacral region
Sacrococcygeal region
Sacroiliac region

739.5 Pelvic region
Hip region
Pubic region

739.6 Lower extremities

739.7 Upper extremities
Acromioclavicular region
Sternoclavicular region

739.8 Rib cage
Costochondral region
Costovertebral region
Sternochondral region

739.9 Abdomen and other

Somatic dysfunction is treatable using osteopathic manipulative procedures,[19] and diagnoses can be coded in the *International Classification of Diseases, Ninth Clinical Modification* (ICD-9CM) controlled vocabularies (Table 25.1).

Almost all physicians who administer osteopathic manipulative treatments (OMT) have treated patients with one procedure and observed "miraculous" cures.[16] This occurs usually when the etiology of the malady is acute somatic dysfunction, such as an occipitoatlantal dysfunction causing a muscle tension headache[21,22] or a sacroiliac dysfunction causing sciatica.[23]

Likewise, they have seen patients who have a recurrent problem. These patients respond favorably to treatment, but as time passes, the problem returns to its pretreatment state, only to respond again and again to treatment. Possible causes are inaccurate or incomplete diagnosis or some outside factor. Outside factors include ongoing misuse, as in repetitive use injuries, ongoing nociceptive perception, either central or peripheral, or something as simple as a short lower extremity.

There has been much discussion[24,25] about prolonged recurrent use of OMT for the same problem. When a patient presents with polyuria, polydipsia, and polyphagia, a blood sugar of 350, and a hemoglobin A1C of 10.2, the prescription might include dietary control, an exercise program, and a blood sugar–lowering agent. When that patient's blood sugar and hemoglobin A1C return to normal, the managing physician does not discontinue therapy. Likewise, when a patient's hypertensive blood pressure returns to normal, the physician does not discontinue the antihypertensives. A subset of patients require recurrent OMT to maintain optimal functionality. Patients in this category include some of those with chronic recurrent headaches[26,27] or chronic recurrent back pain[28] and those with chronic disease states with somatic dysfunction components, such as diabetes, hypertension, and chronic obstructive pulmonary disease.[29,30] It is appropriate to evaluate and treat such patients every 3 or 4 weeks to 2 or 3 times per year.

There is no paucity of studies evaluating manual medicine for the treatment of back pain.[28,30-31] Such studies are viewed as comparable to studies evaluating the efficacy of antibiotics in controlling fever or leukocytosis. OMT is not used to treat back pain; OMT is used to treat somatic dysfunction that may be the cause of back pain.

KINDS OF PAIN

To alleviate pain effectively, it is essential to adequately assess its source or sources. Pain falls into three physiological types, each with differing underlying mechanisms that can occur independently or in combination.

Nociceptive Pain

The nervous system possesses specialized nociceptive pain receptors on the tips of nerve cells that react to extreme temperatures (hot or cold), pressure, and substances released by other cells. These nerves can respond to burns, cuts, infections, inflammation, a severe lack of oxygen, or excessive pressure within or stretching of an organ.

Neuropathic Pain

When nerves become abnormally active, the sensation of pain can result. This neuropathic pain occurs, for instance, in diabetic neuropathy and in the postherpetic neuralgia that accompanies a shingles outbreak. Another example is the pain associated with the phantom limb phenomenon, in which abnormal nerve activity causes pain to persist long past the time expected for healing of the injury.

In other cases, the etiology of the pain can be very difficult to identify and treat. Diagnostic protocols are not standard. Neuropathic, nociceptive, and idiopathic pain may coexist. There is no consensus on the optimal management of neuropathic pain. Treatment may involve drug therapies, invasive therapies (ablative surgery, nerve blocks), and alternative therapies.[34–37]

Psychogenic Pain

When no physical cause of pain can be identified, psychologic causes should be explored.[38–40] No matter what the cause, the subjective sensation of pain varies with every person and can be influenced by an individual's attention to the pain, cultural learning, the perceived meaning of the situation, and any number of other psychological variables.[41]

MODALITIES IN PAIN TREATMENT

Numerous modalities, including pharmaceuticals, physical measures, physical therapy modalities, motion therapies, OMT, dietary measures, behavior modification, and invasive procedures, are available to treat pain (Table 25.2).

Reflecting this range of options is the fact that comprehensive pain management is evolving as a multidisciplinary team approach. The team may include practitioners from many diverse specialty areas. One such team includes 19 providers from the following areas: primary care, neurology, anesthesiology, pain management psychology, osteopathic manipulative medicine, physical therapy, pharmacy, occupational medicine, and acupuncture. There is also a nurse practitioner, who manages medications, and appointment coordinators. The team meets formally weekly to discuss selected new and/or difficult patients. The osteopathic physicians function as an intake portal and administer OMT to patients with somatic dysfunction when indicated.

The OMT practitioners were selected to serve as the intake portal for a number of reasons. Many chronic pain patients have back pain or headache. Approximately 85% of back pain is idiopathic to the allopathic profession.[42] The etiology of pain in many of these patients is somatic dysfunction. Manipulative medicine expertise in evaluating and treating somatic dysfunction that is causing the patient's pain makes the osteopathic physician a valuable front-end asset to the team. These team members are able to identify and treat pain patients and frequently can avoid the expensive workups and interventions, such as invasive injection procedures and surgeries. The use of OMT as an intervention, when effective, is extremely cost effective, eliminating the need for the more invasive procedures. Also, in a subset of patients OMT appears to be synergistic with invasive injections, such as epidural steroid injection or lysis of epidural adhesions. Some who did not initially respond to OMT begin to respond after injections. An unanticipated benefit is the realization that a fair number of patients at the pain clinic have pain that is secondary to previously undiagnosed and untreated systemic disease, such as diabetes, thyroid disease, and the like. This benefit is believed to be the consequence of osteopathic training, whose physicians are instructed in primary care with OMT. After treatment, patients are returned to their primary provider for further evaluation and treatment of their disorders.

TABLE 25.2	

Modalities in Pain Treatment

Pharmacologic	**OMT**
Opioid analgesics	**Dietary measures**
Nonopioid analgesics	Improved nutrition
Nonsteroidal anti-inflammatory drugs	Weight loss
Muscle relaxants	**Behavior modification**
Antiseizure medications	Psychotherapy
Tricyclics	Biofeedback
Serotonin-specific reuptake Inhibitors	Hypnosis
Gabapentin	**Invasive procedures**
Anxiolytics	Trigger point injections
Physical measures	Prolo injections
Heat	Nerve blocks
Ice	Epidural steroids
Traction	Epidural lysis of adhesions
Physical therapy modalities	Facet injections
Ultrasound	Sympathetic blocks
Short-wave diathermy	IDET
E-stim	Acupuncture
Transcutaneous electrical nerve stimulation	Nucleoplasty
Whirlpool	Opioid pumps
Motion therapies	Intrathecal opioids
Stretching exercises	Intrathecal baclofen
Strengthening exercises	Radio frequency ablation
Yoga	Implantable cord and nerve stimulators
Tai chi	Surgery
Aquatic therapy	**Rolfing**
	Reiki

THE OSTEOPATHIC MODEL

The role of osteopathic philosophy and medicine can be illustrated using headache as a model. The osteopathic philosophy dictates that osteopathic physicians treat the whole person. There are many good references on the treatment of headache. Only the aspects of evaluation and treatment that are distinctively osteopathic are discussed here.

Classification of Headaches

The International Headache Society has classified headaches into 14 types with more than 60 subtypes.[43–45] Generally, these may be broken down into primary,

TABLE 25.3

International Classification of Headache Disorders (ICHD-2)

Primary headaches

1. Migraine
2. Tension type
3. Cluster headache and other trigeminal autonomic cephalalgia
4. Other primary headaches

Secondary headaches

5. Headache attributed to head and/or neck trauma
6. Headache attributed to cranial or cervical vascular disorder
7. Headache attributed to nonvascular intracranial disorder
8. Headache attributed to a substance or its withdrawal
9. Headache attributed to infection
10. Headache attributed to disorder of homoeostasis
11. Headache or facial pain attributed to disorder of cranium, neck, eyes, ears, nose, sinuses, teeth, mouth, or other facial or cranial structures
12. Headache attributed to psychiatric disorder

Cranial neuralgias, central and primary facial pain, and other headaches

13. Cranial neuralgias and central causes of facial pain
14. Other headache, cranial neuralgia, central or primary facial pain

secondary, and other headaches (Table 25.3). The American Academy of Osteopathy includes, in a level II course, training instruction on the osteopathic treatment of headache.[46] The following is a description of some procedures developed over the years that have been found to be useful in the manipulative treatment of muscle tension, migraine, and cluster headache secondary to somatic dysfunction and other headaches secondary to visceral disease.

Primary Versus Secondary Causes

When diagnosing any headache, one should first distinguish whether it is primary, secondary, or both. Headache with a close temporal relation to another disorder known to cause headache, a marked worsening of a preexisting headache with the onset of the disorder, good evidence that the disorder can cause or aggravate tension headache, and improvement or resolution of tension headache after relief from the disorder may be considered as being secondary. Disorders to consider include head or neck trauma; cranial or cervical vascular disorders; nonvascular intracranial disorders; substance use or withdrawal; infection; disorders of homeostasis; disorders of the cranium, neck, eyes, ears, nose sinuses, teeth, mouth or other facial or cranial structures; and psychiatric disorders. As part of the complete history and physical, it is important to search for and note the red flags (Table 25.4), as OMT to the head and neck is contraindicated in many of these conditions.

TABLE 25.4

Contraindications to OMT for the Head and Neck

Red Flag	Possible Cause	Diagnostic Test
Sudden-onset headache	Subarachnoid hemorrhage Bleed into a mass or AVM Mass lesion (especially posterior fossa)	Neuroimaging Lumbar puncture (after neuroimaging evaluation)
Worsening headache	Mass lesion Subdural hematoma Medication overuse	Neuroimaging
Headache with systemic illness (fever, neck stiffness, cutaneous rash)	Meningitis Encephalitis Lyme disease Systemic infection Collagen vascular disease Arteritis	Neuroimaging Lumbar puncture Biopsy Blood tests
Focal neurologic signs or symptoms other than typical visual or sensory aura	Mass lesion AVM Collagen vascular disease	Neuroimaging Collagen vascular evaluation
Papilledema	Mass lesion Pseudotumor Encephalitis Meningitis	Neuroimaging Lumbar puncture (after neuroimaging evaluation)
Triggered by cough, exertion or Valsalva maneuver	Subarachnoid hemorrhage Mass lesion	Neuroimaging Consider lumbar puncture
Headache during pregnancy or postpartum	Cortical vein, cranial sinus thrombosis Carotid dissection Pituitary apoplexy	Neuroimaging
New headache type in a patient with		
Cancer	Metastasis	Neuroimaging Lumbar puncture
Lyme disease	Meningoencephalitis	Neuroimaging Lumbar puncture
HIV	Opportunistic infection Tumor	Neuroimaging Lumbar puncture

AVM, arteriovenous malformation.
Adapted from Lipton RB, Bigal ME, Steiner TJ, et al. Classification of primary headaches. Neurology 2004;63:427–435.

Muscle Tension Headache

Tension headaches are the most common type of primary headache, having affected as many as 90% of adults, and they have the highest socioeconomic cost. Tension headaches affect both sides of the head, are typically steady rather than throbbing, and may be triggered in response to stressful events or a hectic day. Previously, this type of headache was considered to be psychogenic, but studies strongly suggest a neurobiological basis, especially for the more severe subtypes. The ICHD-2 (International Classification of Headache Disorders, second edition[45]) has divided this class of headache into infrequent and frequent, episodic, and chronic, with each class subdivided by whether or not they are associated with pericranial tenderness.

In the absence of evidence for a known causative disorder, a tension headache should be considered primary and can be episodic or chronic. Infrequent episodic tension headaches are typically bilateral and last anywhere from 30 minutes to 7 days. To be considered episodic, there should be at least 10 episodes averaging less than 1 day per month and fewer than 12 days per year. These headaches are of mild to moderate intensity unaccompanied by nausea. The pain is pressing or tightening in quality (not pulsating) and does not worsen with routine physical activity, such as walking or climbing stairs, but photophobia or phonophobia may be present. These headaches may or may not be accompanied by increased pericranial tenderness on manual palpation. The presence of increased tenderness is the most significant abnormal finding in tension headache. It is detected by small rotating movements and a firm pressure with the second and third finger on the frontal, temporal, masseter, pterygoid, sternocleidomastoid, splenius, and trapezius muscles.

Frequent episodic tension headache is identical to infrequent episodic tension headache, the difference being that at least 10 episodes occur on more than one but fewer than 15 days per month for at least 3 months (at least 12 and fewer than 180 days per year). This type of headache frequently coexists with migraine without aura. Patients should be taught to differentiate between the two types so as to select the right procedure and to prevent medication overuse headaches. A diagnostic headache diary is useful in identifying coexisting frequent episodic tension headaches in migraine patients.

Chronic tension headaches gradually evolve from episodic tension headaches. These occur on more than 15 days per month for more than 3 months (more than 180 days a year) and are slightly more severe in that they may last hours or be continuous and may be accompanied by photophobia, phonophobia, or mild (not moderate or severe) nausea.

Look for somatic dysfunction as part of the comprehensive structural examination. Anything from flat feet to occipitoatlantal compression associated with tension headache may be the primary etiology of the headache. Look at the occipital and suboccipital areas. The greater occipital nerve traverses the suboccipital triangle. Increased tension in this group of muscles can compress the nerve, causing severe pain in the distribution of the nerve and exquisite tenderness over the nerve. Typical findings are dysfunction at the occipitoatlantal joint, C1 to C2, and/or C2 to C3. For the patient without contraindications, high-velocity, low-amplitude (HVLA) treatment is preferred. Generally, HVLA may not be recommended in this area for geriatric patients. The positioning of the patient should not increase the headache or cause neck pain. If it does, select a different treatment procedure. Treatment using HVLA is preferred because the relief of pain is usually immediate. Be careful using HVLA to C2, particularly on the left side, on the nauseated patient. It is possible to make the nausea severe and precipitate vomiting because a branch of the vagus innervates this area.

The use of cervical and suboccipital HVLA has recently been controversial. (The American Osteopathic Association and the American Academy of Osteopathy have studied the issue and released a position paper that is included in its entirety in the Appendix.)

Sutherland's occipitoatlantal decompression procedure is a cranial procedure that is commonly useful prior to HVLA.[47] Soft tissue treatment to the cervical area along with myofascial release and counterstrain are also useful procedures in this area.

Rarely is cervical dysfunction found without related dysfunction in the upper thoracic area. T2 to T4 dysfunctions are common, as the sympathetic nerves to the head and neck originate in the upper thoracic region. The upper four ribs are also commonly involved, with the first and second ribs held in inhalation and the third and forth held in exhalation. Remember that the insertion of the scalenes is on the first and second ribs. It is usually better to treat thoracic dysfunctions prior to treating cervical dysfunctions. Other areas of attention include the thoracolumbar junction, the sacral base, and the feet.

During a headache or an initial visit, it is usually not necessary to treat more than the upper thoracic region, the cervicals, and the occipitoatlantal joint. It is very easy to overtreat. Treat other areas on follow-up visits as needed. When recurring dysfunctional patterns in the cervical and thoracic areas are encountered, look lower for the primary cause. Remember, the osteopathic physician facilitates healing, but the healing comes from within. Two old adages apply here: "Find it, fix it, and leave it alone," and "Treat what you find, not what you expect to find." The use of OMT to treat somatic dysfunction associated with tension headache is not to be done to the exclusion of other modalities, such as medications, exercise, and addressing any psychosocial issues. Myofascial release procedures that can be performed at home can be taught to many patients with muscle tension headaches (Fig. 25.1). It is imperative that the procedure be done exactly as described. It is not recommended that these procedures be taught to the elderly patient or to patients with cerebral or vertebral basilar artery disease or severe cervical joint disease.

Migraine Headache

By definition migraine headaches are recurrent and are one-sided, pulsating or throbbing. They produce moderate to severe pain that interferes with or prevents normal activity and that worsens during ordinary daily activities. They are accompanied by nausea or vomiting, photophobia, and phonophobia. Frequently, migraines are foretold by symptoms that include various combinations of fatigue, difficulty in concentration, sensitivity to light or sound, neck stiffness, blurred vision, nausea, yawning, or pallor. These premonitory symptoms generally occur hours to a day or two before a migraine attack.

An aura is a complex of neurological symptoms that occurs just before or at the onset of a migraine headache. The aura may manifest itself as fully reversible visual symptoms, such as flickering lights, spots or lines, or loss of vision, fully reversible sensory symptoms, such as pins and needles or numbness, or fully reversible dysphasic speech disturbance. These may develop over more than 5 minutes and may occur in succession, each lasting less than 60 minutes. Migraine headache is categorized as being with or without aura. A genetic form of migraine,

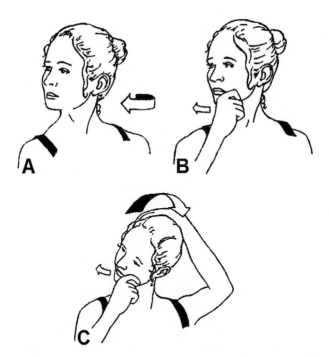

FIGURE 25.1   Myofascial release procedures that can be self-administered by the patient at home. These procedures are also used to test for abnormal muscle contraction associated with chronic headache. **(A)** The first step consists of simple rotation of the head through its full range. There should be no tilting of the head, and the chin should be kept on the same plane throughout the rotation. **(B)** The second step consists of placing the thumb under the chin and holding the head in full rotation by pressing against the chin with the flexed fingers. Then the chin should be elevated 1 or 2 inches. **(C)** The third step consists of lateral bending of the fully rotated head and neck. This maneuver should be done slowly and gently and should not cause pain or dizziness; it should be done in the area where the head and neck join, not in the lower or mid portion of the neck. If this maneuver is done correctly, there will be a stretching pulling sensation just below the superior nuchal line. (Reprinted with permission from Peterson DI. Headache: Modern concepts of diagnosis and management. Primary Care 1984;11:707–721.)

familial hemiplegic migraine, is accompanied by both an aura and motor weakness. The ICHD-2 identifies further subtypes of migraine as well.

In diagnosing migraine, it is particularly important to rule out other underlying somatic causes, because presenting symptoms between primary and secondary migraines may be indistinguishable. A particularly striking example is a report of two patients with identical presentations appearing as migraines. One was secondary to a patent foramen ovale in the heart. The other was associated with increased paravertebral muscle tension of the mid to lower cervical and upper thoracic spine bilaterally and a somatic dysfunction at the atlantoaxial area that was revealed upon osteopathic examination and almost completely resolved by OMT.[48] New oral abortive pharmacotherapeutic agents (triptans) have been successfully used to treat migraine attacks and provide an addition to the armamentarium of the osteopathic physician.[49]

Migraine headache is produced by constriction followed by dilation of the intracranial vessels. Besides being responsive to drugs, such as nitrates and alpha-blockers, the arteries are under the control of the sympathetic nervous system. The headache associated with consumption of nitroglycerine is in a sense a migraine. The sympathetic innervation of the blood vessels in the cranium reaches the vessels by way of multiple ganglia and the trigeminal nerve. The trigeminal nerve supplies three-fourths of the sensory fibers to the meninges.[50] The middle meningeal artery crosses the sphenosquamous articulation and is in approximation to the sphenosquamous pivot. Impaction of the sphenosquamous pivot is a fairly common finding in migraine patients. Any dysfunction of the temporal bone can result in migraine attacks because of its relationship with the trigeminal ganglion and trigeminal nerve. Nausea and vomiting with migraine may be due to vagal involvement at the jugular foramen accompanied by tension on the dural sleeve.[50]

When evaluating patients with migraine, pay attention to the cranium, particularly the sphenobasilar area, the temporal bone, the sphenosquamous pivot, and the jugular foramen. Also look at the suboccipital area, C2 (vagus involvement), and the upper thoracic spine and associated ribs. The role of the sympathetic nervous system in many pain states is supported by the observation that sympathectomies can attenuate the anomalous pain states leading to the diagnosis of sympathetically dependent pain.[51–53] Cranial OMT is best left to visits between migraine attacks, using appropriate procedures to free the sphenobasilar and the temporal regions.[50] Treat the cervical dysfunctions with indirect procedure, balanced ligamentous tension, or very gentle direct myofascial release so as not to further stimulate the vagus. Any appropriate procedure can be used to normalize the function of the upper thoracic and rib dysfunctions. Do not neglect Jones's counterstrain points for the suboccipital area and the inion point. Also, recall that the inion point is frequently a maverick, and the position of treatment is just the opposite of what one would expect.[54] Remember, the last thing patients want during a migraine attack is someone cranking their head around. It is not recommended that the HVLA procedure be used for cervical or suboccipital dysfunction during the acute phase of a migraine, as it frequently aggravates the headache. The use of OMT to treat somatic dysfunction associated with migraine headache is not to the exclusion of other modalities, such as avoidance of triggers, medications, exercise, and addressing any psychosocial issues.

Cluster Headache

Cluster headaches are grouped with other trigeminal autonomic cephalalgias. They are characterized by severe to very severe unilateral pain in and around one eye. Attacks are brief (30 minutes to 2 hours) and happen from once every other day up to eight times per day in clusters that typically last for a few months. Episodic cluster headaches may occur in periods lasting 7 days to a year separated by pain-free periods lasting a month or longer. Chronic cluster headaches occur for more than a year without remission or with remissions lasting less than a month. This type of headache is often accompanied by tearing and redness of the affected eye, a stuffy nose, or ipsilateral forehead or facial swelling. The attacks may be provoked by alcohol, histamine, or nitroglycerine. Most patients are restless or agitated during an attack because the pain is so excruciating that they are unable to lie down. Men are affected six times as frequently as women.

The findings of somatic dysfunction and the osteopathic manipulative procedures for cluster headaches are similar to those of migraine. One additional pearl:

In a patient who reports the sensation of an ice pick behind the eye and who does not have optic neuritis, brain tumor, or other anatomic lesion, look for a C1 to C2 dysfunction, anterior on the side of the pain. Treating this dysfunction can have a dramatic response (Habenicht AL. Personal communication, August 2004).

Headache Tertiary to Secondary Somatic Dysfunction

Many osteopathic physicians who use manipulative procedures have seen patients with headache whose etiology is somatic dysfunction secondary to organ disease. An example of this is the headache associated with gallbladder disease, also known as a bilious headache. The physiologic basis for headache secondary to somatic dysfunction is described here, using biliary dyskinesia as a model. Sympathetic afferent nerves from the biliary tree return to the spinal cord in the T6 to T9 segments. The hyperactivity of the sympathetic afferents causes facilitation of the T6 to T9 dermatome, resulting in increased muscle tone in the muscles innervated by the T6 to T9 somatic afferent nerves, which may result in a type II somatic dysfunction at that level.[55,56] The dysfunction is usually T8 extended with side bending and rotation right. The result frequently is increased muscle tension cephalad to the suboccipital area. The parasympathetic efferents and afferents are with the vagus nerve.[56] A branch of the vagus is given off at C2. This can lead to increased tension of the muscles of the suboccipital triangle, which can in turn cause compression of the vertebral artery and the greater occipital nerve as they pass through the triangle. The result can be both muscle tension and migraine headache. Anticholinergic medication can be specific for treating some muscle tension and migraine headaches using this model. Treatment of headache initiated by visceral pathology begins by treating the underlying cause. Then treat the associated somatic dysfunction.

CONCLUSION

The overall effects of chronic pain on personal and societal health cannot be overstated. A multidisciplinary team approach to comprehensive pain management is evolving as one of the most cost effective and beneficial means to address chronic pain cases. Osteopathic physicians should play a lead role by functioning as an intake portal, administering OMT to patients with somatic dysfunctions that underlie the cause of pain when indicated, possibly avoiding costly workups and allopathic interventions. The successful manipulative treatment of major forms of otherwise idiopathic headache is a case in point. With the use of complementary and alternative medicines on the rise in the United States and the increasing recognition of the potential benefits of such approaches by the allopathic medical establishment, osteopathic physicians stand in a good position to play a vital role in lessening the burden of chronic pain to society.

Procedures

Selected Osteopathic Manipulative Procedures Useful in Treating Headache

In treating the cervical spine, it is important to diagnose and treat the upper thoracic region first.

Muscle Energy, Upper Thoracic Spine

This procedure is employed to treat Fryette type II dysfunction, either flexed or extended, in the upper thoracic spine. (For diagnosis, see the procedure in Chapter 16 and Figure 16.1.)

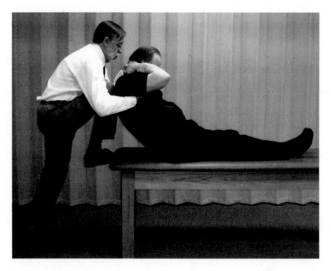

FIGURE 25.2   Knee in the back HVLA procedure for T3 on T4 extended, side bent right, and rotated right.

Knee in the Back, Upper Thoracic Type II Extended Dysfunction (HVLA) (Fig. 25.2)

This procedure is employed to treat type II articular somatic dysfunction of the thoracic spine. The patient position described below specifically allows access to the upper thoracic region. (For diagnosis, see Chapter 3.)

Patient position: seated upon the treatment table with the knees extended and the legs resting lengthwise on the table. Physician position: standing behind the patient at the end of the table. In this position, the patient can comfortably lean back to bring the upper thoracic spine into contact with the physician's knee, even if the physician has relatively short legs.

Procedure (Example: T3 on T4 Extended, Side Bent Right, and Rotated Right)

1. Place a pillow or other small pad over the relatively posterior right transverse process of T3.
2. Place your right foot upon the table and your knee firmly against the pillow or pad in contact with the right transverse process of T3. Your knee must remain tightly in contact with T3 throughout the remainder of the procedure.
3. Instruct the patient to place the hands behind the neck and to lace the fingers together.
4. With both of your hands, reach beneath the patient's axillae on either side and fully extend both of your wrists so that your fingers can contact the dorsal (extensor) surface of the patient's forearms bilaterally at the wrists.
5. Instruct the patient to bring the elbows together in front, laterally displacing the scapulae.
6. Instruct the patient to slump forward; assist by pushing gently downward against the wrists with your fingers and pulling posteriorly against the axillae with your forearms. This will introduce flexion of the upper spine down to and including T3 upon T4.

7. Maintaining the firm contact between your right knee and the right transverse process of T3, use both of your arms to translate the patient's upper torso to the right, thereby introducing left side bending between T3 and T4. Be certain to keep both of the patient's ischial tuberosities solidly in contact with the table during this process.

8. Introduce left rotation of T3 upon T4 by pulling posteriorly with your left forearm against the patient's left axilla.

9. By applying flexion, left side bending, and left rotation through the patient's pectoral girdle with your forearms while maintaining firm contact with your right knee upon the right transverse process of T3, you should be able to localize forces to T3 upon T4.

10. Apply the final corrective force as a quick thrust directed upward and anteriorly against the right transverse process of T3 with your right knee by abruptly plantar-flexing your right ankle in combination with a simultaneous slight increase in flexion of the patient's torso (T3 upon T4) through your fingers in contact with the forearms.

11. Reassess the motion between T3 and T4.

Knee in the Back, Upper Thoracic Type II Flexed Dysfunction (HVLA) (Fig. 25.3)

This procedure is employed to treat type II articular somatic dysfunction of the thoracic spine. The patient position specifically allows access to the upper thoracic region. (For diagnosis, see Chapter 3.)

Patient position: seated upon the treatment table with the knees extended and the legs resting lengthwise on the table. Physician position: standing behind the patient at the end of the table. In this position, the patient can comfortably lean back to bring the upper thoracic spine into contact with the physician's knee, even if the physician has relatively short legs.

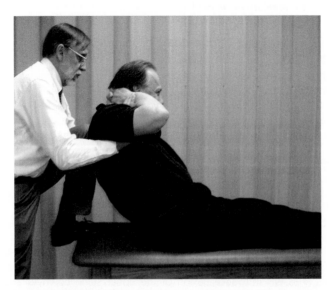

FIGURE 25.3 Knee in the back HVLA procedure for T3 on T4 flexed, side bent right, and rotated right.

Procedure (Example: T3 on T4 Flexed, Side Bent Right, and Rotated Right)

1. Place a pillow or other small pad over the left transverse process of T4.
2. Place your left foot upon the table and your knee firmly against the pillow or pad in contact with the left transverse process of T4. Your knee must remain tightly in contact with T4 throughout the remainder of the procedure.
3. Instruct the patient to place the hands behind the neck and to lace the fingers together.
4. With both of your hands, reach beneath the patient's axillae on either side and fully extend both of your wrists so that your fingers can contact the dorsal (extensor) surface of the patient's forearms bilaterally at the wrists.
5. Instruct the patient to bring the elbows together in front, laterally displacing the scapulae.
6. Instruct the patient to relax; then pull posteriorly against the axillae with your forearms. This will introduce extension of the upper spine down to and including T3 upon T4.
7. Maintaining the firm contact between your right knee and the left transverse process of T4, use both of your arms to translate the patient's upper torso to the right, thereby introducing left side bending between T3 and T4. Be certain to keep both of the patient's ischial tuberosities solidly in contact with the table.
8. Introduce left rotation of T3 upon T4 by pulling posteriorly with your left forearm against the patient's left axilla.
9. By applying extension, left side bending, and left rotation through the patient's pectoral girdle with your forearms while maintaining firm contact with your left knee upon the left transverse process of T4, you should be able to localize forces to T3 upon T4.
10. Apply the final corrective force as a quick upward traction with your hands and forearms through the patient's shoulders against the holding force of your left knee upon the left transverse process of T4.
11. Reassess the motion between T3 and T4.

Reverse Rib (HVLA) (Fig. 25.4)

This procedure is employed to treat costovertebral somatic dysfunction that can affect the second, third, or fourth ribs. The dysfunctional relationship occurs

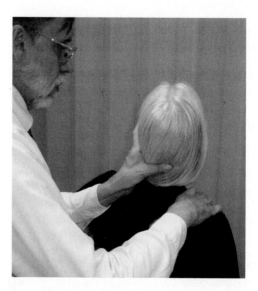

FIGURE 25.4 Reverse rib (HVLA) procedure for treating the dysfunctional relationship between T1 and the second rib on the right.

between a thoracic vertebra and the rib of the segment below. Rotation of the vertebra causes the inferior hemifacet to impinge upon the head of the rib. This in turn drives the rib posterior, impinging upon the costotransverse articulation and causing palpable prominence, tissue texture change, and tenderness over the angle of the dysfunctional rib. This is a secondary dysfunction, the result of a primary thoracic type II vertebral dysfunction. As such, the primary thoracic dysfunction should be treated before this procedure is employed.

Patient position: seated upon the side of the treatment table. Physician position: standing behind the patient.

Procedure (Example: Dysfunction Between T1 and the Second Rib on the Right)

The rib angle is prominent, with tissue texture change and resistance to an anteroinferior force.

1. Place your left foot upon the table just to the left of the patient's pelvis.
2. Place the patient's left arm over your left knee. You may wish to place a pillow between your knee and the patient's axilla.
3. With your left hand, reach in front of the patient, grasp the right wrist, and pull the right arm across the lap to protract the right scapula, exposing the angle of the second rib.
4. Place your right hand upon the patient's right shoulder so that your fingers are directed anteriorly and your thumb points inferiorly, contacting the angle of the dysfunctional second rib.
5. With your right hand, apply an inferomedial force, holding the patient's torso firmly between your right hand and left knee. This holding force must be maintained throughout the remainder of the procedure.
6. With your left hand, grasp the left side of the patient's head so that your widespread fingers are directed anteriorly, contacting the left cheek, and your thumb contacts the posterior skull at or just inferior to the external occipital protuberance.
7. Using your left hand, posteriorly translate the patient's head to straighten the upper thoracic and cervical spine. This spinal positioning must be maintained throughout the remainder of the procedure.
8. Next, with your left hand, introduce rotation of the head and cervical spine to the left until forces accumulate at the level of T1.
9. The final corrective force is a high-velocity, low-amplitude increase in left rotation of the patient's head and cervical spine against the holding force of your right thumb upon the second rib angle.
10. Reassess the motion between T1 and the second rib on the right.

Elevated First and Second Ribs, Patient Prone (HVLA) (Fig. 25.5)

This procedure is employed to treat elevated first or second ribs to restore normal respiratory excursion. Any vertebral somatic dysfunction should be treated before rib dysfunction. (For diagnosis, see Chapter 16.)

Patient position: prone. The chin should be in contact with the table, and the head and cervical spine should be in the midline, with no rotation to either the right or left. Physician position: standing at the patient's head on the side opposite the dysfunctional rib.

Procedure (Example: Elevated Second Rib on the Left)

1. With your right hand, grasp the left side of the patient's head and introduce side bending to the right down to T1 upon T2 by moving the patient's head to the

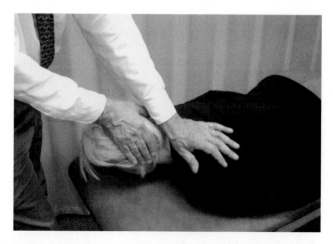

FIGURE 25.5 The HVLA procedure to treat an elevated second rib on the left.

right while keeping the chin in contact with the table and not rotating the head or cervical spine. It is important to maintain this side bending with your right hand against the patient's head throughout the remainder of the procedure.

2. With the thenar eminence of your left hand, contact the angle of the dysfunctional second rib and apply a caudal and somewhat lateral force.
3. Instruct the patient to take a deep breath.
4. As the patient begins to exhale, apply the final corrective force as an HVLA thrust downward, anteriorly and laterally through your left hand against the angle of the dysfunctional second rib.
5. Reassess the motion of the second rib on the left.

Posterior Occiput, Muscle Energy

This procedure is employed to treat articular somatic dysfunction of the occiput relative to C1, the atlas, to establish symmetric motion between the occiput and the atlas. (For diagnosis, see Chapter 3, and the description of the procedure in Chapter 16 and Figure 16.10.)

C1 Posterior (Counterstrain) (Fig. 25.6)

This procedure is employed to reduce discomfort associated with a tender point. The C1 posterior, or inion, tender point is on either side of the midline approximately 3 cm inferior to the external occipital protuberance, inion, in the most medial aspect of the insertion of the splenius capitis onto the occiput. This tender point is found frequently in association with occipital headaches. This is an atypical or maverick counterstrain point.

Patient position: supine. Physician position: seated at the head of the treatment table.

Procedure (Example: Posterior C1 Tender Point Located to the Left of the Midline)

1. Cradle the posterior aspect of the patient's head with your left hand, placing the tip your index finger in contact with the posterior C1 tender point. Your finger should remain in contact with the tender point throughout the treatment procedure.

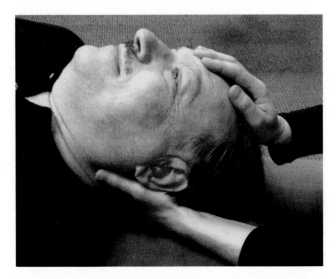

FIGURE 25.6   The position for counterstrain to treat a posterior C1 tender point to the left of the midline.

2. Palpate the point to establish the patient's awareness of the degree of tenderness present and assign a value of 100% to the tenderness.
3. Grasp the top of the patient's head with your right hand so that your palm is in contact with the vertex of the skull and your fingers extend anteriorly toward or onto the forehead.
4. Apply a caudally directed force with your right hand, thereby introducing extension of the occiput upon the atlas, until you feel decreased tension in the tissues surrounding the tender point beneath your left index finger. It may be necessary to position the patient so that the head and neck are off the head of the treatment table in order to introduce the degree of extension necessary to obtain relaxation.
5. It also may be necessary to introduce small amounts of side bending and/or rotation of C1, most often to the left, until you feel further decreased tension in the tissue beneath your index finger. As tissue tension decreases, if asked, the patient will report a proportionate decrease of tenderness.
6. The final position is that in which no more than 30% of the patient's subjective tenderness remains. This position should be held until complete tissue relaxation, a release, occurs. This often requires up to 90 seconds after the final position is obtained.
7. While monitoring the tender point, return the patient's head and neck to the neutral resting position. This process should be done slowly so that the tissue tension in the region of the tender point does not return.
8. Again, palpate the tender point to determine whether any residual tenderness remains.

Sutherland's Occipitoatlantal Decompression (Cranial) (Fig. 25.7)

This procedure is employed to reduce ligamentous articular strain between the occiput and atlas. This is a dysfunction in which the condyles of the occiput are anterior relative to the atlas.

Patient position: supine. Physician position: seated at the head of the treatment table.

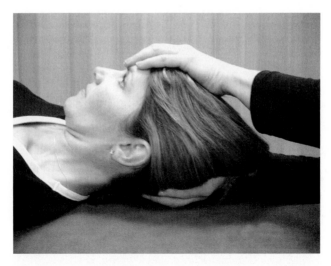

FIGURE 25.7   Sutherland's occipitoatlantal decompression.

Procedure

1. Place one hand palm up beneath the patient's head along the longitudinal axis of the patient's body and with your fingers pointing caudally so that the tip of your middle finger contacts the most inferior aspect of the occiput in the midline.
2. Place the other hand lightly in contact with the patient's forehead to stabilize the head upon the posterior hand.
3. Have the patient minimally tuck the chin, to introduce occipitoatlantal flexion without flexing the remainder of the cervical spine. This will bring the posterior tubercle of the atlas into contact with the tip of the middle finger of the hand cradling the patient's head. This position can be augmented by applying a caudally directed force, lightly applied with the hand in contact with the patient's forehead.
4. Support the atlas with the tip of the middle finger of your posterior hand, thereby allowing the occipitoatlantal ligaments to rebalance the joint as the occiput disengages and moves posteriorly upon the atlas.
5. Reassess the relationship between the occiput and the atlas.
6. This procedure may then be followed with occipital condylar decompression, as dictated by the palpable symmetry of the occiput.

Occipital Condylar Decompression (Cranial) (Fig. 25.8)

This procedure should be used only by individuals experienced with cranial manipulation.

This procedure is employed to reduce intraosseous dysfunction of the occiput involving the squamous, lateral, and basilar parts of the occipital base. These dysfunctions can be very complex, consisting of compression between the basilar and one or both lateral parts, with anteroposterior and mediolateral deviation of the lateral parts and rotational stress upon the squamous portion of the occiput. The procedure is conducted as an indirect treatment method whose goal is to reduce palpable tension asymmetry of the occiput. The example provides a basic hand placement and the approach to a specific pattern example. The procedure as employed clinically should be dictated by the pattern palpated in the individual patient's skull.

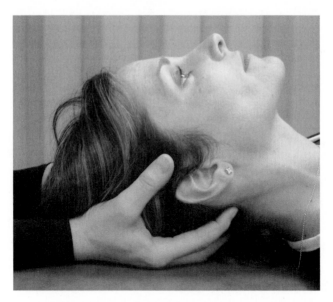

FIGURE 25.8 Occipital condylar decompression.

Patient position: supine. Physician position: seated at the head of the treatment table.

Procedure (Example: Anteroposterior Compression Between the Right Lateral and the Basilar Parts of the Basiocciput)

1. Cradle the patient's occiput in both hands.
2. Place your right hand palm up beneath the patient's head along the longitudinal axis of the patient's body with your fingers pointing caudally so that the tip of your middle finger contacts the most inferior aspect of the occiput in the midline and your index finger is directed toward the right occipital condyle.
3. Have the patient minimally tuck the chin to introduce occipitoatlantal flexion without flexing the remainder of the cervical spine.
4. Use the tip of your right index finger to hold the right lateral part in place.
5. With your left hand, apply gentle, posterosuperior traction to the left side of the squamous portion and left lateral part of the occipital base.
6. Direct the holding force of your right index finger laterally to the patient's right while applying a medially directed force with your right middle finger.
7. Lightly adjust the tensions applied with both hands until you feel the occiput release.
8. The efficacy of this procedure is greatly enhanced by working in synchrony with the cranial rhythmic impulse (CRI).
9. Reassess the occiput.

Frontal Lift (Cranial)

This procedure is employed to treat somatic dysfunction of the frontal bone.
    Patient position: supine. Physician position: at the head of the table.

DIAGNOSIS

Note the frontal bone. Although this bone is a single osseous structure in most adults, it moves like the paired bones of the skull, reflecting its origin as paired bones on either

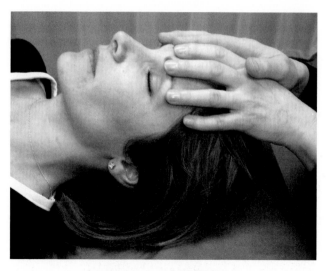

FIGURE 25.9   Frontal diagnosis.

side of the metopic suture; frontal motion should occur in synchrony with the biphasic CRI. Thus, during cranial flexion, the frontal bone or bones externally rotate, widening laterally, and during cranial extension, the frontal bone(s) internally rotate, narrowing laterally. Dysfunction can occur in the symmetry of this motion from many sources. These include dural membrane tension, articular or intraosseous dysfunction at the metopic suture, and articular restriction between the frontal bone and adjacent structures, in this case particularly the greater wings of the sphenoid bone and the paired parietal bones.

Diagnostic Procedure (Fig. 25.9)

1. Place both hands in contact with the frontal bone such that the index fingers are aligned on either side of the metopic suture and the other fingertips contact the brow ridges bilaterally.
2. Palpate the motion between the left and right halves of the frontal bone as you palpate the rate and amplitude of the inherent motion of the CRI. As the head moves into flexion, the frontal bone or bones should be felt to flatten anteriorly and widen laterally in external rotation. As the cranial base moves into extension, the frontal bone or bones should be felt to narrow laterally in internal rotation.
3. Identify motion restriction.

Treatment Procedure

1. Place your elbows upon the table bilaterally on either side of the patient's head and interlace your fingers in front of the patient's forehead. Your fingers should not touch the frontal bone.
2. Contact the lateral angles of the frontal bone or bones bilaterally with your hypothenar eminences.
3. Palpate the CRI.
4. As the head moves into extension and the frontal bone or bones internally rotate, follow with your hands by applying gentle medial pressure with your hypothenar eminences and by attempting to draw your interlaced fingers apart. In internal rotation, you will be able to disengage the frontal bone from adjacent cranial (not facial) structures.

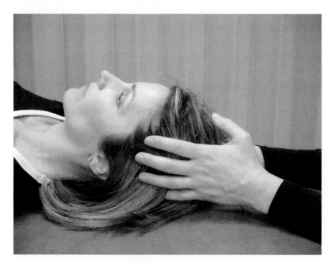

FIGURE 25.10   Parietal lift.

5. During external rotation, lift the frontal bone or bones anteriorly until they are felt to move freely into external rotation.
6. Follow the CRI and return the frontal bone or bones to the starting position.
7. Reassess frontal bone motion.

Parietal Lift (Cranial) (Fig. 25.10)

This procedure is used to treat somatic dysfunction of the parietal bones.
   Patient position: supine. Physician position: seated at the head of the table.

Procedure

Diagnosis of parietal dysfunction is performed in a fashion similar to that of frontal bone diagnosis (described earlier in the chapter), with the exception of hand placement, which should follow the description of hand placement in the treatment procedure here.

1. Place both hands in contact with the parietal bones so that your index fingers are just posterior to the coronal suture and above the sphenoparietal sutures, your middle and ring fingers are slightly separated above the squamous temporoparietal sutures, and your little fingers lie anterior and superior to the lambdoid suture. Your wrists should be lightly approximated, and unless your hands are very small, your palms will not be in contact with the patient's head.
2. Palpate the motion between the left and right parietal bone as you palpate the rate and amplitude of the inherent motion of the CRI.
3. As the cranial base moves into extension and the parietal bones internally rotate, follow with your hands by applying gentle medial pressure with the pads of your fingers. In internal rotation, you will be able to disengage the parietal bones from adjacent cranial structures.
4. During external rotation, draw the parietal bones superiorly toward you until you feel them moving freely into external rotation. The forces applied during the lift may be accentuated through one or more of your finger contact points as the sensation of motion restriction dictates.
5. Follow the CRI and return the parietal bones to the starting position.
6. Reassess the cranial motion of the parietal bones.

References

1. Fox CD, Berger D, Fine PG, et al. Pain assessment and treatment in the managed care environment. A position statement from the American Pain Society. 2000. Available at http://www.ampainsoc.org/managedcare/pdf/aps_position.pdf. Accessed April 17, 2005.
2. Stewart WF, Ricci JA, Chee E, et al. Lost productive time and cost due to common pain conditions in the US workforce. JAMA 2003;290:2443–2454.
3. Barnes PM, Powell-Griner E, McFann K, Nahin RL. Complementary and alternative medicine use among adults: United States, 2002. CDC Advance Data From Vital and Health Statistics; report no 343. Hyattsville, MD: National Center for Health Statistics. May 27, 2004.
4. Astin JA. Why patients use alternative medicine: Results of a national study. JAMA 1998;279:1548–1553.
5. Eisenberg DM, Davis RB, Ettner SL, et al. Trends in alternative medicine use in the United States, 1990–1997: Results of a follow-up national survey. JAMA 1998;280:1569–1575.
6. Oldendick R, Coker AL, Wieland D, et al. Population-based survey of complementary and alternative medicine usage, patient satisfaction, and physician involvement. South Carolina Complementary Medicine Program Baseline Research Team. South Med J 2000;93:375–381.
7. Paramore LC. Use of alternative therapies: Estimates from the 1994 Robert Wood Johnson Foundation National Access to Care Survey. J Pain Symptom Manag 1997;13(2):83–89.
8. Lipton RB, Stewart WF, Diamond S, et al. Prevalence and burden of migraine in the United States: Data from the American Migraine Study II. Headache 2001;41:646–657.
9. Yelin E, Herrndorf A, Trupin L, Sonneborn D. A national study of medical care expenditures for musculoskeletal conditions: The impact of health insurance and managed care. Arthritis Rheum 2001;44:1160–1169.
10. Deyo RA, Weinstein JN. Low back pain. N Engl J Med 2001;344:363–370.
11. Turk DC. Clinical effectiveness and cost-effectiveness of treatments for patients with chronic pain. Clin J Pain 2001;18:355–365.
12. Centers for Medicare and Medicaid Services. 1997 National Health Expenditures Survey. Available at http://222.cms.hhs.gov/statistics/nhe/. Accessed April 17, 2005.
13. Verhaak PF, Kerssens JJ, Dekker J, et al. Prevalence of chronic benign pain disorder among adults: A review of the literature. Pain 1998;77:231–239.
14. Brantingham JW. A critical look at the subluxation hypothesis. J Manip Physiol Ther 1988;11:130–132.
15. Van Buskirk RL. Nociceptive reflexes and the somatic dysfunction: A model. J Am Osteopath Assoc 1990;90:792–809.
16. Wax CM, Abend DS, Pearson PH. Chest pain and the role of somatic dysfunction. J Am Osteopath Assoc 1997;97:347–352, 355.
17. Williams N. Managing back pain in general practice: Is osteopathy the new paradigm? Br J Gen Pract 1997;47:653–655.
18. Irvin RE. The origin and relief of common pain. J Back Musculoskeletal Rehabil 1998;11(2):89–130.
19. Sun C, Desai GJ, Pucci DS, Jew S. Musculoskeletal disorders: Does the osteopathic medical profession demonstrate its unique and distinctive characteristics? J Am Osteopath Assoc 2004;104:149–155.
20. McPartland JM, Goodridge JP. Counterstrain diagnostics and traditional osteopathic examination of the cervical spine compared. J Bodywork Movement Therap 1997;1:173–178.
21. Makofsky H. The effect of head posture on muscle contact position: The sliding cranium theory. Cranio 1989;7:286–292.
22. Stitzel CJ, Morningstar MW, Paone PR. The effects of bite line deviation on lateral cervical radiographs when upper cervical joint dysfunction exists: A pilot study. J Manip Physiol Ther 2003;26(7):E17.
23. Diez F. Chiropractic management of patients with bilateral congenital hip dislocation with chronic low back and leg pain. J Manip Physiol Ther 2004;27(4):E6.
24. Lesho EP. An overview of osteopathic medicine. Arch Fam Med 1999;8:477–484.
25. Bledsoe BE. The elephant in the room: Does OMT have proved benefit? J Am Osteopath Assoc 2004;104:405–406.

26. Biondi DM. Cervicogenic headache: Mechanisms, evaluation, and treatment strategies. J Am Osteopath Assoc 2000;100(9 suppl):S7–S14.

27. Dowling DJ. Progressive inhibition of neuromuscular structures (PINS) technique. J Am Osteopath Assoc 2000;100:285–286, 289–298.

28. Licciardone JC. The unique role of osteopathic physicians in treating patients with low back pain. J Am Osteopath Assoc 2004;104(11 suppl 8):S13–S18.

29. Spiegel AJ, Capobianco JD, Kruger A, Spinner WD. Osteopathic manipulative medicine in the treatment of hypertension: An alternative, conventional approach. Heart Dis 2003;5:272–278.

30. Spaeth DG, Pheley AM. Use of osteopathic manipulative treatment by Ohio osteopathic physicians in various specialties. J Am Osteopath Assoc 2003;103:16–26.

31. Jermyn RT. A nonsurgical approach to low back pain. J Am Osteopath Assoc 2001;101 (4 suppl pt 2):S6–S11.

32. Burton AK, McClune TD, Clarke RD, Main CJ. Long-term follow-up of patients with low back pain attending for manipulative care: Outcomes and predictors. Manip Ther 2004;9(1):30–35.

33. McPartland JM. Travell trigger points: Molecular and osteopathic perspectives. J Am Osteopath Assoc 2004;104:244–249.

34. Harden N, Cohen M. Unmet needs in the management of neuropathic pain. J Pain Symptom Manag 2003;25(5 suppl):S12–S17.

35. Chong MS, Bajwa ZH. Diagnosis and treatment of neuropathic pain. J Pain Symptom Manag 2003;25(5 suppl):S4–S11.

36. Pasero C. Pathophysiology of neuropathic pain. Pain Manag Nurs 2004;5(4 Suppl 1):3–8.

37. Namaka M, Gramlich CR, Rublen D, et al. A treatment algorithm for neuropathic pain. Clin Ther 2004;26:951–979. Erratum in Clin Ther 2004;26:2163.

38. Wang SJ, Juang KD. Psychiatric comorbidity of chronic daily headache: impact, treatment, outcome, and future studies. Curr Pain Headache Rep 2002;6:505–510.

39. Merikangas KR. Association between psychopathology and headache syndromes. Curr Opin Neurol 1995;8:248–251.

40. Merikangas KR, Stevens DE, Angst J. Psychopathology and headache syndromes in the community. Headache 1994;34(8):S17–S22. Erratum in Headache 1995;35(1):precedi.

41. Katz J, Melzack R. Measurement of pain. Surg Clin North Am 1999;79:231–252.

42. Abraham I, Killackey-Jones B. Lack of evidence-based research for idiopathic low back pain: The importance of a specific diagnosis. Arch Intern Med 2002;162:1442–1444; discussion 1447.

43. Taylor FR. Diagnosis and classification of headache. Prim Care 2004;31:243–259.

44. Lipton RB, Bigal ME, Steiner TJ, et al. Classification of primary headaches. Neurology 2004;63:427–435.

45. Headache Classification Subcommittee of the International Headache Society. The international classification of headache disorders. Cephalalgia 2004;24(S1):1–151.

46. American Academy of Osteopathy. Integrating manual medicine into patient care through hands-on workshops, 2005. Flow chart of AAO course offerings. Available at http://www.academyofosteopathy.org. Accessed April 17, 2005.

47. Sutherland WG. Teachings in the Science of Osteopathy. Portland, OR: Rudra, 1990;112.

48. Giatis IZ, Garwood RM. Diagnosing migraines the osteopathic way: Case studies overviewing the importance of recognizing and treating the musculoskeletal components of migraine headaches. Osteopath Fam Physician News 2004;4:1, 10–12.

49. Mueller L. Triptans have revolutionized acute migraine therapy: The osteopathic family physician's migraine armamentarium has greatly expanded over the last decade. Osteopath Fam Physician News 2004;4:14–16.

50. Magoun HI. Osteopathy in the Cranial Field. 3rd ed. Kirksville, MO: Journal Printing, 1976;184, 282.

51. Waldman SD. Interventional Pain Management. 2nd ed. New York: Saunders, 2001;27.

52. Larson NJ. Functional vasomotor hemiparesthesia syndrome. Academy of Applied Osteopathy 1970 Yearbook. Carmel, CA: Academy of Applied Osteopathy, 1970:39–44. (Available through the American Academy of Osteopathy, Indianapolis.)

53. Nelson KE. Osteopathic medical considerations of reflex sympathetic dystrophy. J Am Osteopath Assoc 1997;97:286–289.
54. Yates HA, Glover JC. Counterstrain: A Handbook of Osteopathic Technique. Tulsa, OK: Y Knot, 1995;52.
55. Kuchera WA, Kuchera ML. Osteopathic Principles in Practice. 2nd ed. Columbus, OH: Greyden, 1993;33–34, 229.
56. Walton WJ. Textbook of Osteopathic Diagnosis and Technique Procedures. 2nd ed. Chicago: Chicago College of Osteopathic Medicine, 1972;139–140.

CHAPTER 26

The Patient with Back Pain: Short Leg Syndrome and Postural Balance

Kenneth E. Nelson and Anette K. Schilling Mnabhi

INTRODUCTION

Low back pain is very frequently encountered. It affects most individuals at some time during the course of their life. This chapter discusses the mechanics of unequal leg length and postural balance in the coronal plane. Chapter 27 considers dysfunctional mechanics in the sagittal plane. This is an artificial division, and the material covered in these two chapters should be considered together. A thorough understanding of these mechanics will help with diagnosis and treatment of a significant number of patients with low back pain and individuals with a myriad of other musculoskeletal complaints. Because of the physical stresses that postural accommodation places upon the patient, treatment of dysfunctional balance mechanics proves to be useful adjunctive therapy for most cases of chronic medical conditions that affect the ambulatory patient. Elderly patients with progressive loss of the ability to perform the activities of daily living may regain significant function when the effects of somatic dysfunction are eliminated or reduced.

Inequality of leg length is extremely common.[1,2] Of 105 members of the 1968 to 1971 classes of the Chicago College of Osteopathic Medicine (CCOM) who had postural radiographs done, 58, or 55%, had an inequality of leg length of one-quarter inch or greater. (Serrecchia F, Nelson KE. Survey: CCOM alumni who had postural radiographs as freshman medical students. Unpublished data, 1994.) Studies of schoolchildren show that differences in leg length tend to increase as children grow.[3-5] The diagnosis of short leg syndrome is based upon a constellation of musculoskeletal and general body symptoms and upon physical findings that may be confirmed by radiography. It is necessary to recall one's understanding of sacropelvic mechanics,[6,7] since inequality of leg length is a common cause of pelvic unleveling with resultant sacropelvic dysfunction.

THE PRESENTATION OF THE PATIENT

Typical patients are middle-aged or older. They commonly present with a chief complaint of midline lumbosacral pain that is most often described as dull or aching. Frequently, the pain radiates to one buttock, usually on the side of the short leg. Patients may also have a myriad of other pelvic complaints and myalgias anywhere along the spine. Sometimes they complain of a general feeling of fatigue (bringing such things as anemia and hypothyroidism into your differential diagnosis). Often, when questioned, patients say they awake in the morning with little or no discomfort, but as the day progresses, they become more and more symptomatic. Sometimes they note that their symptoms develop at the same time every day.

An Explanation of the Chief Complaint

If an individual has equal leg length and there is no primary sacropelvic dysfunction, the pelvis and sacral base should be level. With a level pelvis, the spine above should be straight (Fig. 26.1). If one leg is short, the straight spine might be expected to tip to the side of the short leg (Fig. 26.2). This obviously does not occur. Rather, in an attempt to maintain one's center of gravity over the pelvis, a compensatory (Type I) curve develops (Fig. 26.3). A single curve (Fig. 26.3A) can develop, or additional

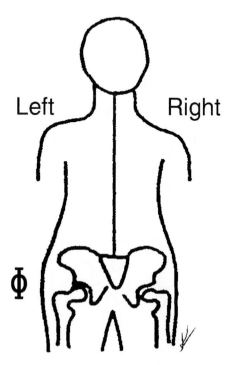

FIGURE 26.1   Level pelvis with a straight spine above.

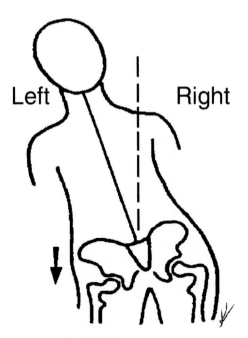

FIGURE 26.2   If one leg is short, the straight spine might be expected to tip to the side of the short leg. This obviously does not occur.

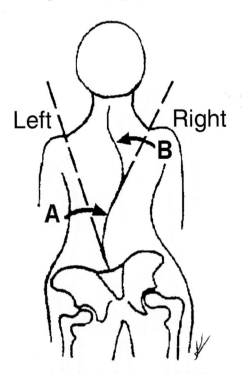

FIGURE 26.3   In an attempt to maintain one's center of gravity over the unleveled pelvis, a compensatory (type I) curve develops. A single curve (**A**) can develop, or additional compensatory curves (**B**) may occur.

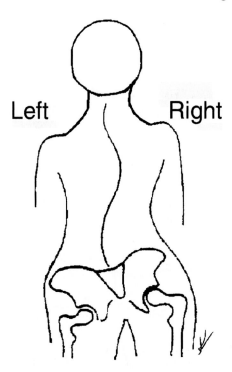

FIGURE 26.4   A short left leg with a compensatory lumbar curve (convex left) and additional thoracic and cervical compensatory curves.

compensatory curves (Fig. 26.3B) may occur. The individual in Figure 26.4 has a short left leg with a compensatory lumbar curve (convex left) and additional thoracic and cervical compensatory curves. These curves are not just balanced above the pelvis, they are the result of and are maintained by asymmetric paravertebral muscle contraction (Fig. 26.5).

Under certain circumstances, the sacrum shifts so that it rotates upon either the left or right oblique axis.[8] Weight bearing on one leg engages the ipsilateral oblique axis, with resultant sacral rotation. Side bending of the lumbar spine also engages the oblique sacral axis on the side toward which the lumbar spine is side bent. Figure 26.6 shows how, because of the short left leg, the compensatory lumbar curve engages the right oblique axis. Also, because of the inequality of leg length, individuals walk and bear weight asymmetrically. As patients walk, they must step up during stance phase upon the long leg and step down during stance phase on the short leg side. This asymmetric workload tends to chronically engage the sacral oblique axis on the long leg side. Since standing and walking tend to occur under neutral circumstances, if, as in Figure 26.6, the right oblique axis is chronically engaged, the sacrum is chronically rotated right on the right oblique axis. Lumbosacral mechanics in this circumstance will be a right-on-right forward torsion. The sacrum, although anatomically part of the pelvis, functions physiologically as if it were part of the lumbar spine.[9] As such, the sacrum is functionally the lowest segment in the compensatory lumbar curve. The curve (Type I mechanics) as a group is side bent right and rotated left. The fifth lumbar vertebra, being below the apex, is side bent right and rotated left relative to the sacrum. Therefore, the left

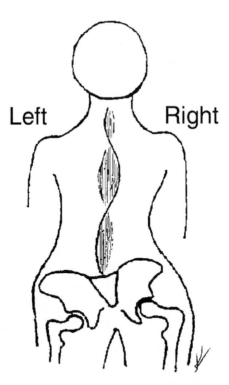

Left   Right

FIGURE 26.5   The compensatory spinal curves above an unleveled pelvis are not just balanced above the pelvis; they are the result of and are maintained by asymmetric paravertebral muscle contraction.

side of the sacral base is relatively anterior to the left transverse process of L5. This is right-on-right forward sacral torsion.

Sacroiliac mechanics are equally logical. If the sacrum is chronically rotated right on the right oblique axis, the mechanics favor either an anterior sacrum on the left or a posterior sacrum on the right. That is, because of sacral rotation to the right between the ilia, the sacrum will be anterior to the ilium at the superior pole of the left sacroiliac articulation and posterior to the ilium at the inferior pole of the right sacroiliac articulation. Anterior and posterior sacrum are dysfunctions of articular motion restriction. So with sacral rotation right on the right oblique axis, if articular motion of left sacroiliac joint is restricted, it is called an anterior sacrum on the left. If articular motion of right sacroiliac joint is restricted, it is called a posterior sacrum on the right. With accommodation to a short leg most commonly there is an anterior sacrum on the short leg side.[10] An anterior sacrum is associated with ipsilateral gluteal (gluteus medius) spasm and pain. A posterior sacrum is associated with ipsilateral piriformis muscle spasm, pain, and often sciatica.

Dysfunctional sacropelvic mechanics twist the three bones of the pelvis so that asymmetric stresses are placed upon the abdominal wall and myofascial tissues of the pelvic floor, which may result in symptoms resembling proctitis, prostatitis, cystitis, and/or a myriad of gynecologic problems.[11] The allopathic diagnoses levator ani syndrome and proctalgia fugax often may be manifestations of sacropelvic dysfunction.

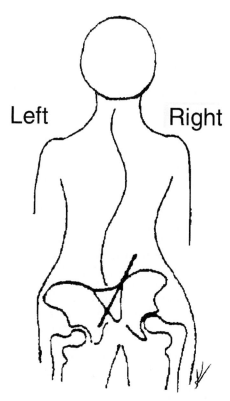

FIGURE 26.6   A short left leg with a compensatory lumbar curve side bent to the right will cause the sacrum to be chronically rotated right on the right oblique axis.

Musculoskeletal complaints above the pelvis result from asymmetric muscle contraction associated with type I mechanics and the fact that soft tissues on the side of the convexity of a type I curve are constantly being stretched.

Type II mechanics are frequently found at transitional points within the patient's type I pattern. Type I curves are frequently associated with increases in the sagittal plane (lordotic, kyphotic) curves. Intersegmental rotational mechanics change at the apex of a type I curve. As such, type II (flexion mechanics) might be expected at the level of the spinal segment immediately above the apex of a type I thoracic curve and type II (extension mechanics) at the level of the segment immediately above the apex of a type I lumbar curve. At the crossover point between two type I curves, the anteroposterior (AP) curve is flattened, making these areas more vulnerable to type II extension dysfunctions in the thoracic region and to type II flexion dysfunction in the lumbar region. Spinal facilitation at these levels can affect the patient in many ways through somatovisceral reflexes. (See Chapter 5.)

Rib complaints may be produced by the side bending and rotational mechanics of a type I thoracic curve. Frequently, a patient has discomfort merely because of the crowding of the ribs on the concave side of a thoracic group curve or the approximation of the lower ribs and iliac crest on the concave side of a lumbar curve. Costotransverse dysfunctions are often found in association with type II vertebral dysfunctions.

Figure 26.4 shows how the compensatory pattern can extend up into the cervicothoracic and upper cervical region. This can produce shoulder pain, cervical pain, muscle tension cephalalgia, and even temporomandibular joint dysfunction.

Muscle contraction (white fiber) is fueled by glycolysis. Initially, muscle contraction (red fiber) is fueled by efficient aerobic glycolysis, in which glucose is oxidized completely to carbon dioxide and water; however, when glucose is incompletely oxidized, such as after prolonged muscle contraction when available oxygen is depleted (the rule of the artery), the system shifts to anaerobic glycolysis. Anaerobic glycolysis results in the production of excess reducing equivalents (hydrogen as reduced nicotinamide adenine dinucleotide [NADH]) and the consequent accumulation of lactic acid within the muscles with resultant myalgia. Asymmetries in postural mechanics result in stress on the musculature, leading to prolonged muscle contraction in the stressed muscle.

With this information in mind, one must reconsider the presentation of the patient with short leg syndrome. The chief complaint is most often midline lumbosacral pain that is the result of altered lumbosacral mechanics. The pain is dull and aching, it is absent or less severe early in the morning, when the patient awakens refreshed after a night's sleep. As the day progresses and the patient fatigues, the pain develops. The asymmetric mechanics of the compensatory curves and sacroiliac dysfunction determine the pain pattern. Since younger individuals have high physical reserve, they tend to have a greater tolerance for the stresses of asymmetric postural mechanics. As patients age, tolerance decreases until eventually symptoms appear. Typically this does not occur until after age 35. If a young patient has what appears to be short leg syndrome, a thorough search should be made for complicating factors. If the patient is younger than 20, a thorough search should be made for significant local pathology (spinal anomalies, discitis, osteomyelitis) or distant pathology resulting in a viscerosomatic reflex. Individuals younger than age 20 rarely present with short leg syndrome.

THE PHYSICAL EXAMINATION

First, consider the apparent leg length and differentiate between functional (i.e., appears to be) and anatomic (i.e., actually is) inequality of leg length. The evaluation of leg length with the patient supine by comparison of the relative positions of the medial malleoli by itself does not adequately differentiate between functional and anatomic leg length discrepancies. Causes of functional leg length discrepancy include the following:

Lumbar curve (Fig. 26.7). In a supine patient, the presence of lumbar group curve (type I mechanics) will tend to pull the hemipelvis on the side of the concavity of the curve cephalad. This will in turn pull the lower extremity cephalad, creating the appearance of (i.e., functional) leg length inequality.

Anterior or posterior rotation of the ilium (Fig. 26.8) is said to occur as rotation of the ilium about the hypothetical inferior transverse sacral axis, as proposed by Mitchell.[8] Because the hip joint is anterior to the sacroiliac joint, posterior rotation of the ilium draws the hip joint cephalad (Fig. 26.8A). With the patient lying down, this creates an ipsilateral functional short leg. Conversely, anterior rotation of the ilium causes the hip joint to move in a caudal direction (Fig. 26.8C). This, with the patient supine, produces a ipsilateral functional long leg.

Some clinicians attempt to measure leg length with a tape measure by determining the distance between the most inferior aspect of the anterior superior iliac

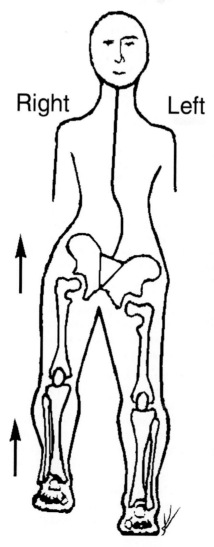

FIGURE 26.7   With the patient supine, the lumbar group curve (type I mechanics) tends to pull the hemipelvis on the side of the concavity of the curve cephalad, causing a functional short leg on that side.

spine (ASIS) and the most distal point on the homolateral medial malleolus. This is done with the patient supine, and although it may suffice for determining orthopedic (measured in inches) anatomic inequalities of leg length, the inequalities dealt with when treating anatomic short leg mechanics are measured in increments of one-eighth inch or in millimeters. The act of placing the tape measure upon the ASIS or malleolus has an inherent error potential of at least one-eighth inch, which invalidates this measurement for assessing minor leg length inequalities. Consider also the effect of pelvic dysfunction upon the position of the ASIS. It can be seen how a posterior ilium will produce a functional short leg (Fig. 26.8A). As the ilium rotates posteriorly, however, it displaces the ASIS superiorly. This increases the distance between the ASIS and

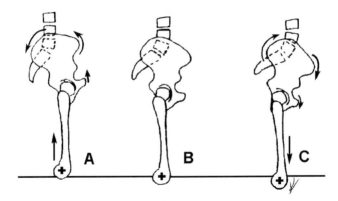

FIGURE 26.8   **(A)** Posterior rotation of the ilium draws the hip joint cephalad, with a resultant functionally short leg on that side. **(B)** Relationship between the normally positioned ilium and the lower extremity. **(C)** Anterior rotation of the ilium displaces the hip joint caudally, with a resultant functionally long leg on that side.

the medial malleolus, causing the functional short leg to measure long. The converse would be true in the presence of an anterior ilium (Fig. 26.8C). These considerations obviously limit the effectiveness of this procedure for the evaluation of the majority of patients.

Anatomic leg length discrepancy is the result of actual inequality of the length of the legs.[10] It can result from actual inequality of the length of the long bones of the legs, or it can be the result of asymmetric mechanics of the knees, valgus or varus deformity, or pronation or supination of the ankles and feet.

It is apparent how asymmetric valgus or varus of the knees can unlevel the pelvis. Dysfunctional mechanics of the ankles and feet are more complex. If the foot is pronated, the foot is abducted, dorsally flexed, and everted; this leads to internal rotation and shortening of the lower extremity. If the foot is supinated, it is adducted, plantar flexed, and inverted. This leads to external rotation and lengthening of the lower extremity. The most common asymmetric foot position is the pronated foot, often found as compensation on the side of the anatomic long leg[12,13] (Fig. 26.9).

After the knees, ankles, and feet have been evaluated for asymmetry, anatomic leg length discrepancy is best assessed with the patient standing, knees fully extended and bearing weight on both legs equally. This uses the floor as a fixed reference point. Observation of a constellation of anatomic landmarks is performed by comparing them bilaterally.

These landmarks include the following:

- Posterior superior iliac spines (PSIS), the landmark many clinicians feel is the best indicator of sacral base plane
- Sacral dimples
- Most lateral aspect of the iliac crests
- Tops of the greater trochanters, the most direct indicator of leg length (They are, however, often obscured by overlying soft tissue and fail to account for inequalities of femoral neck angles or morphologic asymmetries of the trochanters.)

Typically, all of these landmarks are low on the side of the short leg.

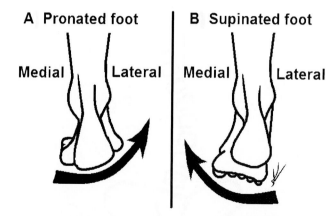

FIGURE 26.9   **(A)** A pronated foot demonstrates abduction, dorsiflexion, and eversion, resulting in internal rotation and functional shortening of the lower extremity. **(B)** A supinated foot demonstrates adduction, plantar flexion, and inversion, hence internal rotation and functional lengthening of the lower extremity.

The standing structural examination may be completed by checking for the following:

- Pelvic side shift (discussed later in the chapter)
- Lateral curves: have the patient bend forward and observe for asymmetric paravertebral prominence, the result of the rotational component of type I mechanics
- Symmetry of anatomic landmarks above the pelvis (i.e., scapulae, acromion processes, mastoid processes)
- Symmetry of anatomic landmarks of the lower extremity (i.e., popliteal creases and medial malleoli)

In addition, observe for asymmetry of skin folds on the torso and the way the patient's garments (e.g., belt line) are positioned.

This complete constellation of observations should give an idea of the patient's neutral weight bearing pattern. If this information is added to that obtained from the supine examination, discussed previously, one can draw conclusions as to the presence and clinical significance of anatomic versus functional leg length mechanics.

Now consider pelvic side shift, or lateral deviation of the pelvis to the right or left of the midline when the patient is standing. It is tested while stabilizing the upper torso by holding the shoulder with one hand and then pushing medially over the lateral aspect of the opposite hemipelvis with the other hand. The test is positive when the pelvis moves freely in one direction and resists movement in the opposite direction. A positive pelvic side shift is designated as either left or right as an indication of the direction of unrestricted pelvic motion. Figure 26.10 illustrates a positive pelvic side shift right.

Since pelvic side shift moves the center of the pelvis away from the midline and a person will attempt to maintain the center of gravity in the midline, the torso above the pelvis will move in the direction opposite the side shift. Under neutral circumstances this results in a compensatory lumbar curve (type 1 mechanics), convex on the side opposite the side shift. In Figure 26.10, the right pelvic side shift is associated with a thoracolumbar curve, convex left. The lumbar side

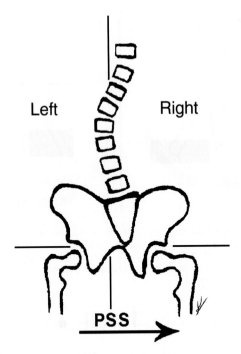

FIGURE 26.10   Level pelvis with a side shift to the right. PSS, pelvic side shift.

bending is to the right (the side of the group concavity), which will engage the sacral right oblique axis. Since conditions are neutral, a right-on-right forward torsion (lumbosacral) results. Because the sacrum is rotated right on the right oblique axis, if sacroiliac dysfunction is present, one would expect to find an anterior sacrum on the left or a posterior sacrum on the right in association with a pelvic side shift to the right.

Pelvic side shift may be the result of conditions affecting the pelvis from below. Inequality of leg length is associated with pelvic shift toward the long leg side.[10] The pelvis functions symmetrically most readily when the sacral base is level. Shifting the pelvis toward the long leg side tends to level the sacral base (Fig. 26.11).

Pelvic side shift may be the result of conditions affecting the pelvis from above. Group curve mechanics (type 1 mechanics) may produce a pelvic side shift.

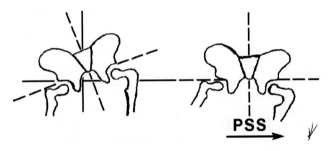

FIGURE 26.11   Inequality of leg length affecting the pelvis from below. The effect of leveling the pelvis is a pelvic side shift toward the long leg side. PSS, pelvic side shift.

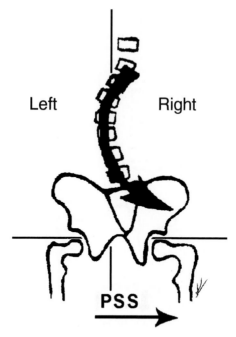

Left   Right

PSS

FIGURE 26.12   A group curve (type 1 mechanics) affecting the pelvis from above and resulting in a pelvic side shift. PSS, pelvic side shift.

Idiopathic scoliosis commonly presents as a primary fixed (i.e., will not straighten when side bending is introduced toward the convex side) thoracic curve that is convex right. There is often a smaller lumbar compensatory curve, convex left. This latter curve will shift the pelvis toward the right (Fig. 26.12). (*Scoliosis* refers to lateral curvature of the spine greater than 10 degrees. The lateral curves associated with short-leg mechanics should not be referred to as *scolioses* or *scoliotic* unless they exceed 10 degrees because of the disquieting effect of these terms upon patients.)

The contribution of type 1 lumbar mechanics to pelvic side shift can be readily seen when a patient has a short leg and the entire compensation occurs between L5 and S1 (Fig. 26.13). Because the spine is straight, the center of gravity is centered over the pelvis, and therefore, no pelvic side shift results. Under these circumstances, the unequal leg length allows the pelvis to tend to shift toward the long leg side, but the side shift is not maintained during normal weight-bearing activity.

Muscle pull mechanics from above can also produce a pelvic side shift. This occurs in the presence of asymmetric spasm of psoas major.[14] Spasm of the left psoas major will produce a side shift to the right in an otherwise level pelvis (Fig. 26.14). Psoas spasm may overcome the compensatory spinal curve from a short leg, eliminating pelvic side shift (Fig. 26.15), or it may augment short leg mechanics (Fig. 26.16). Before short leg mechanics can be effectively diagnosed or treated, dysfunctional muscle pull mechanics must be eliminated.

Spasm on the long leg side can negate the compensatory lumbar curve and pelvic side shift.

Spasm on the short leg side can augment the compensatory lumbar curve and pelvic side shift.

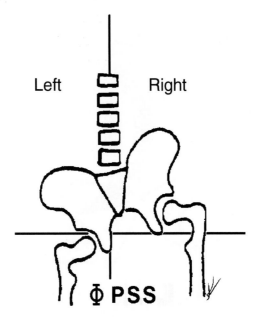

FIGURE 26.13   A short leg with all of the spinal compensation between L5 and S1. PSS, pelvic side shift.

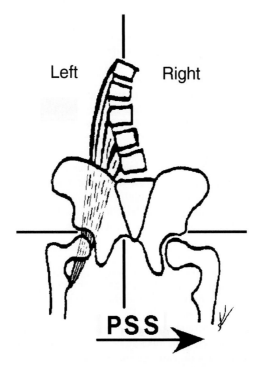

FIGURE 26.14   A level pelvis with pelvic side shift to the right as the result of spasm of the left psoas major muscle. PSS, pelvic side shift.

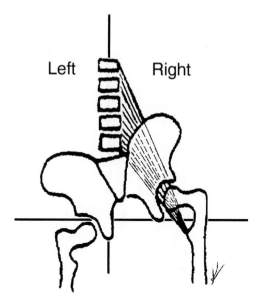

FIGURE 26.15   One combined effect of psoas spasm and unequal leg length.

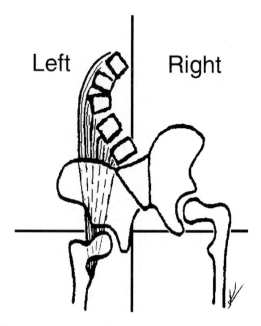

FIGURE 26.16   One combined effect of psoas spasm and unequal leg length.

ASSESSMENT

The diagnosis of short leg syndrome is based upon the pain complaint (pattern, quality, and incidence) and the findings of the musculoskeletal examination.

The pain complaint associated with short leg syndrome is described previously. It is worthwhile to iterate, however, that short leg syndrome is the result of weight bearing upon essentially normal anatomy (since most individuals have leg length inequality). The patient tends to awaken in the morning pain free, or at least with decreased symptoms. The pain complaint increases as the day progresses. Complaints associated with anatomic pathology (herniated nucleus pulposus, spondylolisthesis) are affected similarly by rest and weight bearing; however, they tend to become intensely symptomatic after briefer periods of weight bearing.

Muscle pull mechanics produce pain patterns similar to short leg mechanics. The incidence of the pain differs. Low back pain resulting from psoas spasm is worse after periods of immobility because the offending muscles become set abnormally short when they are resting. The patient has significant discomfort on first walking in the morning. As the patient moves around and the muscles warm up, the symptoms abate.

The musculoskeletal findings typically associated with short leg syndrome are as follows (Fig. 26.17):

1. Anatomic landmarks (PSIS, iliac crest, greater trochanter) low on short leg side (example: on left)
2. Pelvic side shift toward long leg side (example: toward the right)
3. Pelvic rotation toward the long leg side due to forward torsion (example: right on right forward torsion, pelvic rotation right)

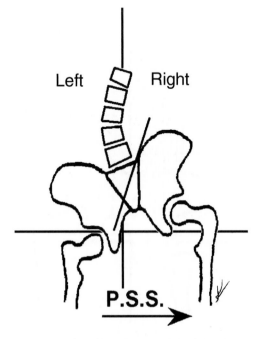

FIGURE 26.17   The musculoskeletal findings typically associated with a short left leg. PSS, pelvic side shift.

4. Anterior sacrum on short leg side (example: on left)
5. Compensatory spinal curve convex on short leg side (example: convex left)

Postural Radiographs

The findings on physical examination may be confirmed by a postural radiographic series.[15,16] The postural series is the gold standard for determining weight-bearing mechanics. It was developed in Chicago by Hoskins[17] and Schwab in the 1920s. The series consists of three films taken with the patient standing:

1. AP pelvis and lumbar spine
2. Lateral pelvis
3. AP thoracic spine

When the postural series is properly performed, measurements obtained from it are accurate to within one-eighth of an inch. Measurements typically obtained from the AP pelvis film include the following (Fig. 26.18):

Femoral head height discrepancy
Sacral base unleveling
Pelvic side shift (static deviation of the pelvis from the weight bearing midline, also called the mid-heel line)
Iliac crest height discrepancy (occasionally measured)

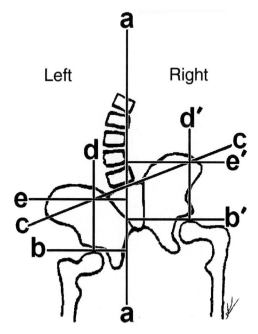

FIGURE 26.18 Marking and interpreting the AP pelvis film of the postural series: (*a*) Vertical reference, the mid-heel line. (*b and b'*) Horizontal lines demarcating the femoral head heights. (*c*) Plane of the sacral base. (*d and d'*) Two vertical lines that demarcate the sacral base relative to the position of the femoral heads. (*e and e'*) Horizontal lines demarcating the amount of sacral base unleveling relative to the position of the femoral heads.

The AP thoracic film gives information regarding the type I spinal compensatory pattern. The lateral pelvic film offers information that cannot be obtained readily by physical examination.

The procedure for taking the postural radiographic series has been described elsewhere.[15,18,19]

The films are viewed with the patient's left on the left side of the radiographic view box (Fig. 26.18), that is, as from behind. The AP films indicate balance mechanics in the coronal plane and are discussed here. The interpretation of the lateral film is discussed at length in Chapter 27.

The first step is to identify a true vertical reference, the mid-heel line (Fig. 26.18, line *a*). This is often obtained by hanging a radiopaque plumb line between the patient and the radiograph cassette. Once the vertical reference mid-heel line has been identified, femoral head heights, that is, true anatomic leg length, should be measured (Fig. 26.18, lines *b* and *b'*). The next step is to locate the top of the femoral heads on either side and draw two horizontal lines, one from the uppermost aspect of each femoral head, that intersect the mid-heel line at 90 degrees and to measure the distance between the points where the horizontal femoral head lines intersect the mid-heel line. This establishes the difference in anatomic leg length.

To measure the amount of sacral base unleveling, one must identify and mark bilaterally symmetric points on the sacral base, like the sacral notches. These two points establish a line that parallels the sacral base (Fig. 26.18, line *c*). This is the sacral base plane. If the sacral notches cannot be identified, it is necessary to draw a line down the center of the sacrum connecting the spinous processes and a second line 90 degrees to the line connecting the sacral spinous processes. This second line approximates the sacral base plane.

The sacral base plane line should extend over the femoral heads bilaterally. The next step is to draw two vertical lines, each 90 degrees to the femoral head lines, directly over the highest point on each femoral head (Fig. 26.18, lines *d* and *d'*) and extend them to transect the sacral base plane. From these two points of intersection, one can draw two horizontal lines that intersect the mid-heel line at 90 degrees (Fig. 26.18, lines *e* and *e'*). The distance between where these two lines intersect the mid-heel line is the amount of sacral unleveling relative to the femoral heads.

Leg length inequality and short leg syndrome are treated by functionally balancing the sacrum. Sacral unleveling, which contributes to sacral dysfunction, is addressed by placing a heel pad in the patient's shoe. The measurement of sacral unleveling obtained over the femoral heads is proportionate to the inequality of leg length. Consequently, it is a better indication of the size of the therapeutic lift.

Up to this point, postural balance has been considered in terms of left–right bilateral mechanics. The standing lateral pelvic radiograph gives important data about balance mechanics in the sagittal plane. This topic is covered in depth in Chapter 27.

Treatment

Having made the diagnosis of anatomic short leg, the physician formulates a treatment plan. The objective is functional balance, that is, leveling, of the patient's sacral base, eliminating the propensity for chronic engagement of either the right or left oblique axis. Dysfunction of the knee, ankle, or foot that affects the distance between the floor and femoral heads during weight bearing should be addressed. Knee bracing may be appropriate, as may be the use of laterally wedged orthotics to address foot and ankle mechanics, but these subjects are beyond the scope of this chapter. If the short leg is, as is commonly the case, the result of unequal length of the long bones of the leg, this may be managed by employing lift therapy.[20] A simple heel pad, typically no larger than one-quarter of an inch, is placed in the patient's shoe on the side of the short leg and then adjusted upward (or downward) in increments of one-eighth inch about every 2 weeks. As long as the anterior sacrum persists on the short leg side, the thickness of the heel pad should continue to be increased. If sacral mechanics invert so that the sacrum becomes anterior on the side opposite the anatomic short leg, an artificial long leg has been created, and the thickness of the heel pad should be reduced to what it was before the sacral mechanics inverted. Heel pads larger than three-eighths of an inch usually are too thick to fit comfortably into the patient's shoe and therefore should be added to the exterior heel of the shoe. Heel pads greater than one-half inch may require building up the sole of the shoe as well as the heel. For older patients, a rough estimate of how much lift will ultimately be required can be obtained by dividing the radiographically measured inequality of sacral base unleveling in half. The size of the initial heel pad and the rate by which the heel pad thickness is increased are determined by the flexibility of the patient. This may be determined by having the patient place the heel of the short leg upon pads of various thicknesses and observing the effect upon the pelvic side shift and the compensatory lumbar type I curve. The adult postural pattern is usually established by the middle of the second decade of life. The longer the leg length inequality has been present, the more fixed the patient's accommodation is likely to be and the more slowly the lift therapy should progress. When treating leg length inequality of recent onset (i.e., fracture or hip surgery), it is appropriate to attempt to correct the difference immediately.

Placing a heel pad in a patient's shoe necessitates that the individual shift the pattern of accommodation accordingly. This shift in accommodation may be facilitated by specifically treating all existent somatic dysfunction before initiating lift therapy or when making changes in the size of the heel pad.

Adjunctive exercise should also be employed. Active stretching exercise will increase the patient's overall range of motion. Passive, lazy-person exercises (see Chapter 28) may be used specifically to stretch the concave side of type I accommodative spinal curves. In general, it is a good principle to stabilize as well as mobilize. Most of these patients have some degree of lumbosacral instability, and actively strengthening the paravertebral and abdominal muscles is always a good idea. Strengthening the abdominal musculature will tend to decrease the lumbar lordosis, Ferguson's angle, and consequently lumbosacral decompensation in the sagittal plane. The Levitor, an orthotic device, may also be used for this purpose. (See Chapter 27.)

CONCLUSION

This chapter provides the information necessary to solve problems of patients with laterally asymmetric postural balance problems. The discussion is essentially limited to the typical pattern of accommodation to leg length inequality. Patients may present with variations in the accommodative pattern, and although the initiation of lift therapy may occasionally be trial and error, these principles still apply.

When a patient's chief complaint is lumbosacral pain, the most common etiologies are functional disorders. For young adults, the likely diagnosis is psoas spasm. In middle-aged patients, short leg syndrome is encountered with increasing frequency.

The pain complaint associated with short leg syndrome is the result of weight bearing upon normal anatomy. Typically, the patient wakes in the morning without discomfort or with decreased symptoms. The pain gets worse as the day progresses. Complaints associated with anatomic pathology (herniated nucleus pulposus, spondylolisthesis) are affected similarly by rest and weight bearing; however, they tend to become intensely painful after brief periods of weight bearing.

Psoas spasm results in pain similar to short leg mechanics. The incidence of the pain differs. Low back pain resulting from psoas spasm is worse after periods of immobility because the offending muscles become set abnormally short when they are resting, and the patient has significant discomfort on first walking in the morning. As the patient moves around and the muscles warm up, the symptoms decrease. The typical patient with acute psoas spasm is a man in his mid 20s with pain upon arising. Many give a history of similar episodes in the past that have resolved spontaneously. This is also, of course, the presentation of a patient with ankylosing spondylitis.

The incidence of psoas spasm and short leg syndrome is higher than that of ankylosing spondylitis or spondylolisthesis; however, their potential to result in lumbosacral pain necessitates a complete history and physical examination. In case one inadvertently misdiagnoses organic pathology as somatic dysfunction, it is important to recognize that organic pathology does not resolve when treated with OMT. Should a patient fail to significantly improve after three to five treatments with OMT, one should look again for underlying organic pathology.

Procedures

Please note: The procedures that follow are examples of manipulative treatment that you may wish to employ. The actual choice of procedures used should be determined by the unique circumstances of each individual patient.

Constant Rest Position (Fig. 26.19)

This position, used to relieve acute low back pain, may be employed while waiting for an analgesic to take effect. It reduces stress on the back by removing the weight transmitted through the lumbar spine during weight bearing. It reduces the lumbar and cervical lordotic curves and relaxes the paraspinal musculature. This position also unloads spastic psoas major muscles, approximating their origin and insertion by flexing the hips.

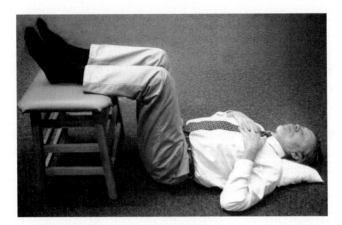

FIGURE 26.19   Constant rest position used to relieve acute low back pain; it may be employed during the wait for an analgesic to take effect. It reduces stress on the back by removing the weight transmitted through the lumbar spine during weight bearing. It reduces the lumbar and cervical lordotic curves and relaxes the paraspinal musculature. It also unloads spastic psoas major muscles by approximating the origin and insertion.

Procedure

1. The patient lies supine on a firm surface with a small pillow beneath the head and neck for comfort.
2. The patient places the feet and legs upon a chair, bench, or similar structure, such that the hips are flexed to 90 degrees or more.
3. This position may be maintained as long as necessary.

Anterior Sacrum, Muscle Energy

This procedure is employed to introduce motion to a dysfunctional sacroiliac articulation (For diagnosis, see Chapter 3, and for a description of this procedure, see Chapter 9 and Figure 9.5.)

Posterior Sacrum, Trunk Rotation (HVLA) (Fig. 26.20)

This procedure is employed to treat specific sacroiliac articular dysfunction found in association with sacral forward torsion. Considering a posterior sacrum, the innominate is anterior to the sacrum, so this procedure moves the ilium posterior to meet the sacrum.

Patient position: supine. Physician position: standing at the level of the patient's pelvis opposite the side of the posterior sacrum.

Procedure (Example: Posterior Sacrum on the Right)

1. Pull the patient's pelvis toward you so that the left hip is at the edge of the table.
2. Move the patient's upper torso away from you to introduce side bending to the right from above down to the sacrum between the ilia. The patient's left shoulder should be lying in the midline of the table.
3. Move the patient's feet away from you to introduce side bending to the right from below up to the sacrum. Steps 1 to 3 combine to introduce sacral side bending to the right between the ilia.
4. Instruct the patient to place the hands behind the neck and to interlace the fingers.
5. Reach across the patient, and coming in from the patient's right, slide your right hand through the triangle formed by the patient's right arm. In this position, your

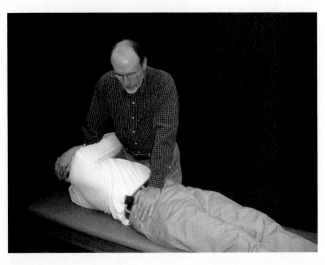

FIGURE 26.20   Trunk rotation to treat a posterior sacrum on the right.

right hand should be directed back at you so that it rests palm up in contact with the patient's sternum.

6. Place your left hand on the patient's right ASIS to hold the right side of the pelvis against the table.
7. Draw your right arm toward you, pulling the patient up onto the left shoulder to rotate the torso to the left. It is important to keep the patient's left shoulder in the center of the table throughout this portion of the procedure to produce rotation to the left coupled with the side bending to the right, introduced in steps 1 to 3.
8. The final corrective force is simultaneous rotation from above with your right arm and a quick thrust posteriorly on the right ASIS, moving the ilium posteriorly upon the sacrum on the right.
9. Reassess right sacroiliac motion.

Lumbar Walk-Around (HVLA or Muscle Energy) (Fig. 26.21)

This procedure is employed to treat lumbar and low to mid thoracic type II somatic dysfunction. (For diagnosis, see Chapter 3.) A similar procedure is described elsewhere for type I, group curve, dysfunction. (See Chapter 28 and Figure 28.4.)

Patient position: seated astride the end of the treatment table with the pelvis as close to the edge of the table as possible and the back toward the physician. Physician position: standing behind the seated patient and slightly toward the side opposite the rotation of the dysfunction.

Procedure (Example: L2 upon L3, Flexed, Rotated Right and Side Bent Right)

1. The patient is instructed to clasp the hands behind the neck and to allow the elbows to drop forward.

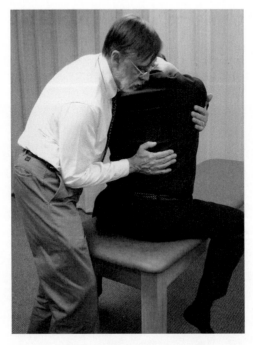

FIGURE 26.21   Walk-around, HVLA or muscle energy, employed to treat lumbar and low to mid thoracic type II somatic dysfunction.

2. Standing behind and slightly to the left of the patient, reach over the patient's left shoulder and across the chest anteriorly with your left arm. Grasp the lateral chest inferior to the right axilla with your left hand.
3. Palpate the interspinous space between L2 and L3 with your right hand.
4. To introduce extension, have the patient sit up straight as you lift the torso with your left arm until you palpate approximation of the spinous processes of L2 and L3. You may wish to place a small pillow between your left forearm and the patient's anterior chest wall. To introduce flexion, when treating an extension dysfunction, instruct the patient to slump forward until you palpate gapping between the spinous processes of L2 and L3.
5. Move your right hand so that your proximal palm is in contact with the posterior right transverse process of L2 and tuck your right elbow into your torso just medial to your right ASIS.
6. Introduce left side bending between L2 and L3 by laterally translating the patient's torso to the right and by applying pressure with your left axilla against the left shoulder while lifting the right shoulder with your left hand.
7. Keep the patient's ischial tuberosities firmly upon the table.
8. Introduce rotation of the patient's torso to the left with your left arm and hand in combination with pressure through your right hand until the barrier is engaged. Apply the force through your right hand by moving your entire body against your right elbow, which is firmly fixed against your right ASIS.
9. Apply a final HVLA force through your right arm by walking (shifting your torso to the right) farther around the end of the table to the right.
10. This procedure may be modified to a muscle energy procedure by instructing the patient to turn to the right against your holding force for 3 to 5 seconds to treat rotation or to raise the left shoulder to treat side bending.
11. Pause for 1 to 2 seconds, and then rotate the patient's torso further to the left or depress the patient's left shoulder and lift the right shoulder to engage the new barrier.
12. Repeat steps 10 and 11 until the best possible increase of motion is obtained.
13. Reassess motion between L2 and L3.

Psoas Spasm (Muscle Energy) (Fig. 26.22)

This procedure is employed for isometric stretch of dysfunctionally tight hip flexors, particularly psoas major. It may also be employed to treat a posteriorly displaced ilium.

Patient position: prone. Physician position: standing on the side of the tight psoas muscle.

Procedure (Example: Tight Right Psoas Major)

1. With your left hand, grasp the patient's right thigh proximal to the knee.
2. Place your right hand on the patient's lumbosacral junction and hold the pelvis firmly against the table.
3. Lift the right thigh from the table, extending the right hip until the dysfunctional barrier is engaged. At this point, you may wish to place your left knee between the tabletop and the patient's thigh to facilitate holding the thigh off the table.
4. Maintain this position and instruct the patient to gently push the right knee back toward the table into your left hand for 3 to 5 seconds.
5. Instruct the patient to relax and pause for 1 to 2 seconds.
6. Lift the right thigh, further extending the right hip to engage the new barrier.
7. Repeat steps 4 to 6 until the desired increase of hip extension is obtained.
8. Reassess ease of extension of the hip as an indicator of psoas tension.

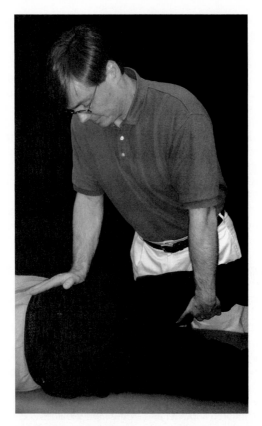

FIGURE 26.22   Psoas muscle energy employed for isometric stretching of dysfunctionally tight hip flexors, particularly psoas major. It may also be employed to treat a posteriorly displaced ilium.

Psoas Stretch Exercises

The following exercises may be employed to stretch tight iliopsoas muscles to stabilize the low back and maintain the therapeutic effects obtained with OMT.

PSOAS STRETCH, STANDING (EXERCISE) (FIG. 26.23)

This exercise is employed to stretch hip flexors, particularly psoas major. It accomplishes this in two ways: It physically stretches the muscles by increasing the distance between the origins and insertions, and it reflexively induces relaxation through reciprocal inhibition, by actively contracting hip extensors. This procedure is particularly useful in that once the patient masters it, it can be performed essentially anywhere. This is a preventive procedure, and the patient who is prone to recurrent episodes of psoas spasm should be encouraged to stretch daily.

   Patient position: standing.

Procedure

1. The patient stands approximately 1 to 2 feet away facing a wall or other solid structure.
2. The patient places the palms upon the wall at shoulder height and keep them there throughout the exercise to maintain balance.

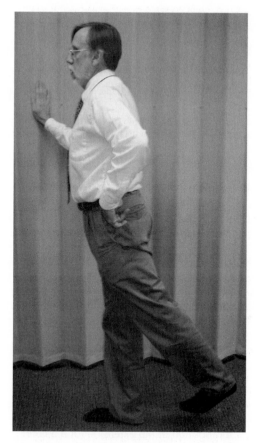

FIGURE 26.23   Psoas stretch, standing, to stretch hip flexors, particularly psoas major.

3. The patient stands erect with the knees locked in full extension throughout the exercise.
4. The patient tightens the lumbar paravertebral musculature and buttocks.
5. The patient places the weight upon one leg and extends the other hip, lifting the foot from the floor and bringing the entire lower extremity, with the knee straight, behind. The degree of hip extension, 10 to 20 degrees from the vertical, is not as important as is keeping a straight back and knee while maintaining lumbar paravertebral and gluteal tension and taking the hip into the fullest possible extension.
6. The patient switches the weight to the other leg and repeats step 5.
7. This procedure may be repeated 5 to 10 times on a side, according to tolerance, and should be performed a minimum of twice daily, before retiring at night and upon arising in the morning. It can be performed as many times a day as necessary and is appropriate before and after prolonged periods of sitting. Patients who sit for long periods or who assume chronic positions that involve lumbar flexion, like automotive mechanics who have to bend over continuously, should be encouraged to stretch frequently.

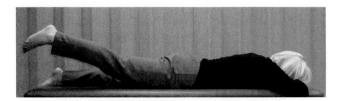

FIGURE 26.24   Prone psoas stretch to stretch hip flexors, particularly psoas major, while strengthening the antagonists, the erector spinae muscles.

PSOAS STRETCH, PRONE (EXERCISE) (FIG. 26.24)

This exercise is employed to stretch hip flexors, particularly psoas major. It accomplishes this in two ways: It physically stretches the muscles by increasing the distance between the origins and insertions, and it reflexively induces relaxation through reciprocal inhibition by actively contracting hip and lumbar extensors.

The procedure consists of repetitive contraction of the lumbar paravertebral musculature and the hip extensors. Each repetition has 3 steps and each step takes about 5 seconds, for a total of 15 seconds per repetition. Having the patient count to 5 out loud during each step prevents the Valsalva maneuver and reduces stress upon the abdominal wall. The sequence typically begins with 10 repetitions. This procedure does more to strengthen the paravertebral musculature than does the standing psoas stretch.

Patient position: prone.

Procedure

1. The patient slowly lifts one thigh from the floor or treatment table by extending the hip while keeping the knee straight for a 5 count.
2. The patient holds this position of hip extension for a 5 count.
3. The patient slowly returns the thigh to the floor for a 5 count.
4. The patient repeats steps 1 to 3 with the other leg.

This procedure may be repeated 5 to 10 times on a side, according to patient tolerance, and may be performed a minimum of twice daily instead of the standing stretch procedure, before retiring at night and upon arising in the morning.

ADDITIONAL PROCEDURES

- Dry-land swim to strengthen paravertebral musculature (See the description of the procedure in Chapter 27 and Fig. 27.17.)
- Back hyperextensions to strengthen paravertebral musculature (See the description of the procedure in Chapter 28 and Fig. 28.5.)
- Torso curls to strengthen abdominal musculature (See the description of the procedure in Chapter 28 and Fig. 28.6.)
- Reverse torso curls to strengthen abdominal musculature (See the description of the procedure in Chapter 28 and Fig. 28.7.)

References

1. Bailey HW, Beckwith CG. Short leg and spinal anomalies. J Am Osteopath Assoc 1937;36: 319–327. Reprinted in American Academy of Osteopathy 1983 Yearbook. Indianapolis: American Academy of Osteopathy, 1983;63–70.

2. Schwab WA. Principles of manipulative treatment: III. The low back problem. J Am Osteopath Assoc 1932. Reprinted in: Academy of Applied Osteopathy 1965 Yearbook. Vol. 2. Indianapolis: American Academy of Osteopathy, 1965;2:30–38.

3. Pearson WM et al. A progressive structural study of school children. J Am Osteopath Assoc. 1951;51:155–167.

4. Klein KK. A study of the progression of lateral pelvic asymmetry in 585 elementary, junior and high school boys. AM Correct Ther J 1969;23:171–173.

5. Klein KK, Redler I, Lowman CL. Asymmetries of the growth in the pelvis and legs of children: A clinical statistical study 1964–1967. J Am Osteopath Assoc 1968;68:153–156.

6. Heinking KP, Kappler RE. Pelvis and sacrum. In: Ward RC, ed. Foundations for Osteopathic Medicine. 2nd ed. Philadelphia: Lippincott Williams & Wilkins, 2002;762–783.

7. Nelson KE. The sacrum: A bone of contention. AAO J 1997;7(4):17–24.

8. Mitchell FL Sr. Structural pelvic function. In: Academy of Applied Osteopathy 1965 Yearbook. Vol. 2. Indianapolis: American Academy of Osteopathy, 1965;2:178–199.

9. Fryette HH. Principles of Osteopathic Technic. Indianapolis: American Academy of Osteopathy, 1954; 1980;30.

10. Kappler RE. Postural balance and motion patterns. J Am Osteopath Assoc 1982;81:598–606. Reprinted in: American Academy of Osteopathy 1983 Yearbook. Indianapolis: American Academy of Osteopathy, 1983;6–12.

11. Jungmann M. Abdominopelvic pain caused by gravitational strain. Southwestern Med 1961;42:501–508.

12. Donatelli R. The Biomechanics of the Foot and Ankle. 2nd ed. Philadelphia: Davis, 1996; 55–59.

13. Pope RE. The Common Compensatory Pattern: Its Origin and Relationship to the Postural Model. AAO Journal 2003;13(4):19–40.

14. Kappler RE. Role of psoas mechanism in low back complaints. J Am Osteopath Assoc 1973;72:794–801.

15. Denslow JS, Chace JA, Gutensohn OR, Kumm MG. Methods in taking and interpreting weight-bearing radiograph films. J Am Osteopath Assoc 1955;54:663–670. Reprinted in American Academy of Osteopathy 1983 Yearbook. Indianapolis: American Academy of Osteopathy, 1983;144–151.

16. Willman MK. Radiographic technical aspects of the postural study. J Am Osteopath Assoc 1977;76:739–744. Reprinted in American Academy of Osteopathy 1983 Yearbook. Indianapolis: American Academy of Osteopathy, 1983;140–143.

17. Hoskins ER. Determining unequal leg length using standing radiographs. J Am Osteopath Assoc. 1933–1934. Reprinted in American Academy of Osteopathy 1983 Yearbook. Indianapolis: American Academy of Osteopathy, 1983;154–155.

18. Beilke M. Roentgenological spinal analysis and the technic for taking standing radiograph plates. J Am Osteopath Assoc 1936;35:414–418.

19. Kuchera ML, Kuchera WA. Radiographic aspects of the postural study. In: Ward RC, ed. Foundations for Osteopathic Medicine. 2nd ed. Philadelphia: Lippincott Williams & Wilkins, 2002;591–602.

20. Heilig D. Principles of lift therapy. J Am Osteopath Assoc 1978;77:466–472. Reprinted in American Academy of Osteopathy 1983 Yearbook. Indianapolis: American Academy of Osteopathy, 1983:113–118.

CHAPTER 27

The Patient with Back Pain: Postural Decompensation in the Sagittal Plane

Nils A. Olson

INTRODUCTION

Chapter 26 discusses leg length discrepancies and their relation to back pain. This chapter deals with an additional type of postural decompensation and its association with back pain. This syndrome is referred to as sagittal plane decompensation. This chapter describes how postural decline and gravitational strain contribute to chronic back pain and reviews some therapies that are useful in treating this problem.

In postural health, the center of gravity in an erect person follows a line that extends from the external auditory canal down through the head of the humerus, the center of the body of the third lumbar vertebra, the greater trochanter, the lateral condyle of the knee, and the lateral malleolus.[1] This weight-bearing line allows the weight and forces of the body to rest upon structures that are designed to support that weight (Fig. 27.1).

In sagittal plane decompensation, these weight-bearing areas do not support the body as they should. Gravity exerts forces on areas not meant to be support structures. This causes the body to compensate in an attempt to maintain that proper structural alignment. This stress causes tension on ligaments and strain on muscles. As ligaments stretch in response to the abnormal weight bearing and the compensatory reaction, muscles must work overtime to maintain posture, actually attempting to provide structural integrity that was originally expected of ligaments.

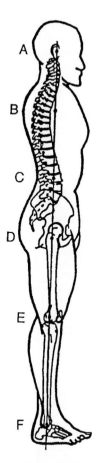

FIGURE 27.1 Least stressful postural alignment of body in relation to the gravitational line. (**A**) External auditory canal. (**B**) Head of the humerus. (**C**) Center of the body of L3. (**D**) Greater trochanter. (**E**) Lateral condyle of the knee. (**F**) Lateral malleolus.

This leads to commonly found somatic dysfunctions and pain, which can become chronic. If the abnormal weight bearing is not addressed, commonly used therapies to relieve pain may not produce the desired long-term effect.

As part of the standing structural portion of the physical examination, the patient should be observed for increase or decrease of the anterior and posterior spinal curves. The postural alignment of the superficial anatomic landmarks of the line of gravity (Fig. 27.1) should also be noted. If indicated, these physical findings may be further evaluated using the lateral standing exposure of the postural series of radiographs. (See Chapter 26.)

THE LATERAL RADIOGRAPH

The spatial relationships of the pelvis to the sacrum and lumbar spine can be analyzed in a lateral pelvic radiograph. To establish a line of reference in the radiograph, one must use a radiopaque wire plumb line suspended behind the standing patient during filming. This reference line should merely be somewhere near the center of the spinal column; it is unimportant if it is slightly off center. This line is useful for making sure that drawn lines are truly vertical or horizontal.

The Pelvic Index

A vertical line is drawn from the anterior tip of the sacrum inferiorly, paralleling the gravitational line, and is labeled Y. A horizontal line is drawn posteriorly from the anterior edge of the pubic bone until it intersects with line Y. This line is labeled X. The pelvic index is found by dividing X by Y (Fig. 27.2).

The spatial relationships of the pelvis to the sacrum and lumbar spine change considerably with age. It is thought that this change is affected by gravitational pull.[2] If one studies the anatomic relationships of the spine to the pelvis in youth, adulthood, and old age, the changes become quite obvious. In the adult, a pelvic

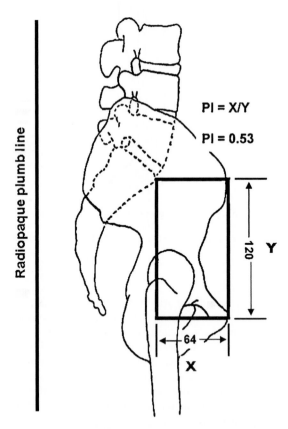

FIGURE 27.2   The pelvic index (PI) determined from a lateral radiograph and measured in reference to anatomic points of the pelvis and sacrum in relation to the gravitational plumb line. (Reprinted with permission from Gallant RA, ed. The Jungmann Concept and Techniques of Anti-Gravity Leverage: A Clinical Handbook. 2nd ed. Rangeley, ME: Institute for Gravitational Strain Pathology, 1992.)

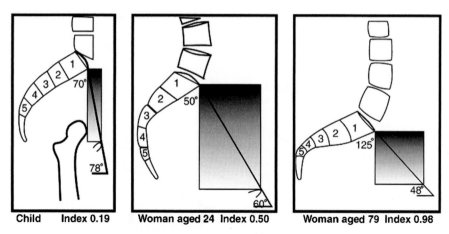

| Child   Index 0.19 | Woman aged 24 Index 0.50 | Woman aged 79 Index 0.98 |

FIGURE 27.3   Typical change in the pelvic index with age. (Reprinted with permission from Schubert EV. Roentgenuntersuchungen des knoechernen Beckens im Profilbild: Exakte Messung der Beckenneigung beim Lebenden [Radiographic investigation of the pelvic bones in sagittal view: Precise measurement of the pelvic inclination in living persons]. Zentralbl Gynakol 1929;17:1064.

index of about 0.5 is considered reasonable for good structural health. In youth, the pelvic index is less than 0.5, and in older age, it is more than 0.5 (Fig. 27.3). This age-related shift in pelvic index is not necessarily accompanied by sagittal decompensation and low back pain. A high pelvic index relative to any given age, however, can be associated with either chronic back pain or vertebral dislocation (Fig. 27.4).

The Spinal Center of Gravity

Weight bearing of the spine as it relates to the base of the sacrum contributes to sagittal decompensation. In health, the center of the third lumbar vertebra is considered the spinal center of gravity. A line drawn inferiorly from the center of L3 and parallel to the vertical line of reference should end within the anterior third of the base of the sacrum. Displacement of this weight-bearing line anterior (most commonly encountered) or posterior to the anterior third of the sacral base can cause muscular and ligamentous strain and shear stress (Fig. 27.5).

Ferguson's Sacral Angle

The third parameter one must evaluate is the sacral angle. This angle is determined by radiography, as in the last example. The plumb line again is a useful tool for making accurate lines and measurements. A line is drawn across the base of the sacrum and extended past the plumb line several inches. Another line is drawn horizontally at a 90-degree angle from the plumb line and extends to the line that was drawn across the base of the sacrum. That intersecting angle is measured (Fig. 27.6). In the adult, this angle is normally between 34 and 44 degrees.

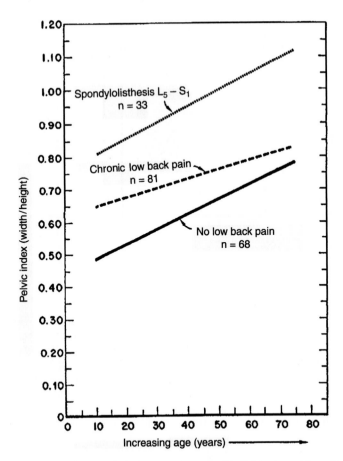

FIGURE 27.4   Pelvic index in relation to age in normal individuals and in patients with chronic low back pain or vertebral dislocation (spondylolisthesis). (Reprinted with permission from Gallant RA, ed. The Jungmann Concept and Techniques of Anti-Gravity Leverage: A Clinical Handbook. 2nd ed. Rangeley, ME: Institute for Gravitational Strain Pathology, 1992.)

Gravitational Pull, Sagittal Plane

Decompensation and How it Produces Pain

When any or all three of these measurements of postural health are abnormal, the result is increased stress on the ligaments and muscles that are attempting to compensate for this abnormality. If the spinal center of gravity is anterior to the sacral promontory, for example, the lumbar muscles are exposed to chronic increased tone as they attempt to pull the torso back toward balance. This attempt at compensation is somewhat like the cervical spine's compensatory action to keep the eyes level in the presence of scoliosis.

Nonsurgical Treatment of Sagittal Plane Decompensation

Multiple modalities aimed at relieving pain and improving function, including exercises, osteopathic manipulation, proliferative therapy, physical therapy, orthotic

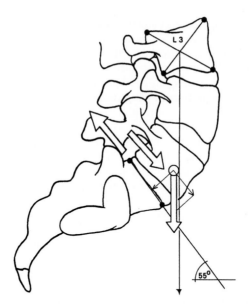

FIGURE 27.5   The third lumbar vertebra spinal center of gravity. Here the L3 weight-bearing line falls anterior to the sacral base, causing shear stress, especially in the posterior elements, the erector spinae muscles, and ligamentous tissues. (Reprinted with permission from Kuchera ML. Gravitational stress, musculo-ligamentous strain, and postural alignment. Spine: State of the Art Reviews 1995;9:463–490.)

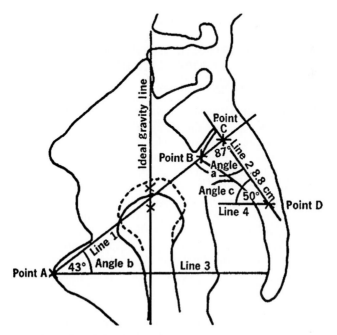

FIGURE 27.6   Determination of the sacral angle (angle B) in relation to the ideal gravity line. (Reprinted with permission from Gallant RA, ed. The Jungmann Concept and Techniques of Anti-Gravity Leverage: A Clinical Handbook. 2nd ed. Rangeley, ME: Institute for Gravitational Strain Pathology, 1992.)

devices, and when appropriate, medications, such as nonsteroidal anti-inflammatory agents and sometimes even opioids, may be used in treatment of this syndrome. The primary exercises used should strengthen the lumbar and abdominal musculature. These include torso curls, reverse torso curls, and the pelvic tilt.

The pelvic tilt may be employed to alter the relationship between the lumbar spine and the pelvis. It is performed lying supine on a firm surface. In this position the patient forces the lumbar spine to flatten against the firm surface. This repetitive series of exercises is usually done twice a day. Once the patient has mastered this maneuver and has begun to strengthen the lumbar musculature, adding bilateral straight leg raising while maintaining the flattened lumbar spine will further improve muscular strength in the lumbar region. However, during straight leg raises, it is important that the patient lift the feet no more than 6 to 8 inches to prevent activation of the psoas muscle during exercise. The torso curls and reverse torso curls will primarily improve the abdominal musculature that secondarily assists the lumbar muscles.

Osteopathic manipulation is useful in treating this syndrome. It is not important which modalities are used as long as the goal is to increase function by improving motion, reducing spasm, and relieving pain. Whether high-velocity, low-amplitude, muscle energy, functional technique, counterstrain, or soft tissue release is chosen is not important. The goal remains the same.

Orthotic devices are continually being developed for use in adjusting spinal misalignments. One such orthotic is the Levitor (U.S. Patent No. 4, 275, 718). In contrast to the full-torso Milwaukee brace or the shorter thoracolumbosacral orthoses (e.g., Boston, Miami, Wilmington, and Rosenberger orthoses) used to treat scoliosis and associated lordosis and kyphosis, the Levitor is a much less cumbersome device designed specifically to correct sagittal plane decompensation.

USE OF THE LEVITOR ORTHOTIC IN THE TREATMENT OF SAGITTAL PLANE DECOMPENSATION

A Brief History of the Levitor Orthotic

Martin Jungmann was a physician in Vienna in the 1930s. He conducted extensive studies on chronic back pain and the effects of gravitational pull on posture and how that related to chronic back pain.[2] He developed the concept of the Levitor orthotic, which changes the postural alignment of the spine as it relates to the sacrum and pelvis, thus relieving pain. In 1939, he moved to New York City, where he continued his research and in 1957 established the Institute for Gravitational Strain Pathology. As he taught his theories and lectured to interested physicians, he formed a particular relationship with the osteopathic community because its practitioners seemed particularly receptive to his concepts and theories. Jungmann died in 1973. Today training in the clinical use of this orthotic is continued in Kirksville College of Osteopathic Medicine in Kirksville, Missouri, and is available through regional Levitor centers throughout the United States and overseas.

Description

The Levitor orthotic is a dynamic brace. It applies various amounts of pressure and may be adjusted using a scale specifically devised to measure the pounds of pressure produced. It changes weight bearing and the effects of gravity upon the spine. It is not a static brace like traditional lumbosacral supports that are made with Velcro, straps, and staves. It is made of aluminum and is custom formed to

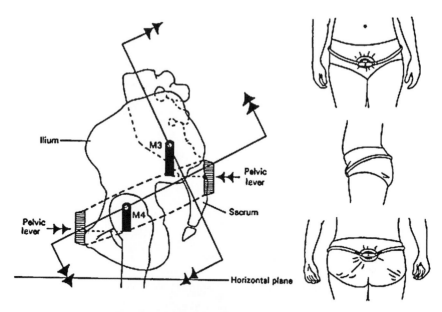

FIGURE 27.7 The pelvic lever action of the Levitor orthotic. (Reprinted with permission from Kuchera ML. Postural considerations in the sagittal plane. In: Ward RC, ed. Foundations for Osteopathic Medicine. Baltimore: Williams & Wilkins, 1997;999–1014.)

each patient. It must be partially fabricated in the physician's office. Semi-firm pads are attached to the front and back of the device. These pads, when properly fitted, rest against the patient over the pubic symphysis and the sacrum (Fig. 27.7).

It is necessary to measure the anteroposterior diameter of the orthotic while it is being worn by using a caliper similar to the obstetric calipers that were used in the past to determine maternal pelvic dimensions (Fig. 27.8). The caliper is placed upon the front and rear pad of the orthotic and a measurement is taken.

The orthotic is then placed on the special scale that measures the amount of pressure exerted on the pelvis by the orthotic. The orthotic must be stretched over the scale to the exact measurement that was taken while the device was on the patient. These pressures are manipulated by bending the metal with a set of specifically designed tools (Fig. 27.9). When properly fitted, the Levitor will produce a pressure in the sagittal plane of 6.5 to 7.5 pounds.

At first, the orthotic will have to be adjusted fairly often, sometimes every 4 or 5 days, to maintain that pressure. As it exerts pressure, the sagittal plane usually narrows, sometimes by several centimeters. This causes the orthotic to produce less pressure and become less effective and necessitates readjustment. The 6.5 to 7.5 pounds of pressure is required to change the pelvic index, center of weight bearing, and sacral angle. Less pressure is not effective. More pressure produces discomfort not usually tolerated by patients and increases the risk of pressure ulcers where the pads touch the body. Eventually, adjustments are needed only every few months, and sometimes the patient can go as long as 6 months between adjustments. Once prescribed, the orthotic must be worn at all times while the patient is up and around (Figs. 27.10 and 27.11). It is taken off only to lie down, bathe, swim, and sometimes to sit. The more the device is removed while the patient is

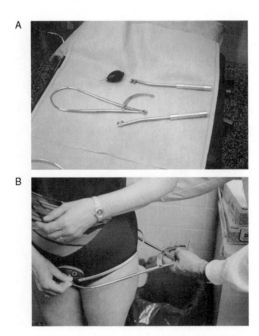

FIGURE 27.8   **(A)** Caliper used to measure the anteroposterior measurement of the Levitor orthotic. **(B)** Proper position on the patient.

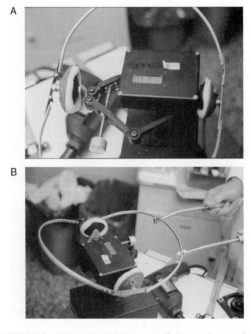

FIGURE 27.9   Pressure adjustment of the Levitor orthotic.

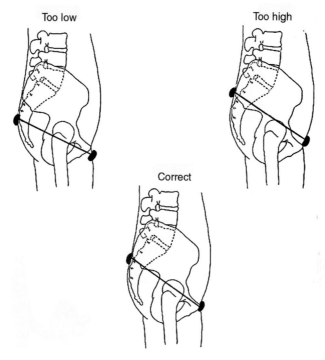

FIGURE 27.10   Proper placement of the Levitor orthotic.

upright, the more gravitational forces will tend to return the anatomy to its previous decompensated position.

Choosing a Candidate for This Treatment

Because of the required commitment to use the orthotic continually, candidates must be chosen carefully, or the physician's time and the patients' money will be wasted, and the patients will be unhappy. Typical patients are middle aged or older and have

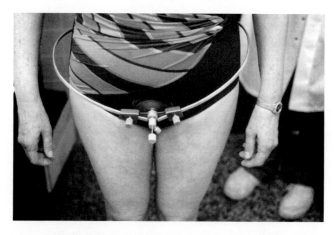

FIGURE 27.11   Properly adjusted Levitor orthotic.

had chronic back pain that may or may not include radicular pain. Many have had several treatments with different modalities—physical therapy, medicinal intervention, osteopathic manipulative therapy (OMT), trigger point injections, or epidural injections—without success. For success with the Levitor, the pain must be significant enough for the patient to be committed to wearing the orthotic continually while awake. This is not to say that it would not work on lesser pain; it is just this author's experience that if the pain is not significant, the patient will abandon the device after a few months. Further, the sacroiliac joint must be mobile enough to move under the pressure produced by the Levitor. Previous surgery does not preclude candidacy. This device has been used successfully even by people who have had lumbar fusion or lumbosacral fusion, both bone graft and internal hardware fixation. It worked in those patients because the sacroiliac joint was mobile enough to respond.

Patients who have symptomatic isthmic spondylolisthesis are good treatment candidates. Pain from this disorder can be relieved with the use of the Levitor.[3] Further study is needed to determine whether use of the Levitor will prevent progression of spondylolisthesis. The Levitor shifts the weight-bearing forces from the posterior lumbosacral structures, thereby removing tissue strain.[4] If spondylolisthesis is found incidentally, however, the patient may not have the pain pattern necessary to impel commitment to use the device. About 5% of the population is thought to have spondylolisthesis, and perhaps only half of these individuals are symptomatic.[5-7] Other investigators have concluded that sagittal plane decompensation is implicated in spondylolysis and spondylolisthesis.[8,9] They use a different method of measurement, spinal incidence, to define sagittal plane decompensation, but it is a similar concept.

The Levitor is not a substitute for appropriate surgical intervention when warranted, such as in a significantly symptomatic herniated lumbar disc or severe spinal stenosis. The Levitor may be used in patients who have chronic pain from postlaminectomy syndrome. This author has, however, found that these patients, while receiving a degree of relief, frequently do not get the desired satisfactory results.

When the typical patient has presented, one must obtain the radiographs, or dynamic films, discussed earlier in the chapter. The patient may then be deemed an appropriate candidate if some or all of the radiographic abnormalities of sagittal plane decompensation are found. In this author's experience, the two most important findings are passing of the weight-bearing line anterior to the sacral promontory and a pelvic index of 1.0 or greater.

As with any modality, the end results vary. Some patients who are ideal candidates do not respond well at all, while some with marginal qualifications do very well. It is difficult to determine who will or will not respond well. Since these patients have had pain for some time and have had multiple unsuccessful interventions before, many are willing to try this therapy. As a general rule, the more of the criteria they meet, the more likely to respond favorably they are.

Manipulation and the Levitor

The Levitor is only one option in the treatment of certain chronic back problems. It is a part of general structural care. It is not a replacement for OMT. OMT should be an integral part of the care of patients with chronic low back pain. The exact modality is not as important as is a plan to maintain mobility and relieve spasm and ligamentous strain. So whether one chooses high-velocity, low-amplitude, muscle energy, soft tissue, counterstrain, functional technique, or any other manipulative modality is not important. What is important is maintaining mobility. Therefore, no specific category of manipulation will be recommended in connection with the Levitor orthotic.

Case Presentations

Case 1

This patient was 55 years old when she presented with chronic back pain. She had a lumbar laminectomy 5 years earlier, followed by a lumbosacral fusion 1 year prior to her initial visit. The fusion was accomplished using plates and screws and included the sacrum and the bottom three lumbar vertebral bodies. A year post fusion, she had only a little relief and complained of muscle spasm and pains to the point of nausea. She had received chiropractic treatment and had gone through two courses of physical therapy and used a TENS unit (transcutaneous electrical nerve stimulator). She had worn a 1-inch lift in her right shoe since a short leg was diagnosed after a motor vehicle accident when she was 25 years old. She had multiple compensatory somatic dysfunctions of the thoracic and cervical spine. Dynamic films revealed a sacral angle of 67 degrees, pelvic index of 1.1, and a weight-bearing line 6.6 cm anterior to sacral promontory (Fig. 27.12).

She was fitted with the Levitor orthotic and was followed for several years. She had the Levitor adjusted periodically and received OMT in the form of myofascial procedures to the lumbar area and a combination of muscle energy, soft tissue, and high-velocity procedures to the thoracic and cervical areas. Within a year of initiation of treatment, she had marked improvement of her symptoms. She carried her body more upright and had subjective relief of pain approaching 80%. Interestingly, she had been bothered by shortness of breath, which also resolved with the treatment, probably from the reduction in compensatory response in the thoracic spine and rib cage caused by the previous imbalance and decompensation. She specifically noted that if she failed to wear the Levitor for any length of time, her symptoms would begin to resurface. The Levitor worked in this woman in spite of her lumbosacral fusion because her sacroiliac joints were still mobile.

Case 2

This patient was 40 years old when she was first seen. She feared that she was "heading down the same path" as her mother. They both had spondylolisthesis of L5 on S1. Her mother had gone through a spinal fusion but was still in pain and was having significant difficulties with activities of daily living. If the patient was invited to a social event, to guarantee that she would have a chair throughout the evening, she and her husband would go early or not go at all. She would not get out of the chair for the entire evening for fear that someone else would take it. Dynamic films revealed a leg length discrepancy of just 8 mm, low on the left. Her weight bearing was 4.2 cm anterior to the lip of the sacrum. The pelvic index was 1.2, and her sacral angle was 72 degrees (Fig. 27.13).

She was given a one-eighth-inch (3 mm) lift to wear in her left shoe and was fitted for a Levitor. She also received manipulative treatments. She continues to wear the Levitor more than 10 years after the treatment was initiated. She has minimal pain in spite of the fact that she is an active professional who must spend much of her day working on her feet.

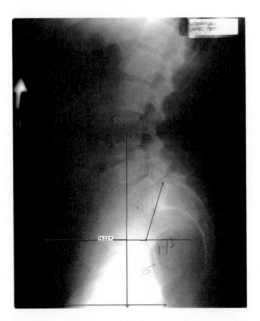

FIGURE 27.12   Dynamic film of a 55-year-old woman, 5 years post laminectomy and 1 year post lumbosacral fusion. Sacral angle, 67 degrees; pelvic index, 1.1; weight-bearing line, 6.6 cm anterior to the sacral promontory.

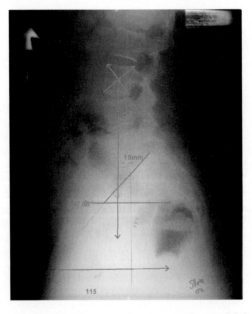

FIGURE 27.13   Dynamic film of a 40-year-old woman with spondylolisthesis of L5 on S1. Sacral angle, 72 degrees; pelvic index, 1.2; weight-bearing line, 4.2 cm anterior to the sacral promontory.

SUMMARY

When treating musculoskeletal pain due to postural decompensation, one must recognize the significance of dysfunctional mechanics in the sagittal plane. Several modalities are useful in treating this decompensation, and these modalities are often used together to improve function by reducing strain and muscle spasms and thereby reducing pain. The Levitor orthotic is one of these useful modalities in the treatment of selected individuals. It requires a commitment on behalf of the patient to wear the device routinely and to come in for timely follow-up and readjustment. It is useful when other modalities, such as physical therapy, manipulation, or surgery, have failed to produce long-lasting results. It does not replace manipulation in these patients, and ongoing evaluation and proper use of OMT can lead to significant improvement in the patient's quality of life.

Procedures

Please note: The procedures that follow are examples of manipulative treatment that you may wish to employ. The actual choice of procedures used should be determined by the unique circumstances of each individual patient.

Lumbosacral Release (Direct Myofascial Release) (Fig. 27.14)

This procedure is employed sequentially to diagnose and then to treat muscular and fascial tension in the area of the lumbosacral junction.

Patient position: prone. Physician position: at either side of the treatment table.

Procedure

1. Place one hand upon the patient's sacrum with the most proximal portion of your palm at the level of the lumbosacral junction and with your fingers pointing toward the patient's coccyx.
2. Place your other hand upon the patient's lumbar spine with your fingers extending up over the thoracolumbar spine and paravertebral muscles.
3. Apply gentle traction to load the muscles and fascia of the lumbosacral junction by pulling cephalad with your thoracolumbar hand and pushing caudad with your

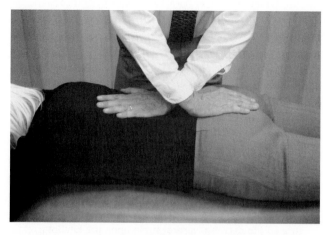

FIGURE 27.14   Direct myofascial release sequentially employed to diagnose and then to treat muscular and fascial tension in the area of the lumbosacral junction.

sacral hand. Use enough pressure to create tension in the soft tissue but stop short of force that will move the sacrum between the ilia.

4. Use your hands alternately now to assess soft tissue tension and with incrementally more force articular compliance.
5. Hold with your sacral hand, and with your thoracolumbar hand actively test motion by introducing lateral translation left and right as well as clockwise and counter-clockwise twisting. Observe directions of tension and ease.
6. Hold with your thoracolumbar hand, and with your sacral hand, actively test lateral translation left and right, sacral flexion and extension, and rotation right and left, on both the right and left oblique axes. Observe directions of tension and ease.
7. Move both hands in the combined directions of tissue tension, hold and wait for a release, the perception of relaxation of tension in tissues between your hands.
8. Reassess the lumbosacral junction and repeat steps 3 to 7 again as necessary to obtain the optimal effect.

Pelvic Tilt (Exercise) (Fig. 27.15)

This exercise is employed to strengthen abdominal and lumbar paravertebral musculature and to decrease vertical strain upon the lumbosacral junction by decreasing the lumber lordosis, shifting the center of the body of L3 posteriorly, and decreasing the sacral angle.

The patient lies supine or stands with the back against a wall. It may be easier to demonstrate pelvic tilt to the patient supine on the treatment table and then demonstrate the procedure standing. Ultimately, it is desirable that patients learn to stand and walk with some degree of pelvic tilt.

Procedure

1. Have the patient lie supine upon the treatment table with the hips and knees flexed and the feet flat upon the tabletop.
2. The patient places the hands upon the lower abdomen so as to monitor rectus abdominus contraction.
3. The patient tightens the buttocks and contracts the anterior abdominal muscles, to push the lumbar spine flat against the tabletop. You may wish to place your hand, palm up, beneath the low back to monitor the process and give feedback.
4. The patient holds the contraction for 30 seconds and repeats the process as tolerated.

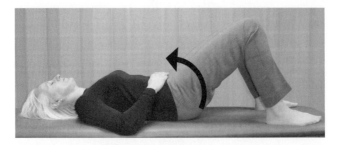

FIGURE 27.15   Pelvic tilt to strengthen abdominal and lumbar paravertebral muscula-ture and to decrease vertical strain upon the lumbosacral junction by decreasing lumbar lordosis, shifting the center of the body of L3 posteri-orly, and decreasing the sacral angle.

5. When the patient understands the procedure, have him or her stand with back to wall. Place your hand between the back and the wall and have the patient repeat steps 3 and 4.
6. Instruct the patient to stand and walk while maintaining this posture.

Psoas and Quadriceps Stretch Kneeling (Exercise) (Fig. 27.16)

This exercise is employed to stretch hip flexors, particularly psoas major. It accomplishes this in two ways: it physically stretches the muscles by increasing the distance between the origins and insertions, and it reflexively induces relaxation through reciprocal inhibition by actively contracting hip extensors. Although psoas spasm often occurs as a primary dysfunction, it is also encountered as a splinting mechanism to stabilize an unstable lumbosacral junction.

Procedure (Example: Tight Left Hip Flexors)

1. The patient kneels upon the left knee with the left hip in slight internal rotation. The right hip and knee should be flexed to 90 degrees, and the right foot is flat on the floor, approximately 18 inches in front of the left knee. The patient may wish to hold onto a chair or some other stable object with the right hand to maintain balance during the procedure.
2. The patient keeps the back straight to tighten the abdominal muscles and buttocks and to perform a pelvic tilt as described earlier in the chapter. The patient maintains this posture throughout the remainder of the procedure.
3. The patient places the left hand upon the left buttock to monitor and maintain gluteal tension.
4. The patient flexes the right knee, pulling the pelvis forward and extending the left hip until tension is felt in the left hip and thigh.
5. The patient maintains this position for a minimum of 30 seconds and repeats as tolerated.
6. The procedure should be repeated on the other side.

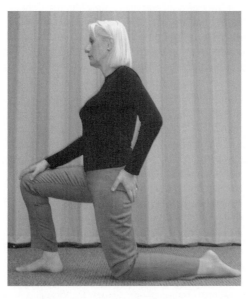

FIGURE 27.16   Kneeling psoas and quadriceps stretch to stretch hip flexors.

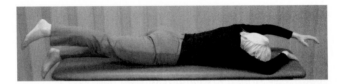

FIGURE 27.17   Dry-land swim to strengthen weak paravertebral musculature.

Psoas, Indirect Release

This procedure is employed to reflexively reduce hypertonicity of the psoas major muscle. (See the procedure described in Chapter 9 and Fig. 9.3)

Dry-Land Swim (Exercise) (Fig. 27.17)

This exercise may be employed to strengthen weak paravertebral musculature. It consists of repetitive contraction of the paravertebral musculature. Each repetition has three steps and each step takes about 5 seconds, for a total of 15 seconds per repetition. Having the patient count to 5 out loud during each step prevents Valsalva and reduces intra-abdominal stress upon the abdominal wall. The sequence typically is initiated with five repetitions on each side. The number of repetitions may be increased as back strength improves.

The patient lies prone upon a firm surface with the legs straight and the shoulders and elbows fully extended so that the arms project above the head along the longitudinal axis of the body. During the entire exercise, the patient must keep the neck flexed by holding the chin against the upper chest to prevent hyperextension strain of the mid to low cervical and upper thoracic regions.

Procedure

1. The patient flexes the neck, bringing the chin to the chest (this should be maintained throughout the exercise) and alternately lifts the right arm and left leg slowly from the floor for a 5 count.
2. The patient holds this position for a 5 count.
3. The patient slowly returns the right arm and left leg to the floor for a 5 count.
4. Alternating, the patient repeats steps 1 to 3 with the left arm and right leg.

ADDITIONAL EXERCISES THAT MAY PROVE USEFUL

- Back extension exercises (See the description of the procedure in Chapter 28 and Fig. 28.5.)
- Torso curls (See the description of the procedure in Chapter 28 and Fig. 28.6.)
- Reverse torso curls (See the description of the procedure in Chapter 28 and Fig. 28.7.)

References

1. Kuchera ML. Gravitational stress, musculo-ligamentous strain, and postural alignment. Spine: State of the Art Reviews 1995;9:463–490.
2. Jungmann M. Backaches, Postural Decline, Aging and Gravity-Strain. Revised ed. Rangeley, ME: Institute for Gravitational Strain Pathology, 1988.
3. Kuchera ML. Gravitational strain pathophysiology. In: Vleeming A, Mooney V, Dorman T, Snijders CJ, eds. Second Interdisciplinary World Congress on Low Back Pain: The Integrated

Function of the Lumbar Spine and Sacroiliac Joint. Parts 1 and 2. Rotterdam: ECO, 1995;659–693.

4. Kuchera ML, Jungmann M. Inclusion of Levitor orthotic device in the management of refractive low back pain. J Am Osteopath Assoc 1986;86:673–674.

5. Kuchera ML. Postural considerations in the sagittal plane. In: Ward RC, ed. Foundations for Osteopathic Medicine. Baltimore: Williams & Wilkins, 1997;999–1014.

6. DiGiovanna EL, Kuchera ML, Greenman PE. Efficacy and complications. In: Ward RC, ed. Foundations for Osteopathic Medicine. Baltimore: Williams & Wilkins, 1997;1015–1023.

7. Willman MK, Kuchera ML, Kuchera WA. Radiographic technical aspects of the postural study. In: Ward RC, ed. Foundations for Osteopathic Medicine. Baltimore: Williams & Wilkins, 1997;1025–1034.

8. Huang RP, Bohlman HH, Thompson GH, Poe-Kochert C. Predictive value of pelvic incidence in progression of spondylolisthesis. Spine 2003;28:2381–2385.

9. Hanson DS, Bridwell KH, Rhee JM, Lenke LG. Correlation of pelvic incidence with low- and high-grade isthmic spondylolisthesis. Spine 2002;27:2026–2029.

10. Gallant RA, ed. The Jungmann Concept and Techniques of Anti-Gravity Leverage: A Clinical Handbook. 2nd ed. Rangeley, ME: Institute for Gravitational Strain Pathology, 1992.

CHAPTER 28

The Patient with Scoliosis

Kenneth E. Nelson

INTRODUCTION

Scoliosis is defined as a rotational deformity of the spine, best observed on forward bending, and associated with a persistent lateral curvature of the spine measuring greater than 10 degrees on weight-bearing radiography.[1]

The diagnosis of scoliosis is based upon a constellation of history and physical findings that must be confirmed radiographically. The radiographs must be taken with the patient standing. The spinal lateral curvature in question must exceed 10 degrees as measured by the Ferguson[2] or Cobb[3] methods (Fig. 28.1).

The diagnosis of scoliosis must not be made lightly. The term *scoliosis* has a prejudicial connotation implying a deforming disease of the spine. Either the noun *(scoliosis)* or the adjective *(scoliotic)* can be very frightening to patients or the parents.

Recording the diagnosis code for scoliosis (ICD-9CM 737.30, idiopathic scoliosis[4]) permanently links this diagnosis with the patient in the computer database of the health history. Alternatively, the term *lateral curve* or *spinal curve* may be used when discussing the subject with the patient. A diagnosis such as myositis (ICD-9CM, 729.1[4]) may be employed if the patient is being treated for associated myalgia. This does not imply that the diagnosis should be withheld when appropriate. Rather, one must be fully aware of the power to affect patients' lives in areas outside of medicine. One must perform one's duties as a physician appropriately but with vigilance and respect for one's influence on patients.

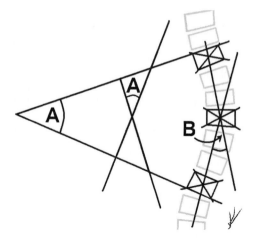

FIGURE 28.1   Methods for measuring the angles of spinal curves. **(A)** Cobb's method (preferred): Place lines parallel with the upper end plate of the upper vertebra and the lower end plate of the lower vertebra of the curve. Extend these lines and measure the angle of intersection. Because in small curves this intersection may not occur within the limits of the radiograph, the same angle can be obtained by measuring the angle formed by the intersection of lines drawn perpendicular to the end plate lines.
(B) Ferguson's method: Place central points in the apical vertebrae of the curvature and in the vertebrae that define the highest and lowest margins of the curve. Connect them with two lines forming an angle. This is the angle of the curve; it is measured as the divergence from 180 degrees.

The treatment of uncomplicated scoliosis is a life-long intervention. This type of continuity of care requires the special skill offered by osteopathic medicine. It is not the purpose of osteopathic medicine to cure the scoliosis. The osteopathic physician treats the patient. The physician, however, must pay special attention to the scoliosis, addressing how it affects the functional status of the otherwise healthy individual. The physician must consider the effect of the scoliosis upon the patient's activities of daily living, upon cardiovascular and pulmonary systems, upon pregnancy, and upon the chronic conditions of aging.

The treatment protocol outlined in this chapter is intended both to mobilize and to stabilize the spine. This may initially seem to be paradoxic. It is directed at selectively addressing the spinal motion restriction that results from somatic dysfunction while strengthening muscles that stabilize the spine to eliminate spinal instability.

ETIOLOGIES OF SCOLIOSIS

Inequality of leg length with resultant pelvic unleveling is present in most adults. (See Chapter 26.) This condition is by far the most commonly encountered etiology of spinal type I group curve mechanics. The amount of pelvic unleveling necessary to produce a compensatory curve large enough (more than 10 degrees) to qualify as scoliosis, however, is rare.

The most commonly encountered scoliosis is idiopathic. The etiology of idiopathic scoliosis is, as the name implies, unknown. Most persons (80%) with idiopathic scoliosis are female. Idiopathic scoliosis demonstrates high incidence in some families, suggesting a genetic origin. It is probably a sex-linked trait. The gene is thought to be on the X chromosome. As such, it can be transmitted from a mother to both sons and daughters. It can be transmitted from a father only to his daughters. The trait demonstrates incomplete penetrance and may not manifest in every generation. It is variably expressive. A mother with severe scoliosis may have a daughter with mild scoliosis. If one parent has scoliosis, even if it is not manifest, the chance that their child will have scoliosis is approximately 33%.

The most commonly encountered scoliotic spinal pattern (90%) is a thoracic curvature convex on the right.[5] It begins developing in early adolescence, often in association with the prepuberty growth spurt.

Infantile scoliosis, a non–weight-bearing spinal curvature that becomes apparent between birth and age 3, is generally considered to be the result of molding due to intrauterine position. Arbuckle,[6] Magoun,[7] and Sergueef[8] suggest that an intraosseous occipital dysfunction is responsible for this condition. The occiput is formed from seven growth centers, five cartilaginous and two membranous. The occipital condyles are at the point of conjuncture between the three anterior cartilaginous centers. (See Chapter 8.) Asymmetric compression of these condylar parts will result in the occiput resting asymmetrically upon the atlas. Asymmetry of the occiput upon the atlas produces a compensatory scoliosis from above downward.

Scoliosis may result from congenital malformation of vertebral segments, wedging, hemivertebra formation, or failure of segmentation. These malformations, of course, cannot be treated with osteopathic manipulative treatment (OMT); however, the logic of mobilization and stabilization, described later, apply to the compensatory mechanics that the anomalies produce.

Myopathic scoliosis can result from asymmetric muscular strength seen in conditions like muscular dystrophy.

Neuropathic (paralytic) causes of scoliosis include poliomyelitis, cerebral palsy, and spinal tumors.

Von Recklinghausen's neurofibromatosis is an autosomal dominant genetic disease that is associated with scoliosis in approximately 40% of cases. This is due to developmental failure of the spine. It can produce severe deformity quite rapidly during periods of growth. These patients also demonstrate the following:

- Neurofibromatous tumors, essentially 100%, a minimum of 2, as a diagnostic criterion, which may affect skin, peripheral nerves, blood vessels, and the gastrointestinal tract
- Areas of cutaneous hyper pigmentation spots, called café au-lait, almost 100%
- Hamartomas of the iris, called Lisch nodules, 90%
- Optic glioma, 15%

Impaired integrity of connective tissue can result in spinal instability and scoliosis. Marfan's syndrome is such a congenital condition. Patients with Marfan's syndrome demonstrate cardiac valvular disease (mitral and aortic regurgitation), aortic aneurysm, dislocation of the optic lenses, and high arched palate. They are tall, with elongated extremities. Ligamentous laxity results in hypermobility, spinal instability, and scoliosis.

Other congenital connective tissue diseases that can result in scoliosis include various types of dwarfism.

Juvenile rheumatoid arthritis is an acquired connective tissue disease. These patients occasionally develop scoliosis.

Physical Examination

Idiopathic scoliosis begins insidiously and can progress to a catastrophic degree. Although it may be difficult for the untrained observer to recognize the anatomic asymmetry of the early stages of scoliosis, the trained examiner can readily identify scoliosis by recognizing asymmetry of normally symmetric anatomy. The structural examination is an integral component of the osteopathic physical examination. It should be performed with appropriate modifications on every patient from neonate to geriatric, and scoliosis screening should be part of the health maintenance program in all school systems.

Scoliosis is pathological Fryette type I (group or neutral) spinal mechanics. The scoliosis screening examination is the same as the osteopathic structural examination with emphasis upon the identification of this type I spinal mechanics. It is performed by standing behind the individual. The first step is to observe the position of bilaterally symmetric structures: mastoid processes, acromion processes, scapulae, iliac crests, sacral sulcae, and greater trochanters. Next is the test for pelvic side shift. Type I mechanics and consequently the severity of scoliosis are specifically identified by having the patient forward bend. The physician should look for the asymmetric paravertebral prominence, which results from the rotational component of spinal group curves. At the thoracic level, it is termed an osseous gibbosity because of the rotation of the ribs; at the lumbar level, it is a muscular gibbosity. It is important to observe standing posture laterally for abnormal mechanics of the kyphotic and lordotic spinal curves. Spinal anteroposterior mechanics increase in the presence of type I curves. Significant findings should be further delineated by regional and segmental diagnosis. Physical findings consistent with scoliosis should then be confirmed and quantified radiographically.

Spinal Mechanics of Scoliosis and Somatic Dysfunction

In type I spinal mechanics, the involved group of vertebrae demonstrates a coupled relationship between side bending and rotation. Under neutral circumstances (absence of spinal flexion or extension engaging the zygapophyseal articulations), when side-bending forces are applied to a group of typical vertebrae, the entire group rotates toward the side of the produced convexity. Side bending and rotation of the entire group are coupled in opposite directions.

Because scoliosis is a rotational deformity, it is named according to the direction of the rotation (the side of the convexity of the curve). Therefore, a curve that is side-bent left (concave left, convex right) and rotated right is described as right scoliosis.

Type II (not neutral) somatic dysfunction is found at the transitional points of group mechanics. The vertebrae of maximum rotation, where rotational mechanics change direction, is called the apex of the curve. The conjuncture of two curves, where side-bending mechanics change, is called the crossover point.

Anterior and posterior spinal mechanics are affected by type I mechanics. The presence of a group curve increases the existing spinal kyphosis or lordosis. Therefore, a thoracic type I curve will demonstrate increased kyphosis, and a lumbar curve will demonstrate increased lordosis. At a crossover point, the existing anteroposterior curve is decreased.

Fryette[9] noted that type II dysfunction most commonly occurs when force decreases the existing anteroposterior curve. The preexisting anteroposterior flattening at the crossover point between two type I curves makes this area most vulnerable for the development of type II dysfunctions.

The rotational relationship between individual segments changes between the apex of a group curve and the segment immediately above it. That is, although the entire curve is side bent and rotated in opposite directions relative to the anatomic position, when the mechanics between individual segments of the curve are considered, this

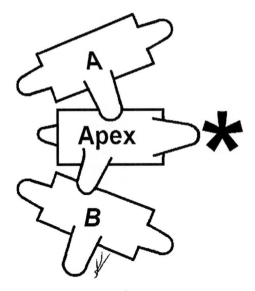

FIGURE 28.2 Coupled side bending and rotation in a type I spinal curve. The entire curve is side bent to the left and rotated to the right relative to the anatomic position. The apex is rotated maximally to the right. Therefore, relative to segment B, the apical segment is side bent to the left and rotated to the right, and relative to the apical segment, segment A is side bent to the left but also rotated to the left.

relationship changes. At the apex of the curve and below, if a vertebral segment is considered relative to the vertebral segment immediately below it, side bending and rotation occur in opposite directions. Above the apex, however, if a segment is considered relative to the segment below it, side bending and rotation occur in the same direction (Fig. 28.2). For this reason, the upper half of a group curve behaves as a series of type II dysfunctions. Because a group curve produces an increase in the normal anteroposterior curve, resultant type II dysfunctions tend to be flexed in the thoracic region and extended in the lumbar region.

Pain Associated with Scoliosis

As idiopathic scoliosis is developing, the spine is laterally unstable. The vertebral segments of such a functional curve maintain unrestricted motion, although there is asymmetric position. There is rarely pain. Consequently, the lateral instability shifts the positions of the anatomic and physiologic barriers of vertebral motion. No restrictive (dysfunctional) barriers are present, however. This is why idiopathic scoliosis is usually first recognized by someone other than the patient. The lateral instability can allow the developing scoliosis to progress fairly rapidly over a few months, making this time insidiously dangerous.

Scoliotic curves that will not straighten when side-bending forces are applied are called structural (fixed) curves. Scoliotic curves that do straighten when side-bending forces are applied are nonstructural or functional curves. Typically, the curve becomes structural in late adolescence. Because of a young adult's ability to compensate (tolerance), there is usually no pain.

Pain complaints more often begin to manifest as the adult with scoliosis reaches middle age. Commonly, areas of chronically restricted motion are not painful.

Pain tends to develop in the segments adjacent to the restricted area. These segments must compensate for the restricted motion of their neighbors. The mechanical stress of this compensation produces pain. These compensatory areas are commonly found at the crossover points above and below the structural curve. The flattening of the anteroposterior curve at the crossover point allows the development of type II mechanics that oppose the anteroposterior curve of the region, that is, extension type II dysfunction, often found at a crossover point in the thoracic region, and flexion type II dysfunction, found in the lumbar region. The presence of an extension dysfunction within a kyphotic curve (or flexion within lordosis) results in the opposition of flexion and extension weight-bearing forces in adjacent segments. The resulting mechanical stress, augmented by the increased motion necessary to compensate for the adjacent structural curve, is particularly painful.

Diagnostic Testing

Further evaluation of the spine is done radiographically. A scoliosis series is the appropriate radiographic evaluation. The radiographs are taken with the patient standing. The exposure should include the entire spine and pelvis. Three such exposures are taken. The first is taken with the patient standing normally, with weight equally distributed upon both lower extremities. This film is used to measure the spinal curves, and if properly taken, it can be used to measure pelvic unleveling and leg length. (See Chapter 26.) The second and third exposures are taken while the patient bends the torso to the left and right. These films are used to differentiate structural (fixed) curves from nonstructural (functional) curves. A fourth radiograph, often of the hand, is taken to evaluate the status of epiphyseal fusion in adolescents. The evolving scoliosis tends to stabilize with the cessation of bone growth. One additional radiograph is necessary to fully evaluate the weight-bearing mechanics of a patient with scoliosis. A standing lateral lumbosacral spine film is required for measurement of the sacral angle and pelvic index. This last film is included in the postural series.[10,11] (See Chapter 27.) However, the side-bending films and the film to determine epiphyseal status are not part of the postural series and should be employed for initial evaluation of scoliosis. As such, a combination of the scoliosis series and postural series is appropriate.

Treatment Protocol

The treatment of a patient with scoliosis is directed at maintaining function and preventing sequelae. The initial identification of a spinal curve of 20 degrees or greater is indication for referral to a consultant who specifically treats scoliosis.

Underlying causes, if identifiable, should be addressed. Treatment protocols for rare conditions like Marfan's syndrome should be initiated. It is here that the recognition of unequal leg length (static scoliosis) and chronic occupational posture (habit scoliosis) can be useful. In most cases of idiopathic scoliosis, leg length has no relationship to the scoliotic pattern. Occasionally, the pelvic unleveling associated with short leg is consistent with the spinal scoliotic pattern. These patients may benefit from lift therapy. Rarely an individual has scoliosis because of accommodation to unequal leg length. These patients can be "cured" with lift therapy. (See Chapter 26.)

Occupational postural stresses may contribute to discomfort. Hairdressers and violinists adopt chronic positions that induce a spinal curvature in an otherwise normal back. Where change of occupation is unrealistic, individualized stretching and strengthening exercises can be prescribed.

Infantile scoliosis can be treated with cranial manipulation. The occiput should be examined with attention to the condylar parts. Sphenobasilar synchondrosis dysfunction and the remaining cranial pattern should be identified. The total body pattern, with particular attention to the cervicothoracic region, sacrum and pelvis, should be defined. Identified dysfunctional and accommodative patterns can be treated, frequently with profound results. (See Chapter 8.)

The treatment of adolescent idiopathic scoliosis has two prongs, mobilization and stabilization. It is necessary that the patient develop proprioception, body awareness of good posture, and at the same time work in building self-esteem. The protocol must be individualized to the requirements of the specific patient. Patients must become actively involved in development of their protocol. This ensures that they will continue (and continually adjust) the treatment throughout life. This is particularly difficult with adolescents, yet they are the individuals who will benefit the most from treatment.

Mobilization and continued mobility are a significant part of treatment. Mobilization procedures are directed at stretching the concave side of the spinal curves.

Passive stretching—lazy person—exercises are appropriate (Fig. 28.3). The patient is instructed to lie on the side so that the convex side of the curve being treated is down. A firm but compliant roll approximately 6 inches in diameter is placed beneath the patient at the level of the apex of the curve. This passive exercise must be timed carefully to avoid painful overdosing. Initially, 1 or 2 minutes daily is sufficient. This can be increased gradually to 5 or more minutes daily, according to tolerance.

Active stretching exercises should also be done. Patients should participate in the selection of exercise type. The exercise must be bilateral, but again, stretching of the concavity of the curve or curves is the focus of the activity. The mobilization of specific areas of somatic dysfunction with OMT should be done judiciously. Gentle direct stretching, articulation, muscle energy, and direct and indirect myofascial procedures are most appropriate.

It may seem inappropriate to mobilize a potentially unstable condition. In fact, it is, unless stabilization exercises are a major part of the treatment protocol. Here again, it is important to encourage the patient to participate in the selection and development of the exercise program. Predominantly asymmetric exercise, such as tennis, is contraindicated. The exercise should be bilateral, but pounding weight-bearing exercises, such as jogging, should also be discouraged. Swimming, being both symmetric and non–weight bearing, is an example of an ideal choice. The program should pay particular attention to strengthening core musculature (i.e., abdominal and paravertebral muscles) along with development and implementation of both mobilization and stabilization exercises. Consultation with a physical therapist can be beneficial.

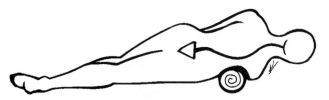

FIGURE 28.3   Lazy person exercise. The patient lies on the side with the convexity of the scoliotic curve down upon a firm roll 5 to 6 inches in diameter. This is a passive form of exercise employed to stretch the concave side of the curve.

Progress should be monitored closely. Regularly checking height is an easy way for patients to monitor themselves at home. Any decrease in height should be considered to be increase of the scoliotic curve.

Following the initial visit, the patient should be seen in the office at 2-week intervals once or twice to ensure efficacy of the exercise program and monitor progress. Follow-up visits may be extended to about one a month for the first 6 months and every 3 to 6 months thereafter.

For office documentation, the use of a Polaroid or digital camera to take serial photographs of the patient is worthwhile. Patients should stand with their back toward the camera, ideally against a wall marked in such a way that changes in height are apparent. The photo should be taken with the camera always in the same position. A tripod is useful for this purpose. The neutral standing radiograph of the scoliosis series should be repeated for comparison if there is any indication of increase of the scoliosis as demonstrated by two or more consecutive decreases in height. Radiographs can be repeated annually until it is apparent that the curve has stabilized. Progression of the curve necessitates referral to a spine surgeon for possible bracing or surgical stabilization.

Adult patients with idiopathic scoliosis typically seek medical help in middle age, when their ability to functionally compensate for their asymmetric weight-bearing pattern declines and they begin having persistent pain. The pain, as described earlier, is typically in functional areas that are under stress because they compensate for adjacent areas of restricted motion.

The therapeutic approach is, as for the adolescent patient, a combination of mobilization and stabilization. The mobilization component for the adult scoliotic is stressed more than for the adolescent. The adult patient will typically tolerate more aggressive forms of OMT well. The focus of treatment is the maintenance of functional articular mobility. With sensitivity to tolerance, the primary area of restricted motion (the structural primary curve) should be treated with the intention of maintaining intervertebral range of motion. Stretching the concavity of the primary curve and gentle mobilization of compensatory secondary (nonstructural, nonfunctional) curves and crossover points should be done in close association with stabilization exercises.

As the scoliotic spine ages, the effects of the thoracic curve affect mobility of the thoracic cage and consequently cardiac and pulmonary physiology. The maintenance of mobility of the ribs is an important therapeutic goal for the care of anyone with scoliosis. It becomes ultimately important for the geriatric patient.

As mentioned earlier, the mechanics of the scoliotic curves and the existence of pelvic unleveling from unequal leg length are rarely consistent with one another. Inequality of leg length is present in most adults. The mechanical interface between the scoliosis and short leg mechanics is commonly found at the lumbosacral junction. This stress results in an increased incidence of lumbosacral degenerative disc disease, arthritic change, and radiculopathy. Heel pads may be used empirically to reduce lumbosacral stress. Occasionally, the lift must be placed on the side of the long leg. The use of lift therapy under these circumstances is directed at reduction of weight-bearing stress. The effect of the use of a lift upon the lumbosacral consequences of scoliosis must be weighed against its effect upon sacropelvic mechanics. The goal is to reduce lumbosacral stress while maintaining comfort.

More Aggressive Therapies

Failure to prevent progression of the spinal curvature is indication for more aggressive therapies. This is why it is important to monitor the patient's progress closely until the curve or curves are stable. The use of braces that stimulate active core muscle contraction (Milwaukee brace) is a consideration under these circumstances.

Surgical intervention for spinal fusion and implantation of metal (as in the Cotrel-Dubousset procedure) paraspinal rods is indicated where bracing fails to arrest curve progression. It is also indicated if the curve remains unstable and the brace cannot be discontinued. Other indications for surgery include progressive loss of pulmonary function, pain, and severe cosmetic issues.

Long-Term Consequences of Scoliosis

The asymmetric weight-bearing stresses of scoliosis have long-term consequences. Forces transmitted through bone modify osteoclastic and osteoblastic activity in such a way that the architecture of the bone adjusts to the stress (Wolff's law). The shape of the vertebrae and ribs change, which changes the neutral position of the axial skeleton without necessarily resulting in the establishment of a dysfunctional barrier. It is circumstances like these that invalidate the use of positional asymmetry alone in the diagnosis of somatic dysfunction.

These asymmetric positional mechanics facilitate the development of somatic dysfunction. They also have additional mechanical implications.

Idiopathic scoliosis typically is stable during adult life. Pregnancy, however, can pose significant problems. Mechanical asymmetry of the lumbar spine and pelvis can greatly affect the birth process. For management of pregnant patients, the maintenance of spinal stability as described earlier is a prime objective. Here, as when managing the adolescent with scoliosis, vigilance for progression of spinal curves is important; however, radiographic studies are inappropriate for pregnant women. The status of the curves must be determined by physical findings. Serial photos may also be used.

CONCLUSION

The therapeutic goals for treating a patient with scoliosis are the same as those for treating any other patient with a chronic disorder. They are to empower the patient to deal effectively with a lifelong condition, to maintain optimal function and prevent progression of the condition, and not necessarily to decrease the degree of the spinal curvature. Any reduction in curvature, although desirable, should be considered as fortuitous secondary gain. An effective protocol begins with specific identification of the body mechanics of the individual patient, with recognition of the spinal level of crossover points between group curves and the level and side of the apices of curves. Standing postural radiographs are useful for this purpose.[10,11] Patients should be apprised of these mechanics since a personal understanding of their postural asymmetries will assist greatly in the development of a treatment protocol. Often it is desirable to provide patients with a drawing of their spinal apices and crossover points.

The individualized therapeutic protocol will include both mobilization and stabilization. Mobilization may be accomplished with stretching exercises and OMT. Any manipulative procedures may be appropriate, although aggressive mobilization should not be employed in younger patients before their curves have stabilized. The choice of OMT to be employed is dictated by the criteria discussed in Chapter 4. Stabilization is accomplished with strengthening exercises, and its importance cannot be overemphasized. The following are examples of mobilization procedures and stabilization exercises.

Procedures

Please note: The procedures that follow are examples of manipulative treatment that you may wish to employ. The actual choice of procedures used should be determined by the unique circumstances of each individual patient.

Lazy Person Exercise (Mobilization) (See Fig. 28.3)

This is a passive exercise. Its purpose is to stretch the contracted soft tissues on the concave side of a type I group curve. Certain precautions that must be taken for this exercise. Because scoliosis is a potentially unstable condition and it is the purpose of this exercise to stretch soft tissue, it is probably not appropriate to begin this activity until after the curve has become fixed. Consequently, this exercise is appropriate for adults and can be considered as an activity to help maintain mobility as opposed to something to reverse the curve. Further, because this is a passive activity, dosage (duration of time spent doing the exercise) is often deceptively short. Spending more time than tolerated may not prove to be harmful to an individual with a fixed curve, but it can be very uncomfortable.

Patient position: lying on the side with the convexity of the curve down.

Procedure

1. A firm yet pliable roll should be constructed. A tightly rolled bed sheet is about the correct consistency. Rolled newspaper wrapped in a terry cloth towel is also functional. The roll should be 5 or 6 inches in diameter.
2. The patient lies on a firm surface on the side with the convexity of the curve down and with the roll its long axis oriented anteroposterior to the patient, beneath the patient at the level of the apex of the curve.
3. The patient lies on the roll initially for no longer than 1 minute.
4. The time spent on the roll may be increased gradually in 30-second increments according to tolerance. The maximum time that the patient need spend doing the exercise is probably 3 to 5 minutes.
5. The procedure can be repeated daily.

Group Curve Mobilization (Articulation, HVLA, or Muscle Energy) (Fig. 28.4)

This procedure is employed to enhance spinal motion and to keep a type I group curve flexible. It is useful for curves with apices from the mid thoracic region through the lumbar spine. Because of the way spinal rotation is addressed, the entire curve may be treated in a single procedure. (For diagnosis, see the discussion earlier in this chapter and also Chapter 3.)

Patient position: seated astride the end of the table with the back toward the end.
Physician position: standing behind the patient on the concave side of the curve.

Procedure (Example: Convex Right, Thoracic Type I Group Curve, T4 to T12, with the Apex at T8)

1. Instruct the patient to clasp the hands behind the neck.
2. Standing behind and to the left of the patient, place your left arm in front of the patient's chest so that your left shoulder is beneath the patient's left axilla and your hand is grasping the right shoulder.
3. Place the heel of your right hand upon the apex (T8) of the curve on the side of the convexity (right).
4. Side-bend the patient's spine to the right. The correct placement of your right arm in step 2 will allow you to do this easily by lifting the patient's left axilla with your shoulder while depressing the right shoulder with your left hand.

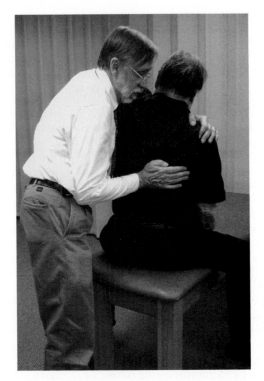

FIGURE 28.4   Group curve, articulation or HVLA to enhance spinal motion to keep a type I group curve flexible. It is useful for curves with apices from the mid thoracic region through the lumbar spine.

5. Hold the patient in this fashion throughout the remainder of the procedure. With this position, the curve has been straightened with upward traction, the lower end of the curve is held by the patient's pelvis, and the upper end is immobilized by your hold on the patient's pectoral girdle.
6. To address the rotational component of the curve, press your right hand upon the apex (T8 right) while maintaining the holding force upon the upper end of the curve as described in steps 4 and 5.
7. The spinal segments of the curve may now be articulated by repeatedly applying the rotational force with your right hand against the holding force of your left arm. Or you may wish to apply a final HVLA thrust to the apex with the heel of your right hand against the holding force of your left arm.
8. Reassess for symmetry of spinal motion.

ALTERNATIVE PROCEDURES

This procedure may be modified as a muscle energy procedure as follows:

1. To correct the side-bending component, maintain the patient and physician positions described earlier. Have the patient actively try to side-bend the upper torso to the left for 3 to 5 seconds against your holding force. The patient may do this by lifting the right shoulder against your left hand, or bringing the left axilla down against your left shoulder. Relax for 1 to 2 seconds, and then engage the new barrier by lifting the left shoulder with your left upper arm. Repeat this procedure three to five times.

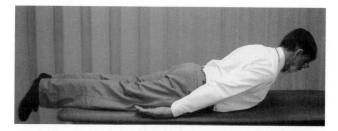

FIGURE 28.5 Back extension exercise to strengthen weak paravertebral musculature.

2. To correct the rotational component, have the patient actively try to rotate the upper torso to the right for 3 to 5 seconds against your holding force. Relax for 1 to 2 seconds, and then engage the new barrier by increasing the force applied to the apical vertebral segment with your right hand while continuing the holding force from above with your left arm. Repeat this procedure three to five times.

Back Extension Exercises (Stabilization) (Fig. 28.5)

These exercises may be employed to strengthen weak paravertebral musculature. They consist of repetitive contraction of the paravertebral musculature. Each repetition has three steps; each step takes about 5 seconds, for a total of 15 seconds per repetition. Having the patient count to 5 out loud during each step prevents the Valsalva maneuver and reduces intra-abdominal stress upon the abdominal wall. The sequence typically is initiated with 10 repetitions. The number of repetitions may be increased as back strength improves.

The patient lies prone upon a firm surface with the legs fully extended. If tolerated, the patient may employ ankle weights or hook the ankles beneath a piece of furniture to stabilize the torso from below. When first performing this exercise, the patient should place the arms at the sides with the elbows fully extended and the hands palm up. As the patient becomes accustomed to the exercise, he or she may wish to lace the fingers together behind the neck and thereby increase the work load on the back muscles. During the entire exercise, the patient must keep the neck flexed by holding the chin against the upper chest to prevent hyperextension strain of the mid to low cervical and upper thoracic regions.

Procedure

1. The patient flexes the neck, bringing the chin to the chest (this should be maintained throughout the exercise), and slowly lifts the head and upper torso off the floor for a 5 count.
2. The patient holds this position for a 5 count.
3. The patient slowly returns the upper torso to the floor for a 5 count.

Torso Curls Exercises (Stabilization) (Fig. 28.6)

These exercises may be employed to strengthen weak core musculature, particularly the upper rectus abdominis. Torso curls consist of repetitive contraction of the musculature of the anterior abdominal wall. Each repetition has three steps; each step takes about 5 seconds, for a total of 15 seconds per repetition. Having the patient count to 5 out loud during each step prevents the Valsalva maneuver and reduces intra-abdominal stress upon the abdominal wall. The sequence typically is initiated with 10 repetitions. The number of repetitions may be increased as abdominal strength improves.

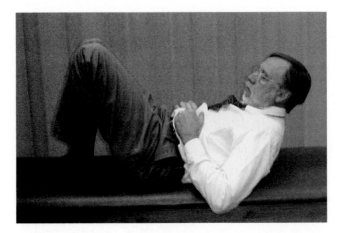

FIGURE 28.6 Torso curl to strengthen weak core musculature, particularly the upper rectus abdominis.

The patient lies supine on a firm surface with the hips and knees flexed and the feet flat on the floor. The patient places the fingers upon the upper abdomen to monitor muscular contraction and keeps the abdominal muscles tight during the entire exercise. The patient should be cautioned to keep the thoracolumbar function in contact with the floor to avoid contracting psoas major.

Procedure

1. The patient flexes the neck, bringing the chin to the chest (this should be maintained throughout the exercise), and slowly lifts the head and upper torso off the floor for a 5 count.
2. The patient holds this position for a 5 count.
3. The patient slowly returns the upper torso to the floor for a 5 count.

Reverse Torso Curls Exercises (Stabilization) (Fig. 28.7)

These exercises may be employed to strengthen weak core musculature, particularly the lower rectus abdominis. Reverse torso curls consist of repetitive contraction of the musculature of the anterior abdominal wall. Each repetition has three steps; each step takes about 5 seconds, for a total of 15 seconds per repetition. Having the patient count to 5 out loud during each step prevents the Valsalva maneuver and reduces intra-abdominal stress upon the abdominal wall. The sequence typically is initiated with 5 repetitions. The number of repetitions may be increased as abdominal strength improves. This is a difficult exercise to master.

The patient lies supine on a firm surface with the hips and knees flexed upon the abdomen, and with the arms resting at either side, forearms pronated, palms down. The patient keeps the abdominal muscles tight during the entire exercise.

Procedure

1. Slowly lift the buttocks until the entire lumbar spine is off the floor for a 5 count.
2. The patient holds this position for a 5 count.
3. The patient slowly returns the hips to the floor for a 5 count, taking care not to drop the hips to the floor quickly.

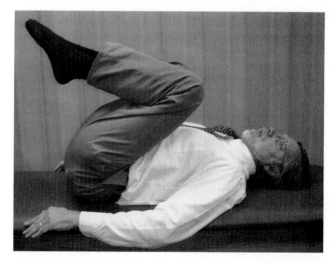

FIGURE 28.7 Reverse torso curl to strengthen weak core musculature, particularly the lower rectus abdominis.

References

1. Keim H, Hensinger R. Spinal deformities: Scoliosis and kyphosis. Clin Symp 1989;41(4):3–32.
2. Ferguson AB. Roentgen diagnosis in the extremities and spine. American Academy Orthopaedic Surgery Instructional Course Lectures. Ann Arbor, MI: J W Edwards, 1948;2:214–224.
3. Cobb JR. Outline for the study of scoliosis. American Academy of Orthopaedic Surgery Instructional Course Lectures. Ann Arbor, MI: J W Edwards, 1948;5:261–275.
4. ICD-9CM International Classification of Disease, 9th Revision, Clinical Modification. 5th ed. Salt Lake City: Medicode, 1999.
5. Reamy BV, Slakey JB. Adolescent idiopathic scoliosis: Review and current concepts. Am Fam Physician 2001;64:111–116.
6. Arbuckle BE. The selected writings of Beryl E. Arbuckle. Chapter 22. Indianapolis: American Academy of Osteopathy. 1977.
7. Magoun HI. Osteopathy in the Cranial Field. 3rd ed. Kirksville, MO: Journal Printing, 1976;143, 235, 291–292.
8. Sergueef N. Le B.A. BA du cranien, Spek ed. Paris, 1986.
9. Fryette HH. Principles of Osteopathic Technic. Carmel, CA: Academy of Applied Osteopathy, 1954;24.
10. Willman MK. Radiographic technical aspects of the postural study. J Am Osteopath Assoc 1977;76:739–744. Reprinted in 1983 Yearbook. Indianapolis: American Academy of Osteopathy, 1983;140–143.
11. Kuchera ML, Kuchera WA. Radiographic aspects of the postural study. In: Ward RC, ed. Foundations for Osteopathic Medicine. 2nd ed. Philadelphia: Lippincott Williams & Wilkins, 2002;591–602.

Practice Issues

CHAPTER 29

The Office

Dean Raffaelli

INTRODUCTION

Contrary to popular belief, a new office can be very straightforward to set up, needing only six modest rooms and totaling approximately 800 to 1000 square feet: a waiting room, a hallway, two examination or osteopathic manipulative treatment (OMT) rooms, one procedure room, a bathroom, and a storage closet. I will begin by describing each room as the patients will see them, going over furniture and equipment needed for a bare-bones but efficient operation that can be set up for a reasonable amount of money and some sweat equity.

The waiting room is the first room most patients encounter. It need not be large; about 150 square feet should suffice. Two to four chairs; a small table for a couple of magazines or better yet, health information; a desk for the phone and appointment book; and two five-drawer file cabinets are all that is required. This room contains the front desk (receptionist's area).

The most important concern at the front desk is managing appointments. It is important not to skimp on the appointment book. It should be as big as will fit on the desk. A physician's practice requires a lot of space to record all of the information needed and to make changes. Of course, a computer equipped with a quality office management program can facilitate efficiency. The basics are the same for either an electronic or a paper office system.

The physician must decide how long office visits will be and whether to incorporate OMT and procedures into regular office hours or to assign these activities to different days. Obviously, it is necessary first to define office hours: which times to see patients for general concerns and which hours to set aside, if desired, for doing OMT and other procedures.

The length of office visits can evolve over time. To start, 15-minute visits work fine and allow enough flexibility to add new patients without special scheduling. At 10 minutes per patient, it is important to allow two slots for each new patient. New patients are the lifeblood of any practice and should not be frustrated in obtaining prompt appointments.

This is the twenty-first century, and computers can take the place of most of the paper functions in the office. However, it may be wise not to make a large outlay of capital for practice management software until the practice has been operating for a while and the practitioner's needs are clearly defined. If all goes well, the practitioner can automate quickly and efficiently.

The next area the patient encounters is the hallway. Probably the only things visible should be a scale with a height measure, possibly a wall phone, and chart containers on the examination room doors. In this author's office, colored plastic flags denote which room to enter, but this is hardly necessary in a small space with two or three rooms. If the practitioner is caring for infants, an infant scale is necessary.

This author's office plan assumes that there will be two examination and OMT rooms and one procedure room. Room sizing is an art, but examination rooms used for OMT have to be bigger than the size needed for other primary care practice because of the necessity of moving about the patient on all sides. Approximately 8 by 10 feet for the examination rooms and 10 by 10 feet for the procedure room should be large enough. Many practitioners mix and match these rooms to suit their particular style of practice.

The location of a practice often defines its needs. A practice in the outer collar counties of a large city may serve primarily children and their pregnant mothers. A practice in a central urban area may be full of 20 year olds and older, with an emphasis on sport injuries and sexually transmitted diseases. A practice near an industrial site is likely to deal with workers compensation cases. Depending on the scenario, it may be necessary to emphasize one use over another.

The examination room should have the following attributes: good lighting; an examination and OMT table; adjustable stool on rollers; blood pressure cuff; mirror; writing surface; storage cabinet; oto-ophthalmoscope; clothes rack or hooks; a hard, easily cleaned tile floor; and if there is room, a chair. A sink is nice but not necessary and can be replaced by a soapless hand cleaner.

Lighting usually is not easily changed without spending a lot of money that could be put to better use elsewhere. A solution to poor lighting is to supplement it with floor lamps; a lamp with an adjustable neck is helpful.

The examination tables can be simple or complex, hence cheap or expensive. The table should do double duty, serving for both physical examination and OMT. Most osteopathic physicians were trained on sturdy flattop tables, which at the right height work just fine. These are inexpensive and will last an entire career.

One of the benefits of OMT is that it is a procedure and can be billed as such. It requires no more equipment than is found in the examination room plus the physician's two hands.

Tables to consider have a slot for the patient's face and a place on either side for the patient's arms to lie comfortably. This author purchased such a table for approximately $400 in 2002, and prices have not significantly changed over the past few years. Tables at this price level usually require some simple assembly but are adjustable for the practitioner's height and ordinarily are quite durable.

A common mistake when one is setting up the examination room is not to consider the needed space surrounding the treatment table. Adequate space for the physician is essential for efficiency and for comfortably performing manipulation. Having too little space is like playing pool with no room to swing the cue stick. Being cramped increases fatigue, chips away at efficiency, opens the door to work-related injuries, and eventually cuts down on use of OMT simply because of the hassle factor. A good rule of thumb is to be able to scoot around the table on the stool without running into any obstruction.

Most practitioners acquire a blood pressure cuff and an oto-ophthalmoscope while they are students. Initially, these can be used instead of new ones for each room. One caveat is the need for a full size range, from child to adult XXL, of blood pressure cuffs.

If patients are to disrobe, they need a place to hang their clothes. Coat racks and hooks on the wall with several hangers will suffice. A mirror allows patients to repair their appearance after a disheveling procedure.

A surface to write or type on—or both—is essential. For a small room, a shelf that folds flat against the wall when not in use can be helpful, but a small table will suffice. Most of the office furniture can be obtained at stores that offer simple Scandinavian-style pieces with clean lines that are durable and reasonably priced.

Patients requiring procedures such as Pap smears (the Papanicolaou test), pelvic examinations, dermatologic care, physical therapy modalities, flexible sigmoidoscopy, and blood draws need a separate room with more specialized equipment. It is important to define carefully the type of services the practice will offer. Such procedures provide services to your patient on site and provide another revenue stream, but they must be balanced against increased equipment and malpractice cost.

Procedure room equipment includes everything from a sharps container to a table designed for gynecological procedures. Most family practices do Pap and pelvic examinations on a regular basis. The necessary equipment includes gowns of various sizes, a selection of stainless steel specula (or disposable plastic specula), microscope slides, cover slips, potassium hydroxide (KOH) and saline solutions, and a bright floor lamp. Use of steel specula will save the cost of disposables but necessitate an autoclave or other sterilizer.

A microscope is required for the practitioner who will read slides. This is definitely a device to buy used if at all possible. Very good used scopes can be found for reasonable prices, although they may need a little cleaning.

Other devices include electrocautery for dermatologic procedures, electrotherapy and ultrasound to help with the treatment of acute and chronic musculoskeletal disorders, and possibly a scope for performing colon cancer screening sigmoidoscopy. Another flat table is necessary so patients can lie comfortable while having therapy applied.

Two other areas that are often overlooked are a separate storage space and the bathroom. A lockable supply room is helpful for all of the disposables, medication samples, linens, forms and everything else that needs a home if space is available. If not, lockable cabinets in each room will suffice.

The bathroom can be a real budget buster if the office space does not already meet the codes for accessibility. A priority while shopping for an office is to find a space already modified to the proper standards. A renter should come to an arrangement with the owners for making the necessary modifications before signing the lease.

Telecommunications can eat up a lot of cash. Most offices need two phone lines, a fax machine, and a copier. Fax and copier combinations are reasonably priced, and for phones, wireless handsets or headsets negate the need for running wires throughout the office. Answering machines can replace answering services; however, because most physicians need to be reachable, an answering service may prove to be an inescapable cost.

Finally, is a private office necessary? Probably not. Diplomas and certificates can hang in the treatment rooms for the patients to see. Charts can be done promptly in the room with the patient. Phone inquiries can be handled as they come in. Each day's paperwork should be done before the physician leaves the office because there will just be more to do the next day.

CONCLUSION

This chapter provides the basics of what it takes to set up an office. With a bare-bones approach, it is not an insurmountable or prohibitively expensive task. Each locality has different requirements, such as handicap access and zoning restrictions. It is important to know these matters during the search for space.

The less the space must be altered, the more resources available for self-promotion, loan repayments, and a kitty for the first few months before the checks for all that excellent care start to roll in.

CHAPTER 30

Progress Notes and Coding

Douglas J. Jorgensen, Raymond T. Jorgensen,
and Kenneth E. Nelson

This chapter provides guidelines, recommendations, and interpretations that are to be used as a guide for implementation in practice. The actual implementation and interpretation of these guidelines and recommendations for coding and documentation are at the sole discretion of the provider and staff. Therefore, the provider and staff accept sole responsibility for these decisions and any repercussions. Neither the authors, Jorgensen Consulting, nor Priority Management Group accept any liability in this regard.

INTRODUCTION

The medical record is longitudinal documentation of an individual's health care. It contains various pieces of information germane to the patient's health history and current medical problems. From pharmaceutical lists to demographic information, much can be gleaned from an individual's medical record. The bulk of the medical record consists of the encounters between patient and provider, or progress notes. The progress note documents a single encounter, a snapshot in time, between the physician and the patient.

Prior to the 1970s, progress notes were recorded according to the style of the individual attending physician. More individuals became concomitantly involved in the care of the patient as postdoctoral education and subspecialty medicine grew in prominence. To facilitate communication, it became apparent that a universal format for recording progress notes had to be adopted. The most commonly employed sequence was history (subjective information), physical examination (objective information), diagnosis (assessment), and medical decision making (plan for treatment). Lawrence L. Weed of the University of Illinois at Chicago proposed that this sequence be adopted and coined the acronym SOAP note.[1]

The physician–patient encounter consists basically of the evaluation (SOA) and management (P) of the patient. The criteria for the various types and levels of evaluation and management (E&M) have been defined and assigned identifying alphanumeric codes known as current procedural terminology (CPT)[2] codes. The CPT codes are supported or justified by diagnosis codes, or ICD codes. The ICD stands for International Classification of Disease, and the 9th Clinical Modification is in use; hence the abbreviation ICD-9CM. The ICD-9CM and CPT codes must correlate appropriately. Certain ICD-9CM codes (e.g., chest pain, ankle pain) justify certain CPT codes (e.g., electrocardiogram or ankle radiographs, respectively). To justify an electrocardiographic study with ankle pain instead of chest pain would make little to no sense. Thus, the codes assigned for diagnosis (ICD-9CM code) and intervention (CPT code) are critical to a clear understanding of what (CPT code) occurred at the encounter and why (ICD-9CM code) it was necessary.

CURRENT PROCEDURAL TERMINOLOGY

CPT codes describe what clinical services a patient receives from a medical provider. CPT is a component of the national Health Care Financing Administration's (HCFA) nomenclature, HCPCS (pronounced *hickpicks,* HCFA's common procedure coding system), and is owned and copyrighted by the American Medical Association (AMA). A new copy of this text should be purchased and commonly used codes reviewed annually for changes, updates, or deletions. Implementation—or when the codes go into effect and must be used for correct coding and proper reimbursement to occur—as of 2005 begins annually on January 1. Therefore, the late summer or early fall is a good time to review the codes one uses to make certain no changes have been made.

One commonality of the CPT codes among most physicians and midlevel providers is the use of E&M codes. Each E&M code depicts the type of visit that occurred, denotes a place of service, and usually identifies the level of service provided. For the purposes of this chapter, the E&M services provided are inpatient or outpatient and will typically be new (99201–99205 or 99221–99223), consultative visits (99241–99245, 99251–99255, or 99271–99275), or established patient encounters (99212–99215 or 99231–99233). Inpatient or outpatient encounters are classified as being facility or nonfacility visits, respectively.

The physician–patient encounter may also include procedures, such as osteopathic manipulative treatment (OMT), repair of a laceration, cryosurgery, or flexible sigmoidoscopy. Such procedures are considered to be additional to the E&M and are assigned specific CPT codes.

The CPT codes are used to record the extent of the encounter for billing purposes and should describe as specifically as possible what occurred at the visit. There are other types of E&M codes and visits, both facility and nonfacility, that this chapter does not address. This chapter's focus is on the common E&M codes used with osteopathic manipulation codes (98925–98929). These additional categories covering patient care rendered from newborn care to nursing facility services, can be found in the E&M chapter of CPT. Again, CPT is what was done, and the ICD-9CM is why it was done.

ICD-9CM

ICD-9CM coding is responsible for conveying medical necessity, or the reason for the patient's encounter with the health care provider.[3] *Medical necessity* is a federally defined term.* For this chapter's purposes, medical necessity is established in the notes by a complaint or reason for the visit (e.g., back pain, paresthesia, migraines), and the balance of the history and examination result in exact diagnoses (e.g., L4 radiculopathy) or symptoms (e.g., paresthesias) to justify CPT codes, such as magnetic resonance imaging (MRI) to look for a cause of the L4 radiculopathy or perhaps OMT (CPT codes 98925–98929) to treat the complaint. Providers often get focused on diagnoses when symptoms alone can create medical necessity to justify a test, imaging study, or even a procedure, such as a colonoscopy for hematochezia.

Alphanumeric identification of what the physician does and why expedites translation to insurers so that they understand what is going on with the patient, or beneficiary, without having to read the note. In theory, this also expedites care and reimbursement.

Coding Errors and Fraud

In learning and performing this documentation, one wants to be as accurate as possible to avoid misrepresenting what occurred at the visit. To do so haphazardly could result in poor reimbursement or even penal action for not following the federal documentation guidelines. To do so habitually could constitute fraud, and the federal government can prosecute for fraud without proving intent. The government simply has prove that it occurred, and the physician's notes are evidence enough.[4] Therefore, it is important to learn the proper techniques to document and code correctly to be optimally reimbursed and out of harm's way in the event of an audit.

This said, most providers are thought to be following the guidelines, and even when mistakes are encountered, they are not typically labeled as fraud. If one makes an earnest effort to learn the federal documentation guidelines, keeps up to date with the CPT and ICD-9CM changes, and codes and bills only for services provided and documented, one will in all likelihood not have penal action in one's future. (Gerold KB. Program Integrity Update. Lecture delivered at the National Heritage Insurance Company's Carrier Advisory Committee Meeting, Waltham, MA, November 5, 2001.) At this writing, federal, state, and private payer entities are still actively seeking out fraud and abuse in health care, and one must remain ever vigilant. The private payers (e.g., Blue Cross, Cigna, Aetna), except where company memoranda deviate, follow the federal documentation guidelines in determining the levels of CPT coding. The E&M and OMT codes are outlined in this chapter to allow for correct documentation and coding. At the risk of being redundant, however, it is the responsibility of the provider, not the billing staff, medical assistant, nurse, or office manager, to make certain the correct codes are assigned for ICD-9CM and CPT to represent what occurred at each encounter.

---

*Medical necessity is defined as a service that is reasonable and necessary for the diagnosis and treatment of illness or injury or to improve the functioning of a malformed body member.

Evaluation and Management

Per CPT definition, each level of E&M is defined in terms of seven components. The three key components in determining the levels of most E&M visit levels are history (S), examination (O), and medical decision making (A and P). There are three contributory components: the nature of the presenting problem, counseling, and coordination of care.[2] A fourth component that is sometimes used is time. Time is used only if more than 50% of the visit encompassed counseling and coordination of care for the patient's complaints or medical conditions. The nature of the presenting problem is sometimes used in defending why a certain code was picked, but because of its subjective nature, it is not recommended to justify a code. Only the three key components (history, examination, and medical decision making) are outlined in this chapter, as they are the keys to correct E&M coding. Before getting to these, some rules and definitions must be addressed.

New patients are those who have not received face-to-face service by a provider of the same specialty within a group practice during the preceding 3 years.[5] This is important for determining who is considered new and who is considered an established patient. The face-to-face service is a recent change, as it negates telephone calls and other services that do not constitute an inpatient or outpatient E&M visit. The same-group portion of the new patient rule refers to providers who share a federal tax identification number. The same-specialty issue is based upon national boards; this means that in a primary care practice, an internist could technically see a family physician's patient, and because they have different board certifications, the internist could charge the patient as a new patient. Many groups choose not to do this as a cost-saving measure to their patients, but this is a business decision for the practice.

Two more rules must be explained: the three-of-three and two-of-three rules. Understanding these rules and the definition of a new patient are critically important for understanding how E&M codes are chosen. The assignment of three numeric values (e.g., 2, 3, 4 or 2, 2, 3) indicates the scoring for the level of (1) the history, (2) the physical examination, and (3) medical decision making. They will delineate how one identifies the proper E&M codes for both new and established patients. The three-of-three rule, for the purpose of this chapter, applies to new patients and consults. Simply stated, it says go to the lowest number. That is, given three numbers, 2, 3, and 4, the three-of-three rule says pick the number 2, for it is the lowest of the three. If the numbers were 2, 2, and 3, the three-of-three rule says go to the lowest number, so 2 is the number again.

The two-of-three rule says go to the middle number—not the number in the center of the string in your records but the number in the middle of the counting range—such that 3, 2, 4, using the two-of-three rule, makes 3 the correct answer because 3 is the middle number (falls between 2 and 4 in counting). Given the example of 2, 2, and 3 the two-of-three rule would pick 2. In this case, the middle and the lowest number are 2.

HISTORY

The history has four major categories: chief complaint (CC), history of present illness (HPI), past family, medical, and social history (PFSH), and the review of systems (ROS).

The CC creates medical necessity by giving you a reason for the visit. Without it, the visit might not be reimbursed because there would be no documented cause for the visit. The HPI describes the chief complaint or complaints, and the PFSH and ROS are important to evaluate pertinent positive or negative findings that will help in E&M.

If the CC is pain, the HPI can be broken down into the following elements:

Location (where is the pain)
Quality (type of pain: sharp, burning, lancing)
Severity (scale of 1 to 10)
Duration (how long has the problem persisted)
Timing (time of day or frequency)
Context (what the patient did to cause problem or was doing when problem occurred)
Modifying factors (what made the problem better, worse, and so on)
Associated signs and symptoms

One scores this as Brief or Extended depending upon how many of the elements are present in the HPI. A brief HPI has one to three elements, whereas an Extended HPI has four or more. The score is cumulative, so if the patient has more than one complaint, two elements about each problem are acceptable to achieve an extended HPI. This is a typical history one might encounter that consists of more than four elements: 36 yo WDWNWHF c/o back pain. Mid back × 24 hours. Tylenol helped. Worse today. Sneezed and it hurt her. No W/A, NSD, BBI.

This is the type of history you might find in a chart, but the acronyms may or may not be familiar. It describes a patient who is a 36-year-old well-developed, well-nourished, well-hydrated female with a complaint of back pain in the mid back, present for 24 hours, relieved by Tylenol, worse today, and aggravated by sneezing. She denies weakness or atrophy, neurosensory deficits, and bowel or bladder incontinence. If one uses acronyms that are not standard (even if one thinks they are, an auditor might not understand them), keep an acronym list so it can be used as a key to interpret the notes. Would this list of acronyms be considered associated signs and symptoms or a review of systems? The differentiation between the two is considered in the next section.

The ROS is an extremely important component of the history that often is not given proper credit in documentation. It is necessary to include all pertinent positives and negatives in the appropriate systems. There are up to 14 systems to be reviewed. For new patients, it may make sense to review all of them to determine a comprehensive picture of the patient's problem or problems. For established patients seen in follow-up, however, it is necessary only to review the germane systems. Here are the ROS body areas and organ systems (BA/OS) as defined by Medicare:

1. Constitutional
2. Eyes (Head, eyes, ears, nose, and throat should be delineated into each body area or organ system.)
3. Ears, nose, mouth, and throat (See comment in item 2.)
4. Cardiovascular
5. Respiratory
6. Gastrointestinal
7. Genitourinary
8. Musculoskeletal
9. Integumentary
10. Neurological
11. Psychiatric
12. Endocrine
13. Hematologic, lymphatic
14. Allergic, immunologic

There are three ROS levels dependent on BA/OS reviewed:

Pertinent: 1 BA/OS
Extended: 2–9 BA/OS
Complete: 10+ BA/OS

Under the HPI, it is advisable to avoid using the associated signs or symptoms, as most patients give more than enough history to achieve four elements in the HPI. Thus, one can put in the ROS the balance of the positive and negative questions employed to narrow the diagnostic focus to receive appropriate and legitimate credit for obtaining and evaluating this information.

The PFSH is rather straightforward and can even be referenced in notes once it is part of the permanent medical record. Simply list relevant past medical history (PMH) with diabetes, hypertension, asthma, and so on as it pertains to the patient. If the information is noncontributory, but one still wants credit for asking, simply document PMH: NC. Not documenting leaves the assumption that the question was not asked, so the practitioner receives no credit in terms of scoring the history section of the visit. The social history and family history are treated just like the PMH; list what is germane, and if it is not, list NC. The PFSH score is based upon how many of these questions were asked and documented. Only one from any of the three (family, medical, or social) need be present for a pertinent PFSH score and two for a complete score in an established patient. In a new patient, three of these must be covered to get a complete score.

The medical assistant or nurse can take and document the history for every visit, or a form that the patient fills out before the visit may be employed. To do this, date and initial the form at least semiannually and initial and date any new information that might be acquired during subsequent visits. If you wish to reference a document to get credit for it in the history, document the date and what specifically you are referencing, such as "For the balance of PFSH, please see H&P from 6/25/04."

The last step in the history is scoring it. Table 30.1 outlines that process using the three-of-three rule. The numbers in parentheses are the scores associated with the different history levels and used to calculate the E&M codes. If the ROS is not clearly designated in the progress note, there may be no credit for it. Therefore, regardless of the length or extent of the history, it cannot be designated as anything other than a level 1 problem-focused history.[†] Similarly, to achieve a comprehensive history (4) you must include 10 of the 14 systems in the ROS. Without a complete ROS on new patients or consults, level 4 or 5 cannot be achieved, nor can higher than a level 1 initial hospital visit be achieved.

This is a good time to review the example, restated here, labeling the different components. It is apparent that a detailed history was achieved with little effort and a small but relevant amount of documentation: 36 yo WDWNWHF c/o back pain. Mid back × 24 hours. Tylenol helped. Worse today. Sneezed and afterwards it hurt her.

ROS: No W/A, NSD, BBI
PMH: Allergic rhinitis
Social/FMH: NC

[†]The 1995 federal documentation guidelines defined only problem-focused and comprehensive examinations and left the expanded-problem-focused (EPF) and detailed examinations open to interpretation regarding the number or BA/OS. Thus, by convention, the 2-4 and 5-7 designations for EPF and detailed, respectively are national, commonly understood and accepted standards, since problem focused is ≤BA/OS and comprehensive is ≥8 BA/OS.

TABLE 30.1

Billing and Coding

History Type and Level	HPI	ROS	PFSH
Problem focused (1)	Brief	None	None
Expanded problem focused (2)	Brief	Problem Pertinent	None
Detailed (3)	Extended	Extended	Pertinent
Comprehensive (4)	Extended	Complete	Complete

1995 and 1997 federal documentation guidelines. Adapted with permission from Jorgensen DJ, Jorgensen RT. A Physician's Guide to Billing and Coding. Columbus, OH: Greyden, 2004.

From the scoring table (Table 30.1), it is apparent that this brief description is a detailed history. The only thing keeping it from being a comprehensive history is the ROS, as it needs 10 ROS to get to this level. Although the provider did not think the social or family histories were relevant, rather than just not documenting it, he or she wrote NC (noncontributory). This makes it part of the note and proves that it was asked, not forgotten or omitted. The above are designated the Subjective portion of the SOAP note.

Physical Examination

The physical examination is the Objective portion of the SOAP note. There are two sets of guidelines regarding documentation of the physical examination, and either may be used. The choice even varies from patient contact to patient contact. It is the authors' recommendation that the 1995 system be preferentially used for most specialties, as it is more forgiving.[‡] To compare and contrast the two systems, go to the Medicare Web site (http://cms.hhs.gov/).[6] The physical examination itself is defined in terms of the number of body areas and/or organ systems examined. These must be germane to the complaint. When a physician is trying to establish a diagnosis or find the etiology of a new patient's complaint, it is likely that a multisystem examination will be performed. In most cases, this will include a thorough osteopathic musculoskeletal structural examination. There are 10 body areas (BA) and 11 organ systems (OS) listed next. The examination may include both body areas and organ systems, but credit cannot be obtained for redundant examination.

The CPT recognizes 10 body areas:

1. Head (including the face)
2. Neck
3. Chest (including breasts and axillae)
4. Abdomen
5. Genitalia, groin, and buttocks

[‡]In April 1998, there was a "fly-in" meeting in Chicago, due to unrest by the physician community at the stringent nature of the 1997 guidelines. At that meeting, the 1997 system was indefinitely suspended, leaving providers with a choice to use either the 1995 or 1997 guidelines. However, an outcome is that if you use the 1995 system and try to use the complete single system examination to achieve a comprehensive examination score, you must defer to the 1997 guidelines definition of what that single system examination should be. Prior to 1997, the federal government allowed providers to determine what constituted a complete single system examination, but now that the more strict 1997 exists, we are urged to default to its rules for this portion of the 1995 examination.

6. Back

7–10. Each of the four extremities (four separate body areas)

The CPT recognizes eleven organ systems:

1. Eyes
2. Ears, nose, mouth, and throat
3. Cardiovascular
4. Respiratory
5. Gastrointestinal
6. Genitourinary
7. Musculoskeletal
8. Skin
9. Neurologic
10. Psychiatric
11. Hematologic, lymphatic, and immunologic

Using these body areas and organ system designations, the 1995 scoring is as follows:

Problem focused	$\leq$1 BA/OS
Expanded problem focused	2–4 BA/OS
Detailed	5–7 BA/OS
Comprehensive	$\geq$8 BA/OS or 1 complete single systemic

As can be seen, the levels of the History and Examination use identical terminology and are based on a four-tiered system with the same point assignment. Medical Decision Making does not use this same terminology but instead uses descriptors as to the complexity of the Medical Decision Making provided.

Going back to the example for mid back pain, the following physical examination documentation would be sufficient, using the 1995 federal guidelines, for a detailed examination:

PE: WDWNWHF in mild distress on examination

Eyes: PERRLA w/EOMI

ENT: Negative

MS: Mid thoracic trapezius and iliocostalis strain. Pain with mid thoracic extension approximately T8

Neuro: No neurosensory deficits noted. No reproducible pain with spinal compression

Skin: No ecchymoses noted over site of pain

T6-7NRRSL with ribs 6–8 locked in inhalation

T8FRSR

T9-10NRRSL

T11-L2NRLSR

Key: PE, physical examination; WDWNWHF, well-developed, well-nourished, well-hydrated female; PERRLA, pupils equal, round, and reactive to light and accommodation; EOMI, extra-ocular muscles intact; ENT, ears, nose, and throat; MS, musculoskeletal; NRRSL, neutral, rotated right, side bent left; NRLSR, neutral, rotated left, side bent right.

This example has six areas or systems examined and documents well the areas of somatic dysfunction (thorax [ICD-9CM designation, 739.2], ribs [739.8], and lumbar [739.3]) that will likely be addressed with OMT and/or other medical management.

Medical Decision Making

The Medical Decision Making portion of the E&M involves a review of the assessment and plan, the A and P of the SOAP note. At first glance this section, as compared to the history or physical examination, is the most daunting. However, in daily practice, the practitioner develops more of a gestalt mode for Medical Decision Making. This takes practice and experience, but coupled with quarterly audits to determine whether the coding that is being submitted is accurate, it is not difficult to learn this skill. The assessment is the result of the History and Physical Examination, with a tally of the number of diagnoses or undiagnosed issues (symptoms) and with clarification regarding their status, such as new versus established or chronic and stable, improved, or worsening.[2,3] The Plan (P of SOAP) is the recommended course and type or types of treatment associated with each item in the assessment. There are four levels of Medical Decision Making:

1. Straightforward
2. Low complexity
3. Moderate complexity
4. Comprehensive

   Determining the final level of Medical Decision Making is done by scoring three independent areas of the assessment and plan:

1. The number of diagnoses or management options
2. The amount or complexity of the data
3. The degree of risk of complications, morbidity, and/or mortality

Number of Diagnoses and Management Options (Table 30.2)

Table 30.2 allows one to tally the number of diagnoses; whether the diagnosis, problem, or symptom is new or chronic; and whether it is improved, stable, or worsening.

TABLE 30.2

Diagnosis or Diagnoses and Management

Options

Problem Categories	Number (X) of Problems	Possible Points	Score
Self-limited, minor	(Max = 2)	1	
Established problem; stable or improved; resolving or resolved; well controlled		1	
Established problem; inadequately controlled or worsening		2	
New problem; no additional workup	(Max = 1)	3	
New problem; additional workup planned		4	
		Total	

Federal E&M documentation guidelines.

Straightforward problems are just that; they require no additional workup. However, a questionable deep tendon reflex at L4 could warrant an MRI, and if the problem is new, the MRI is the additional workup noted in the table. The maximum score possible for this table is 4, so even if one exceeds this number with diagnoses, problems, acuity, and so on, it is not possible to get extra credit in the final medical decision making table.

In the column headed Number (X) of Problems, the Max = 2 and Max = 1 statements apply only to the line item to the left, not up or down the column. For example, a patient presenting with two or more new problems that will not require any diagnostic studies receives a maximum of three points. This is because the maximum credit for this line is three points, as the directive is Max = 1.

The following examples more clearly demonstrate the use of Table 30.2:

1. A patient presents with an exacerbation of chronic obstructive pulmonary disease (COPD) and an axillary mass that is discovered during the examination. This patient receives two points for the COPD as an established problem; worsening, and an additional four points for the axillary mass as a new problem; additional workup planned. The total for this encounter would be six. The maximum required for any of the medical decision-making tables is four, because four points equals the highest of the four possible levels.

2. A patient presents with ankle sprain and also mentions having contact dermatitis that developed over the weekend after work in the garden. Assuming no diagnostic procedures for either, both issues fall under the category of new problem, no workup planned. This category affords three points per issue but has a maximum credit per patient encounter of only one new problem. Therefore, while one may be tempted to show a total of six points for this encounter, (three points for the sprain plus an additional three points for dermatitis), credit is afforded for only one of the two issues, that is, a maximum of three points for this example.

Again, category points are totaled with a maximum score of four points. Once the maximum of four total points has been achieved, there is no need to continue adding points.

Amount or Complexity of Data

Table 30.3 allocates points for ordering or reviewing laboratory tests, reviewing data, deciding to obtain old records, or even discussing results with another doctor. Points cannot be obtained by both ordering and reviewing tests on the same date of service for the same appointment. On a given date, credit is given for one or the other. Further, no additional credit is given for ordering more than one diagnostic procedure from the same CPT chapter in the radiology (i.e., 70,000 range), clinical laboratory (i.e., 80,000 range) or medicine (i.e., 90,000 range) sections. However, if tests are ordered or reviewed from different sections or a test is ordered and discussed with another provider in consultation about the patient, the points are cumulative.

The Type of Data column determines what data are being reviewed or ordered as well as sources of information. Most of the credit for this table is afforded from the Plan element of the SOAP note. Occasionally, these data may be in the subjective portion or in a referenced note. Here it is important to be familiar with what tests are commonly ordered and from which section they are taken so that points can be appropriately allocated. The numeric classification should make this a simple exercise. The decision to obtain medical records or to obtain a medical

TABLE 30.3

Amount and/or Complexity of Data to be Reviewed

Amount of Data to be Reviewed or Complexity

Type of Data	Indicate Credit (X)	Possible Points	Score
Review and/or order tests in CPT 8XXXX (clinical laboratory tests)		1	
Review and/or order tests in CPT 7XXXX (radiology)		1	
Review and/or order tests in CPT 9XXXX (medicine section)		1	
Discuss test results with performing doctor		1	
Independent review of image, tracing, or specimen		2	
Decision to obtain old records and/or obtain history from others		1	
Review and summarize old records, and/or obtain history		2	
		Total	

Federal E&M documentation guidelines.

history from others simply should be documented as from whom the records were obtained and/or who was spoken with to get the history. Family counts, even a wife or husband or a sibling or child. "Review and summarize medical records" requires a written document that the physician or someone else put together, but it could even be the patient's existing medical record that was credited after having been summarized. This source need not come from outside the practice.

Risk

Table 30.4 represents the Level of Risk that is assumed when treating and caring for a patient. There are four Levels of Risk: minimal, low, moderate, and high, again scored 1 to 4. There are three distinct categories: Presenting Problems (level of acuity), Diagnostic Procedures (type of tests that might be ordered or per-formed), and Management Options (e.g., treatments or procedures).

Some aspects of this table make little to no sense. The most obvious is the fourth column (Management Options) in the section on moderate risk, the third item. Prescription drug management is not necessarily prescribing a medication but perhaps considering it or discussing it with the patient. The federal documen-tation guidelines consider the fourth item, therapeutic nuclear medicine, to be analogous in terms of complexity. However confusing this table is, it is the system with which the physician has to work. This is the third and final table to review before calculating the Medical Decision Making total and adding it to the History and Physical Examination to determine the E&M code.

TABLE 30.4

Risk of Complications and/or Morbidity or Mortality; Also Risk of Malpractice

Highest Level in Any Category Is the Level of Risk

Level of Risk	Category One Presenting Problem	Category Two Diagnostic Procedure(s) Ordered	Category Three Management Options Selected
Minimal (1)	One self-limited or minor problem, e.g., cold, insect bite, tinea corporis	Laboratory test requiring venipuncture	Rest
		Chest radiography	Gargles
		ECG, EEG	Elastic bandages
		Urinalysis	Superficial dressings
		Ultrasound, e.g., echocardiography	
		KOH prep	
Low (2)	Two or more self-limited or minor problems	Physiologic tests not under stress, e.g., pulmonary function tests	Over-the-counter drugs
	One stable, chronic illness, e.g., well controlled hypertension, non-insulin dependent diabetes, cataract, BPH	Imaging study (not cardiovascular) with contrast, e.g., barium enema	Minor surgery with no identified risk factors
	Acute uncomplicated illness or injury, e.g., cystitis, allergic rhinitis, simple sprain	Superficial needle biopsies	Physical therapy
		Clinical laboratory testing requiring arterial puncture	Occupational therapy
		Skin biopsy	IV fluids without additives
Moderate (3)	One or more chronic illnesses with mild exacerbation, progression, or side effects of treatment	Physiologic testing under stress, e.g., cardiac stress test, fetal contraction stress test	Minor surgery with identified risk factors
	Two or more stable chronic illnesses	Diagnostic endoscopy with no identified risk factors	Elective major surgery (open, percutaneous, or endoscopic) with no identified risk factors
	Undiagnosed new problem with uncertain prognosis, e.g., lump in breast	Deep needle or incisional biopsy	Prescription drug management

(continued)

TABLE 30.4 (CONT.)

Risk of Complications and/or Morbidity or Mortality; Also Risk of Malpractice

Highest Level in Any Category Is the Level of Risk

Level of Risk	Category One Presenting Problem	Category Two Diagnostic Procedure(s) Ordered	Category Three Management Options Selected
	Acute illness with systemic symptoms, e.g., pyelonephritis, pneumonitis, colitis	Cardiovascular imaging study with contrast, no identified risk factors, e.g., arteriogram, cardiac catheterization	Therapeutic nuclear medicine
	Acute complicated injury, e.g., head injury with brief loss of consciousness	Obtain fluid from body cavity, e.g., lumbar puncture, thoracentesis, culdocentesis	IV fluid with additives
			Closed treatment of fracture or dislocation without manipulation
High (4)	One or more chronic illnesses with severe exacerbation, progression, or side effects or treatment	Cardiovascular imaging study with contrast with identified risk factors	Elective major surgery (open, percutaneous or endoscopic) with identified risk factors
	Acute or chronic illness or injury that threatens life or bodily function, e.g., multiple trauma, acute myocardial infarction, pulmonary embolus, severe respiratory distress, progressive severe rheumatoid arthritis, psychiatric illness with possibility of threat to self or others, peritonitis, acute renal failure	Cardiac electrophysiologic tests Diagnostic endoscopy with identified risk factors	Emergency major surgery (open, percutaneous, or endoscopic) Parenteral controlled substances
	An abrupt change in neurologic status, e.g., seizure, transient ischemic attack, weakness, sensory loss	Discography	Drug therapy requiring intensive monitoring or toxicity
			Decision not to resuscitate or to deescalate care because of poor prognosis

Federal E&M documentation guidelines.

Table 30.4 is scored by picking the single highest item in any of the three categories: Presenting Problem, Diagnostic Procedures Ordered, or Management Option. That highest item is the third Medical Decision Making score.

The best recommendation for individual practitioners is to develop clinical vignettes that work for their practice. Again, consistent usage by clinicians is essential to ensure accurate coding and to minimize risk associated with an audit. A written policy is strongly recommended.

Table 30.4 is taken directly from the 1995 guidelines. Tables 30.2 and 30.3 were jointly developed by the Center for Medicare Standards (CMS) and the Marshfield Clinic. Although Tables 30.2 and 30.3 are not in the 1995 guidelines, they were distributed to all Medicare carriers by CMS for use and implementation of the 1995 guidelines.

Following Table 30.5 by the book each and every visit is impractical. One has to look at the Assessment (diagnosis or diagnoses; A of SOAP) and add them up with the diagnosis table; look at the studies, laboratory findings, and medical record review, and add those points up on that table; and then go to the table of risk to determine which single element is the highest level of risk and assign a point from there. Each table will be tallied 1 to 4. Then take the middle number (two-of-three rule), and that is the Medical Decision Making score, as Table 30.5 shows. Although it is confusing at first, with practice one will begin to see trends in one's medical decision making. Practice will allow a more gestalt-driven pragmatic use of this table, for to use it every time one sees patients is a near impossibility.

Identifying the Evaluation and Management Service

E&M services are specifically identified using five-digit numeric descriptors. To determine the identifying number, the physician must decide upon the general category or type of visit (outpatient versus inpatient, established or follow-up visit, new visit or consult). Next the physician decides upon the level of service that was provided by adding up the History points, Physical Examination points, and Medical Decision Making points, and applying the two-of-three or three-of-three rules as the particular code category dictates. Time, as allocated per code by CPT, can be used only to justify a particular code when counseling or coordination of care constituted more than 50%

TABLE 30.5

Medical Decision Making Scoring Summary

Medical Decision Making Determination (2 of 3)

Decision Making	Straightforward	Low	Moderate	High
1. Number of diagnosis, management options	Minimal (1)	Limited (2)	Multiple (3)	Extensive (4+)
2. Amount of data to be reviewed	Minimal, none (1)	Limited (2)	Multiple (3)	Extensive (4+)
3. Table of risk	Minimal (1)	Low (2)	Moderate (3)	High (4)

of the face-to-face contact in the physician–patient encounter. In such an instance, time may be considered the controlling factor to qualify for a particular level of E&M service. In this instance, Time supersides the three key components.

Compared to the 1997 system, the 1995 system will at times allow for and appear to justify overcoding of a seemingly routine visit. The History and Examination sections revealed that by sticking to the rules, by and large the practicing physician can stay safe in an audit. The greatest reason for the creation of the 1997 system was to remove the ambiguity and ability to overcode that the 1995 system afforded a practitioner for routine patient encounters. Unfortunately, the 1997 system went too far and made it too difficult to achieve legitimate codes with its onerous bulleted examinations. The 1997 system does, however, allow a specialist to achieve a higher-level examination even though only one or two body systems are examined. If one learns from one's practice what the typical codes are, and if the visit is more complex than usual, one can document as is appropriate, and paying particular attention to the three key components, code the visit as allowed. It is important not to undercode out of fear of audits or penalties but equally important to avoid overcoding just because the rules are known and enough history or examination can be added to turn an uncomplicated otitis media into a 99214. Critics of the 1995 system argue that it allows, if not justifies, such coding, but pragmatically, an office visit for an uncomplicated ear infection is likely a 99213 unless other factors complicate matters. The best advice is to document what is found and code the visit accordingly, keeping in mind the level of intensity and acuity.

Levels and Codes

With these rules and tables already presented, the following tables provide the foundation for determining the code selection based upon the type of visit and the documentation of the History, Physical Examination, and Medical Decision Making. If time is used and OMT is done at that visit, the time doing the OMT does not count toward the time for the visit. Many providers talk with patients about various issues during OMT, but this does not count toward the 50% rule, because the physician is already being reimbursed for the time for doing the OMT. In most instances, proper documentation of the History, Physical Examination, and Medical Decision Making will make the use of time as the principal documentation quite unnecessary. As one becomes skilled in documentation methodology, one documents what is needed for the medical record, and it will gel fluidly with what is needed for coding as well.

New Patient Codes (99201–99205)

These codes are used for patients who meet the new-patient definition[§] and are seen in an outpatient setting. Patients in the emergency department or in the hospital for observation have outpatient status, and therefore, outpatient codes may be used in those settings as well. The scope of this chapter does not allow for further discussion. Thus the reader is referred to CPT or one of the referenced texts for further information. These codes are used once, and visits after the first one, assuming it is less than 3 years, are typically billed in the established patient visit code set (99212–99215). Table 30.6 outlines the History, Examination, and Medical Decision Making for the new-patient codes. These, like Consult codes, require the three-of-three rule (go to the lowest number) when determining the codes.

[§]Patient not seen by a provider of the same speciality within a group practice (single EIN/TAX I.D.) during the last three years.

TABLE 30.6

New Patient Visits and Consultation: Three-of-Three Rule

Outpatient Consult	New Patient	History	Physical Examination	Medical Decision Making
99241	99201	Problem focused	Problem focused	Straightforward
99242	99202	Expanded problem focused	Expanded problem focused	Straightforward
99243	99203	Detailed	Detailed	Low complexity
99244	99204	Comprehensive	Comprehensive	Moderate complexity
99245	99205	Comprehensive	Comprehensive	High complexity

Adapted with permission from Jorgensen DJ, Jorgensen RT. A Physician's Guide to Billing and Coding. Columbus, OH: Greyden, 2004.

Consultations

Consult codes also require the three-of-three rule (lowest number), whether they are inpatient (99251–99255) or outpatient (99241–99245), facility or nonfacility, respectively. Care may be initiated at the time of consultation.[7] A written request or at least a specified request or referral from the referring provider is required. For an inpatient, a written order in the chart is needed (a verbal order by a nurse is acceptable) before the patient can be seen. For an outpatient, after the consultation, a letter (not just a carbon copy of the consultation note) must be sent to the referring provider. It can be a form letter thanking the provider for the request and saying that a copy of the consultation note will follow, but it must be a letter. Some providers prefer to dictate the entire visit in letter format for the referring provider. Either method is fine as long as a letter is sent. Consults can be done within the same office and within the same specialty, but the referral and letter rules still apply. Some private insurers have specific rules regarding who can or cannot do consults, but most allow any provider who is qualified to do consultative work.

Once a consult has been done, the subsequent visits use the established patient codes for outpatients (99212–99215) and use hospital care codes (99231–99233) for inpatients. The only time to use another consult code is if the patient presents with a new and unrelated problem, and another referral and evaluation have been requested. If this is done in the inpatient facility setting, use the follow-up consult codes (99261–99263) noted later in the chapter. Do not use follow-up consult codes for routine follow-up from an initial consult; these are only for a new problem that the consultant has been requested to evaluate and possibly treat. See Tables 30.7 to 30.9.

Established Patient Office Visits (99211–99215)

Established patient visit codes are the most commonly used E&M codes. These codes follow the two-of-three rule. Providers should use codes 99212 to 99215, as 99211 is typically allocated to nursing staff. They are used after consults or new patient visits for follow-up visits. Table 30.10 shows the algorithm to determine the code selection.

TABLE 30.7

Initial Hospital (Facility) Consult Codes: Three-of-Three Rule

Initial Inpatient Consult	History	Physical Examination	Medical Decision Making	Time
99251	Problem focused	Problem focused	Straightforward	20
99252	Expanded problem focused	Expanded problem focused	Straightforward	40
99253	Detailed	Detailed	Low complexity	55
99254	Comprehensive	Comprehensive	Moderate complexity	80
99255	Comprehensive	Comprehensive	High complexity	110

Adapted with permission from Jorgensen DJ, Jorgensen RT. A Physician's Guide to Billing and Coding. Columbus, OH: Greyden, 2004.

TABLE 30.8

Subsequent Hospital Care Codes: Two-of-Three Rule

Subsequent Hospital Care	History	Physical Examination	Medical Decision Making	Time
99231	Problem-focused interval	Problem focused	Straightforward, low complexity	15
99232	Expanded problem-focused interval	Expanded problem focused	Moderate complexity	25
99233	Detailed interval	Detailed	High complexity	35

Adapted with permission from Jorgensen DJ, Jorgensen RT. A Physician's Guide to Billing and Coding. Columbus, OH: Greyden, 2004.

TABLE 30.9

Follow-up Inpatient Consults: Two-of-Three Rule

Follow-up Inpatient Consult	History	Physical Examination	Medical Decision Making	Time
99261	Problem-focused interval	Problem focused	Straightforward, low complexity	10
99262	Expanded problem focused	Expanded problem focused	Moderate complexity	20
99263	Detailed interval	Detailed	High complexity	30

Adapted with permission from Jorgensen DJ, Jorgensen RT. A Physician's Guide to Billing and Coding. Columbus, OH: Greyden, 2004.

TABLE 30.10

Established Patient Office Visits: Two-of-Three Rule

Code	History	Physical Examination	Medical Decision Making	Time
99211	Physician not required		Straightforward	5
99212	Problem focused	Problem focused	Straightforward	10
99213	Expanded problem focused	Expanded problem focused	Low complexity	15
99214	Detailed	Detailed	Moderate complexity	25
99215	Comprehensive	Comprehensive	High complexity	40

Adapted with permission from Jorgensen DJ, Jorgensen RT. A Physician's Guide to Billing and Coding. Columbus, OH: Greyden, 2004.

Use of OMT

OMT is defined in CPT as "a form of manual treatment applied by a physician to eliminate or alleviate somatic dysfunction and related disorders." The doctor of osteopathy has been trained to diagnose somatic dysfunction and use OMT. OMT is a therapeutic procedure. Any procedure performed upon a patient must be recorded in the progress note. In the SOAP note format, therapeutic procedures are recorded in the P, or Plan, portion of the note. In the standard osteopathic medical record, developed by the Louisa Burns Osteopathic Research Committee of the American Academy of Osteopathy, a specific area has been allocated for recording both somatic dysfunction and its treatment with OMT. (See Chapter 31.)

Once the physician has examined the patient and decided upon a diagnosis and plan for treatment, an E&M code is identifiable. This code must be recorded in association with all appropriate diagnoses. Diagnoses such as somatic dysfunction are identified numerically. ICD-9CM is the reference in which accepted diagnosis codes are to be found. A diagnostic code for somatic dysfunction, 739, is listed in ICD-9CM. It is subdivided according to the anatomic region where somatic dysfunction is diagnosed as follows:

739.0, somatic dysfunction cranial
739.1, somatic dysfunction cervical
739.2, somatic dysfunction thoracic
739.3, somatic dysfunction lumbar
739.4, somatic dysfunction sacrum/pelvis
739.5, somatic dysfunction ilium/pelvis
739.6, somatic dysfunction lower extremity (one or both)
739.7, somatic dysfunction upper extremity (one or both)
739.8, somatic dysfunction ribs (any or all)
739.9, somatic dysfunction abdomen/other[8]

As a procedure, OMT is carried out in addition to E&M. A fee for service may therefore be submitted for OMT in addition to the fee submitted for E&M. Under these circumstances, a 25-modifier (-25) must follow the appropriate E&M code.

Thus, the E&M code for an established patient level II visit in which OMT has been performed is 99212-25. The 25-modifier is a significantly and separately identifiable service in addition to E&M. A 25-modifier is used to obtain reimbursement for an E&M service by the same provider on the same day as another service or a procedure when an E&M component is significantly and separately identifiable from the other service or procedure. It indicates that an additional procedure code is being submitted in association with the primary E&M code. The diagnosis leading to the decision to provide OMT can be the same as the one used for the E&M, and the AMA, in a letter to the American Osteopathic Association (AOA) legal department, has upheld that OMT does not include any E&M service (letter from Sherry L. Smith, committee secretary, AMA Specialty Society RVS Update Committee, to Yolanda L. Doss, RHIA, assistant director of coding and reimbursement, AOA, March 10, 2003). This means that OMT and E&M are not bundled, and if both services were provided and the documentation supports it, both should be billed and reimbursed.

The 25-modifier does not specifically indicate that OMT was done, as it can be used with any number of other procedures (e.g., flexible sigmoidoscopy, cryotherapy, skin biopsies). It is simply a means to inform the insurer that this is not a straightforward office or hospital visit and the physician submitting the bill wants and expects to be paid for both services.

OMT CPT Codes

A series of five-digit codes (98925–98929) are used to identify OMT. These codes indicate the number of separate body regions in which somatic dysfunction has been diagnosed and OMT has been used. They do not indicate the type of OMT that has been used.

98925: 1 or 2 body regions
98926: 3 or 4 body regions
98927: 5 or 6 body regions
98928: 7 or 8 body regions
98929: 9 or 10 body regions[2]

Each OMT CPT code can be used once per visit. If 7 or 8 areas were treated, the code is 98928. If 9 areas were treated, the code is 98929. Using multiple OMT CPT codes per visit is fraudulent and misrepresents what occurred at the visit. It is also not acceptable to use the term *therapy* in the progress note or any other communications for cranial osteopathy or any other type of OMT. The T in OMT stands for *treatment*. To use the word *therapy* misrepresents what has been done for the patient, and it confuses the issue for insurers, some of whom do not reimburse for craniosacral therapy but do pay for osteopathy in the cranial field or other cranial osteopathic procedures. Semantics are important, and learning the proper terminology and using it is paramount.

When an OMT procedure code is submitted, the number of 739 diagnosis codes submitted must substantiate that procedure code. That is, if 98926 is submitted, indicating the treatment of three or four regions, it must be accompanied by at least three separate 739 diagnosis codes, indicating that somatic dysfunction was diagnosed in at least three separate body regions. It is not appropriate to use physical therapy codes to charge for OMT. Physical therapy is just that—therapy. Physicians, physician assistants, and nurse practitioners perform procedures and specifically do not do therapy in terms of manipulative medicine. Therefore, do not allow OMT to be allocated in this realm, as it is not correct coding.

CONCLUSION

The practice of medicine at the outset of the twenty-first century has become extremely complex. The progress note is an important component of contemporary medical practice. The complexity of contemporary medical practice requires practitioners to adhere to a strict protocol for writing progress notes for medicolegal and reimbursement purposes.

The progress note is the record that allows continuity of care. Subspecialty medical practice with associated diagnostic and therapeutic advances has created an environment wherein patients are regularly cared for by more than one physician. In academic medicine, the presence of students and residents produces additional levels of complexity. To maintain continuity among all of the participants, it is imperative to communicate clearly. To ensure optimal patient care, all physicians must follow the same rules.

In the past, patients personally paid the physician for their health care. They were directly aware of what had been done and consequently could judge whether the fee for service was appropriate. Third-party reimbursement for physician services has changed that relationship. The third party cannot have direct knowledge of what occurs between the patient and physician. The medical record therefore serves as documentation of the extent of service rendered. The progress note justifies the dollar amount requested for E&M services and indicates whether or not diagnostic and therapeutic procedures are reimbursable. If that documentation does not justify what is charged, be prepared to repay the reimbursement, possibly with penalties, in the event of an audit.

It may seem crass to discuss money when talking about the care of patients. Medicine, however, is a business. It is a business of caring for people, but a business nonetheless. Doctors cannot care for their patients if they cannot afford to keep the office open. Worse yet, patients may find their trust in their physician shaken if their physician is accused of fraudulent activity. Having spent many years learning medicine, physicians must also learn the requirements of correct medical record keeping, a continually evolving area of information that is part of their continuing education.

References

1. Sleszynski SL, Glonek T, Kuchera WA. Standardized medical record: A new outpatient osteopathic SOAP form: Validation of a standardized office form against physician's progress notes. J Am Osteopath Assoc 1999;10:516–529.
2. Current Procedural Terminology (CPT) 2004. Chicago: American Medical Association, 2003.
3. Jorgensen DJ, Jorgensen RT. A Physician's Guide to Billing and Coding. Columbus, OH: Greyden, 2004.
4. Section 1128A of SSA, HIPAA of 1996, Public Law 104-91.
5. Medicare Carrier Manual 15502. Paragraph A.
6. Centers for Medicare and Medicaid Services. Documentation Guidelines: Evaluation and Management Services. Available at http://www.cms.hhs.gov/medlearn/emdoc.asp. Last modified October 7, 2004. Accessed February 22, 2005.
7. Medicare Carrier Manual 15506. Paragraph B.
8. International Classification of Diseases, 9th Revision: Clinical Modification. 5th ed. Salt Lake City: Medicode, 1999.

CHAPTER 31

The Standardized Medical Record

Sandra L. Sleszynski and Thomas Glonek

INTRODUCTION

On January 12 to 14, 1996, in a small conference room at the Hamilton Inn O'Hare in Chicago, a group of 14 individuals met for a concentrated weekend to discuss the realm of medical record standardization.* The American Academy of Osteopathy (AAO) Louisa Burns Osteopathic Research Committee (LBORC) of the American Osteopathic Association (AOA) and guests, under the leadership of Sandra Sleszynski and funded by the AAO, gathered to develop an instrument that could be used efficiently and effectively for specific osteopathic clinical, educational, and research purposes. This new progress note would follow the SOAP format (subjective, objective, assessment, plan), be simple, guide in coding for reimbursement, allow tracking for education, and facilitate research data collection with little effort. Out of this private group of clinicians, educators, and researchers, the single-page Outpatient Osteopathic SOAP Note Form was created.[1]

---

*Invitees included 38 doctors of osteopathy and doctors of philosophy and 2 administrative staff. (Committee listed in acknowledgment.)

SOAP NOTES AND CURRENT PROCEDURAL
TERMINOLOGY CODING GUIDELINES: 1995 OR 1997?

Coding for reimbursement and the ease of coding are key issues in any clinical practice. The current 1995/1997 Medicare documentation guideline ruling[2] is problematic,[3,4] particularly if one's intention is to standardize and simplify medical reporting, which is what SOAP notes and electronic medical records are supposed to be all about. Needless to say, it is impossible to create a one-size-fits-all reporting instrument in an atmosphere of federal and medical community squabbling and indecision. Nevertheless, it is important to try since regulatory issues continually evolve and inaction invites Chaos.

At the time the first SOAP note form was being created, the 1997 CPT coding guidelines were in force. Since this new set of guidelines also was compatible with the use of standardized forms and electronic medical records, it was decided to meet the new guidelines and create the SOAP notes consistent with the 1997 reporting system. For once, it was thought, we were ahead of the game. How foolish.

The medical community howled! Not only were the new guidelines more complicated, demanding still more documentation per patient visit, they were more restrictive, resulting in undercoding and decreased practice revenues. The federal government reconsidered. In an April 1998 fly-in-to-the-AMA in Chicago, the 1997 system was indefinitely suspended, making it one option and the 1995 system another.[2,4] This is still the case.

Most nonmedical personnel, such as lawyers and consultants, of course, prefer the 1997 system, as it requires counting bullets, and one doesn't need to know much about medicine. The 1997 guidelines also facilitate the development and use of electronic medical records. It is thought by many, however, that the 1995 system far outweighs the 1997 system in simplicity of implementation in the clinic.[3] This system is familiar to clinicians and more protective of the practice in the event of a state, federal, or penal audit or any other payment review process.

Meanwhile, back at SOAP note headquarters (spread all over the country but linked via the Internet) and on the heels of this switch to the dual-reporting system, SOAP notes were being designed, content was being decided, and validation programs were being written and carried out. It was decided to continue following the 1997 guidelines, since they were in force at the time, and the intent of the SOAP note instrument was creation of consistent documentation for care of the patient and ease of review and data collection (patient, educational tracking, and research information). Moreover, the history and the medical decision-making sections of progress notes were virtually identical for the 1995 and 1997 guidelines, so one need only know the physical examination differences to implement either one of them. The osteopathic manipulative treatment (OMT) tables in the SOAP notes were designed to facilitate this. During this time, the LBORC was aware of the brewing discontent within the medical practice community but reasoned that increased restrictions, the need for increased documentation, and standardization were inevitable. It was then and still is believed that compatibility with the 1997 system was the safe option and that with time reporting would drift in the direction of more and more rigorous documentation and standardization in the medical record.

Some practitioners use the 1997 system in practice but request that the 1995 system be used in the event of an audit. This provides more than ample documentation. The downside is that physicians can find themselves not billing at legitimate higher-level codes, because the 1997 system disallows some coding.[2,4] In either case, physicians are well known to down-code levels of service and not sufficiently document the care they give. The SOAP notes provide tools to help remedy these inherent traits of physicians. On the upside, because of their design, use of SOAP notes has done the following:

- Made practice more efficient by requiring less thinking about what is included in the note and making it easier to find the diagnosis, the treatments prescribed, the techniques that are working, the procedures that were done, and the degree of patient compliance, with follow-up appointments to improve care and to justify coding choices
- Made it obvious how many and which regions of the body were treated
- Reduced the incidence of failure to reimbursement due to unclear notes
- Decreased confusion as to whether the patient was improving
- Yielded payment when charges look suspicious, such as with Medicare, prolonged visits, counseling visits, and any time there are higher charges than appear warranted from the diagnoses or procedure codes listed on the insurance form

RAISONS D'ÊTRE

Have you ever wondered why osteopathic medicine exists and persists? To retain its professional identity, osteopathic medicine must address concerns critical to the future of the profession. It must provide information on concepts that are central to treatment and on how the disturbances it professes to treat, almost uniquely in the health care field, are distributed among the population. In this regard, the most characteristic component is "the role of palpatory diagnosis and manipulative treatment in osteopathic teaching and practice."[5]

Third-party payers are demanding that medical practices be evidenced based. This poses a particular dilemma for osteopathic medicine because the multiple variables encountered in holistic medical practice necessitate that one deal with large and diverse volumes of information, a good portion of which is difficult to quantify.

There have been many clinical reports of the efficacy of osteopathic evaluation and manipulative treatment in the management of a host of diseases and disorders of structure and function. The corresponding basic science data involving human subjects that support the clinical studies, however, are relatively few, primarily because of a lack of appropriate investigative technologies. The scientific solution to these deficiencies and the key to professional survival for osteopathic manipulative medicine lie in the generation of clinical outcomes data on a national scale. Implicit in this statement are the requirements for standardized nomenclature and a standardized method of reporting, involving trained investigators.

The development of a vehicle for the establishment of an accessible database of clinical information would greatly facilitate and accelerate osteopathic outcomes research. Consider, for example, the Danish "Better Health for Mother and Child" cohort study. The goal of this national outcomes program is the creation of a databank that generations of investigators can mine and/or use as a starting point for studies on the effects of medical treatment.[6]

In contrast to pure outcomes studies, however, Americans prefer to design their studies to answer specific questions or to conduct long-term follow-ups. The goals of the osteopathic SOAP note program incorporate both outcomes and clinical trials philosophies: to begin the creation of an osteopathic medical databank for research mining, as in the Danish program, but also to conform to the American model and answer specific clinical questions using the mined data. Once created, the database itself will facilitate the training of family medicine residents by providing hard data for both retrospective and prospective resident research papers.

With the growing call for outcomes-based research,[7,8] there is an increasingly urgent need for a standardized format for reporting the incidence, severity, treatment, and outcomes related to family practice and particularly musculoskeletal somatic dysfunction. If osteopathic medicine is to continue in the increasingly competitive arena of health care provision, it must provide information on the concepts that are central to its treatment and how the disturbances it professes to treat, almost uniquely in the health care field, are distributed among the population. Moreover, to be reimbursed by third-party payers, physicians must document all aspects of evaluation and management (E&M). The level of complexity of E&M determines the level of reimbursement. If interaction with a patient is highly complex but the physician fails to document that level of complexity, the physician will be reimbursed only for what was documented rather than what was actually done in the clinic.

One of the persistent problems that has faced osteopathic medicine, however, is the lack of reliable and easy-to-use methods for recording clinical findings and treatments in a format that is usable for subsequent data collection. This has been in part responsible for the lack of a referable database from the practitioners of the profession on the general parameters of osteopathic family practice; on the prevalence, frequency, and severity of somatic dysfunction in various classes of patients, and on the effects of treatment. There have been attempts to present a standardized format for such examinations.[9] In addition, standardization for research protocols has been discussed in various forums.[10–18] Most of these attempts, however, have been to provide complete guides to the documentation of osteopathic diagnosis and somatic dysfunction and may be too cumbersome for outcomes research involving large groups of participating family physicians.

A standardized medical record nevertheless is essential for documentation of osteopathic practice. Standardization will provide an efficient profession-wide national database of outcomes information that will find use in documenting the efficacy of osteopathic medical practice for the public as well as for medical, legal, insurance, and other third parties. It will also facilitate postdoctoral education in family medicine by providing the data required for resident tracking.

PAPER SOAP NOTES

Only through valid and consistent documentation can osteopathic physicians hope to obtain the outcomes information needed for providing quality patient care, full reimbursement, and quality postdoctoral education programs. The establishment of a common record-keeping system for osteopathic physicians was suggested more than 20 years ago.[19] More recent studies have recommended the development of such a system in hospitals, based on evidence that there was a lack of osteopathic evaluation on inpatients in osteopathic hospitals along with incorrect recording of findings when such evaluations were performed.[20] The original SOAP note was developed by Weed.[21–24] SOAP notes essentially cover the range of the physician's activity during an encounter with a patient. (A further development of the SOAP note is the problem-oriented note based on the patient's chief complaint.) The presentation of a SOAP note can vary significantly from a series of check boxes to a full narrative. A SOAP note form pioneered by the LBORC was developed specifically for osteopathic medicine (Fig. 31.1). The original form, named the Outpatient Osteopathic SOAP Note Form, has been in use in physicians' offices nationwide since 1998. This form has been formally validated against physicians' progress notes through a grant from the AOA.[1]

Outpatient Health Summary

wak SOAP version 5: 091102b

Patient's Name			Date		Update:			
Date of Birth		Sex	Phone Numbers:		Home			
Marital Status:	M S D W				Work			
Significant Others:			DNR Status: Resuscitate?		Yes	No	Qualifications:	
Religion:			Next of Kin:					

Social History:	Employment		Occupation		Education			
	Tobacco	ETOH		Drugs			Sex Hx	
Family History:	M		Siblings		Others:			
	F							

Past Medical History

CPT#	Start Date	Problem / Diagnosis	Medications	Start	Stop

Allergies, Adverse Drug Reactions: _____

Health Maintenance

Parameter	Dates							
DPT/DT/TD								
OPV								
MMR								
HIB								
Influenza								
Hepatitis								
PPD/Tine								
Pneumovax								
H & P								
Eye exam								
Dental exam								
PAP smear								
Mammogram								
Urinalysis								
Hemoccult								
Cholesterol								
Sigmoidoscopy								
Others								

Past Surgical History

Date	Type

Consultants

Funded by a grant from the Bureau of Research. © 2002 American Academy of Osteopathy.
Designed to coordinate with the Established Outpatient Osteopathic SOAP Note Form. Recommended by American Association of Colleges of Osteopathic Medicine.

FIGURE 31.1   The Outpatient Osteopathic SOAP Note Form series. **(A)** Page 1, outpatient health summary.

The two-page revised version of this form (Fig. 31.2) is secured by copyright and is being distributed to interested physicians and schools through the American College of Osteopathic Family Physicians (ACOFP)[25] as well as the AAO.[25] (The more comprehensive four-page version of this note also is available (Fig. 31.1). This SOAP note was the first step in providing standardized documentation for osteopathic family practice. Sufficient data have been collected since its creation that the form is now ready to be used for outcomes research.

Outpatient Osteopathic SOAP Note History Form

wak SOAP version 5: 091102b

Patient's Name _____   Date _____   Age _____

Office of:	
For office use only:	

HISTORY

S   (See Outpatient Health Summary Form for details of history)

Patient's Pain Analog Scale: ☐ Not done

NO PAIN   WORST POSSIBLE PAIN

CC

History of Present Illness   **Level: HPI**

		Elements			
	☐	Location	OR Status of ≥ 3 chronic or inactive conditions	☐	**II**
	☐	Quality			**III** 1-3 elements reviewed
	☐	Severity		☐	**IV**
	☐	Duration			**V** ≥ 4 elements OR status of ≥ 3 chronic conditions
	☐	Timing			
	☐	Context			
	☐	Modifying factors			
	☐	Assoc. Signs and Sx			

Review of Systems (Only ask / record those systems pertinent for this encounter.)   ☐ Not done   **Level: ROS**

☐	Constitutional (Wt loss, etc.)	☐	**II**	None
☐	Eyes	☐	**III**	1 system pertinent to the problem
☐	Ears, nose, mouth, throat			
☐	Cardiovascular	☐	**IV**	2-9 systems
☐	Respiratory	☐	**V**	≥ 10 systems
☐	Gastrointestinal			
☐	Genitourinary			
☐	Musculoskeletal			
☐	Integumentary (skin, breast)			
☐	Neurological			
☐	Psychiatric			
☐	Endocrine			
☐	Hematologic/lymphatic			
☐	Allergic/immunologic			

Past Medical, Family, Social History   ☐ Not done   **Level: PFSH**

☐	Past history / trauma	☐	**II** / **III**	None
☐	Allergies:	☐	**IV**	1 history area
☐	Medications:	☐	**V**	≥ 2 history areas
☐	Family history			
☐	Social history			

Overall History = Average of HPI, ROS or PFSH: ☐ II (1-3 HPI)   ☐ III (1-3 HPI, 1 ROS)   ☐ IV (4+ HPI, 2-9 ROS, 1 PFSH)   ☐ V (4+ HPI, 10+ ROS, 2+ PFSH)

Signature of transcriber: _____   Signature of examiner: _____

Funded by a grant from the Bureau of Research. © 2002 American Academy of Osteopathy.
Designed to coordinate with the Established Outpatient Osteopathic SOAP Note Form. Recommended by American Association of Colleges of Osteopathic Medicine.

FIGURE 31.1   **(B)** Page 2, history. (Continued)

CLINICAL OUTCOMES AND EVIDENCE-BASED MEDICINE

Clinical outcomes have become an important buzzword in the lexicon of managed care. Outcomes are measured to predict the course of an illness and to analyze the effects of various treatment options. Outcomes data can be divided into three groups: input (stratification of patients based on diagnosis), intervention (treatment options), and outcomes (results of treatment on the course of the process).[26] Measuring outcomes has been facilitated by the addition of symptom data (chief

Outpatient Osteopathic SOAP Note Exam Form

wak SOAP version 5: 091102b

O ☐ Not done

Patient's Name _____		Date _____		Sex: Male ☐ Female ☐	
* Vital Signs (3 of 7) Wt. _____		Ht. _____		Temp. _____	
	Reg. ☐	Pt. position for recording BP:			
Resp. ____ Pulse ____	Irreg. ☐	Standing _____ Sitting _____ Lying _____			

Office of: ____

For office use only: ____

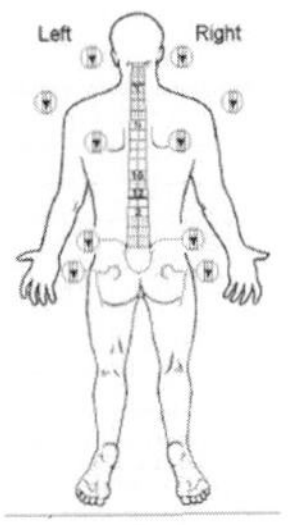

Level of GMS		
☐	**II**	1-5 elements
☐	**III**	6+ elements
☐	**IV**	2+ from each or 6 areas OR 12+ elements in 2+ areas
☐	**V**	Perform all elements ≥ 9 areas

Key to the Severity Scale	0 = No SD or background (BG) levels	2 = Obvious TART (esp. R and T), +/- symptoms
	1 = More than BG levels, minor TART	3 = Key lesions, symptomatic, R and T stand out

	Methods Used For Examination					Region Evaluated	Severity				Somatic Dysfunction and Other Systems MS / SNS / PNS / LYM. / CV / RESP. / GI / FAS. / etc.
	All	T	A	R	T		0	1	2	3	
*1	☐	☐	☐	☐	☐	Head and Face	☐	☐	☐	☐	
	☐	☐	☐	☐	☐	Neck	☐	☐	☐	☐	
	☐	☐	☐	☐	☐	Thoracic T1-4	☐	☐	☐	☐	
	☐	☐	☐	☐	☐	T5-9	☐	☐	☐	☐	
*2	☐	☐	☐	☐	☐	T10-12	☐	☐	☐	☐	
	☐	☐	☐	☐	☐	Ribs	☐	☐	☐	☐	
	☐	☐	☐	☐	☐	Lumbar	☐	☐	☐	☐	
	☐	☐	☐	☐	☐	Sacrum / Pelvis	☐	☐	☐	☐	
	☐	☐	☐	☐	☐	Pelvis / Innom.	☐	☐	☐	☐	
	☐	☐	☐	☐	☐	Abd. / Other	☐	☐	☐	☐	
*3	☐	☐	☐	☐	☐	Upper R	☐	☐	☐	☐	
*4	☐	☐	☐	☐	☐	Extremity L	☐	☐	☐	☐	
*5	☐	☐	☐	☐	☐	Lower R	☐	☐	☐	☐	
*6	☐	☐	☐	☐	☐	Extremity L	☐	☐	☐	☐	

Signature of transcriber: _____   Signature of examiner: _____

Funded by a grant from the Bureau of Research. © 2002 American Academy of Osteopathy.
Designed to coordinate with Outpatient Osteopathic SOAP Note Form. Recommended by American Association of Colleges of Osteopathic Medicine.

FIGURE 31.1   (C) Page 3, physical examination. (Continued)

complaint, or the problem[24]), as well as functional assessments, such as the Rand SF-36.[27] Analysis of outcomes and incorporation into the clinical setting leads to the practice of evidence-based medicine.

Over the past several years, there has been an increasing emphasis on outcome measures in the practice of medicine. Medical outcomes research investigates how a process used in providing health care services affects the outcome of the patient's disease or health status. This type of research does not look at mechanisms or causes of the change in outcome, but only the end result of the procedure. Outcomes can include physical data, treatment results, practice encounter characteristics, types and

Outpatient Osteopathic Assessment and Plan Form

wek SOAP version 5: 091102b

				Office of:	
A Patient's Name _____ Date _____				For office use only:	

Dx No.	ICD Code	Written Diagnosis	Dx No.	ICD Code	Written Diagnosis
	739.0	Somatic Dysfunction of Head and Face		739.4	Somatic Dysfunction of Sacrum
	739.1	Somatic Dysfunction of Neck		739.5	Somatic Dysfunction of Pelvis
	739.2	Somatic Dysfunction of Thoracic		739.9	Somatic Dysfunction of Abd / Other
	739.8	Somatic Dysfunction of Ribs		739.7	Somatic Dysfunction of Upper Extremity
	739.3	Somatic Dysfunction of Lumbar		739.6	Somatic Dysfunction of Lower Extremity

Physician's evaluation of patient prior to treatment: First visit ☐   Resolved ☐   Improved ☐   Unchanged ☐   Worse ☐

P ☐ All not done

Region	OMT		Treatment Method														Response			
	Y	N	ART	BLT	CR	CS	DIR	FPR	HVLA	IND	INR	LAS	ME	MFR	ST	VIS	OTH	R	I	U	W
Head and Face	☐	☐	☐	☐	☐	☐	☐	☐	☐	☐	☐	☐	☐	☐	☐	☐	☐	☐	☐	☐	☐
Neck	☐	☐	☐	☐	☐	☐	☐	☐	☐	☐	☐	☐	☐	☐	☐	☐	☐	☐	☐	☐	☐
Thoracic T1-4	☐	☐	☐	☐	☐	☐	☐	☐	☐	☐	☐	☐	☐	☐	☐	☐	☐	☐	☐	☐	☐
T5-9	☐	☐	☐	☐	☐	☐	☐	☐	☐	☐	☐	☐	☐	☐	☐	☐	☐	☐	☐	☐	☐
T10-12	☐	☐	☐	☐	☐	☐	☐	☐	☐	☐	☐	☐	☐	☐	☐	☐	☐	☐	☐	☐	☐
Ribs	☐	☐	☐	☐	☐	☐	☐	☐	☐	☐	☐	☐	☐	☐	☐	☐	☐	☐	☐	☐	☐
Lumbar	☐	☐	☐	☐	☐	☐	☐	☐	☐	☐	☐	☐	☐	☐	☐	☐	☐	☐	☐	☐	☐
Sacrum	☐	☐	☐	☐	☐	☐	☐	☐	☐	☐	☐	☐	☐	☐	☐	☐	☐	☐	☐	☐	☐
Pelvis	☐	☐	☐	☐	☐	☐	☐	☐	☐	☐	☐	☐	☐	☐	☐	☐	☐	☐	☐	☐	☐
Abdomen/Other	☐	☐	☐	☐	☐	☐	☐	☐	☐	☐	☐	☐	☐	☐	☐	☐	☐	☐	☐	☐	☐
Upper Extremity	☐	☐	☐	☐	☐	☐	☐	☐	☐	☐	☐	☐	☐	☐	☐	☐	☐	☐	☐	☐	☐
Lower Extremity	☐	☐	☐	☐	☐	☐	☐	☐	☐	☐	☐	☐	☐	☐	☐	☐	☐	☐	☐	☐	☐

Meds: _____   PT: _____

Exercise: _____   Other: _____

Nutrition: _____

Complexity / Assessment / Plan (Scoring) *Default to level 2—same criteria

Problems		Risk (presenting problem(s), diagnostic procedure(s), Management options)		Data	Maximum Points
Self-limiting	1 (2 max.)	Minimal = Min.		Lab	1
Estimated problem improved / stable	1	Low		Radiology	1
Estimate—worsening	2	Moderate = Mod.		Medicine	1
New—no workup	3 (1 max.)	High		Discuss with performing physician	1
New—additional workup	4			Obtain record or Hx from others	1
				Review records, discuss with physician	2
				Visualization of tracing, specimen	2

Level I	Level II	Level III	Level IV	Level V	Level I	Level II	Level III	Level IV	Level V	Level I	Level II	Level III	Level IV	Level V
≤1 pt.	2 pt.	3 pt.	≥4 pt.			Min.	Low	Mod.	High		≤1 pt.	2 pt.	3 pt.	≥4 pt.
☐	☐	☐	☐			☐	☐	☐	☐		☐	☐	☐	☐

Requires only 2 above 3 (problems, risk and data).   Level of complexity = average of included areas.

Traditional Method—Coding by Components						Optional Method—Coding by Time					
						When majority of the encounter is counseling / coordinating, the level is determined by total time					
History	I	II	III	IV	V		I	II	III	IV	V
Examination	I	II	III	IV	V	New patients (minutes)	10	20	30	45	60
Complexity / Assessment Plan	I	II	III	IV	V	Established patients (minutes)		10	15	25	40
Final level of service	☐	☐	☐	☐	☐	**Final level of service**	☐	☐	☐	☐	☐
All these areas required. Average of three levels of service.						Dictate total time and counseling / coordinating time plus a brief description of topics discussed					

Minutes spent with the patient:	☐	☐	☐	☐	☐	☐	Follow-up:												Units:	☐	☐	☐	☐
	10	15	25	40	60	>60		1	2	3	4	5	6	7	8	9	10	11	12		D	W	M	Y	PRN

OMT performed as Above:	0 areas ☐	1-2 areas ☐	3-4 areas ☐	5-6 areas ☐	7-8 areas ☐	9-10 areas ☐

Other Procedures Performed:	CPT Codes:										
	Written Dx:										

E/M Code:	New	☐	☐	☐	☐	EST	☐	☐	☐	☐	☐	Consults	☐	☐	☐	☐	☐
Write 992 plus ...		02	03	04	05	...	11	12	13	14	15	...	41	42	43	44	45

Signature of transcriber: _____   Signature of Examiner _____

Funded by a grant from the Bureau of Research. © 2002 American Academy of Osteopathy.
Designed to coordinate with Outpatient Osteopathic SOAP Note Form. Recommended by American Association of Colleges of Osteopathic Medicine.

FIGURE 31.1 **(D)** Page 4, assessment, treatment plan, and determination of E&M level.

frequency of procedures used, frequency of disease, psychological data, satisfaction with treatment, quality of life and function, health care costs, or a combination of these factors.

As managed care organizations and government agencies increasingly rely on clinical outcomes measurements for development of clinical practice guidelines, increasing demands will be placed upon physicians to conform to these guidelines in their practices.[28,29] It has been suggested that a central resource, such as a professional organization, be used to develop practice guidelines, with practitioners within that organization contributing to their development.[30] By participating in

Outpatient Osteopathic SOAP Note—Follow-up Form

wak SOAP Follow-up version 2:011403b

Patient's Name _____ Date _____ Sex: Male ☐ Female ☐ | Office of: | |

Age _____ * Vital Signs (3 of 7) Wt. _____ Ht. _____ Temp. _____

Reg. ☐ Pt. position for recording BP | For office use only: |

Resp. ____ Pulse ____ Irreg. ☐ Standing_____ Sitting_____ Lying_____

S **Patient's Pain Analog Scale:** ☐ Not done

NO PAIN | WORST POSSIBLE PAIN

CC: HPI: (Location, Quality, Severity, Duration, Timing, Context, Modifying factors, Associated Signs and Sx)
PFSH: ROS: (Constitutional, Eyes, Ears/Nose/Mouth/Throat, Cardiovascular, Respiratory, GI, GU, Musculoskeletal, Integumentary, Neurological, Psychiatric, Endocrine, Hematologic/Lymphatic, Allergic/Immunologic)

Meds:

Level: HPI

II	1-3HPI
III	1-3 HPI
IV	4+ HPI
V	4+ HPI

Level ROS

II	None
III	1 ROS
IV	2-9 ROS
V	10+ ROS

Level of PFSH

II	None
III	None
IV	1 PFSH
V	2+ PFSH

Overall History = Average of HPI, ROS or PFSH: ☐ **II** (1-3 HPI) ☐ **III** (1-3 HPI, 1 ROS) ☐ **IV** (4+ HPI, 2-9 ROS, 1 PFSH) ☐ **V** (4+ HPI, 10+ ROS, 2+ PFSH)

O

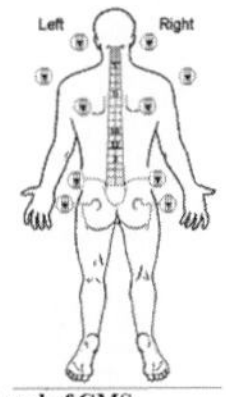

Left | Right

Level of GMS

☐	II	1-5 elements
☐	III	6+ elements
☐	IV	2+ from each of 6 areas OR 12+ elements in 2+ areas
☐	V	2+ elements from each of 9 areas

Signature of transcriber: _____ Signature of examiner: _____

Funded by a grant from the Bureau of Research. © 2002 American Academy of Osteopathy.
Designed to coordinate with the Initial Outpatient Osteopathic SOAP Note Form. Recommended by American Association of Colleges of Osteopathic Medicine.

FIGURE 31.2 The Outpatient Osteopathic SOAP Note, Follow-up Form. **(A)** Page 1, space allocated for demographics, vital signs, and narratives of the subjective and objective portions of the note. (Continued)

this process, not only do clinicians become de facto researchers, but they also of necessity develop lifelong learning skills (and help control their own destiny). The creation of outcomes-based clinical practice guidelines for osteopathic medicine will not only have the effect of standardizing osteopathic medical care on a national basis but will also significantly streamline the process of professional educational assessment. Curricula in undergraduate and graduate programs will change to more accurately reflect the practice of medicine, that is, an integrated, problem-oriented approach.

Outpatient Osteopathic SOAP Note—Follow-up Form   *wak SOAP Follow-up version 2:011403b*

	Office of:
	For Office use only:

Patient's Name _____   Date _____

O (continued)

Exam Method Used					Severity Scale:	**0** = No SD or background (BG) levels **1** = More than BG level, minor TART				**2** = Obvious TART (esp. R and T), +/- symptoms **3** = Key lesions, symptomatic, R and T stands out				

						☐ All not done	Severity				Somatic Dysfunction / Other	OMT		Treatment Method	Response			
	All	T	A	R	T	Region	0	1	2	3	MS/SNS/PNS/LYM/CV/RESP/GI/FAS/ etc.	Y	N	(Circle Method Used)	R	I	U	W
*1						Head and Face	☐	☐	☐	☐		☐	☐	ART / BLT / CR / CS / DIR / FPR / HVLA IND / INR / LAS / ME / MFR / ST / VIS	☐	☐	☐	☐
						Neck	☐	☐	☐	☐		☐	☐	ART / BLT / CR / CS / DIR / FPR / HVLA IND / INR / LAS / ME / MFR / ST / VIS	☐	☐	☐	☐
						Thoracic T1-4	☐	☐	☐	☐		☐	☐	ART / BLT / CR / CS / DIR / FPR / HVLA IND / INR / LAS / ME / MFR / ST / VIS	☐	☐	☐	☐
						T5-9	☐	☐	☐	☐		☐	☐	ART / BLT / CR / CS / DIR / FPR / HVLA IND / INR / LAS / ME / MFR / ST / VIS	☐	☐	☐	☐
						T10-12	☐	☐	☐	☐		☐	☐	ART / BLT / CR / CS / DIR / FPR / HVLA IND / INR / LAS / ME / MFR / ST / VIS	☐	☐	☐	☐
*2						Ribs	☐	☐	☐	☐		☐	☐	ART / BLT / CR / CS / DIR / FPR / HVLA IND / INR / LAS / ME / MFR / ST / VIS	☐	☐	☐	☐
						Lumbar	☐	☐	☐	☐		☐	☐	ART / BLT / CR / CS / DIR / FPR / HVLA IND / INR / LAS / ME / MFR / ST / VIS	☐	☐	☐	☐
						Sacrum / Pelvis	☐	☐	☐	☐		☐	☐	ART / BLT / CR / CS / DIR / FPR / HVLA IND / INR / LAS / ME / MFR / ST / VIS	☐	☐	☐	☐
						Pelvis / Innom.	☐	☐	☐	☐		☐	☐	ART / BLT / CR / CS / DIR / FPR / HVLA IND / INR / LAS / ME / MFR / ST / VIS	☐	☐	☐	☐
						Abd ./ Other	☐	☐	☐	☐		☐	☐	ART / BLT / CR / CS / DIR / FPR / HVLA IND / INR / LAS / ME / MFR / ST / VIS	☐	☐	☐	☐
*3						Upper R	☐	☐	☐	☐		☐	☐	ART / BLT / CR / CS / DIR / FPR / HVLA IND / INR / LAS / ME / MFR / ST / VIS	☐	☐	☐	☐
*4						Extremity L	☐	☐	☐	☐		☐	☐	ART / BLT / CR / CS / DIR / FPR / HVLA IND / INR / LAS / ME / MFR / ST / VIS	☐	☐	☐	☐
*5						Lower R	☐	☐	☐	☐		☐	☐	ART / BLT / CR / CS / DIR / FPR / HVLA IND / INR / LAS / ME / MFR / ST / VIS	☐	☐	☐	☐
*6						Extremity L	☐	☐	☐	☐		☐	☐	ART / BLT / CR / CS / DIR / FPR / HVLA IND / INR / LAS / ME / MFR / ST / VIS	☐	☐	☐	☐

Physician's evaluation of patient prior to treatment: First visit ☐   Resolved ☐   Improved ☐   Unchanged ☐   Worse ☐

A

Dx No.	Written Diagnosis	ICD Code	Dx No.	Written Diagnosis	ICD Code	Dx No.	Written Diagnosis	ICD Code
_____	_____	_____	_____	SD Head and Face	739.0	_____	SD Sacrum	739.4
_____	_____	_____	_____	SD Neck	739.1	_____	SD Pelvis	739.5
_____	_____	_____	_____	SD Thoracic	739.2	_____	SD Abd / Other	739.9
_____	_____	_____	_____	SD Ribs	739.8	_____	SD Upper Extremity	739.7
_____	_____	_____	_____	SD Lumbar	739.3	_____	SD Lower Extremity	739.6

P   Meds: PT:

Exercise: Other:

Nutrition:

Minutes spent with the patient:	☐ 10	☐ 15	☐ 25	☐ 40	☐ 60	☐ >60	Follow-up:	☐ 1	☐ 2	☐ 3	☐ 4	☐ 5	☐ 6	☐ 7	☐ 8	☐ 9	☐ 10	☐ 11	☐ 12	Units:	☐ D	☐ W	☐ M	☐ Y	☐ PRN

Complexity / Assessment / Plan (Scoring) Requires only 2 of the 3 below (Problems, Risk and Data).   Level of complexity = average of the 3 categories recorded

Problems		Risk (presenting problem(s), diagnostic procedure(s), management options)		Data	Maximum Points
Self-limiting	1 (2 max.)	Minimal = Min.	1	Lab	1
Established problem improved / stable	1	Low		Radiology	1
Established—worsening	2	Moderate = Mod.		Medicine	1
New—no workup	3 (1 max.)	High	4	Discuss with performing physician	1
New—additional workup	4			Obtain records or Hx from others	1
				Review records, discuss with physician	2
				Visualization of tracing, specimen	2

Level I	Level II	Level III	Level IV	Level V		Level I	Level II	Level III	Level IV	Level V		Level I	Level II	Level III	Level IV	Level V
-----	≤1 pt.	2 pt.	3 pt.	≥4 pt.		-----	Min.	Low	Mod.	High		-----	≤1 pt.	2 pt.	3 pt.	≥4 pt.
	☐	☐	☐	☐			☐	☐	☐	☐			☐	☐	☐	☐

Traditional Method—Coding by Components						**Optional Method—Coding by Time**					
Average of three levels **equals final** level of service.						When majority of the encounter is counseling / coordinating, the level is determined by total time Dictate total time and counseling / coordinating time plus a brief description of topics discussed					
History	I	II	III	IV	V		I	II	III	IV	V
Examination	I	II	III	IV	V	New patients (minutes)		10	20	30	45	60
Complexity / Assessment / Plan	-----	II	III	IV	V	Established patients (minutes)	-----	10	15	25	40
Final level of service	☐	☐	☐	☐	☐	**Final level** of service	☐	☐	☐	☐	☐

OMT performed as Above:	0 areas ☐	1-2 areas ☐	3-4 areas ☐	5-6 areas ☐	7-8 areas ☐	9-10 areas ☐

Other Procedures Performed:	CPT Codes: _____ Written Dx: _____								

E/M Code:	New	☐	☐	☐	☐	EST	☐	☐	☐	☐	☐	Consults	☐	☐	☐	☐	☐
Write 992 plus ...		02	03	04	05	...	11	12	13	14	15	...		41	42	43	44	45

Signature of transcriber: _____   Signature of examiner: _____

Funded by a grant from the Bureau of Research. © 2002 American Academy of Osteopathy.
Designed to coordinate with the Initial Outpatient Osteopathic SOAP Note Form. Recommended by American Association of Colleges of Osteopathic Medicine.

FIGURE 31.2   (B) Page 2, areas designated to record the diagnostics and treatment of somatic dysfunction, assessment, treatment plan, and determination of E&M level.

In the present medical environment, it is essential that the medical professions be able to conduct outcomes research. To enable medical professions to investigate and validate their treatment, diagnostic, and prevention modalities, methods of clinical data collection in practice-based settings must be developed and validated. This process has begun using the Outpatient Osteopathic SOAP Note Form to collect and report incidences of different disease entities within a family practice.[31]

PREAMBLE TO AN ELECTRONIC MEDICAL RECORD: THE VALIDATED SOAP NOTE FORM

The long-term goal of LBORC's progress note work, defined at the inaugural meeting in 1996, has been the creation of an electronic version of the Outpatient Osteopathic SOAP Note Form for use by all family practitioners, American Academy of Family Physicians (AAFP) as well as ACOFP. Since that meeting, the federal government has mandated that within a decade nearly all Americans must have an electronic medical record.

Recognizing the impending change, the LBORC, in association with Institutional Computing at Des Moines University under the leadership of Bryan Larsen, set out to create an online version of the osteopathic SOAP note form. Named eSOAP, this prototypical online data collection form incorporates an attractive Web interface that resembles the paper SOAP note form but exists on the World Wide Web. The system allows users to log on to a Web site and have a blank SOAP note that can be completed with deidentified patient data. This electronic note is available for use by interested investigators.[32†]

The original purpose of developing eSOAP was to allow the creation of a national osteopathic database that could provide information on practice patterns and efficacy of the diagnostic and therapeutic measures employed by physicians practicing manual medicine. The current design, however is much more flexible, in that additional modules may be incorporated as needed for specific projects or applications.[32‡] This flexibility permits the capabilities of eSOAP to be enhanced. From the research perspective, the current system has successfully completed beta test trials and is considered scientifically validated.[36]

Because the purpose of eSOAP was primarily research, not medial record keeping, it was decided to eliminate private health information (PHI) from the database, since the inclusion of PHI would necessitate specific authorization from each patient represented in this database. The Health Insurance Portability and Accountability Act (HIPAA) requires that specific authorization to use PHI for research must be obtained from research participants. Because it was not certain that such authorization would be collected in every instance, the database was constructed without the inclusion of PHI. eSOAP retains utility for practicing physicians as a chart note, since the physician can, upon completion of the record, print it and affix the patient's identifying information to it for inclusion in the chart.

While the Web-based eSOAP was functional and attractive, its one key drawback was that physicians could not readily complete the eSOAP while seeing patients, since data input required being online. Thus, for most practices, a separate session to input data would be needed. It was concluded that this would reduce participation, a consideration that suggested a new version of eSOAP was needed.

In view of the foregoing, LBORC/IT (Des Moines) began development of a stand-alone personal computer (PC) version of the eSOAP. This has been implemented on a tablet computer that can be used in the examination room during an office visit. The interface for this stand-alone eSOAP product has been redesigned so that many pull-down menus and check boxes are employed to keep the user from having to scroll down long pages of information. The record can contain PHI, since the record will reside on the physician's computer. A hard copy can be printed to go into the patient's permanent record. The inaugural demonstration of

---

†Email: bryan.larsen@dmu.edu. Dean of university research, Des Moines University Osteopathic Medical Center.
‡Email: tglonek@rcn.com. Past chair, LBORC.

"Stand-alone eSOAP" has been announced for the Fall 2006 AOA Convention in Las Vegas, Nevada.

In the course of development of the stand-alone eSOAP, it became apparent that this instrument could be used to document items needed for the AOA's Clinical Assessment Program (CAP). As a result, additional fields have been incorporated into the latest version of the stand-alone eSOAP that will support CAP. As development continues, it will be possible to add increasing levels of functionality as future versions of eSOAP are developed. Ultimately, an interface will be available for the stand-alone eSOAP that will allow upload of deidentified data to the national osteopathic database for major interinstitutional studies of efficacy and practice patterns.

Within the clinic, physicians can use computer progress notes linked to decision support systems to modify their practice patterns in response to a quickly changing environment.[33,34] Third-party payers actually prefer electronic records over handwritten notes or even paper SOAP notes. Keeping electronic medical records (EMRs) is nearly effortless. They tend to be complete, providing thorough documentation for the medical practice with fewer resubmissions, less hassle, and greater reimbursement: the perfect remedy for rising practice costs.

One of the principal advantages of using multisite computer patient records is the capability of recording large quantities of data within a central repository over a relatively short time. With HIPAA-compliant oversight, these data may be analyzed in clinical research studies, vastly increasing efficiency over conventional (analog) methods. The advantages to osteopathic postgraduate training institutions and family medicine residency programs are enormous.

Studies already completed have shown substantial economic advantages. As a group, no matter whether paper notes or electronic media, family physicians habitually undercode. In one small study carried out in 2002, a private physician switched practice recording to use of the SOAP notes, and the estimated yearly revenue increase amounted to $12,000. The increased revenue was due primarily to a 50% increase in the use of level 3 codes over level 2 (Table 31.1). Add computer aids and reminders to this mix to facilitate accurate coding, and reimbursement can only go up.

In addition to providing economic advantages, in the context of outcomes research, EMRs provide a formidable data-handling instrument. It is expected that

TABLE 31.1

Estimated Yearly Revenue Increase Following Use of the SOAP Note Form in a Private Family Practice

Average Yearly Breakdown		January 2002	February 2002[a]
Code Level	Usage (%)	Usage (%)	Usage (%)
2	70	63	38
3	25	33	50
4	4	3	11
5	1	1	1

Estimated yearly increase in revenue: $12,000–14,000

[a]New SOAP note form.

the use of computer records will greatly facilitate the availability of large amounts of standardized, centralized data, addressing the need for outcomes research more efficiently while effectively producing validated practice guidelines for osteopathic family practice.

The Paper SOAP Note Forms

The original SOAP note form, the Outpatient Osteopathic SOAP Note Form, was created and validated with the intent that the note would be as follows:

1. A standardized recording instrument
2. Used by physicians worldwide
3. Easy to use as well as useful in the clinical setting
3. Used to standardize education and the tracking of training;
5. Able to be modified for different research topics
6. Capable of collecting reliable research data quickly

To date, the SOAP notes are standardized, used by physicians worldwide, and have been shown to be easy to use and useful in the clinical setting. Recent retrospective studies have shown the note's ability to collect reliable research data quickly on many topics and to track the training of residents.[35,36]

Imagine trying to get 14 osteopathic physicians to agree on the perfect note for everyone. Difficult? Indeed yes. Impossible? Well, not really. To facilitate consensus prior to the actual creation of the SOAP note, three broad areas of need were identified: clinical practice, education, and research.

- Professional and clinical needs involve providing improved quality patient care, developing practice guidelines, and providing justification for reimbursement in an easy-to-use efficient format.
- Educational needs involve tracking captured experiences, ensuring that distinctively osteopathic educational requirements for accreditation and graduation are met, and providing a training tool for documentation and coding.
- Research needs involve gathering large amounts of quality research data in a standardized format by physicians worldwide using validated instruments, with a framework easily modified for a variety of topics and types of research designs (e.g., retrospective, prospective).

Advantages of Using the Outpatient Osteopathic SOAP Note Forms

Why use a form rather than scribbling on a blank piece of paper? A form is simpler and faster to use, standardized, and it provides unambiguous hardcopy proof of what was done. Further, it saves the practice a great deal of money through coding reminders and by providing proper, easily reviewed documentation. Outlined next are other advantages.

Educational Advantages

- Provides tracking of patient encounters for physicians, students, interns, and residents, including diagnoses, treatments, and procedures. Patient encounters using the SOAP note forms are being analyzed for educational tracking purposes.[35] The use of these forms in training institutions will improve quality by clarifying the accreditation and graduation process.

- Documents whether competency requirements are being met. The series is recommended for use by American Association of Colleges of Osteopathic Medicine (AACOM).
- Provides training and reminders with regard to documentation. Students, interns, and residents who have used the initial SOAP note form found it easy to use and helpful in reminding them of items they were forgetting during patient encounters.[1]
- Provides training in coding. Physicians in training who have used the form in the past now request to use it because of its training value.
- Reminds the author that there may be a musculoskeletal component to consider.
- Provides for a uniform educational tracking infrastructure.

Research Advantages

- Facilitates retrospective chart review[36]
- Facilitates outcomes research[31,35,36]
- Adapts easily for use in prospective studies
- Accepts additional study-specific modules as required
- Allows data to be archived in a nationwide database for access by investigators addressing other research questions. Such an archive also may provide the natural history of a disease or assist in finding anomalous regional health patterns useful in fighting the war on bioterrorism.
- Provides a uniform research infrastructure among cooperating groups
- Has been validated in published studies funded by the AOA[1,35–37]

Profession Advantages

- Uniform notes make auditing and peer review easier on the reviewer.
- Clear coding justification promotes reimbursement.
- The condensed note format promotes documenting more of what occurred during the patient encounter, leading to higher coding levels.
- It minimizes lack of reimbursement or claim rejection due to unclear notes.
- It yields payment when charges look suspicious for diagnoses used, such as with Medicare, prolonged visits, and counseling.
- It renders obvious how many and what body regions are treated.
- It eases credentialing of hospitals, schools, and programs, especially with regard to the musculoskeletal component.
- It provides tracking of patient encounters for improved clinical practice.
- CME credit is available for training in the use of the form.
- A variety of forms are available for specific kinds of patient visits.
- It is time efficient.
- It allows for less thinking about reporting format, hence more thinking about the patient.

Patient Advantages

- Promotes easy tracking of patients' progress overall and progress with respect to pain management through the pain analog scale
- Facilitates clinical guideline development
- Identifies findings that are out of the ordinary to prompt early intervention
- Facilitates quality assurance by peer review
- Makes items in the note, such as diagnoses, treatment, and procedures, easy to find from visit to visit
- Aids in identification of procedures that are helping or not helping the patient and that should be continued or discontinued

The SOAP note forms are effective data-gathering instruments for answering outcomes questions facing osteopathic medicine today. In published outcomes analyses,[31,35,36] questions were answered based on frequencies, averages, correlations, and comparisons. All questions asked could be answered using data from the SOAP note forms. For example, the severity of somatic dysfunction, the number of regions treated with OMT, procedures used, and responses to treatment could all be explored. Questions on averages, such as age, duration of visit, and follow-up time, were answered. Questions on correlations between disease entities and specific OMT procedures used and between severity of somatic dysfunction and OMT treatment response were answered. Questions on differences among doctors, such as the top four diagnoses of each attending physician, were addressed. In addition to answering these kinds of outcomes questions, the SOAP notes provided the following functions: postdoctoral and predoctoral tracking, additional outcomes research into the efficacy of osteopathic intervention, medical science research, autonomic correlation with disease entities, documentation on the natural history of musculoskeletal dysfunction, and billing information. Further, the data permitted internal comparisons among osteopathic physicians.

The Forms

General

Basic information needed for educational and research purposes for tracking and data gathering as determined by LBORC and confirmed by a retrospective study[36] includes the following:

1. First and last name and date of visit on each page
2. Age
3. Patient's pain analog scale
4. Chief complaint
5. Musculoskeletal table(s) to include either checking a box that states "all not done" or some combination of methods used for examination or examination method used (tissue texture change, asymmetry, range of motion, and tenderness [TART]), severity of somatic dysfunction, description of somatic dysfunction findings, whether OMT was performed, what OMT procedures were used, and response to treatment
6. Physician's evaluation of the patient prior to treatment (first visit or resolved or improved or unchanged or worse)
7. Prioritized diagnoses, written out and ICD-9CM-coded
8. Minutes spent with the patient
9. Follow-up recommended in number of days, weeks, months, years or as needed
10. Number of areas on which OMT was performed
11. Other procedures performed, including Current Procedural Terminology (CPT) code and written description
12. E&M code
13. Signatures of examiner and transcriber (if one is used) at the bottom of each page

This basic information includes only information pertinent to the chief complaint and excludes the complete general history, such as the past medical history, health maintenance information, and other data that are not needed for every follow-up visit.

Three versions of the SOAP note form are recommended for use and can be downloaded from the ACOFP and AAO Web sites:[25]

1. Outpatient Osteopathic SOAP Note Form (1998), one page
2. Outpatient Osteopathic SOAP Note—Follow-up Form (revised 2002), two pages (Fig. 31.2)
3. Outpatient Osteopathic SOAP Note Form Series (revised 2002), three or four pages (Fig. 31.1)

Specialty Forms Developed from the Original SOAP Note Forms

1. Outpatient Osteopathic Single Organ System Musculoskeletal Form Series
2. Outpatient Osteopathic Cranial SOAP Note Form[§]
3. Osteopathic Musculoskeletal Examination of the Hospitalized Patient, a one-page inpatient form for only the examination portion of a patient encounter[**]

All of the SOAP notes developed since 1996 are recommended for use by the AOA, AACOM, ACOFP, and AAO. The original one-page note, Outpatient Osteopathic SOAP Note Form, was validated in 1997, with the copyright secured in 1998 and the validation study published in 1999. Although it was adequate at the time, 2 years later a revision process began. This expanded the form to two pages and became the Outpatient Osteopathic SOAP Note Follow-up Form, copyright secured in 2002. Through interaction and feedback from the osteopathic community, it was determined that several notes were needed. An initial-visit form was deemed necessary, and the form was further expanded to become the four-page Outpatient Osteopathic SOAP Note Form Series.

The Outpatient Osteopathic SOAP Note Form Series is intended for use in primary care practice and manipulative medicine specialty practices other than osteopathic practices. The Outpatient Osteopathic Single Organ System Musculoskeletal Form Series (SOS) was validated in 2004.[37] This series is intended for use in osteopathic manipulative medicine specialty practices or whenever a complete musculoskeletal examination is needed, such as during an initial history and physical. The main difference between the SOAP note series and the SOS is the examination form. In the SOS, the examination form is detailed to include items needed for a comprehensive examination for coding. In addition, it suggests items that the physician may want to track or that are useful in osteopathic treatment. The Outpatient Osteopathic Cranial SOAP Note Form D is designed specifically for osteopathic physicians who primarily use cranial osteopathy or for patients who have a head disorder or dysfunction.

All of these forms can be used together or separately in an outpatient office in any manner the practitioner chooses. For example, on an initial visit one could use the Outpatient Osteopathic SOAP Note Form Series. At the first visit, the physician finds that the patient has low back pain, and on a return visit, a complete musculoskeletal examination is given. For this return visit, one could use the Outpatient Osteopathic Single Organ System Musculoskeletal Form Series. For subsequent follow-up visits for OMT, the Outpatient Osteopathic SOAP Note–Follow-up Form will work well for recording the encounters. All of these forms contain the basic information needed for clinical, educational, and research purposes. The original Outpatient Osteopathic SOAP Note Form was designed so

---

[§]Spearheaded by LBORC member Miriam Mills.
[**]Spearheaded by LBORC member Michael Kuchera.

that physicians could make up their own expanded versions for clinical or research purposes so as long as they contained the basic required information and appeared in the same general format of the original note. The basic information and formatting are important for ease of data extraction.

In 1998, for the inpatient arena, the Osteopathic Musculoskeletal Examination–Hospital Form and Instruction Manual was developed. Shortly thereafter, the AOA House of Delegates recommended the form for use by osteopathic students and residents in the hospital setting.[38] The principles and basic information of the Outpatient Osteopathic SOAP Note Form were put to yet another use.

The salient feature of all of these forms is the uniquely osteopathic musculoskeletal table. This table includes TART for regions examined, presence and severity of somatic dysfunction, and sometimes, depending on the form, whether OMT was done, what modalities were used, and what the response to treatment was.

The Forms: Detail

The original Outpatient Osteopathic SOAP Note Form, now obsolete, was a one-page note. It was the simplest paper version and was easy to use in clinical practice but was limited in the amount of space available for charting. It was designed for use in the outpatient setting, usually for a follow-up or return visit. From the research perspective, it already has been applied successfully to outcomes research in family practice.[31] However, it collected minimal data and was very deficient in gaining useful information about diagnoses. It also has been used for educational tracking.[1,31]

The revised Outpatient Osteopathic SOAP Note–Follow-up Form, the preferred established-patient note for private practice, is a two-page note[25] (Fig. 31.2). This form is an expanded version of the original SOAP note form that provides additional space for handwritten notes in the subjective and objective sections and a more structured and detailed way of listing diagnosis. In addition, there is considerably greater detail with regard to coding, particularly in the subjective, assessment, and plan sections of the form. When copied front to back, the form may be placed on a single sheet of paper, making it easier to manipulate during the patient encounter while reducing pages in the patient's chart, two features that are readily appreciated in busy practices.

The revised Outpatient Osteopathic SOAP Note Form Series, the preferred note for a new patient visit and physicians in training, is a three- to four-page note[25] (Fig. 31.1). This series includes an outpatient health summary (filled in mostly during the first visit) and three pages for the progress note, the history form, examination form, and assessment and plan form. It contains more information but is still simple and easy to use once one is familiar with its format. It has more room to write subjective and objective findings and an increase in coding training information. Because of this it is designed for use in the outpatient setting, usually for a new patient. With more coding guidelines included, this is the ideal note for physicians in training to use with new-patient and follow-up visits. From the educational tracking and research perspectives, these notes are considered equally competent, as they both contain the essential information deemed necessary by the LBORC.

The SOS form is a three- to four-page note (with summary page) designed to complement the SOAP note form.[25,37,39] Its use at the initial visit allows the other SOAP note forms to be used most effectively as follow-up forms. In addition to the information in the musculoskeletal table, the SOS form includes such items as gait and station, spinal curves, examination positions, leg lengths, levelness of landmarks, reflexes, and motor evaluation that is required in a comprehensive examination of the musculoskeletal system. Other areas of the form include the general appearance, cardiovascular, lymphatic, skin and neurologic/psychiatric examinations. These specific areas were included for coding purposes and are listed in box form for easy use. The SOS form is structured so that if all areas and boxes are filled, the physician will have met all coding criteria for reimbursement for a level 5 comprehensive examination as set forth by the May 1997 Health Care Financing Administration.

The Outpatient Osteopathic Cranial SOAP Note Form is a specialty form for use with outpatients who have significant cranial dysfunction. It simplifies documentation of cranial findings and the results of treatment.[25]

The Osteopathic Musculoskeletal Examination of the Hospitalized Patient is the inpatient form recommended by the AOA for the standardized hospital structural examination in all osteopathic hospitals.[25,38] It is a one-page form with an optional worksheet that has many of the features of the SOAP note series form, most notably the presence of the musculoskeletal somatic dysfunction table. This form is limited in that it contains the examination portion but no history, assessment, plan, or treatment given during a patient encounter.

Outpatient Osteopathic SOAP Note Form Series: Form Pages

Of the three SOAP note forms available, this version is the most comprehensive. It includes the Outpatient Health Summary Form, the Outpatient Osteopathic SOAP Note History Form (page 1 of 3), the Outpatient Osteopathic SOAP Note Examination Form (page 2 of 3), and the Outpatient Osteopathic Assessment and Plan Form (page 3 of 3) (Fig. 31.1, A–D). On these forms, bold black boxes are provided for many of the entries that indicate the data critical to research and required to be filled in. The format of these forms was designed so that data could easily be collected and analyzed by computer and so that additions to the form could be made without disruption of basic data gathering. All definitions are obtained from the standard CPT and ICD-9CM books and the Glossary of Osteopathic Terminology.[40] This valid, standardized, and easy-to-use form is our best recommendation for research and training in osteopathic medicine.

Outpatient Health Summary is the front left-hand page of a two-section chart system or the front page of a one-section chart (Fig. 31.1A). This page is reviewed at each patient visit, and all sections are kept current. It is divided into six sections:

I. Identification and disposition
II. Social and family history
III. Past medical history
IV. Health maintenance
V. Past surgical history
VI. Consultants

At each patient visit, this section provides rapid retrieval of past medical, surgical, social, family, allergy, and medication history and a list of consultants, routine screening dates, and immunizations. This form also contains general demographic information, including date of birth, sex, marital status, significant others, religion, date and updates, phone numbers, do-not-resuscitate status, and whom and how to call in case of an emergency.

The outpatient history form, page 1 of 3, provides the subjective portion of a SOAP note for an outpatient visit (Fig. 31.1*B*). It is divided into two sections:

I. Patient's name, date, age, pain analog scale, and chief complaint
II. History of present illness, review of systems, and past medical, family, and social history

The second section is designed to make the counting of elements easy for billing purposes. Once items in each section are counted, the physician can choose the appropriate level of coding simply by looking to the left of each section. At the bottom of the page, the three sections above are collated to compute a final history level to be used on the last page to determine the E&M service code.

Outpatient Osteopathic SOAP Note Exam Form, page 2 of 3, provides space for the objective, or physical examination, findings section of the SOAP note (Fig. 31.1*C*). It is divided into four sections:

I. The patient's name, date, sex, and vital signs
II. Objective section (continued)
III. Horizontal planes and level of general multisystem examination
IV. Musculoskeletal table

Physical findings for any areas or systems of the general multisystem examination are recorded in the objective section. A diagram is used on this page to indicate levelness of landmarks. The diagram is placed for the convenience of the recorder and can be used in any way the recorder wishes. It is not essential to collect baseline research data. Starred areas on this page are for coding assistance. Key points to remember are that each extremity is counted individually for elements in the examination section but are grouped in the treatment section and that the spine (thoracic, ribs, lumbar, sacrum/pelvis, pelvis/innom., abd./other) is grouped in the examination section but counted separately in the treatment section. Each TART criterion for each examination region is counted as one element. An examination conducted in the usual osteopathic manner would then provide four elements per specified region. The allowed regions—(1) head, face, and neck; (2) spine; (3) right upper extremity; (4) left upper extremity; (5) right lower extremity; (6) left lower extremity—are grouped and starred on the form for easy remembrance. A coding guide for the final examination level is present on the form. The final examination code can then be transferred to the third page for computing the final level of the E&M service code for the visit.

Outpatient Osteopathic SOAP Note Assessment and Plan Form, page 3 of 3, is divided into six sections beginning with the assessment section of the SOAP note (Fig. 31.1*D*).

I. Patient's name and date
II. Diagnosis and evaluation prior to treatment
III. Plan: somatic dysfunction region, OMT done, treatment method(s) used, and response to OMT
IV. Other treatment methods used
V. Coding
VI. Minutes spent with the patient, follow-up, units, OMT performed as above (number of areas), other procedures performed, and E&M codes

The newest forms provide for prioritization of diagnoses and space for both written diagnoses and their associated ICD-9CM codes. Space is provided for other treatment methods, such as medicaments, exercise, nutrition, physical therapy, and anything else that a physician might order. The coding section includes criteria for both coding by components and coding by time, whichever the physician may need for a particular visit. Areas where OMT can be performed include head and face, neck, thoracic, ribs, lumbar, sacrum, pelvis, abdomen/other, upper extremity, and lower extremity. This page also includes the table for figuring the final level of service E&M code, the aggregate of each final level of service for the history, examination, and medical decision making.

All other versions of the SOAP forms are variations on these forms. They all have the basic essential information for research and tracking purposes but have more or less information in specific areas.

Usage Guides, Materials, and Courses Available

Published and bound usage guides (secured by copyright) for three of the SOAP notes, each of which contains blank full-page copies of the forms, may be obtained in hardcopy versions, without charge, from the American Academy of Osteopathy (3500 DePauw Blvd., Suite 1080, Indianapolis, IN 46236-1136). The forms are titled Outpatient Osteopathic SOAP Note Form Series, Outpatient Osteopathic SOAP Note Follow-Up Form, and Outpatient Osteopathic Single Organ System Musculoskeletal Form Series. In addition, each form, including the Outpatient Osteopathic Cranial SOAP Note Form, may be downloaded from the AAO's Web site[25] or the Web site of the ACOFP.[25]

The Osteopathic Musculoskeletal Examination of the Hospitalized Patient is available through the Web site of the ACOFP.[25]

An instructor's kit for training users to be certified (for quality assurance) also is available upon request from the LBORC chair.[††] Participant kits identical to that used in the conventions' certification course are available through the AAO.

The training kit contains the following modules:

1. Participant List Form for certification of the Outpatient Osteopathic Single Organ System (SOS) and SOAP Note Form Series
2. Physician Demographic/Participation Form
3. Training outlines for the Outpatient Osteopathic SOS Musculoskeletal Exam Form Series and Outpatient Osteopathic SOAP Note Form Series
4. Current applications
5. Training objectives for the Outpatient Osteopathic SOS and SOAP Note Forms
6. Usage guides, with blank forms, for the Outpatient Osteopathic SOAP Note Form Series, the SOAP Note Form (short form), the Follow-up Form, and the SOS Musculoskeletal Form Series
7. Documentation guidelines and coding, including E&M coding and documentation guidelines, 1995, 1997
8. Additional data survey tools (Rand 36-Item Health Survey 1.0 [SF36], Rand Health Sciences Program; Musculoskeletal Outcomes Data Evaluation and Management System; Consumer Satisfaction Survey, 2nd edition, GHAA/Davies & Ware; Specialized Osteopathic Questionnaire, LBORC, AOA for Osteopathic Manipulative Medicine Patient Satisfaction)
9. Certification process, including instructions, case studies, and blank forms

---

[††]Contact the LBORC chair, now Michael A. Seffinger, Department of Osteopathic Manipulative Medicine, College of Osteopathic Medicine of the Pacific, Western University of Health Sciences, 309 East Second Street, Pomona, CA 91766-1854.

10. A CD-ROM containing a PowerPoint tutorial on the use of the notes
11. A DVD audio tutorial on the use of the notes

CONCLUDING REMARKS

SOAP note instruments are a set of tools for documenting all aspects of the clinical practice of osteopathic medicine, particularly those that address efficacy in the realm of musculoskeletal diagnosis and treatment. The importance of this cannot be overstated, because it is the diagnosis and treatment of somatic dysfunction that to a great extent distinguish osteopathic medicine from all other medical professions.

When first seen, SOAP note instruments present a daunting obstacle. Like income tax forms, they are horrible, ugly things. These authors, however, are not going to apologize for them because these notes or something very much like them will soon be here for every overworked practicing physician to complete.

But really, honorable colleagues—come on. Adapt. Let young postdoctoral students lead the way. Let the students teach the teachers! They are the new century's experts at filling out forms and computer data entry sheets, and they can demonstrate that it's not so bad. It is not necessary to fill out the whole form, only what has been done. Within a brief time, after the physician is accustomed to the positions of items on the form, the forms actually will facilitate an organized approach to clinical practice. This approach will be consistent among otherwise independent family practitioners, and this consistency will defeat much of the chaos in daily practice and in osteopathic research.

Independent family practitioners may not wish to submit themselves to practicing in such a regimented fashion, but in point of fact, third-party payers already require them to do so to get paid.

Certain aspects are common to any variety of the practice of family medicine. Anatomy is common. The physical examination is common. These are fairly easy to deal with in a standardized progress note. Other aspects are a jumble of constantly changing items that continually must be sorted out: medicaments, the formulary, laboratory tests, coding, and psychosocial issues (home life, culture, poverty, level of education, compliance, support systems). These are difficult—some say impossible—to deal with. Nevertheless, the pressure to yield to standardization will continually mount. The only practical course of action is for all to participate. Jump in, give it a good try, and watch the money, quality training, and research evidence fly.

ACKNOWLEDGMENTS

We thank the SOAP Committee of 01-12-96, Sandra L. Sleszynski, DO, Chairman; Jane Carreiro, DO; Thomas Glonek, PhD; Rebecca Harris, DO; William Johnston, DO; Robert Kappler, DO, FAAO; Albert Kelso, PhD' Michael Kuchera, DO, FAAO; Kim Sing Lo, DO; Kenneth Nelson, DO, FAAO, FACOFP; Lynn Newlun; Stephen Noone, CAE; Michael Patterson, PhD; David Yens, PhD.

References

1. Sleszynski SL, Glonek T, Kuchera WA. Standardized medical record: A new outpatient osteopathic SOAP form: Validation of a standardized office form against physician's progress notes. J Am Osteopath Assoc 1999;10:516–529.

2. Draft E & M documentation guidelines. Centers for Medicare and Medicaid Services. Available at http://cms.hhs.gov. June 2000. Accessed February 23, 2005.

3. Jorgensen DJ. How to examine the examination and decide on medical decision making. 2003. American College of Osteopathic Family Physicians web publication. Available at http://www.acofp.org/member_publications/examination.htm. Accessed February 23, 2005.

4. Jorgensen DJ, Jorgensen RT. A Physician's Guide to Billing and Coding. Manchester, ME: Authors, 2004:61–65. (Available through American Academy of Osteopathy, Indianapolis.)

5. Gevitz N. 'Parallel and distinctive': the philosophic pathway for reform in osteopathic medical education. J Am Osteopath Assoc 1994;94:328–332 [review].

6. Frank L. Epidemiology. The epidemiologist's dream: Denmark. Science 2003;301(5630): 163–EOA.

7. Korr IM. Osteopathic research: The needed paradigm shift. J Am Osteopath Assoc 1991;91:161–168.

8. Ross-Lee B, Weiser MA. Healthcare regulation, past, present and future. J Am Osteopath Assoc 1994;94:74–78.

9. Seffinger MA, Friedman HD, Johnston WL. Standardization of the hospital record for osteopathic structural examination: Recording of musculoskeletal findings and somatic dysfunction diagnosis. J Am Osteopath Assoc 1995;95:90–96.

10. Chila AG. Aspects of osteopathic clinical research. Osteopath Ann 1983;11:292–293.

11. Chila AG. Research in manipulative therapy. Osteopath Ann 1983;11:294–295.

12. Ward RC. Research in osteopathic practice: Many dilemmas and some opportunities. Osteopath Ann 1983;11:296–299.

13. Patterson MM. Osteopathic research: Wither or whither? Osteopathic Ann 1983;11:300–305.

14. Harakal JH. Research and practice: A common ground. Osteopath Ann 1983;11:306–307.

15. Chila AG. Somatic dysfunction as the independent variable in clinical research. Osteopath Ann 1983;11:308–311.

16. Measel JW Jr. A team approach to clinical research. Osteopath Ann 1983;11:312–314.

17. Sinclair RJ. Conducting research with an osteopathic physician: Problems and possible solutions. Osteopath Ann 1983;11:315–317.

18. Upledger JE. Craniosacral function in brain dysfunction. Osteopath Ann 1983;11:318–324.

19. Kelso AF. Records to assist osteopathic physicians. J Am Osteopath Assoc. 1975;74:751–754.

20. Friedman HD, Johnston WL, Kelso AF, Schwartz FN. Effects of an educational intervention on quality and frequency of osteopathic structural documentation on hospital admitting examination. J Am Osteopathic Assoc 1990;90:840-EOA.

21. Weed LL. Medical records, patient care, and medical education. Ir J Med Sci 1964;17: 271–282.

22. Weed LL. Medical records that guide and teach. N Engl J Med 1968;278:593–600, 652–657.

23. Weed LL. Medical Records, Medical Education, and Patient Care. Cleveland, OH: Case Western Reserve University, 1969.

24. Weed LL. Implementing the Problem-Oriented Medical Record. 2nd ed. Seattle: Medical Computer Services, 1976.

25. SOAP Note availability expands. American Academy of Osteopathy. May 2004;9:EOA. Available as a .pdf file on download from http://www.academyofosteopathy.org or contact the American Academy of Osteopathy, 3500 DePauw Boulevard, Suite 1080, Indianapolis, IN 46236-1136; Tel. (317) 879-1881. Also available through the ACOFP web site, http://www.acofp.org.

26. Dolin RH. Outcome analysis: Considerations for an electronic health record. MD Comput Jan–Feb 1997;14(1):50–56 [review].

27. Ware S, Sherbounie C. The MOS 36 Item Short Form Health Survey (SF36): I. Conceptual framework and item selection. Med Care 1992;30:473–483.

28. Carrey RM, Engelhard CL. Academic medicine meets managed care: A high impact collision. Academic Med 1996;71:839–845.

29. McCormick KA, Cummings MA, Kovner C. The role of the Agency for Health Care Policy and Research in improving outcomes of health care. Nurs Clin North Am 1997;32:521–542.

30. Owens DK. Use of medical informatics to implement and develop clinical practice guidelines. W J Med 1998;168:166–175.

31. Nelson KE, Glonek T. Computer/outcomes: Hardcopy SOAP Note preliminary report: Family physician. Fam Physician 1999;3(8):8–10.
32. http://www.red-c.dmu.edu. Users must be certified and authorized.
33. Evidence-Based Medicine Workgroup. Evidence-based medicine: A new approach to teaching the practice of medicine. JAMA 1992;268:2420–2425.
34. Michaud GC, McGowan SL, Van Der Jagt RH, et al. The introduction of evidence-based medicine as a component of daily practice. Bull Med Libr Assoc 1996;84:478–481.
35. Licciardone JC, Nelson KE, Glonek T, et al. Osteopathic manipulative treatment of somatic dysfunction among patients in the family clinic setting: A retrospective analysis. J Am Osteopath Assoc 2005;105(12):537–544.
36. Sleszynski SL, Glonek T. Outpatient Osteopathic SOAP Note Form: Preliminary results in osteopathic outcomes-based research. J Am Osteopath Assoc 2005;105:181–205.
37. Sleszynski SL, Glonek T, Kuchera WA. Outpatient Osteopathic Single Organ System Musculoskeletal Examination Form Series: Validation of the Outpatient Osteopathic SOS Musculoskeletal Examination Form, a new standardized medical record. J Am Osteopath Assoc 2004;104:423–438.
38. Ettlinger H. Treatment of the acutely ill hospitalized patient. In: Ward RC, ed. Foundations for Osteopathic Medicine. 2nd ed. Philadelphia: Lippincott Williams & Wilkins, 2002;1115–1142.
39. Sleszynski SL, Glonek T, Kuchera WA. Outpatient Osteopathic Single Organ System Musculoskeletal Examination Form: Training and certification. J Am Osteopath Assoc 2004;104:76–81.
40. ECOP. Glossary of osteopathic terminology. In: Ward RC, ed. Foundations for Osteopathic Medicine. 2nd ed. Philadelphia: Lippincott Williams & Wilkins, 2002;1229–1253.

American Osteopathic Association Position Paper on Osteopathic Manipulative Treatment of the Cervical Spine

Adopted by AOA House of Delegates, July 17, 2004[*]

BACKGROUND AND STATEMENT OF ISSUE

There has recently been an increasing concern about the safety of cervical spine manipulation. Specifically, this concern has centered on devastating negative outcomes such as stroke. This paper will present the evidence behind the benefit of cervical spine manipulation, explore the potential harm and make a recommendation about its use.

BENEFIT

Spinal manipulation has been reviewed in meta-analysis published as early as 1992, showing a clear benefit for low back pain.[1] There is less available information in the literature about manipulation in regards to neck pain and headache, but the evidence does show benefit.[2-6] There have been at least 12 randomized controlled trials of manipulative treatment of neck pain. Some of the benefits shown include relief of acute neck pain, reduction in neck pain as measured by validated instruments in sub-acute and chronic neck pain compared with muscle relaxants or usual medical care. There is also short-term relief from tension-type headaches.[7]

---

[*]From American Osteopathic Association position paper on osteopathic manipulative treatment of the cervical spine, Adopted by AOA House of Delegates, July 17, 2004. AAO Newsletter 2004 (August): 15–17.

Manipulation relieves cervicogenic headache and is comparable to commonly used first line prophylactic prescription medications for tension-type headache and migraine.[8] Meta-analysis of 5 randomized controlled trials showed that there was a statistically significant reduction in neck pain using a visual analogue scale.[9]

HARM

Since 1925, there have been approximately 275 cases of adverse events reported with cervical spine manipulation.[10–13] It has been suggested by some that there is an under-reporting of adverse events.[10] A conservative estimate of the number of cervical spine manipulations per year is approximately 33 million and may be as high as 193 million in the US and Canada.[14,15] The estimated risk of adverse outcome following cervical spine manipulation ranges from 1 in 400,000 to 1 in 3.85 million manipulations.[16–19] The estimated risk of major impairment following cervical spine manipulation is 6.39 per 10 million manipulations.[20] Most of the reported cases of adverse outcome have involved "Thrust" or "High Velocity/Low Amplitude" types of manipulative treatment.[11] Many of the reported cases do not distinguish the type of manipulative treatment provided. However, the risk of a vertebrobasilar accident (VBA) occurring spontaneously is nearly twice the risk of a VBA resulting from cervical spine manipulation.[7] This includes cases of ischemic stroke and vertebral artery dissection. A concern has been raised by a recent report that VBA following cervical spine manipulation is unpredictable.[10] This report is biased because all of the cases were involved in litigation. The nature of litigation can lead to inaccurate reporting by patient or provider. However, it did conclude that VBA following cervical spine manipulation is "idiosyncratic and rare." Further review of this data showed that 25% of the cases presented with sudden onset of new and unusual headache and neck pain often associated with other neurologic symptoms that may have represented a dissection in progress.[21] In direct contrast to this concern of unpredictability, another recent report states that cervical spine manipulation may worsen preexisting cervical disc herniation or even cause cervical disc herniation. This report describes complications such as radiculopathy, myelopathy, and vertebral artery compression by a lateral cervical disc herniation.[12] The authors concluded that the incidence of these types of complications could be lessened by rigorous adherence to published exclusion criteria for cervical spine manipulation.[12] The current literature does not clearly distinguish the type of provider (i.e., MD, DO, DC, or PT) or manipulative treatment (manipulation vs mobilization) provided in cases associated with VBA. This information may help to understand the mechanism of injury leading to VBA, as there are differences in education and practice among the various professions that utilize this type of treatment.

COMPARISON OF ALTERNATIVE TREATMENTS

NSAIDs are the most commonly prescribed medications for neck pain. Approximately 13 million Americans use NSAIDs regularly.[32] 81% of GI bleeds related to NSAID use occur without prior symptoms.[32] Research in the United Kingdom has shown NSAIDs will cause 12,000 emergency admissions and 2,500 deaths per year due to GI tract complications.[22] The annual cost of GI tract complications in the US is estimated at $3.9 billion, with up to 103,000 hospitalizations and at least 16,500 deaths per year.[23,24,32] This makes GI toxicity from NSAIDs the 15th most common cause of death in the United States.[32] Epidural steroid injection is a popular treatment for neck pain. Common risks include subdural injection, intrathecal injection and intravascular injection.[35] Subdural injection occurs in ~1% of procedures.[35] Intrathecal injection occurs in ~0.6–10.9% of procedures.[35] Intravascular injection is the most significant risk and occurs in ~2% of procedures and ~8% of procedures in pregnant patients.[35] Cervical epidural abscess is rare, but has been reported in the literature.[36]

PROVOCATIVE TESTS

Provocative tests such as the DeKline test have been studied in animals and humans. This test and others like it were found to be unreliable for demonstrating reproducibility of ischemia or risk of injuring the vertebral artery.[25–30]

RISK FACTORS

VBA accounts for 1.3 in 1000 cases of stroke, making this a rare event. Approximately 5% of patients with VBA die as a result, while 75% have a good functional recovery.[33] The most common risk factors for VBA are migraine, hypertension, oral contraceptive use and smoking.[31] Elevated homocysteine levels, which have been implicated in cardiovascular disease, may be a risk factor for VBA.[34] A study done in 1999 reviewing 367 cases of VBA reported from 1966–1993 showed 115 cases related to cervical spine manipulation; 167 were spontaneous, 58 from trivial trauma and 37 from major trauma.[31] Complications from cervical spine manipulation most often occur in patients who have had prior manipulation uneventfully and without obvious risk factors for VBA.[7] "Most vertebrobasilar artery dissections occur in the absence of cervical manipulation, either spontaneously or after trivial trauma or common daily movements of the neck, such as backing out of the driveway, painting the ceiling, playing tennis, sneezing, or engaging in yoga exercises."[10] In some cases manipulation may not be the primary insult causing the dissection, but an aggravating factor or coincidental event.[21] It has been proposed that thrust techniques that use a combination of hyperextension, rotation and traction of the upper cervical spine will place the patient at greatest risk of injuring the vertebral artery. In a retrospective review of 64 medical legal cases, information on the type of manipulation was available in 39 (61%) of the cases. 51% involved rotation, with the remaining 49% representing a variety of positions including lateral flexion, traction and isolated cases of non-force or neutral position thrusts. Only 15% reported any form of extension.[21]

CONCLUSION

Osteopathic manipulative treatment of the cervical spine, including but not limited to High Velocity/Low Amplitude treatment, is effective for neck pain and is relatively safe, especially in comparison to other common treatments. Because of the very small risk of adverse outcomes, trainees should be provided with sufficient information so they are advised of the potential risks. There is a need for research to distinguish the risk of VBA associated with manipulation done by provider type and to determine the nature of the relationship between different types of manipulative treatment and VBA. Therefore, it is the position of the American Osteopathic Association that all modalities of osteopathic manipulative treatment of the cervical spine, including High Velocity/Low Amplitude, should continue to be taught at all levels of education, and that osteopathic physicians should continue to offer this form of treatment to their patients.

References

1. Shekelle, P, Adams, A, et al. Spinal manipulation for low-back pain. Annals of Internal Medicine 1992;117(7):590–598.
2. Koes, BW, Bouter, LM, et al. The effectiveness of manual therapy, physiotherapy, and treatment by the general practitioner for nonspecific back and neck complaints, a randomized clinical trial. Spine 1992;17(1):28–35.
3. Koes, B, Bouter, L, et al. Randomised clinical trial of manipulative therapy and physiotherapy for persistent back and neck complaints: results of one year follow up. BMJ 1992;304: 601–605.
4. Koes BW, Bouter LM van Marmeren H, et al. A randomized clinical trial of manual therapy and physiotherapy for persistent neck and back complaints: sub-group analysis and relationship between outcome measures. J Manipulative Physio Ther 1993;16:211–219.
5. Cassidy JD, Lopes AA, Yong-Hing K. The immediate effect of manipulation versus mobilization on pain and range of motion in the cervical spine: A randomized controlled trial. J Manipulative Physio Ther 1992;15:570–575.
6. Jensen OK, Nielsen FF, Vosmar L. An open study comparing manual therapy with the use of cold packs in the treatment of posttraumatic headache. Cephalgia 1990;10:241–250.
7. Hurwitz EL, Aker PD, Adams AH, Meeker WC, et al. Manipulation and Mobilization of the Cervical Spine. A systematic review of the literature. Spine 1996;21(15):1746–1756.
8. Bronfort G, Assendelft WJ, Evans R, Haas M, Bouter. Efficacy of spinal manipulation for chronic headache: a systematic review. J of Manip & Physio Ther 2001;27(7):457–466.
9. Gross AR, Aker PD, Goldsmith CH, Peloso P. Conservative management of mechanical neck disorders. A systematic overview and meta-analysis. Online J Curr Clin Trials. 1996; Doc No 200–201.
10. Haldeman S, Kohlbeck FJ and McGregor M. Unpredictability of cerebrovascular ischemia associated with cervical spine manipulation: A review of 64 cases after cervical spine manipulation therapy. Spine 2002;27:49–55.
11. Assendelft WJJ, Bouter LM and Knipschild PG. Complications of spinal manipulation: A comprehensive review of the literature. J Fam Pract 1996;42:475–480.
12. Malone DG, Baldwin NG, Tomecek FJ, Boxell CM, et al. Complications of cervical spine manipulation therapy: 5-Year retrospective study in a single-group practice. Neurosurg Focus 13(6), 2002.
13. Vick DA, McKay C, Zengerle CR. The safety of manipulative treatment: review of the literature from 1925 to 1993. JAOA 1996;96(2):113–115.
14. Haldeman S, Carey P, Townsend M, Papadopoulos C. Arterial dissection following cervical manipulation. The chiropractic experience. CMAJ 2001;165:905–906.
15. Hurwitz EL, Coulter ID, Adams AH, Genovese BJ, Shekelle PG. Use of chiropractic services from 1985 through 1991 in the United States and Canada. Am J Public Health 1998;88: 771–776.
16. Jenson et al. Complications of cervical manipulation, General Forensic Science 1987;32(4): 1089–1094.
17. Koss RW. Quality assurance monitoring of osteopathic manipulative treatment. JAOA 1990;90(5):427–433.
18. Dvorak J, Orelli F. How dangerous is manipulation to the cervical spine? Case report and results of a survey. Manual Med 1985;2:1–4.
19. Carey P. A report on the occurrence of cerebral vascular accidents in chiropractic practice. J Can Chiropract Assoc 1993;37:104–106.
20. Coulter ID, Hurwitz EL, Adams AH, et al. The appropriateness of manipulation and mobilization of the cervical spine. Santa Monica CA: Rand, 1996.
21. Haldeman S, Kohlbeck FJ, McGregor. Stroke, cerebral artery dissection, and cervical spine manipulative therapy. J of Neurol 2002;249:1098–1104.
22. Blower Al, Brooks A, Fenn CG et al. Emergency Admissions for Upper Gastrointestinal Disease and Their Relation to NSAIDs Use. Alimart. Pharmacology Ther, 1997;11:283–291.
23. Fries JF, Miller SR, Spitz PW, Williams CA, Hubert HB, Bloch DA. Toward an epidemiology of gastropathy associated with nonsteroidal anti-inflammatory drug use. Gastroenterology. 1989;96:647–655.

24. Bloom BS. Direct medical costs of disease and gastrointestinal side effects during treatment for arthritis. Am J Med 1988;84(suppl 2A):20–24.

25. Licht PB et al. Vertebral artery flow and cervical manipulation: an experimental study. J Manipulative Physiol Ther 1999;Sep; 22(7):431–435.

26. Cote P, Kreitz BG, Cassidy JD, et al. The validity of extension-rotation tests as a clinical screening procedure before neck manipulation: A secondary analysis. J Manipulative Physio Yher 1996;19:159–164.

27. Refshauge KM. Rotation: A valid premanipulative dizziness test? Does it predict safe manipulation? J Manipulative Physio Ther 1994;17:15–19.

28. Stevens A. A functional doppler sonography of the vertebral artery and some considerations about manual techniques. J Manual Med 1991;6:102–105.

29. Theil H, Wallace K, Donat J, et al. Effect of various head and neck positions on vertebral artery blood flow. Clin Biomech 1994;9:105–110.

30. Weingart JR, Bischoff HP. Doppler sonography of the vertebral artery with regard to head positions appropriate to manual medicine. J Manual Medicine 1992;6:62–65.

31. Haldeman S, Kohlbeck FJ, McGregor M. Risk factors and precipitating neck movements causing vertebrobasilar artery dissection after cervical trauma and spinal manipulation: Spine 1999;24:785–794.

32. Wolfe M, Lichtenstein D, Singh G. Gastrointestinal Toxicity of Nonsteroidal Antiinflammatory Drugs. N Engl J Med June 17, 1999;340(24):1888–1899.

33. Schievink W. Spontaneous Dissection of the Carotid and Vertebral Arteries. N Engl J Med March 22, 2001;344(12):898–906.

34. Rosner A. Spontaneous Cervical Artery Dissections and Implications for Homocysteine. Journal af Manip and Phys Thera February 2004;27(2):124–132.

35. Mulroy M, Norris M, Spencer L. Safety Steps for Epidural Injection of Local Anesthetics: Review of the Literature and Recommendations. Anesth Analg, Vol 85(6). Dec 1997: 1346–1356.

36. Huang RC Cervical epidural abscess after epidural steroid injection. Spine Jan 2004;29(1): E7–9.

Index

Page numbers followed by f denote figures; those followed by t denote tables